METHODS IN MOLECULAR MEDICINE™

Cystic Fibrosis Methods and Protocols

Edited by

William R. Skach, MD

*Division of Molecular Medicine,
Oregon Health Sciences University,
Portland, OR*

Humana Press ✳ Totowa, New Jersey

© 2002 Humana Press Inc.
999 Riverview Drive, Suite 208
Totowa, New Jersey 07512

www.humanapress.com

This publication is printed on acid-free paper. ∞
ANSI Z39.48-1984 (American Standards Institute) Permanence of Paper for Printed Library Materials.

Cover design by Patricia F. Cleary.

Production Editor: Mark J. Breaugh.

For additional copies, pricing for bulk purchases, and/or information about other Humana titles, contact Humana at the above address or at any of the following numbers: Tel.: 973-256-1699; Fax: 973-256-8341; E-mail: humana@humanapr.com; Website: http://humanapress.com

Printed in the United States of America. 10 9 8 7 6 5 4 3 2 1

Library of Congress Cataloging in Publication Data

Cystic fibrosis methods and protocols / edited by William R. Skach.
    p. ; cm. -- (Methods in molecular medicine ; 70)
  Includes bibliographical references and index.
  ISBN 0-89603-897-1 (alk. paper)
   1. Cystic fibrosis--Laboratory manuals. I. Skach, William. II. Series.
  [DNLM: 1. Cystic Fibrosis Transmembrane Conductance Regulator--Laboratory Manuals. 2. Cystic Fibrosis--genetics--Laboratory Manuals. QU 25 C997 2002]
  RC858.C95 .C974 2002
616.3'7--dc21

                                  2001039467

METHODS IN MOLECULAR MEDICINE™

John M. Walker, Series Editor

Cystic Fibrosis Methods and Protocols

Preface

Since the cloning of the cystic fibrosis transmembrane conductance regulator (CFTR) nearly a decade ago, cystic fibrosis (CF) research has witnessed a dramatic expansion into new scientific areas. Basic researchers, clinicians, and patients increasingly rely on fundamental techniques of genetics, molecular biology, electrophysiology, biochemistry, cell biology, microbiology, and immunology to understand the molecular basis of this complex disease. Research into the pathophysiology of CF has established numerous paradigms of ion channel dysfunction that extend from inflammation and infection in the airways of patients to basic mechanisms of protein processing and regulation in intracellular components.

With these rapid advances has come an increasing need for research scientists to understand and utilize a growing array of basic laboratory tools. This volume of Methods in Molecular Medicine, *Cystic Fibrosis Methods and Protocols* satisfies that need by providing detailed protocols for the laboratory techniques used throughout CF research. From electrophysiology and cell biology, to animal models and gene therapy, the comprehensive set of methods covered here provide step-by-step instructions needed for investigators to incorporate new approaches into their research programs. Contributions have been chosen to reflect the rich diversity of techniques and to provide a cohesive framework for understanding challenges that are currently at the forefront of CF research. It is hoped that this volume will serve as a valuable reference that will not only foster interdisciplinary investigations into current problems encountered in CF, but also facilitate the translation of new scientific discoveries into clinical solutions.

I would like to sincerely thank all of the contributing authors for their cooperation, patience, and invaluable contributions to this volume. I would also like to thank those investigators, physicians, caregivers, patients, and their families whose continuous dedication has contributed to the rapid advance in our understanding of this devastating disease. Particular thanks go to the Cystic Fibrosis Foundation and its many supporters for their encouragement and assistance to the CF research community. Finally, I would like to thank Nancy Clark and Linda Delacy in the OHSU Molecular Medicine Division and the production staff at Humana Press for their advice and assistance.

William R. Skach, MD

Contents

Contributors

FRANK J. ACCURSO • *Department of Pediatrics, The Children's Hospital, University of Colorado Health Sciences Center, Denver, CO*

MYLES H. AKABAS • *Department of Physiology and Biophysics, Albert Einstein College of Medicine, Bronx, NY*

JUAN G. ALVAREZ • *Department of Obstetrics/Gynecology, Beth Israel Deaconess Medical Center, Harvard Medical School, Boston, MA*

ISABEL AZNAREZ • *Department of Genetics, The Hospital for Sick Children, Toronto, Ontario, Canada*

SONIA BACONNAIS • *Unite de Recherche, INSERM Unit 314, Reims, France*

GÉRARD BALOSSIER • *Unite de Recherche, INSERM Unit 314, Reims, France*

CHRISTINE E. BEAR • *Programme in Cell Biology, Research Institute, Hospital for Sick Children and the Department of Physiology, Faculty of Medicine, Toronto, Ontario, Canada*

MOHAMED BENHAROUGA • *Program in Lung and Cell Biology, The Hospital for Sick Children; Department of Laboratory Medicine and Pathobiology, University of Toronto, Toronto, Ontario, Canada*

MELVIN BERGER • *Department of Pediatrics, Rainbow Babies and Children's Hospital and Case Western Reserve University School of Medicine, Cleveland, OH*

PAOLA G. BLANCO • *Department of Medicine, Beth Israel Deaconess Medical Center, Harvard Medical School, Boston, MA*

RICHARD C. BOUCHER • *Cystic Fibrosis/Pulmonary Research and Treatment Center, University of North Carolina, Chapel Hill, NC*

NEIL A. BRADBURY • *Cystic Fibrosis Research Centre, Department of Cell Biology and Physiology, University of Pittsburgh School of Medicine, Pittsburgh, PA*

ROBERT J. BRIDGES • *Department of Cell Biology and Physiology, University of Pittsburgh, Pittsburgh, PA*

JEFFREY L. BRODSKY • *Department of Biological Sciences, University of Pittsburgh, Pittsburgh, PA*

RUTH BRYAN • *College of Physicians & Surgeons, Columbia University, New York, NY*

SENG H. CHENG • *Genzyme Corporation, Framingham, MA*

KYE A. CHESNUT • *Powell Gene Therapy Center, University of Florida, Gainesville, FL*

JAMES F. CHMIEL • *Department of Pediatrics, Rainbow Babies and Children's Hospital and Case Western Reserve University School of Medicine, Cleveland, OH*

ALEXANDER M. COLE • *Department of Medicine and the Will Rogers Institute Pulmonary Research Laboratory, UCLA School of Medicine, Los Angeles, CA*

MICHAEL J. CORBOY • *Department of Physiology, The University of Texas Southwestern Medical Center, Dallas, TX*

CALVIN U. COTTON • *Departments of Pediatrics, Physiology and Biophysics, Case Western Reserve University, Cleveland, OH*

KIMBERLY V. CURLEE • *Departments of Medicine and Physiology and Biophysics, Gregory Fleming James Cystic Fibrosis Research Center, University of Alabama–Birmingham, Birmingham, AL*

DOUGLAS M. CYR • *Department of Cell and Developmental Biology, University of North Carolina School of Medicine, Chapel Hill, NC*

DAVID DAHAN • *Department of Physiology, McGill University, Montréal, Québec, Canada*

PAMELA B. DAVIS • *Department of Pediatrics, Rainbow Babies and Children's Hospital and Case Western Reserve University School of Medicine, Cleveland, OH*

MICHAEL DEAN • *Human Genetics Section, Laboratory of Genomic Diversity, National Cancer Institute–Frederick Cancer Research and Development Center, Frederick, MD*

DANIEL C. DEVOR • *Department of Cell Biology and Physiology, University of Pittsburgh, Pittsburgh, PA*

SCOTT H. DONALDSON • *Cystic Fibrosis/Pulmonary Research and Treatment Center, University of North Carolina, Chapel Hill, NC*

ELAINE B. DOWELL • *Department of Pediatrics, The Children's Hospital, University of Colorado Health Sciences Center, Denver, CO*

MARIE E. EGAN • *Yale University School of Medicine, New Haven, CT*

OFER EIDELMAN • *Department of Anatomy, Physiology and Genetics; Institute for Molecular Medicine, USU School of Medicine, USUHS, Bethesda, MD*

JOHN F. ENGELHARDT • *Departments of Anatomy & Cell Biology and Internal Medicine, and Center for Gene Therapy of Cystic Fibrosis and Other Genetic Diseases, College of Medicine, The University of Iowa, Iowa City, IA*

ALEXANDRA EVAGELIDIS • *Department of Physiology, McGill University, Montréal, Québec, Canada*

MOHAMMED FILALI • *Department of Anatomy & Cell Biology, College of Medicine, The University of Iowa, Iowa City, IA*

HORST FISCHER • *Children's Hospital, Oakland Research Institute, Oakland, CA*

TERENCE R. FLOTTE • *Powell Gene Therapy Center, University of Florida, Gainesville, FL*

J. KEVIN FOSKETT • *Department of Physiology, University of Pennsylvania, Philadelphia, PA*

STEVEN D. FREEDMAN • *Department of Medicine, Beth Israel Deaconess Medical Center, Harvard Medical School, Boston, MA*

RAYMOND A. FRIZZELL • *Department of Cell Biology and Physiology, University of Pittsburgh, Pittsburgh, PA*

TOMAS GANZ • *Departments of Medicine and Pathology and the Will Rogers Institute Pulmonary Research Laboratory, UCLA School of Medicine, Los Angeles, CA*

DAMJAN GLAVAC • *Laboratory of Molecular Pathology, University of Ljubljana, Ljubljana, Slovenia*

BARBARA R. GRUBB • *Cystic Fibrosis/Pulmonary Research and Treatment Center, University of North Carolina, Chapel Hill, NC*

KENNETH R. HALLOWS • *Department of Medicine, University of Pennsylvania, Philadelphia, PA*

JOHN W. HANRAHAN • *Department of Physiology, McGill University, Montréal, Québec, Canada*

JAY B. HILLIARD • *Department of Pediatrics, Rainbow Babies and Children's Hospital and Case Western Reserve University School of Medicine, Cleveland, OH*

DEBORAH A. R. HINKSON • *Department of Physiology, McGill University, Montréal, Québec, Canada*

MARYBETH HOWARD • *Department of Surgery, University of California, San Francisco, CA*

TZYH-CHANG HWANG • *Department of Physiology and Dalton Cardiovascular Research Center, University of Missouri, Columbia, MO*

SUJATHA JAYARAMAN • *Departments of Medicine and Physiology, Cardiovascular Research Institute, University of California, San Francisco, CA*

ILANA KOGAN • *Programme in Cell Biology, Research Institute, Hospital for Sick Children and the Department of Physiology, Faculty of Medicine, Toronto, Ontario, Canada*

MICHAEL W. KONSTAN • *Department of Pediatrics, Rainbow Babies and Children's Hospital and Case Western Reserve University School of Medicine, Cleveland, OH*

PATRICIA L. KULTGEN • *Department of Cell and Molecular Physiology, University of North Carolina, Chapel Hill, NC*

CANHUI LI • *Programme in Cell Biology, Research Institute, Hospital for Sick Children and the Department of Physiology, Faculty of Medicine, Toronto, Ontario, Canada*

GERGELY L. LUKACS • *Program in Lung and Cell Biology, The Hospital for Sick Children; Department of Laboratory Medicine and Pathobiology, University of Toronto, Toronto, Ontario, Canada*

CHRISTOPHER R. MARINO • *Departments of Medicine and Physiology, University of Tennessee Health Sciences Center, VA Medical Center, Memphis, TN*

DANUTA MARKIEWICZ • *Department of Genetics, The Hospital for Sick Children, Toronto, Ontario, Canada*

JOHN MARSHALL • *Genzyme Corporation, Framingham, MA*

GEOFFREY C. MEACHAM • *Department of Cell Biology and the Gregory Fleming James Cystic Fibrosis Research Center, University of Alabama–Birmingham, Birmingham, AL*

SUSAN MICHAELIS • *Department of Cell Biology, Johns Hopkins School of Medicine, Baltimore, MD*

SHARON L. MILGRAM • *Department of Cell and Molecular Physiology, University of North Carolina, Chapel Hill, NC*

PETER J. MOHLER • *Department of Cell and Molecular Physiology, University of North Carolina, Chapel Hill, NC*

BRYAN D. MOYER • *Department of Cell Biology, The Scripps Research Institute, La Jolla, CA*

GEORG NAGEL • *Max-Planck-Institut für Biophysik; Johann-Wolfgang-Goethe-Universität, Biozentrum, Frankfurt, Germany*

ANJAPARAVANDA P. NAREN • *Department of Physiology, The University of Tennessee Health Science Center, Memphis, TN*

JON OBERDORF • *Division of Molecular Medicine, Oregon Health Sciences University, Portland, OR*

TUNCER ONAY • *Department of Genetics, The Hospital for Sick Children, Toronto, Ontario, Canada*

ELAINE G. POLIGONE • *Cystic Fibrosis/Pulmonary Research and Treatment Center, Department of Cell and Molecular Physiology, University of North Carolina, Chapel Hill, NC*

HARVEY B. POLLARD • *Department of Anatomy, Physiology and Genetics; Institute for Molecular Medicine, Uniformed Services UniversitySchool of Medicine, USUHS, Bethesda, MD*

ALLAN POWE • *Department of Physiology and Dalton Cardiovascular Research Center, University of Missouri, Columbia, MO*
ALICE PRINCE • *College of Physicians & Surgeons, Columbia University, New York, NY*
EDITH PUCHELLE • *Unite de Recherche, INSERM Unit 314, Reims, France*
VISWANATHAN RAGHURAM • *Department of Physiology, University of Pennsylvania, Philadelphia, PA*
MOHABIR RAMJEESINGH • *Programme in Cell Biology, Research Institute, Hospital for Sick Children and the Department of Physiology, Faculty of Medicine, Toronto, Ontario, Canada*
TERESA C. RITCHIE • *Department of Anatomy & Cell Biology and Center for Gene Therapy of Cystic Fibrosis and Other Genetic Diseases, College of Medicine, The University of Iowa, Iowa City, IA*
SCOTT D. SAGEL • *Department of Pediatrics, The Children's Hospital, University of Colorado Health Sciences Center, Denver, CO*
MANU SHARMA • *Program in Lung and Cell Biology, The Hospital for Sick Children; Department of Laboratory Medicine and Pathobiology, University of Toronto, Toronto, Ontario, Canada*
JULIE C. SHEA • *Department of Medicine, Beth Israel Deaconess Medical Center, Harvard Medical School, Boston, MA*
ASHVANI K. SINGH • *Department of Cell Biology and Physiology, University of Pittsburgh, Pittsburgh, PA*
SANGEETA SINGH • *Department of Cell Biology and Physiology, University of Pittsburgh, Pittsburgh, PA*
WILLIAM R. SKACH • *Division of Molecular Medicine, Oregon Health Sciences University, Portland, OR*
ERIC J. SORSCHER• *Departments of Medicine and Physiology and Biophysics, Gregory Fleming James Cystic Fibrosis Research Center, University of Alabama at Birmingham, Birmingham, AL*
MEERA SRIVASTAVA • *Department of Anatomy, Physiology and Genetics; Institute for Molecular Medicine, Uniformed Services UniversitySchool of Medicine, USUHS, Bethesda, MD*
BRUCE A. STANTON • *Department of Physiology, Dartmouth Medical School, Hanover, NH*
RHESA D. STIDHAM • *Department of Physiology, Graduate Program in Molecular Biophysics, The University of Texas Southwestern Medical Center, Dallas, TX*
M. JACKSON STUTTS • *University of North Carolina Cystic Fibrosis/Pulmonary Research and Treatment Center, Chapel Hill, NC*

ROBERT TARRAN • *Cystic Fibrosis/Pulmonary Research and Treatment Center, University of North Carolina, Chapel Hill, NC*

PHILIP J. THOMAS • *Department of Physiology, The University of Texas Southwestern Medical Center, Dallas, TX*

LAP-CHEE TSUI • *Department of Molecular and Medical Genetics, University of Toronto; Department of Genetics, The Hospital for Sick Children, Toronto, Ontario, Canada*

JOHN TZOUNZOURIS • *Department of Genetics, The Hospital for Sick Children, Toronto, Ontario, Canada*

WILLY VAN DRIESSCHE • *Laboratory of Physiology, Katholik Universitat Leuven, Leuven, Belgium*

ALAN S. VERKMAN • *Departments of Medicine and Physiology, Cardiovascular Research Institute, University of California, San Francisco, CA*

ISABEL VIRELLA-LOWELL • *Powell Gene Therapy Center, University of Florida, Gainesville, FL*

KELLY WEIXEL • *Cystic Fibrosis Research Centre, Department of Cell Biology and Physiology, University of Pittsburgh School of Medicine, Pittsburgh, PA*

WILLIAM J. WELCH • *Departments of Surgery and Medicine and Physiology, University of California, San Francisco, CA*

W. CHRISTIAN WIGLEY • *Department of Physiology, The University of Texas Southwestern Medical Center, Dallas, TX*

JEFFREY J. WINE • *Cystic Fibrosis Research Laboratory, Stanford University, Stanford, CA*

JEAN-MARIE ZAHM • *Unite de Recherche, INSERM Unit 314, Reims, France*

YIMAO ZHANG • *Department of Biological Sciences, University of Pittsburgh, Pittsburgh, PA*

YULONG ZHANG •*Department of Anatomy & Cell Biology and Center for Gene Therapy of Cystic Fibrosis and Other Genetic Diseases, College of Medicine, The University of Iowa, Iowa City, IA*

ZHEN ZHOU • *Department of Physiology and Dalton Cardiovascular Research Center, University of Missouri, Columbia, MO*

TANG ZHU • *Department of Physiology, McGill University, Montréal, Québec, Canada*

JULIAN ZIELENSKI • *Department of Genetics, The Hospital for Sick Children, Toronto, Ontario, Canada*

I

GENETICS OF CYSTIC FIBROSIS

1

CFTR Mutation Detection by Multiplex Heteroduplex (mHET) Analysis on MDE Gel

Julian Zielenski, Isabel Aznarez, Tuncer Onay, John Tzounzouris, Danuta Markiewicz, and Lap-Chee Tsui

1. Introduction

Mutation detection in an integral part of disease diagnosis and patient study. For most Mendelian diseases, multiple mutations may be found in a single gene among a patient population. The type of mutations may vary from large deletions to single-base-pair (bp) substitutions, and different diseases may have different predominant types. For example, large deletions are often found in Duchenne muscular dystrophy *(1)* and truncation mutation is the predominant type in BRCA1-associated breast cancer *(2)*. Therefore, different mutation detection strategies are required for different diseases.

Cystic fibrosis (CF) is an autosomal recessive disorder caused by mutations in the cystic fibrosis transmembrane conductance regulator (CFTR) gene *(3–5)*. The gene spans over 210 kb and consists of poorly defined promoter and 27 exons *(6)*. Although the major mutation, ΔF508 (a 3-bp deletion) accounts for about 70% of the mutant alleles worldwide, close to 1000 presumed disease-causing mutations have been identified in the gene (*see* Cystic Fibrosis Mutations Database, http://www.genet.sickkids.on.ca/cftr/). It is also of interest to note that almost 99% of the CFTR mutations identified so far have been point mutations, due to either a single-bp substitution or small insertion or deletion of one or a few base pairs. There are only 10 reported CFTR mutations in which whole exons are deleted.

Searching for mutations in the CFTR gene is generally a two-step process. A standard screening panel of 25 known mutations can detect over 80% of the mutant alleles for an average CF population in North American. In order to identify the remaining unknown CFTR mutations, a number of different screening methods have been implemented; these include single-strand conformation

From: *Methods in Molecular Medicine, vol. 70: Cystic Fibrosis Methods and Protocols*
Edited by: W. R. Skach © Humana Press Inc., Totowa, NJ

polymorphism (SSCP) *(7)*. Denaturing, gradient gel electrophoresis (DGGE) *(8)*, heteroduplex analysis *(9)*, and chemical cleavage *(10)*. These and other methods have been reviewed previously in detail *(11)*. Any indication of DNA sequence change in the screening (e.g., altered mobility in gel electrophoresis) is followed by DNA sequencing analysis to identify the exact nucleotide alteration and confirmed by additional tests.

In this chapter, we describe our multiplex heteroduplex (mHET) protocol, which we have refined for our CF mutation screening over the past 9 yr. Almost 3000 DNA samples, each up to 30 CFTR gene fragments, were screened during this period of time. The sample included patients diagnosed with different forms of cystic fibrosis, patients with other diseases with partial similarity to CF, and control disease or healthy individuals.

The principle of heteroduplex analysis has been reviewed previously *(12,13)*. The factors that may influence the heteroduplex separation process for single nucleotide substitutions have also been discussed *(14)*. We also take advantage of a chemically modified polyacrylamide gel matrices called HydroLink *(9)*, which has been specifically formulated to improve heteroduplex detection (The product known as MDE is available from FMC BioProducts, Rockland, ME). The mHET procedure, as described in this chapter, appears to be highly efficient (high sensitivity and specificity), relatively simple, does not require expensive equipment, is low-cost and flexible (amenable to changes and improvements). The detection rate of heteroduplex is not affected by size of an amplicon in range of 100 to 600 bp. This allows for convenient distribution and identification of DNA fragments of various sizes on the electrophoretic MDE gel. The abnormal patterns reflecting the presence of DNA alterations are usually observed in proximity of a corresponding homoduplex(es). This feature facilitates interpretation of results in terms of assignment of aberrant brands to particular fragments. Also, as the DNA is retained in its double-strand form, the probing of DNA fragments does not require strand-specific probes and offers greater flexibility in selection of more effective probes.

1.1. Overall Design and Characteristics of the mHET Protocol

The layout of the current mHET protocol is outlined in **Fig. 1**. The major steps are (1) extraction and preparation of the genomic DNA from the tissues or cells; (2) multiplex PCR amplification of genomic DNA samples designed to produce fragments spanning all regions of interest; (3) reaction pooling and polymerase chain reaction (PCR) product purification by spin columns; (4) electrophoresis of purified DNA samples on the MDE gel matrix; (5) DNA transfer from gel to nylon membrane; (6) probing and hybridization with fragment specific primers; (7) autoradiography; (8) DNA band pattern interpretation; and (9) direct sequencing analysis of DNA fragments with abnormal

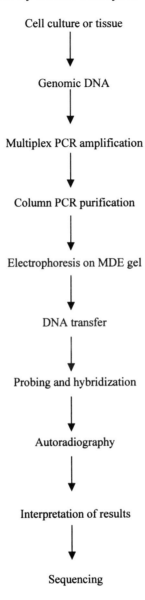

Fig. 1. General stages of the mHET protocol.

electrophoretic migration patterns. Unlike other PCR-based electrophoretic scanning methods which process one fragment at a time, the mHET protocol enables simultaneous analysis of a large number of DNA fragments from multiple patients with one gel. In our current protocol for screening of the CFTR gene we test 32 DNA fragments from 10 patients with one gel. In addition, the PCR amplification was also multiplexed by combining four or five primer pairs per reaction. Using the 8×12 microplate format, 32 fragments for 10 patients were simultaneously amplified in one thermocycling session. The multiplexing of PCR significantly reduced both the time required to generate amplicons for mHET analysis as well as the cost of this screening procedure.

1.1.1. Sensitivity

In order to evaluate a mutation detection rate for the mHET protocol using the HydroLink MDE gel matrix, we tested retrospectively DNA samples heterozygous for 112-nucleotide CFTR variants. These variants represented different DNA alterations including single-nucleotide substitutions, SNA ($n = 83$) and small deletions and insertions ($n = 20$). Of the 83 single-nucleotide substitutions, 77 (93%) were detected using our protocol and all 29 (100%) deletions and insertions were detected. The overall detection rate for any type of mutation in this sample was then 95%. In order to see if there is any bias in detecting particular nucleotide mismatches we examined distribution of various mismatches in the tested sample of single-nucleotide substitutions and compared with previously reported findings from the large mutations *(15)*. The overall difference in proportion of six types of detectable mismatches (A:T/G:C; A:T/C:G; A:T/T:A; C:G/G:C; C:G/T:A, and G:C/T:A) between our sample and that of previously published samples from public databases was not significant ($p < 0.5$), demonstrating that there was no bias in the detection rate by our protocol.

1.1.2. Specificity

Due to the multiplexing, occasionally some nonspecific background can be present when using the mHET protocol. This is sometimes observed in form of additional DNA bands. Although hybridization using nested oligonucleotides as probes usually minimizes the background resulting from nonspecific PCR amplification, there may be some cross-reactivity in the multiprobing cocktails used for hybridization. The occasional background patterns usually do not pose a major problem because they appear identical in all tested patients and can be excluded from further analysis. The rate of false positives in very low (1%) and usually stems from misinterpretation of band appearance (thicker band relative to others; background). On rare occasions a band may be wrongly assigned to specific DNA region based on the distance to the nearest PCR product. It this happens, reprobing of the membrane with specific oligonucleotides may be required to establish the origin of abnormal pattern. False negative results are on the ~6% level for the single-nucleotide substitutions (retrospective study) and 0% for minor deletions and insertions.

1.1.3. Size Effect

Simultaneous running of multiple PCR fragments on one gel requires a convenient size distribution (size range 200–600 bp). We examined an effect of

PCR fragment size on a shifting efficiency in Hydrolink MDE gel matrix under standard conditions. DNA heterozygous for different mutations were amplified using primers producing PCR fragments of different sizes (178–570 bp). We have found that a heteroduplex shifting shown as extra band or unusual band pattern is preserved for PCR fragments carrying the same mismatch in the tested size range, although the extent of shifting and its appearance may vary for different fragments. This finding allowed us to visualize 4- to 6-well-spaced PCR fragments per one probing.

1.1.4. Heteroduplex vs Homoduplex Detection

Although the HET method by definition is based on formation of heteroduplexes and their efficient separation from homoduplexes, we have also observed abnormal band patterns corresponding to DNA homozygous for specific mutant variants. We found that the single-nucleotide substitutions producing clear band patterns (large shift or presence of multiple bands) in a heterozygous state tend to form distinct band shifts in a homozygous state (1540A/G; I336K; -896T/G; R764X; R1066C; M1101K). The capacity to detect homoduplexes from patients homozygous for rare mutations is increased by partial denaturing conditions employed by the mHET protocol (see Materials and Methods subheadings).

1.1.5. Cost

Multiplexing is a cost-saving solution (option) since it reduces both the material cost of the protocol as well as labor time, which can partially be associated to the cost through the technician's salary. Our estimate of cost is based on the present version of the mHET protocol. It is based on generating 5 membranes with the same DNA content from one gel for 10. The cost of this protocol when compared with the simplex approach is reduced about 6.5 times.

2. Materials

2.1. Multiplex PCR

Equipment requirements: Thermocycler (PCR) system with top heating, 8×12 microplate format (trays, racks), and programmable temperature gradient.

1. 10× PCR buffer: 100 mM Tris-HCl, pH 8.3, 500 mM KCl, 17.5 mM MgCl$_2$, 0.01% gelatin.
2. Taq-polymerase (5 U/μL).
3. 2 mM dNTP mix: 2 mM solution of each of four dNTPs (dATP, dGTP, dCTP, and dTTP) in deionized water.

2.2. Column Purification

1. QIAquick Spin Purification kit or equivalent reagent for purification of PCR products.

2. Microcentrifuge (Eppendorf type).
3. SpeedVac or equivalent equipment.
4. 2× loading buffer: 40 g sucrose, 30 g urea, 50 mg Bromophenol blue, and 50 mg xylene cyanol in 100 mL water.

2.3. DNA Electrophoresis on Hydrolink-MDE Gel

1. 1.2× TBE-urea buffer: 0.12 M Tris, 0.11 M boric acid, 2.4 mM ethylenediame-tetraactic acid (EDTA), and 5 M urea.
2. MDE polymerization mix: 1 volume of commercial MDE™ stock solution (BMA, Rockland, ME), 2 parts of 1.2× TBE-urea buffer, and 1 part of deionized formamide (*see* **Note 1**).
3. 10% ammonium sulfate and TEMED.
4. 5× TBE buffer: 54 g Tris, 27.5 g boric acid, 3.7 g EDTA in 1 L of deionized water.
5. 0.6× TBE.
6. Electrophoretic apparatus with glass plates, spacers, and combs (*see* **Note 2**).
7. High-voltage power supply.
8. MDE quality control sample (we use PCR fragment corresponding to exon 3 of the CFTR gene from a patient heterozygous for the R75Q variant. Good-quality MDE gel electrophoresis should produce a distinct pattern of 3 bands for this sample.).

2.4. Transfer of DNA to a Nylon Membrane

1. Hybond-N$^+$ transfer membrane (Amersham).
2. Whatman 3MM filter paper.
3. 0.4 N NaOH.
4. 20× sodium-saline-citrate (SSC): 3 M NaCl, 0.3 sodium citrate, pH 7.0.
5. 2× SSC.

2.5. Hybridization and Probing

1. Amasino buffer for hybridization: 7% sodium dodecyl sulfate (SDS), 10% poly-ethylene glycol (PEG), 0.25 M NaCl, 0.13 M phosphate buffer (pH 7.2).
2. Hybridization oven with flasks (Hybaid).
3. Terminal deoxynucleotidyl transferase (TdT) and enzyme buffer (Gibco-BRL or Amersham).
4. ^{32}Pα-dCTP.
5. Probing oligonucleotides (*see* **Table 1**).
6. Columns with Sephadex™ G25 fine (Amersham Pharmacia Biotechlab).
7. 1% SDS in 3× SSC.
8. 0.2× SSC.
9. Saran wrap.

2.6. Autoradiography

1. X-ray film; Scientific Imaging Film X-OMAT.AR (35 × 43 cm) from Kodak.
2. Autoradiography cassette.
3. Film developing equipment.

Table 1
Primer Mixes for Probing[a]

PCR fragment	Sequence (5'→3')	Primer name	Fragment size (bp)
Probing mix #1			
10	AGTGTGAAGGGTTCATATGC	10i-3s	491
13B	TTTCGGTGAATGTTCTGACC	13i-3sC	428
23	GTAAATACAGATCATTACTG	23i-5s	400
8	AATGCATTAATGCTATTCTG	8i-5s 359	
22	TGTCACCATGAAGCAGGCAT	22i-3 306	
Probing mix #2			
PRO 2	AAGGAGGGTCTAGGAAGCTC	Pi-5sA	644
1	TTAGGAGCTTGAGCCCAGAC	1i-5 553	
13A	TGGTCGAAAGAATCACATCC	13i-3sA	453
6a	GGAAGATACAATGACACCTG	6ai-5s	385
11	CAGGAAATGGTTGCTAGACC	11i-3s	355
3	TGCAACTTATTGGTCCCACT	3i-5s 309	
Probing mix #3			
24	CTTAGACTTGCACTTGCTTG	24i-3s	569
21	GGTAAGTACATGGGTGTTTC	21i-5s	477
14a	TGGCATGAAACTGTACTGTC	14ai-5s	511
5	CCTGAGAAGATAGTAAGCTAG	5i-5s 395	
12	TCTACACTAGATGACCAGGA	12i-5s	368
4	TGTGTTGAAATTCTCAGGGT	4i-5s 314	
6b	TTAAGGACAGAATTACTAAC	6bi-3s	233
Probing mix #4			
9 TGm/Tn	GATTTGGGGAATTATTTGA	9i-5sA	560
PRO 1	GGTGGATTAGTCAAGATGTT	Pi-5 471	
17a	TCTCAAATAGCTCTTATAGC	17ai-3s	449
7	TTCAATAGCTCAGCCTTC	17i-5s	410
18	AAGTCGTTCACAGAAGAGAG	18i-5s	320
2	GTGAATATCTGTTCCTCCTC	2i-5s 294	
9	GATTTGGGGAATTATTTGA	9i-5sa	235
20	GTCACAGAAGTGATCCCATC	20i-5s	213
Probing #5			
16	GCGTCTACTGTGATCCAAAC	16i-5s	570
15	GTGATTATCACCAGCACCAG	15i-5s	485
IVS19	AGGCTTCTCAGTGATCTGTTG	4712 437	
19	GCCAACTCTCGAAAGTTATG	19i-5s	379
17b	TGTGGAACAGAGTTTCAAAG	17bi-3s	344
14b	GAACACCTAGTACAGCTGCT	14bi-5	288

[a]For primer quantities, *see* **Note 10**.

3. Methods

3.1. Multiplex PCR

Genomic DNA was extracted from peripheral blood samples by standard methods (*see* **Note 3**) *(16)*.

3.1.1. Reaction Mixes (see **Note 4**)

1. Arrange required number of thin-wall PCR tubes in the tube rack (tray) with the 8×12 layout (*see* **Note 5**).
2. Distribute components of reaction mixes to the tubes. Each mix should combine the following in a total volume of 25 µL: 13 µL of primer mix (the primer composition and their concentrations are shown in **Table 2**); 1.0 µL of the genomic DNA (~250–500 µg/mL); 2.5 µL of 2 m*M* dNTP mix; 2.5 µL of 10× PCR buffer; 0.5 µL Taq polymerase (5 U/µL); and 5.5 µL of deionized water (*see* **Note 6**).

3.1.2. PCR Program

1. Run the multiplex PCR reactions using the "touchdown" thermocycling program *(17)* (*see* **Note 7**).
2. Examine the quality of PCR amplification for randomly selected reaction mixtures (representing all different combinations) by electrophoresis of 5-µL PSR aliquots on 3% aragose gel. With well-spaced amplicon sizes and similar amplification efficiency, all expected bands should be present upon staining with ethidium bromide.

3.2. Column Purification

1. Pool 20-µL aliquots of each PCR multiplex mix from the same patient to one tube (final volume = number of multiplex mixes × 20 µL).
2. Purify PCR-amplified DNA fragments from PCR reagents using the QIAquick Spin PCR Purification Kit (Qiagen) or any other PCR purification kit (*see* **Note 8**). Collect the final PCR eluate in water (50 µL).
3. Evaporate the water from the PCR preparation using SpeedVac and redissolve a dry residue in 20 µL of the 2× loading buffer.

3.3. DNA Electrophoresis on Hydrolink-NDE Gel

Gloves should be worn at all stages of the method.

1. Assemble the clean glass plates with side and bottom spaces (*see* **Note 2**).
2. Prepare the MDE polymerization mix using slight excess over the required volume for the specific glass plate setup. For polymerization, add 0.7 mL of 10% ammonium persulfate (APS) and 88 µL of TEMED per 100 mL of the MDE mix. Mix and use immediately.
3. Cast the gel slowly, pouring the polymerization mix over the larger plate while holding the plates at a 45° angle. Lower the plates on the bench and insert the comb. Leave undistributed for polymerization. The gel can be used for electrophoresis after 1 h. When the gel is ready for use, remove the bottom spacer.

Table 2
Primer Composition of Multiplex PCR Mixes

PCR fragment[a]	Sequence (5'→3')	Primer name	PCR size (bp)	Amount of primer per mix[b] pmol (μL)
Primer mix #1				
24	GGACACAGCAGTTAAATGTG	24i-5	569	7.6 (0.5)
	ACTATTGCCAGGAAGCCATT	24i-3		7.6 (0.5)
17a	AATGTTTACTCACCAACATG	17ai-5s	449	22.7 (1.5)
	TGTACACCAACTGTGGTAAG	17ai-3		22.7 (1.5)
14a	AAAAGGTATGCCACTGTTAAG	14ai-5	511	22.7 (1.5)
	GTATACATCCCCAAACTATCT	14ai-3		22.7 (1.5)
11	TGAGCATACTAAAAGTGACTC	11I-5s	355	14.4 (1.0)
	GCACAGATTCTGAGTAACCATAAT	11I-3		12.6 (1.0)
Primer mix #2				
16	CAGAGAAATTGGTCGTTACT	16i-5	570	15.1 (1.0)
	ATCTAAATGTGGGATTGCCT	16i-3		15.1 (1.0)
15	GTGCATGCTCTTCTAATGCA	15i-5	485	15.1 (1.0)
	AAGGCACATGCCTCTGTGCA	15i-3		14.4 (1.0)
19	TGTGAAATTGTCTGCCATTC	19i-5sA	379	15.1 (1.0)
	GCTAACACATTGCTTCAGGCT	19i-3		15.1 (1.0)
2	CCAAATCTGTATGGAGACCA	2i-5	294	15.1 (1.0)
	AGCCACCATACTTGGCTCCT	2i-3s		14.4 (1.0)
Primer mix #3				
PRO 1	(AA)GGTGGATTAGTCAAGATGTT	Pi-5	471	7.6 (0.5)
	CTCCTCCTTTTCCCGATGAT	Pi-3		7.6 (0.5)
7	AGACCATGCTCAGATCTTCCAT	7i-5	410	27.5 (2.0)
	GCAAAGTTCATTAGAACTGATC	7i-3		27.5 (2.0)
3	CTTGGGTTAATCTCCTTGGA	3i-5	309	15.1 (1.0)
	ATTCACCAGATTTCGTAGTC	3i-3		15.1 (1.0)
9A	GATTTGGGGAATTATTTGA	9i-5sA	235	23.9 (1.5)
	AAGAGACATGGACACCAAAT	9i-3s		22.7 (1.5)
PRO 2	GACCCTTGCAAACGTAACAG	Pi-5A	644	22.7 (1.5)
	GGCGCTGGGGTCCCTGCTAG	Pi-3A		22.7 (1.5
13A	TGCTAAAATACGAGACATATTGC	13i-5	453	9.9 (0.75)
	AGGGAGTCTTTTGCACAATG	13i-3sB		11.4 (0.75)
6a	TTAGTGTGCTCAGAACCACG	6ai-5	385	7.6 (0.5)
	CTATGCATAGAGCAGTCCTG	6ai-3		7.6 (0.5)
8	TGAATCCTAGTGCTTGGCAA	8i-5	359	11.4 (0.75)
	TCGCCATTAGGATGAAATCC	8i-3		11.4 (0.75)
Primer mix #5				
1	TTAGGAGCTTGAGCCCAGAC	1i-5	553	22.7 (1.5)
	GTTGGCTGAATTCAGTCAAG	1i-3A		22.7 (1.5)
13B	TCAATCCAATCAACTCTATACGAA	X13B-5	428	25.2 (2.0)

(continued)

Table 2 *(continued)*

PCR fragment[a]	Sequence (5'→3')	Primer name	PCR size (bp)	Amount of primer per mix[b] pmol (µL)
	CTACTCAATTGCATTCTGTG	13i-3s		30.3 (2.0)
5	ATTTCTGCCTAGATGCTGGG	5i-5	395	15.1 (1.0)
	AACTCCGCCTTTCCAGTTGT	5i-3		15.1 (1.0)
14b	GAACACCTAGTACAGCTGCT	14bi-5	288	22.7 (1.5)
	ATACAAACATAGTGGATTAC	14bi-3s		22.7 (1.5)
Primer mix #6				
21	AATGTTCACAAGGGACTCCA	21i-5	477	7.6 (0.5)
	CAAAAGTACCTGTTGCTCCA	21i-3		7.6 (0.5)
IVS19	AGGCTTCTCAGTGATCTGTTG	4712	437	10.8 (0.75)
	GAATCATTCAGTGGGTATAAGCAG	3849-3'		9.5 (0.75)
12	TCTACACTAGATGACCAGGA	12i-5s	368	15.1 (1.0)
	CTGGTTTAGCATGAGGCGGT	12i-3		15.1 (1.0)
4	TGTGTTGAAATTCTCAGGGT	4i-5s	314	11.4 (0.75)
	ATGGGGCCTGTGCAAGGAAG	4i-3s		11.4 (0.75)
Primer mix #7				
23	AGCTGATTGTGCGTAACGCT	23i-5	400	15.1 (1.0)
	TAAAGCTGGATGGCTGTATG	23i-3		15.1 (1.0)
22	GAATGTCAACTGCTTGAGTG	22i-5s	306	15.1 (1.0)
	TGTCACCATGAAGCAGGCAT	22i-3		15.1 (1.0)
6b	GATTGATTGATTGATTTACAG	6bi-5sA	233	28.8 (2.0)
	GAGGTGGAAGTCTACCATGA	6ci-3		30.3 (2.0)
20	GTCACAGAAGTGATCCCATC	20i-5s	213	30.3 (2.0)
	CTGGCTAAGTCCTTTTGTTC	20i-3s		30.3 (2.0)
Primer mix #8				
9B	TAATGGATCATGGGCCATGT	9i-5	560	15.1 (1.0)
	ACAGTGTTGAATGTGGTGCA	9i-3		15.1 (1.0)
10	GCAGAGTACCTGAAACAGGA	10i-5	491	15.1 (1.0)
	CATTCACAGTAGCTTACCCA	10i-3		15.1 (1.0)
17b	GTTATTTGCAATGTTTTCTAT	17bi-5sA		22.7 (1.5)
	ATAACCTATAGAATGCAGCA	17bi-3		22.7 (1.5)
18	GTAGATGCTGTGATGAACTG	18i-5	320	45.4 (3.0)
	CATACTTTGTTACTTGTCTG	18i-3s		45.4 (3.0)

*a*The name of each fragment denotes exon or intron (IVS) number in the CFTR gene according to the historical nomenclature. The only exceptions are 9A, 9B, 13A, and 13B, which are overlapping fragments of corresponding exons (9 and 13). In addition, there are two overlapping promoter-containing fragments (PRO1 and PRO2) corresponding to a ~1-kb sequence upstream of exon 1.

*b*After combining the indicated amounts of primers for each mix, the final volume was made up to 13 µL by water.

4. Mount plates with gel on the electrophoretic unit and fill the upper and lower chamber with the 0.6× TBE buffer. Carefully remove the comb and rinse the wells with a syringe. To remove air bubbles trapped in the space left after removing the bottom spacer, purge it with the buffer using a 50-mL plastic syringe with a bent needle.

5. Pre-run the gel for 30 min at 1000 V. *Note:* Wear gloves and operate with caution when operating the unit during electrophoresis.

6. Prior to loading, switch off the power supply and thoroughly flush the wells. Load 3–4 µL of each sample (*see* **Note 9**). To control the quality of electrophoretic separation in some runs we also load DNA carrying the R75Q (356 G/A mismatch) allele in exon 3 of the CFTR gene (the corresponding heteroduplex produces a unique pattern of 3 bands).

7. Run the samples initially for 5–10 min at 1000 V and then overnight (16–18 h) at 500 V (500 V – 7 mA–5 W [constant]). The temperature of the gel should not rise above room-temperature level.

3.4. Transfer of DNA to a Nylon Membrane

1. Pry the glass with metal spatula to part the plates. The gel should stay on one of the plates.

2. Cut the Hybond-N$^+$ membranes according to the size of areas with DNA ~10 cm from the well level and 2 cm from the bottom of the gel (*see* **Note 9**). Typically the membranes are about 30 cm high.

3. Carefully place the membranes (prewetted in 0.6× TBE buffer) on the corresponding areas of the gel. Overlay three pieces of Whatman 3MM filter paper on each membrane. Note: the paper should be shorter than membrane in each dimension by 0.5 cm. The air trapped between the gel and the membrane should be removed by gentle pipet rolling over the paper pad. To increase contact between the gel and membrane and ensure even pressure distribution, place a glass plate on the top of the setup with a light object (reagent bottle) on it. The minimum time for the transfer is 4 h. If convenient, the transfer could be done overnight (no band diffusion has been observed).

4. Remove the membrane(s) from the gel and place in 0.4 *N* NaOH for 10 min to fix the DNA and then transfer to 2× SSC solution for 10 min.

5. Blot the membrane between two pieces of Whatman 3MM filter paper and wrap it in Saran wrap to prevent it from drying if not hybridized immediately.

3.5. Hybridization and Probing

3.5.1. Prehybridization

1. Roll each membrane with the DNA side facing in and place in the hybridization bottle. More than one membrane can be placed in a bottle for hybridization with the same probing mix.

2. Pour 20 mL of the hybridization solution (Amasino buffer) preheated to 42°C and prehybridize for 1 h.

3.5.2. Probe Preparation (Labeling)

1. Label the primers for probing (oligonucleotides) using the terminal deoxynucleotidyl transferase, TdT, and ^{32}P dCTP as a source of radioactivity (*see* **Note 10**).
2. Purify the labeled primers by passing through the 1-mL TE-equilibrated column of the Sephadex G25 and eluting with 100 μL of the TE.

3.5.3. Hybridization and Washing

1. Add the probe to the hybridization buffer in a bottle and hybridize overnight at 42°C.
2. Wash the filters in 3× SSC + 0.1% SDS at room temperature for 20 min and follow with two consecutive washed with 0.2× SSC at 36°C.

3.6. Autoradiography

1. Blot dry membrane and wrap in Saran wrap.
2. Expose the membrane to X-ray film (1–5 h). Occasionally, the exposure may have to be extended overnight or longer, due to the weak signal from some DNA samples.
3. Develop the exposed film.

3.7. Interpretation of Results

1. View the film using a light box and search for abnormal electrophoretic band patterns.
2. Except for deletions and insertions of three or more nucleotides, the band shifts corresponding to heteroduplexes are found typically very near homoduplexes. In some cases, more than one band shift is observed for certain alleles, probably due to separation of both homoduplexes and two types of heteroduplexes. Some examples from screening of the CFTR gene by the mHET protocol are shown in **Fig. 2** (*see* **Note 11**).

3.8. Sequencing Analysis

1. Amplify specific DNA fragment from tested individual as indicated by the mHET analysis.
2. Purify using PCR purification kit.
3. Sequence using thermocycling reaction with the ^{32}P-labeled dideoxy-nucleotides Thermo Sequenase radiolabeled terminator cycle sequencing kit (Amersham-Life Science, Cleveland, OH).

4. Notes

1. To deionize formamide, mix 20 mL of formamide with 3 g of Rexyn 300 (Fisher) or equivalent, gently for 1 h, and filter through Whatman filter paper. After combining all the components in the MDE mix, filter it through a 0.2-μm filter unit (Nalgene or Gelman Scientific VacuCap 90).

2. We use the sequencing electrophoretic unit (model STS) from IBI with commercial (STS45) glass plates (38 × 43 cm and 38 × 43 cm), spacers (0.4 mm) and 64-sharktooth combs (0.4 mm). The dimensions of the gel are 35.4 cm × 41 cm × 0.4 mm. The amount of MDE mix required for this setup is ~60 mL. It is recommended, however, to prepare a slight excess of MDE mix (10–15 mL) in case of leakage.

3. Besides DNA preparations made in our laboratory, we analyze DNA samples from many external sources. The purity of genomic DNA varies among different preparations, affecting the multiplex PCR amplification. DNA samples to be screened should be as pure as possible. To ensure reproducible, high-quality amplification, well-established DNA preparation protocols with phenol–chloroform extraction should be used. The quality of genomic DNA preparations can be monitored both by the OD_{260}/OD_{280} ratio (1.6–2.0) as well as by the aragose gel electrophoresis to test for DNA degradation. Impure DNA samples interfere with the multiplex PCR reaction as well as with subsequent purification and concentration (high salt or protein content). The lack of proper purification tends to increase with the salt concentration in the samples. This will decrease the quality of the electrophoretic separation of PCR fragments and in consequence the mutation detection efficiency.

4. For screening of the CFTR gene, the entire coding region of the gene (27 exons) including flanking intron sequences (50–200 bp), ~1000 bp of the 5'-untranslated region (UTR5'), and part of intron 19 (detection of 3849 + 10 kbC→T) *(18)* were amplified to produce 32 fragments (13A and 13B). Exon 9 and flanking intron sequences were also amplified in two parts (9A and 9B) in order to separate exon 9 sequence from the highly polymorphic acceptor/branch segment of intron 8 (TGmTn) *(19)*. Eight multiplex PCR reactions have been designed (**Table 2**) to the minimize number of amplification reactions. Mixes 1, 3, 4, 5, 6, and 7 amplify four PCR fragments, mix 2 amplifies five fragments, and mix 8 amplifies three fragments.

5. Many thermocyclers currently available on the market (e.g., Perkin-Elmer 9600 or 9700 model; MJ Research PTC-100) use the 8 × 12 format for simultaneous amplification of 98 DNA samples. Typically we run PCR reactions for 12 patients in one tray (12 patients × 8 PCR mixes [#1–8] = 96 tubes). This format is very convenient for efficient PCR and distribution of reaction mix components from premixes using the 8- or 12-channel pipettors. The streamlined distribution of liquid components reduces the possibility of handling errors due to fatigue and misplacing when processing a large number of samples individually. Alternatively, the whole process can be automated using specialized equipment if it is available in a laboratory.

6. To minimize the chance of handling errors, the nonspecific components of the PCR reaction mixtures were dispensed from a premix using a multichannel pipettor. In our protocol, we premix all the shared (common) components (PCR buffer, NTP mix, Taq polymerase and water) and aliquot to tubes using an 8-channel pipettor (11 µL/tube). The primers are added prior to the premix to bettor control distribution of specific reagents.

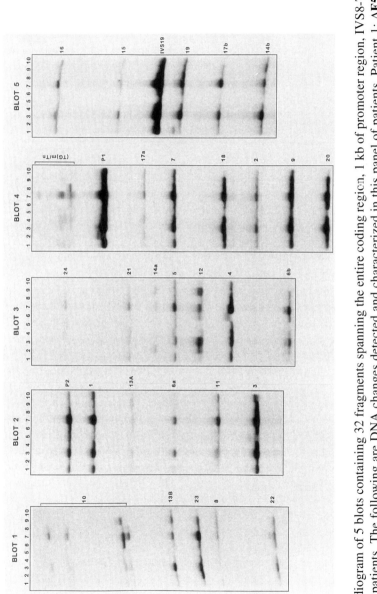

Fig. 2. Autoradiogram of 5 blots containing 32 fragments spanning the entire coding region, 1 kb of promoter region, IVS8-T tract, and IVS19 for 10 CF patients. The following are DNA changes detected and characterized in this panel of patients. Patient 1: **ΔF508** (blot 1, exon 10); **3659delC** (blot 5, exon 19); 1001+11CT/t (blot 3, exon 6b); 1898+152T/A (blot 3, exon 12). Patient 2: ΔF508 (blot 1, exon 10); **185+1G→T** (blot 2, exon 1); 1001+11C/T (blot 3, exon 6b); 1898+152T/A (blot 3, exon 12); 2694T/G (blot 3, exon 14a); 4521G/A (blot 3, exon 24); −896T/G (blot 4, P1). Patient 3: ΔF508 (blot 1, exon 10); **G551D1784C→A** (blot 2, exon 11); 1001=11CT/A (blot 3, exon 6b); 1898+152T/A (blot 3, exon 12); 3014-92G/A (blot 5, exon 16). Patient 4: ΔF508 (blot 1, exon 10); **711+1G→T** (blot 3, exon 5); 1001+11CT/ A (blot 3, exon 6b); 4521G/A (blot 3, exon 24). Patient 5: ΔF508 (blot 1, exon 10); **V1250G3814T→G** (blot 4, exon 20); R75Q356G→A

7. The PCR thermocycling "touchdown" program for amplification of the CFTR gene fragments using the GenAmp PCR System 9600 (Perkin-Elmer) consists of the following:

Segment 1: Initial denaturation; 94°C/2 min

Segment 2: 20 cycles of denaturation 94°C/20 s; annealing with initial temperature 60°C/20 s; decreasing 0.5°C every cycle (to final 50°C); extension 72°C/30 s

Segment 3: 15 cycles of denaturation 94°C/20 s; annealing 50°C/20 s; extension 72°C/30 s

Segment 4: 1 cycle of denaturation 94°C/20 s; annealing 50°C/20 s; extension 72°C/7 min

Segment 5: Denaturation 94°C/5 min

Segment 6: 5°C/5 min and cooling down to 4°C

Additional segments of denaturation and reannealing (segments 5 and 6) were added to maximize a heteroduplex formation.

8. In our protocol, 20 μL of each PCR mix (8 mixes, **Table 2**) from one individual are combined in one tube (total volume 8×20 μL = 160 μL) and purified using QIAquick Spin PCR Purification Kit (Qiagen). 600 μL of buffer PB (from the kit) was added to each tube, vortexed, and processed according to the manufacturer's protocol. After adding the washing solution PE (from the kit), the samples were left on the bench for 5 min before spinning (decreased salt content). The PCR DNA was eluted with 50 μL of deionized water and spun in the microcentrifuge for 60 s. The samples were dried in the SpeedVac and resdissolved in 20 μL of 1× loading buffer.

9. For faster and high-quality results, 10 samples were loaded five times on the same gel for subsequent parallel hybridization with five different probing cocktails (*see* **Subheadings 3.4.** and **3.5.**). Loading many samples (~50) at the same time and producing one membrane probed by five consecutive hybridizations rounds did not produce high-quality results due to incomplete DNA stripping, high background, and DNA loss. Therefore, five membranes with the same DNA content were produced for parallel hybridization with five probing cocktails.

(blot Fig. 2 *(continued)* 2, exon 3)/1001=11CT/t (blot 3, exon 6b). Patient 6: **I148T575T→C** (blot 3, exon 4); **319del6** (blot 4, exon 17a); 1898+152T/A (blot 3, exon 12); 3041-11C/T (blot 3, exon 6b). Patient 7: ΔF508 (blot 1, exon 10); **P574H1853C→A** (blot 3, exon 12); 4224G/A (blot 1, exon 22). Patient 8: ΔF508 (blot 1, exon 10); **N1303K4041C→G** (blot 3, exon 21). Patient 9: **L218X785T→A** (blot 2, exon 6a); **L967S3032T→C** (blot 5, exon 15); 1540G/A (blot 1, exon 10); 1898+152T/A (blot 3, exon 12). Patient 10: ΔF508 (blot 1, exon 10); **G85E386G→A** (blot 2, exon 3). ΔF508, the most common CFTR mutation, is a 3-bp deletion between nucleotides 1652 and 1655. Names in bold are disease-causing mutations. Other alterations are polymorphisms.

10. In our protocol, we used the following components in the primer labeling reaction mixture (quantities per one filter):

Primer(s)	$n*\mu L$
5× TdT buffer (Gibco-BRL)	10.0 μL
TdT (Gibco-BRL)	2.5 μL
^{32}P-dCTP	5.0 μL
water to	50.0 μL

    *1 μL of each primer solution is used in the reaction, so for four primers $n = 4$ μL. We use primers in concentration 100 ng/μL. The actual molar quantities of primers were 16.8 pmol for 18-mer, 15.9 pmol for 19-mer, 15.1 pmol for 20 mer, and 14.4 pmol for 21-mer. For labeling the TdT, enzyme is added just before the ^{32}P-dCTP and the reaction is carried out for 1 h at 37°C. In the CFTR protocol for probing 32 PCR fragments, five probe mixes are used. Their oligonucleotide composition is shown in **Table 1**.

11. **Figure 2** shows an autoradiogram of CFTR mutation screening results for DNA samples from 10 patients using the mHET protocol. The PCR band shifts corresponding to various heteroduplexes range from very minor, appearing as a thicker band, for example, to very clear patterns (e.g., ΔF508 or R75Q).

References

1. Worton, R.G. (1992) Duchenne musclar dystrophy: gene and gene product; mechanism of mutation in the gene. *J. Inherit. Metab. Dis.* **15,** 539–550.
2. Shen, D. and Vadgama, J. V. (1999) BRCA1 and BRCA2 gene mutation analysis: visit to the Breast Cancer Information Core (BIC). *Oncol. Res.* **11,** 63–69.
3. Rommens, J. M., Iannuzzi, M. C., Kerem, B., et al. (1989) Identification of the cystic fibrosis gene: chromosome walking and jumping. *Science* **245,** 1059–1065.
4. Riordan, J. R., Rommens, J. M., Kerem, B., et al. (1989) Identification of the cystic fibrosis gene: cloning and characterization of complementary DNA. *Science* **245,** 1066–1073.
5. Kerem, B., Rommens, J. M., Buchanan, J. A., et al. (1989) Identification of the cystic fibrosis gene: genetic analysis. *Science* **245,** 1073–1080.
6. Zielenski, J., Rozmahel, R., Bozon, D., et al. (1991) Genomic DNA sequence of the cystic fibrosis transmembrane conductance regulator (CFTR) gene. *Genomics* **10,** 214–228.
7. Orita, M., Iwahana, H., Kanazawa, H., et al. (1989) Detection of polymorphisms of human DNA by gel electrophoresis as single-strand conformation polymorphisms. *Proc. Natl. Acad. Sci. USA* **86,** 2766–2770.
8. Myers, R. M., Fischer, S. G., Lerman, L. S., and Maniatis, T. (1985) Nearly all single base substitutions in DNA fragments joined to a GC-clamp can be detected by denaturing gradient gel electrophoresis. *Nucleic Acids Res.* **13,** 3131–3145.
9. Keen, J., Lester, D., Inglehearn, C., Curtis, A., and Bhattacharya, S. (1991) Rapid detection of single base mismatches as heteroduplexes on Hydrolink gels. *Trends Genet.* **7,** 5.
10. Saleeb, J. A., Ramus, S. J., and Cotton, R. G. (1992) Complete mutation detection using unlabeled chemical cleavage. *Hum. Mutat.* **1,** 63–69.

11. Nollau, P. and Wagener, C. (1997) Methods for detection of point mutations: performance and quality assessment. IFCC Scientific Division, Committee on Molecular biology *Techniques. Clin. Chem.* **43,** 1114–1128.
12. Bhattacharyya, A. and Lilley, D. M. (1989) Single base mismatches in DNA. Long-and short-range structure probed by analysis of axis trajectory and local chemical reactivity. *J. Mol. Biol.* **209,** 583–597.
13. Bhattacharyya, A. and Lilley, D. M. (1989) The contrasting structures of mismatched DNA sequences containing looped-out bases (bulges) and multiple mismatches (bubbles). *Nucleic Acids Res.* **17,** 6821–6840.
14. Highsmith, E. W., Nataraj, A. J., Jin, Q., et al. (1994) novel mutation in the cystic fibrosis gene in patients with pulmonary disease but normal sweat chloride concentrations. *N. Engl. J. Med.* **331,** 974–980.
15. Cooper, D. N., Krawczak, M., and Antonarakis, S. E. (1995) The nature and mechanisms of human gene mutation, in *The Metabolic and Molecular Bases of Inherited Disease* (Scriver, C., Beaudet, A., Sly, W., and Valle, D., eds.), McGraw-Hill, New York, pp. 259–291.
16. Gilbert, J. R. and Vance, J. M. (1998) Isolation of genomic DNA from mammalian cells, in *Current Protocols in Human Genetics* (Dracopoli, N. C., Haines, J. L., Korf, B. R., et al., eds.), Wiley, New York, pp. A.3B.1–2.
17. Don, R. H., Cox, P. T., Wainwright, B. J., et al. (1991) "Touchdown" PCR to circumvent spurious priming during gene amplification. *Nucleic Acids Res.* **19,** 4008.
18. Highsmith, W. E., Burch, L. H., Zhou, Z., et al. (1994) A novel mutation in the cystic fibrosis gene in patients with pulmonary disease but normal sweat chloride concentrations. *N. Engl. J. Med.* **331,** 974–980.
19. Chu, C. S., Trapnell, B. C., Curristin, S., et al. (1993) Genetic basis of variable exon 9 skipping in cystic fibrosis transmembrane conductance regulator mRNA. *Nat. Genet.* **3,** 151–156.

2

cDNA Microarrays for Pharmacogenomic Analysis of Cystic Fibrosis

Meera Srivastava, Ofer Eidelman, and Harvey B. Pollard

1. Introduction

Cystic fibrosis (CF) is a single-gene disorder with a complex phenotype, in which multiple organs are affected. The pulmonary complications of CF, including mucous plugging and chronic bacterial infection of the lung, represent the major cause of morbidity and mortality *(1)*. It has long been suggested that mutations in CFTR, localized to the apical membrane of airway epithelia, lead to abnormalities in the fluid lining the airway surface. Accumulating evidence suggests that the inflammatory response in the CF lung may be excessive. However, it is not clear to what extent this reflects unusual persistence of stimulation of this response by bacteria or other pathogens, vs to what extent defects in CFTR might by themselves stimulate or cause dysregulation of inflammatory responses. Changes in the multigene patterns of expression can provide clues about regulatory mechanisms and broader cellular functions and biochemical pathways. In the context of cystic fibrosis disease and treatment, the knowledge gained from these types of measurements can help determine the causes and consequences of disease, how drugs and drug candidates work in cells and organisms, and what gene products might have therapeutic uses themselves or may be appropriate targets for therapeutic intervention.

For our own studies, we have concentrated on HEK-293 cells expressing recombinant wild-type or ΔF508 mutant CFTR *(2)*, and the naturally occurring CFTR mutant IB3 epithelial cells, repaired with wild-type CFTR using an AAV vector *(3)*. We describe here how the cells and cellular processes are studied using DNA arrays that allow complex mixtures of RNA and DNA to be interrogated in a parallel and quantitative fashion. Unlike the recombinant HEK-

From: *Methods in Molecular Medicine, vol. 70: Cystic Fibrosis Methods and Protocols*
Edited by: W. R. Skach © Humana Press Inc., Totowa, NJ

293 system, IB3 cells mirror the high IL8 secretion phenotype typical of the CF airway. Therefore, we have tended in recent times to concentrate in the latter system.

Our own approach has been to appreciate that not every site in the airway is identical physiologically to others, and to take these differences into account when devising and interpreting experiments. For example, CF epithelial cells high in the airway, such as nasal epithelia, secrete much less pro-inflammatory IL8 than those from lower in the airway. Furthermore, there are instances in which immortalized CF airway cells have lost their CF dependent pro-inflammatory phenotype of high IL8 secretion. For example, there are lines of IB3 cells that have lost their high IL8 secretion phenotype. In this case, one may want either to avoid these cells or use them in a knowledgeable manner.

The basic strategy is to grow cells of interest, treat them as dictated by the experiment, isolate messenger RNA, and analyze by cDNA or oligonucleotide array methods. Other approaches are available according to the taste and pocketbook of the investigator. For the academic investigator, cDNA arrays are less expensive than oligonucleotide arrays. These arrays also have the advantage of 25+ years of experience with dot-blot Northern assays.

2. Materials

2.1. Growth of IB3 Cells

1. Serum-free LHC-8 medium.

2.2. For DNase 1 Treatment of Total RNA

1. RNase-free DNase I (Boehringer-Mannheim #776-785, 10 U/μL): dilute to 1 U/μL in 1× DNase I buffer before to use.
2. 10× DNase I buffer: 400 mM Tris-HCl, pH 7.5, 100 mM NaCl, 60 mM MgCl$_2$.
3. Phenol/chloroform/isoamyl alcohol (25/24/1), equilibrated with 0.1 M sodium citrate (pH 4.5), 1 mM EDTA.
4. 95% ethanol.
5. 2 M NaOAc (pH 4.5).
6. 10× termination mix: 0.1 M EDTA, pH 8.0, 1 mg/mL glycogen (Sigma #G1508 or Boehringer-Mannheim #901-393).

2.3. cDNA Probe Synthesis

1. 10× dNTP mix (5 mM each of dCTP, dGTP, dTTP).
2. CDS primer mix.
3. 5× reaction buffer.
4. MMLV reverse transcriptase.
5. DTT (100 mM).
6. 10× termination mix: 0.1 M EDTA, pH 8.0, 1 mg/mL glycogen.
7. C$_0$t-1 DNA (1 mg/mL).
8. Deionized water.
9. (α-^{32}P)dATP (10 μCi/μL; 3000 Ci/mmol; Amersham #PB10204).

2.4. Purification of Probe

1. Nucleospin extraction spin columns (Clontech).
2. 2-mL collection tubes.
3. Buffer NT2 (Clontech).
4. Buffer NT3 (Clontech) (add 15 mL of 95% ethanol before use).
5. Buffer NE (Clonetech).

2.5. Choice of cDNA Microarrays

We have routinely purchased arrays from Clontech and used radiolabeled probes for quantitation. Other companies supply such arrays, and we do not represent any to be better than others.

2.6. Hybridization and Washing

1. Sheared salmon testes DNA (10 mg/mL; Sigma #D7656).
2. 10× denaturing solution: 1 M NaOH, 10 mM EDTA.
3. 2× neutralizing solution: 1 M NaH$_2$PO$_4$, pH 7.0.
4. 20× SSC (1 × SSC=0.15M NaCl and 0.015M sodium citrate).
5. 20% sodium dodecyl sulfate (SDS).
6. Wash solution 1: 2× SSC, 1% SDS.
7. Wash solution 2: 0.1× SSC, 0.5% SDS.

2.7. Analysis of Arrays

Phosphorimager. We happen to use an instrument from Molecular Dynamics. However, other instruments are available that to our knowledge are just as functional.

3. Methods
3.1. Origin of the IB3 Cells

IB3 cells are SV40 transformed cells derived from tracheal epithelial cells of a CF patient who received a lung transplant at Johns Hopkins University *(4)*. The IB3 cells are compound heterozygous mutants for the CFTR locus. One allele is the frequent mutation, ΔF508; the other is the less common mutation W1282X. The only expressed CFTR allele in IB3 cells is the ΔF508 (P. Zeitlin, personal communication). Two kinds of AAV-mediated repairs have been performed on this cell. One repair ("C38") was with a truncated CFTR missing the first 119 residues. The second repair was with a full-length CFTR ("S9").

3.2. Cell Culture

IB3 cells and repaired cell lines were obtained from Dr. Pam Zeitlin, Johns Hopkins University School of Medicine, and cultured in serum-free LHC-8 medium (Gibco, BRL). The cells are grown to confluence, washed with fresh medium, and then replaced in the incubator. Samples of supernatant medium were removed at the times shown and placed at –80°C until assayed for secreted materials, such as IL8. The cells themselves are taken for RNA isolation (*see* **Subheading 3.3.**).

3.3. Treatment of Cells with Bacteria or Drugs

If bacteria are to be included in the experiment, the LHC-8 medium must be modified by omitting the proprietary gentamycin. This allows the bacteria to survive during exposure to the cells. Cells are seeded at 2×10^5/well, and incubated overnight with drugs or carriers. At time zero, cells are washed with fresh medium and mixed with bacteria. In the case of *Pseudomonas aeruginosa* we use a ratio of bacteria/cell of 15/1.

3.4. Preparation of Total RNA

Total RNA is prepared by the method of Chirgwin et al *(5)*.

3.5. Treatment of Total RNA with DNase 1

The quality of the RNA used to make probes is the most important factor influencing the sensitivity and reproducibility of the hybridization pattern. A poor-quality RNA preparation leads to a high background on the membrane and an inaccurate hybridization pattern. These problems are typically caused by residual RNase and genomic DNA contamination. We use the Atlas Pure method to produce high yields of quality total RNA that is virtually free of genomic DNA, nucleases, and other impurities.

1. Combine the following reagents in a 1.5-mL microcentrifuge tube for each sample: 500 μL total RNA (1 mg/mL), 100 μL 10× DNase I buffer, 50 μL DNase I (1 U/μL), 350 μL deionized water, 1.0 mL total volume
2. Incubate the reactions at 37°C for 30 min.
3. Add 100 μL of 10× termination mix.
4. Split each reaction into two 1.5-mL microcentrifuge tubes (550 μL per tube).
5. Add 550 μL of phenol/chloroform/isoamyl alcohol (25/24/1; pH 4.5) to each tube and vortex thoroughly.
6. Spin in a microcentrifuge at 14,000 rpm for 10 min at 4°C to separate phases.
7. Carefully transfer the top aqueous layer to a new 1.5-mL microcentrifuge tube. Avoid pipetting any material from the interface or lower phase.
8. Repeat **steps 5–7** with 550 μL of chloroform
9. Add 1/10 vol (50 μL) of 2 *M* NaOAc (pH 4.5) and 2.5 vol (1.5 μL) of 95% ethanol.
10. After incubating in ice for 10 min, spin in a microcentrifuge at 14,000 rpm for 15 min at 4°C.
11. Wash the pellet with 500 μL of 80% ethanol.
12. Dissolve the precipitate in 250 μL of RNase-free H_2O and check the quality of total RNA by electrophoresing 0.5–2 μg on a denaturing formaldehyde/agarose/ethyl bromide gel.

Total RNA should have the two bright 28S and 18S rRNA bands at approximately 4.5 and 1.9 kb, respectively. The ratio of intensities of these bands should be 1.5–2.5:1.

3.6. Probe Synthesis from Total RNA

1. Prepare a master mix for all labeling reactions plus one extra reaction to ensure that you have sufficient volume. Combine the following reagents in a 0.5-mL microcentrifuge tube at room temperature:

	per rxn	4 rxns
5× reaction buffer	2 μL	8 μL
10× dNTP mix (for dATP label)	1 μL	4 μL
[α-^{32}P]dATP (3000 Ci/mmol, 10 μCi/μL)	3.5 μL	14 μL
DTT (100 mM)	0.5 μL	2 μL
Total volume	7 μL	28 μL

   (NB: ^{32}P or ^{33}P can be used interchangeably)

2. Preheat a polymerase chain reaction (PCR) thermal cycler to 70°C.
3. For each reaction, combine the following in a labeled 0.5-mL PCR tube:

For experimental RNA samples	For control RNA samples
1–2 μL RNA (2–5 mg)	1 μL RNA
1 μL CDS primer mix	1 μL CDS primer mix

   To each tube, add deionized H$_2$O to a final volume of 3 μL (if necessary).
4. Incubate tubes in a preheated PCR thermal cycler at 70°C for 2 min.
5. Reduce the temperature of the thermal cycler to 50°C (or 48°C if you are using an unregulated heating block or water bath) and incubate tubes for 2 min. During this incubation, add 1 μL MMLV reverse transcriptase per reaction to the master mix (add 4 μL MMLV RT for the 4-reaction master mix). Mix by pipetting, and keep the master mix at room temperature.
6. After completion of the 2-min incubation at 50°C, add 8 μL of master mix to each reaction tube.
7. Mix the contents of the tubes by pipetting and immediately return them to the thermal cycler.
8. Incubate tubes in the PCR thermal cycler at 50°C (or 48°C) for 25 min.
9. Stop the reaction by adding 1 μL of 10× termination mix.
10. Proceed with the column chromatography under **Subheading 3.6.** If necessary, store your probe on ice or at 4°C for a few hours.

3.7. Purification of Labeled cDNA from Unincorporated ^{32}P- or ^{33}P-Labeled Nucleotides by Column Chromatography

1. Dilute probe synthesis reactions to 200 μL total volume with buffer NT2.
2. Place a NucleoSpin extraction spin column into a 2-mL collection tube, and pipet the sample into the column. Centrifuge at 14,000 rpm for 1 min. Discard collection yube and flowthrough into the appropriate container for radioactive waste.

3. Insert the NuceloSpin column into a fresh 2-mL collection tube. Add 400 μL of buffer NT3 to the column. Centrifuge at 14,000 rpm for 1 min. Discard collection tube and flowthrough.
4. Repeat **step 3** twice.
5. Transfer the NucleoSpin column to a clean 1.5-mL microcentrifuge tube. Add 100 μL of buffer NE, and allow column to soak for 2 min.
6. Centrifuge at 14,000 rpm for 1 min to elute purified probe.
7. Check the radioactivity of the probe by scintillation counting:
   a. Add 2 μL of each purified probe to 5 mL of scintillation fluid in separate scintillation-counter vials.
   b. Count ^{32}P-labeled samples on the ^{32}P channel, and calculate the total number of counts in each sample.

3.8. Hybridizing cDNA Probes to the cDNA Microarray

1. Prepare a solution of ExpressHyb and sheared salmon testes DNA:
   a. Prewarm 5 mL of ExpressHyb at 68°C.
   b. Heat 0.5 mg of the sheared salmon testes DNA at 95–100°C for 5 min, then chill quickly on ice.
   c. Mix heat-denatured sheared salmon testes DNA with prewarmed ExpressHyb. Keep at 68°C until use.
2. Wet the Atlas array by placing it in a dish of deionized H_2O, and then place the membrane into the hybridization bottle. Pour off all the water from the hybridization bottle. Add 5 mL of the solution prepared in **step 1**. Ensure that the solution is evenly distributed over the membrane. Perform this step quickly to prevent the array membrane from drying (prehybridize for 30 min with continuous agitation at 68°C).
3. Prepare probe for hybridization by following the appropriate steps below.
   a. Mix together:
      Labeled probe (entire pool; 0.5–20 × 10^6 cpm): ~200 μL
      10× denaturing solution (1 M NaOH, 10 mM EDTA): ~22 μL
      Total volume: ~222 μL
   b. Incubate at 68°C for 20 min.
   c. Add the following to your denatured probe:
      C_0t-1 DNA (carrier DNA): 5 μL
      2× neutralizing solution (1 M NaH$_2$PO$_4$, pH 7.0): ~225 μL
      Total volume: ~450 μL
   d. Continue incubating at 68°C for 10 min.
4. Add the mixture prepared in **step 3** directly to the prehybridization solution.
5. Hybridize overnight with continuous agitation at 68°C.
6. The next day, prewarm wash solution 1 (2× SSC, 1 % SDS) and wash solution 2 (0.1× SSC, 0.5% SDS) at 68°C.
7. Carefully remove the hybridization solution and replace with 200 mL of prewarmed wash solution 1. Wash the Atlas array for 30 min with continuous agitation at 68°C. Repeat this step three more times.
8. Perform one 30-min wash in 200 mL of prewarmed wash solution 2 with continuous agitation at 68°C.

9. Perform one final 5-min wash in 200 mL of 2× SSC with agitation at room temperature.
10. Using forceps, remove the Atlas array from the container and shake off excess wash solution.
11. Immediately wrap the damp membrane in plastic wrap and expose the Atlas array to a phosphorimaging screen at room temperature.

3.9. Imaging and Quantitation of the cDNA Microarray

1. The imaged data from the Storm PhosphorImager are subjected to graphical organization with the IMP program, or an equivalent. The exact identification of points is verified by the PSCAN program, or an equivalent. With a limitated number of points (up to 1000) the data can be conveniently downloaded to a Microsoft Excel spreadsheet. Expression of each gene, in duplicate, are ratioed to the ubiquitin standard or to a basket of genes, chosen on the basis of no change under experimental conditions. This is a matter of taste and skill in design.
2. In the glass slide "chip" format with fluorescent labeled cDNAs, a ratio of messages from two conditions is obtained directly. Companies supplying these "chips" have proprietary software for analysis.

3.10. Data Mining Algorithms from cDNA Arrays

3.10.1. Hierarchial Clustering Algorithms

1. Several versions are available for this algorithm. We have had good experience with the Scanalyze software developed at Stanford University.
2. This algorithm can be used to find similarities between cells under different treatment conditions. A discussion of the caveats important in this approach are given by Pollard et al. *(6)*.

3.10.2. The GRASP Algorithm

1. The analytic strategy we have employed routinely is embodied in the GRASP algorithm. In this algorithm, changes in gene expression due to a given set of experimental conditions are quantitated in terms of the number of standard deviations (SDs) from the mean of all the genes in the array (*see* Srivastava et al., 1999). This technique vastly increases the statistical power of the analysis. Following ratioing to the ubiquitin standard, as mentioned above, each gene on each blot is analyzed in duplicate. In the specific case of the 588 Clontech array, the duplicate positions have an error of ca. 1.3%. Duplicate samples on duplicate blots in this system (or other) were found to vary from each other by only ca. 12%. An expression data for a given gene in a treated cell are then ratioed to expression in the parental cell line.The log of this ratio is then graphed against the log of an equivalent ratio of gene expressions for a different treatment to that of the parental cell line. The diagonal of this orthogonal plot is the distribution of equivalently expressing genes. The relationship of different genes to this diagonal can then be expressed as being inside or outside the ±1 SD region around the diagonal. Knowledge of relative positions on the orthogonal plot, outside the ±1

SD region, then allow one to state that the expression of the given gene is or is not related to the mutation or experimental condition. Genes are then assessed as being a given multiple of SDs from the mean of the entire distribution. Mutation on condition-specific genes are then available by inspection.

2. The advantages of the GRASP orthogonal plot is that the specific effects of drugs or other variables can be assessed directly. For example, the place on the plot may vary from the "control" if a drug is added to the cells. The two positions on the graph constitute a "vector," with magnitude and direction. Movements "toward" or "away" from the diagonal can be interpreted in terms of possible medicinal value. We have specifically developed these genomic vectors for the study of the CFTR-mimetic drug CPX in recombinant HEK-293 cells *(2)* and refer the reader to that paper for more details.

3.10.3. GENESAVER Algorithm

The GENESAVER algorithm (gene space vector) allows one to use physiological variables to define genes involved in processes related to the variable. In one conceptual formulation of the fundamental problem in cystic fibrosis, it is thought that the epithelial cells in the lung express an intrinsic inflammatory phenotype. This is manifest by elevated IL8 secretion from the epithelial cells. So, one can use the GENESAVER algorithm to determine which genes are expressed in proportion to IL8 secretion under various conditions *(3)*. More generally, any physiological parameter can be used to evaluate the genomic basis of a biological process or disease.

The GENESAVER algorithm is applied as follows.

3. The first step is to identify a physiological parameter that is causatively related to or is symptomatically indicative of the disease. In the case of CF, one can use IL8 or other pro-inflammatory cytokine in the lung. For diabetes, it might be blood sugar. The choice is limited by the disease of interest. This relevant parameter can also be the expression level of a given gene. The relevant physiological parameter is then measured under the different conditions and the results are used to create a multidimensional mathematical vector. Finally, at the time of the physiological variable, one collects RNA from affected cells or tissues, or surrogates that one hopes might reflect the affected tissue.

4. The next analytic step is to take each gene on the array, to calculate a similar multidimensional vector based on the expression levels of that gene in the various experimental conditions. The components of these vectors should be the logarithm of the ratio between the expression level in each experimental condition and in the control for that given gene. We use one of the conditions (i.e., "control") as a benchmark, and create an $(n-1)$-dimensional vector (where n is the number of experimental conditions). This allows us to compare between different genes with disparate expression levels, and also to eliminate possible effects from dissimilar binding efficiencies for the cDNAs of different genes.

5. The final step in the analysis is to calculate the angle in multidimensional space between the vector for each gene and the vector for the physiological parameter.

Small angles between vectors indicate that there is a correlation between the changes in expression levels of specific genes and the changes in the physiological parameter. Angles close to 180° indicate anticorrelation between the gene and the paramete. This means that in those experimental conditions where the parameter increases, the gene expression is reduced, and vice versa.

6. The advantage of the GENESAVER algorithm is that the approach allows one to identify genes that exhibit a pattern of expression that is similar to a physiological parameter relevant to the studied disease. The advantages of this approach include the ability to test a hypothesis regarding signaling pathway genes involved in the physiological or disease process of interest. In the case of our CF experiments, IL8 secretion is highly correlated with selected genes from the TNFαR/NFκB pathway *(3)*. However, since the algorithm requires no a priori assumptions, it is useful for investigations that are "discovery driven." For those interested in the details of this algorithm, and its application to specific conditions, please contact the authors.

References

1. Welsh, M. J., Tsui, L.-C., Bost, T. F., and Beaudet, A. L. (1995) Cystic fibrosis, in *The Methods and Molecular Bases of Inherited Disease* (Sciver, C. R., Beaudet, A. L., Sly, W. S., and Valle, D., eds.), McGraw-Hill, New York, pp. 3799–3876.
2. Srivastava, M. Eidelman, O., and Pollard, H. B. (2000) Gene expression microarray pharmacogenomics of wt and mutant CFTR, and of the CF drug CPX. *Mol. Med.* **5,** 753–767.
3. Eidelman, O., Srivastava, M., Zhang, J., Murtie, J., Jacobson, K., Metcalf, E., Weinstein, D., and Pollard, H. (2001) Control of the proinflammatory state in cystic fibrosis lung epithelial cells by genes from the TNFαR/NFκB pathway. *Mol. Med.* **7,** 523–534.
4. Zeitlin, P. L., Lu, L., Hwang, T.-C, Rhim, J., Cutting, G. R., Keiffer, K. A., Craig, R., and Guggino, W .B. (1991) A cystic fibrosis bronchial epithelial cell line: immortalization by adeno12-SV40 infection. *Am. J. Respir. Cell Mol. Biol.* **4,** 313–319.
5. Chirgwin, J. M., Przybyla, A. E., MacDonald, R. J., and Rutter, W. J. (1979) Isolation of biologically active ribonucleic acid from sources enriched in ribonuclease. *Biochemistry* **18,** 5294–5299.
6. Pollard, H. B., Eidelman, O., Jacobson, K. A., and Srivastava, M. (2001) Pharmacogenomics of cystic fibrosis. *Mol. Intervent.* **1,** 54–63.

3

Natural Animal Models of Human Genetic Diseases

Jeffrey J. Wine, Michael Dean, and Damjan Glavac

1. Introduction

The earth's organisms are a vast repository of genetic diversity. Each species ($n > 10^6$) is distinguished from every other by a unique genomic sequence that is passed on to successive generations with extremely high, but not perfect, fidelity. Imperfections in DNA replication and repair mean that the genome of each member of a species is also unique. Intraspecific differences are one basis for individuality, including individual differences in susceptibility to disease. The most striking example of such differences is genetic diseases.

1.1. The Need for Animal Models and a New Approach to Obtaining Them

Animal models of genetic diseases have been extremely useful. Models can arise from chance discoveries, such as narcopleptic dogs (1,2), or by intentional screening of inbred animals (3). Most important, actual creation of mouse models of diseases has been made possible by stem cell lines and methods for introducing specific mutations into those cells (4,5), which has led to an explosion of information (6). Unfortunately, mouse models are not ideal for some human diseases. For example, in the mouse model of cystic fibrosis (CF), the mice fail to develop the lung and pancreatic pathology that are hallmarks of the human disease, but have a more severe form of intestinal disease (7,8). Furthermore, even though mice with improved disease features are being developed through selective breeding (9), mice are still not ideal for many purposes, especially those related to the evaluation of clinical interventions. Thus, alternative animal models would be a boon for researchers. However, in animals other than the mouse it has so far been extremely difficult to develop embryonic stem cell lines that routinely give rise to viable offspring (10–12).

From: *Methods in Molecular Medicine, vol. 70: Cystic Fibrosis Methods and Protocols*
Edited by: W. R. Skach © Humana Press Inc., Totowa, NJ

In this chapter we describe an alternative strategy for the discovery of natural animal models of recessive genetic diseases. The strategy is based on the hypothesis that *disease frequencies across human populations offer some guide to disease frequencies in animals.* When disease frequencies are high enough ($>10^{-6}$), the method is feasible using existing methods for genetic screening of genomic DNA.

The key to the feasibility of the method is the ability to screen for unaffected heterozygotes. It is not sufficiently appreciated that even rare, recessive genetic diseases have relatively high heterozygous gene frequencies. For example, a recessive disease frequency of 1/1,000,000 arises from a carrier frequency of only 1/500. This enormous disparity explains why carriers can be detected readily in populations for which the associated recessive disease is apparently "nonexistent."

In this chapter we introduce the general concept, outline two attempts to implement the approach *(13)*, and provide a series of steps that should be followed to allow this approach to become a general and cost-effective alternative to stem cell technology.

1.2. Do Recessive Human Genetic Diseases Have Animal Counterparts?

Some recessive diseases have been documented in both humans and animals *(1,2)*, but how likely is it that a specific human genetic disease will occur in a specific animal species? The human genome is estimated to contain between 30,000 and 40,000 genes *(14)*. However, the Online Mendelian Inheritance in Man lists fewer than 10,000 autosomal entries, and fewer than half of these are recessive. The disparity between gene number and disease number has many explanations, but the contribution of each is unknown. If we consider only recessive mutations, we know from experimental work that some of these cause early embryonic lethality when homozygous, whereas others cause no obvious phenotype. Another consideration is that recessive diseases are usually so rare that the chance of a disease escaping diagnosis is high. That leaves an unknown proportion of genes for which it might be argued that the lack of a known disease state arises simply because the mutation frequency in the associated gene is so low that no human exists who has two copies of the mutated gene. How likely is this?

The human population is estimated to be approaching 6×10^9 individuals. To estimate the number of mutations within this vast gene pool we need to know the mutation rate for human genomic DNA. Unfortunately, estimates of that rate vary widely. Based on extensive experiments with *Drosophila*, Crow gives an estimated mutation rate per nucleotide per generation, of 1.5×10^{-8}, and predicts that the 3×10^9 nucleotide pairs of the human genome will therefore acquire ~100 new mutations in each human zygote, with ~2% of these affecting genes. To avoid the accumulation of an enormous mutational load, it is proposed that heterozygotes are mildly but cumulatively disadvantaged, and that their preferential elimination culls numerous mutations simultaneously to counterbalance the accumulation *(15)*. In contrast, experiments in which 50 independent lines of *Caenorhabditis elegans* were allowed to accumulate spontaneous mutations led to the conclusion that the deleterious mutation rate per haploid genome was 0.0026 *(16)*.

1.3. Carriers Greatly Exceed Affected Individuals

As stated above, the enormous disparity between heterozygote and homozygote frequencies (**Fig. 1**) is not widely appreciated. Cystic fibrosis illustrates some of the consequences of this disparity. CF has an extraordinarily high frequency in the U.S. and northern European Caucasian populations, where about 1/25 individuals is heterozygous for mutations in the causative gene, *CFTR*. Cystic fibrosis is comparatively rare in other populations. One estimate of the incidence rate of cystic fibrosis in Japan gave a rate of 3.1 per million live births from 1969 to 1980 (~1/323,000). The highest rates of CF were in Hokkaido (the most northern Island) and lowest in Okinawa (the most southern island). The mean age at death from CF was 3 years for both sexes during the period 1969 to 1985 *(17)*. A similar estimate of 1/350,000 using different methods was made more recently *(18)*. Inspection of **Fig. 1** or simple calculation shows that the lowest estimate still corresponds to a carrier frequency of ~1/295, suggesting that the Japanese population ($n \approx 10^8$), has ~ 339,000 individuals carrying disease-causing *CFTR* mutations. A similar exercise for China suggests it has > 4 million cystic fibrosis carriers.

The high incidence of cystic fibrosis in Caucasian populations results primarily but not exclusively from the frequency of one very common allele (ΔF508). In the CF population of the United States and Canada, the ΔF508 mutation accounts for ~70% of all alleles. Hence, if ΔF508 were to be subtracted out, the frequency of cystic fibrosis in this population would drop from about 1/2,500 (1/25 carrier frequency) to ~1/28,000 (~1/83 carrier frequency). That is still much higher than the estimates for CF in Japan, and suggests that factors other than the ΔF508 mutation are at work.

1.4. The Hypothesis: The Aggregate "Background" Frequency of Human and Animal Mutations Are Similar

We hypothesize that the *aggregate* frequency of non-ΔF508 CF-causing mutations in human populations offers a rough guide to the *aggregate* CFTR mutation frequencies in non-human primates. This hypothesis does not assume that any specific mutations found in human populations will necessarily be found in nonhuman primates. Correspondingly, of course, the frequency of particular mutations in the human population will not provide information

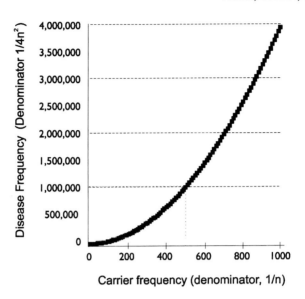

Fig. 1. Relation between carrier and homozygous (disease) frequencies for recessive genetic diseases. The key concept for the natural animal models strategy is based on the relatively high frequency of carriers even for rare recessive diseases. For example, as shown here, a disease that occurs in only 1 per million animals has a disease frequency of 1/500 animals.

about particular mutation frequencies in nonhuman primate populations; that is evident from the different pattern of mutations observed in separated human populations. Thus, it does not make sense to search nonhuman populations for specific mutations. Instead, a method is required that is capable of detecting unknown mutations.

We know of no *a priori* reasoning and certainly no data that would suggest a much different aggregate CF mutation frequency in nonhuman primates. *CFTR* is a large gene, and like any gene it is susceptible to insertions or deletions that cause frame shifts, as well as stop mutations and splicing mutations. *CFTR* is also, for unknown reasons, extremely susceptible to missense mutations that cause it to be misprocessed *(19,20)*. Even wild-type *CFTR* is inefficiently processed. Approximately 75% of wild-type CFTR protein is degraded after core glycosylation and never reaches the plasma membrane—this occurs across a range of cells expressing various levels of CFTR and so is not merely an artifact of high levels of exogenous expression *(21)*. At least four critical regions in *CFTR* (the pore and the two NBFs) are susceptible to missense mutations that interfere with CFTRs ability to function as a Cl^- channel— these also cause cystic fibrosis *(22)*. Finally, recent evidence indicates that some missense mutations that have little affect on processing or chloride channel function can cause CF by altering HCO_3^- transport (*23*).

In sum, the large size of *CFTR* creates many opportunities for mutations, and a high proportion of all mutations render *CFTR* nonfunctional and lead to disease in the homozygous state. In humans and mice, heterozygosity for CF has no detectable disadvantage. Thus, leaving aside the possibility of a heterozygote advantage, and barring some unforeseen feature that powerfully selected against monkey carriers, there is no efficient mechanism to prevent *CFTR* mutations from accumulating in a population at low frequencies, since such frequencies will give rise to homozygotes too infrequently to alter mutation frequencies in the population.

1.5. Which Species Should Be Studied?

The choice of species to be studied is greatly narrowed by several obvious features. Because mice can be genetically manipulated, there is little reason to study any species further removed from humans than mice. Among remaining species, four main criteria determine suitability for discovery of natural animal models. These criteria are (1) *availability*, (2) *experimental tractability*, (3) *similarity to humans*, and (4) *genetic diversity*. The first two criteria need not be elaborated. However, the criterion of human similarity can vary depending on the disease of interest, such that a more closely related species may be less optimal than species that are further removed phylogentically. For example, sheep (*24*) and pigs (*25*) have lungs that may be better experimental models of some human lung diseases than monkeys. Genetic diversity within the target population is a crucial feature. Unfortunately, the need for high genetic diversity excludes most domestic populations of animals, but even wild populations may be unsuitable. For example, cheetahs display an extreme degree of genetic homogeneity, presumably as a result of a severe population bottleneck that occurred ~10,000 years ago (*26*).

Old World monkeys, particularly the genus *Macaca*, rank highly on all four criteria. (1) Availability is good. Wild populations are still large (though declining at an alarming rate) and are extensively distributed throughout Africa and Asia. An estimated 40,000 primates are imported annually into the United States for research purposes. Of greater relevance are the large number of primates (~16,000) maintained at National Institutes of Health (NIH) Regional Primate Research Centers. This population is bred exclusively for research, and the monkeys receive excellent care and typically live for longer than a decade. The last point is critical, because it is essential to be able to retrieve an animal after a mutation has been identified in its DNA. (2) Monkeys are good experimental subjects, and for some experiments are virtually the only suitable animal subjects. (3) Monkeys are in general more similar to humans than any other species except the great apes, and apes have become so endangered that their use is virtually precluded except for the most essential studies. (4) Finally, the evidence suggests that monkeys may be an unusually rich repository of genetic diversity. Studies of six species of macaques *(27)* and of 23 local populations of Rhesus monkeys spread across Vietnam, Burma, and 10 provinces of China *(28)* extended previous estimates of genetic heterogeneity among and within species. Our own studies have confirmed a high degree of genetic diversity even within *Macaca* maintained for many years within Regional Primate Research Centers.

A possible heterozygote advantage. With regard to a possible heterozygote advantage, it may be relevant that monkeys are notoriously susceptible to secretory diarrhea. Human CF heterozygotes are thought to be partially protected against certain diarrheal diseases because CFTR is rate-limiting for Cl^--mediated electrolyte and fluid secretion from intestinal crypts *(29,30)*. In some secretory pathways, fluid secretion by CF heterozygotes is indeed reduced to 50% of normal *(31)*. Hence, diarrheal diseases that stimulate the CFTR-dependent pathway should cause less fluid and electrolyte loss in heterozygotes. This hypothesis has been tested directly by administering cholera toxin to heterozygous CF mice, but results were conflicting *(32,33)*.

A study of serum electrolyte values in 100 Rhesus monkeys with diarrhea observed hyponatremia in 88% and hypochloremia in 80% *(34)*. This strongly suggests that the putative protective effect of CFTR mutations should also apply to nonhuman primates, and could result in positive selection pressure and hence some enrichment of CF alleles in nonhuman primate populations. To give some indication of the magnitude of this potential selection pressure for *CFTR* mutations, in the California Primate Research Center, 34% of nonexperimental deaths in macaques 1 year of age and older were due to gastrointestinal disease *(35)*.

Possible heterozygote disadvantages. The severity of disease caused by *CFTR* mutations is closely related to the extent to which CFTR-mediated Cl^- conductance is lost. Mild mutations can arise for each class of *CFTR* mutation; for example, some trafficking mutations allow a certain proportion of *CFTR* to be processed *(36,37)*, some regulatory mutations do not completely disrupt function *(36,37)*, and all conductance mutations to date produced only a partial loss of conductance.

Within a critical range of residual CFTR function, subjects no longer display the classic cystic fibrosis syndrome, but instead suffer, if they are male, from sterility secondary to congenital bilateral absence of the vas deferens (CBAVD) *(38)*. The extreme susceptibility of the vas deferens to mutations in *CFTR* is not completely understood. However, part of the answer may be that *CFTR* is spliced differently in the vas. A common mutation that contributes to

CBAVD is a reduction in a tract of eight thymidines within intron 8 to a five-thymidine variant that leads to missplicing of *CFTR*. The proportion of misspliced *CFTR* is greater in the vas deferens than in the lung *(39)*. Unlike humans, mice that are homozygous for *CFTR* mutations remain fertile *(40)*. Given this species difference, a possibility that must be considered is that in some species male fertility will be lost or compromised even in the heterozygous state.

1.6. Testing the Approach: the Search for a Monkey CF Carrier

In spite of such arguments, only direct experimental test can provide accurate estimates of the frequency of *CFTR* mutations and polymorphisms in a given species. With no additional information, the chances of mutations being more frequent in nonhuman primates than in human populations is equal to the chance that they are less frequent. For a mutation frequency of 1/500 (for a disease frequency of 1/1,000,000); screening 1500 animals, yields ~95% chance of detecting a mutation if the detection method is perfect. Of course, no detection method is perfect. The single-strand conformation polymorphism (SSCP) method is nearly perfect for detecting small insertions and deletions, and probably detects >90% of point mutations. However, it does not detect intronic mutations or deletions of entire exons. Based on assays of CF populations, the single-strand conformation polymorphism and heteroduplex (SSCP/HD) method we use is estimated to be able to detect ~95% of CF mutations *(41)*. Thus, screening of 1500 primates provides a 95% chance of finding a mutation if mutations occur at a frequency of 1/400 or greater, equal to a disease frequency of ~1/640,000. It is worth emphasizing that even a disease frequency of 1/100,000 would make it unlikely that even a single CF birth would have occurred among the entire primate population in all of the U.S. Primate Research Centers during the last decade. Given the infant mortality rate mentioned above, even if such a rare event occurred, the chance that it would have been detected is remote. This emphasizes the power of heterozygote analysis even among populations in which the disease appears to be "nonexistent."

The general significance of this program will be to determine the feasibility of establishing animal models *for any disease* by screening. If our hypothesis of an approximate correspondence in mutation frequencies among primates is confirmed, a program like the one we propose should be at least as cost-effective as the production of mice by stem cell recombinant methodology.

2. Materials

1. Whole blood (~3 mL) was obtained by venipuncture, mainly during routine medical checkups of primates, and was shipped on ice in ethylenediaminetetraacetic acid (EDTA)-containing (purple-top) tubes.
2. EDTA (Sigma, St. Louis, MO); 1 mL of 10% EDTA solution was used for each blood sample.

3. Puregene DNA isolation kit (Gentra Systems, Research Triangle Park, NC).
4. CFTR Primers, Operon Technologies (for primer sequences, *see* **ref. *42***).
5. AmpliTaq® DNA Polymerase and GeneAmp® 10× polymerase chain reaction (PCR) Buffer was used for PCR amplification (Applied Biosystems, Foster city, CA).
6. GeneAmp 10× PCR buffer: 500 mM KCl, 100 mM Tris-HCl (pH 8.3), 15 mM $MgCl_2$, and 0.01% (w/v) gelatin.
7. GeneAmp® dNTPs: Each four-vial set contains 320 µL of 10 mM dATP, dCTP, dGTP, or dTTP.
8. Isotope α^{32}P dCTP (3000 Ci/mM) (Amersham Pharmacia Biotech, Piscataway, NJ). 0.5 mCi of α^{32}P dCTP (3000 Ci/mM) isotope was included in each 10-µL PCR mixture for labeling.
9. Denaturing mixture: 95% formamide, 20 mM EDTA, 0.05% bromophenol blue, 0.05% xylene cyanol, and 20 mM NaOH.
10. Standard components for vertical polyacrylamide gel electrophoresis (e.g., MDE gel solution or acrylamide/bis-acrylamide mix, glycerol, TEMED, vertical slab gel Kodak Biomax STS 45i apparatus for running 35 × 40 cm, 0.4 mm-thick gels).
    a. Plates (35 × 40cm) for vertical slab gel Kodak Biomax STS 45I apparatus (Eastman Kodak Company, Rochester, NY).
    b. TEMED (N,N,N',N'-tetramethylethylenediamine), >99% (Sigma).
    c. MDE gel (BioWhittaker Molecular Applications, Rockland, ME)
    d. Glycerol >99% electrophoresis reagent (Sigma) 10% added to MDE gel solution.
    e. Polyacrylamide: Bio-Rad Laboratories 40% acrylamide:N,N'-.
    f. Methylenebisacrylamide solution, 37.5:1 (2.6%C).
    g. Tris-Borate–EDTA (TBE) buffer, 5× concentration (Sigma).
    h. 1 L of 1× TBE buffer was used for electrophoresis.
11. Electrophoresis power supply, EPS 1001 (Amersham Pharmacia Biotech, Piscataway, NJ) was used for electrophoresis.
12. Autoradiography was done on Kodak Scientific Imaging Film X-OMAT AR (35 × 43 cm) (Eastman Kodak Company, Rochester, NY).
13. Mutations were made with Stratagene's Quick-change site-directed mutagenesis kit (La Jolla, CA) and verified with restriction enzymes (Life Technologies, Grand Island, NY) or sequencing.
14. Plasmid purification: Qiagen plasmid maxi kit (Valencia, CA).
15. Transfection: SuperFect transfection reagent (Qiagen).
16. Dish coating: fibronectin (Sigma, F2006).
17. DME H21, with 10% fetal bovine serum, 2 mM glutamine, and Pen/Strep (100 U/ mg/mL) (Sigma).
18. Efflux buffer: 50 mM N-2-hydroxy ethylpiperazine-N'-2-ethane sulfonic acid (HEPES), 5.4 mM KCl, 130 mM NaCl, 1.8 mM $CaCl_2$, 1.0 mM sodium phosphate (monobasic), 0.8 mM $MgSO_4$, pH adjusted to 7.4 with NaOH, and glucose 100 mg/100 mL (all from Sigma).

3. Methods

The overall approach is outlined in **Fig. 2**.

Identify Animal Population
Obtain blood
Purify DNA
Design Primers
Amplify and label Exons
Denature-Renature
Run on non-denaturing gel
Identify shifts
Sequence
Identify candidate mutations
Introduce mutations into cDNA
Express mutated cDNA
Assay
Identify candidate carriers and establish breeding groups
Screen offspring for homozygous individuals

Fig. 2. Outline of methods.

1. *Identify an Animal Population.* Our sample consisted of 1500 primates, *Macaca mulatta, M. nemestrina, M. fuscata, M. arctoides, M. fasicularis*, and *P. anubis*. We used different species as a way of increasing genetic diversity. The similarity among species was such that the primers amplified CFTR in all species. The primates are maintained at five NIH Regional Primate Research Centers. Pedigrees are used when available to select maximally outbred animals. A program is now underway to use genetic typing to establish pedigrees for all primates in the Research Centers. That will make future use of these animals more efficient.

2. *Obtain blood.* Blood samples (2 mL in EDTA-containing tubes) are obtained during routine testing of animals and shipped on ice via overnight express.

3. *Purify DNA.* Genomic DNA is purified from the blood samples using a commercially available kit (Puregene, Gentra) and stored at –20°C.

4. *Design primers.* It is necessary to know or to obtain the genomic sequence of the target gene before proceeding. We use intronic primers so that we do not miss mutations in the splice sites and adjacent regions of exons. We start with intronic primers based on the published genomic sequence for human *CFTR (43)*. Because the homology between human and monkey introns is about 90%, this strategy amplified about half of the *CFTR* exons. New primers were designed for 12 exons that did not amplify with human primers *(42)*. To obtain intronic primers for the primate exons that did not amplify with human primers, we reasoned that the high intronic conservation between monkeys and humans *(42)* would allow us to obtain effective primers simply by shifting the primer site to different regions of the introns. That strategy was successful for many exons on the first try. For others, we select yet a different region of each flanking intron and pair it with an

exonic primer. By repeating this process we were able to amplify flanking intron sequences for all remaining exons. Optimal intronic primers were then selected.

5. *Amplify and label exons.* We studied 25 of the 27 *CFTR* exons, omitting the two shortest exons. Genomic DNA is amplified and radioactively labeled with conventional polymerase chain reaction. PCR is carried out with a 10-mL reaction mixture containing 40 ng DNA, 0.2 U *Taq* polymerase, 2.5 pmol of each primer, 50 mM KCl, 2.5 mM MgCl$_2$, 10 mM Tris-HCl (pH 8.3), 200 μM each of dATP, dGTP, dTTP dCTP; 0.5 mCi of $^{\gamma 32}$PdCTP (3000 Ci/mM), and 0.001% gelatin. Amplification parameters: denature 6 min at 94°C, then 30 cycles of: denature for 30 s at 94°C, anneal 30 s at 55°C, extend 1 min at 72°C; followed by 7 min at 72°C. DNA can be amplified from 96 different monkeys in parallel.

6. *Denature–renature.* After amplification each reaction mixture in the 96-well plate is diluted 1:1 with a mixture of 95% formamide, 20 mM EDTA, 0.05% bromophenol blue, 0.05% xylene cyanol, and 20 mM NaOH. The plate is then returned to the PCR machine and heated to 95°C for 4 min, followed by snap-cooling in an ice/water bath.

7. *Run on nondenaturing gel.* Exons are screened using single-strand conformation polymorphism and heteroduplex (SSCP/HD) analysis *(44)*. The principle of this method is illustrated in **Fig. 3**. In brief, after denaturing and renaturing, the single strands refold on to themselves as well as annealing with opposite strands. In the purest case, each single strand will refold into one conformation that will migrate differently from the opposite strand and from the duplex, giving three distinct bands. However, variations of this simplest pattern can be observed if a portion of one or the other strand assumes a second stable configuration. Regardless, if a mutation exists on one chromosome, it almost always alters the migration pattern of one or both strands, as well as forming heteroduplexes with the unmutated opposite strands. The method depends simply on being able to detect this different migration. We use gel conditions that had previously been optimized for *CFTR* and that should be capable of detecting >95% of *CFTR* mutations *(45,46)*. For each exon from each animal, 2–4 μL of PCR reaction mixture is loaded in one well of a 100-lane gel. Lanes are generated with a shark's-tooth comb), polyacrylamide gel consisting of 0.5× MDE (FMC Bioproducts, Rockland, ME) plus 10% glycerol *(47)*. Gels are run in a 4°C cold room for 4–8 h at 50 W. Gels are then adsorbed onto filter paper and the paper with adherent gel is peeled from the glass plates, dried, and autoradiographed for 12–48 h.

8. *Identify shifts.* Each gel contains 96 juxtaposed lanes. The method relies on the majority of exons having identical sequences and hence identical SSCP patterns, against which any shifts are obvious by comparison with the flanking sequences.

9. *Sequence exons of interest.* Amplified and purified DNA from samples displaying different SSCP patterns is then sequenced. Because sequencing is now so commonly used and is often carried out by a separate, dedicated facility, this step is not described further.

10. *Identify candidate disease-causing mutations.* The choice of which missense mutations to pursue via functional analysis is subjective. Obvious criteria include the

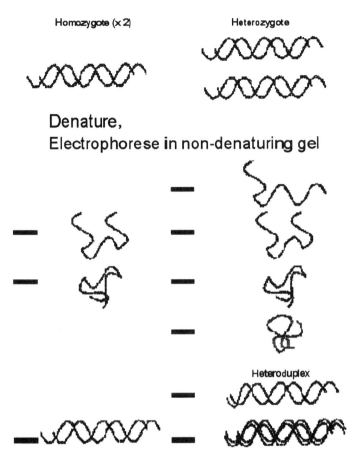

Fig. 3. Schematic of SSCP. A genomic DNA fragment of ~200–500 base pairs is amplified and isotopically labeled, then denatured and run on a nondenaturing gel. With proper dilution, similar proportions of the sense and antisense strands fold onto themselves, assuming different conformations and thus migrating as two distinct bands. If the conditions are chosen correctly, another portion will reanneal with the opposite strand and run as a duplex. Ideally this yields three bands, but many variants are possible because a strand may form more than one stable conformation. When the DNA is from a region that is heterozygous, additional bands are typically observed as both single strands and heteroduplexes.

    frequency of the mutation, whether it changes a conserved amino acid, and whether the change is conservative or nonconservative. Less obvious criteria are based on comparisons with the large number of human missense mutations; certain regions of *CFTR* (e.g., NBD1) appear to be more sensitive to the missense mutations.
11. *Introduce mutations into cDNA.* For functional assays, candidate missense mutations are introduced into human CFTR cDNA using Stratagene's Quick-change

site-directed mutagenesis kit. The presence of the mutation was verified with restriction site analysis as appropriate and direct sequencing.

12. *Express mutated cDNA.* Plasmids are purified with the Qiagen plasmid maxi kit and concentrated to ~1 µg/µL. Human embryonic kidney (HEK) 293 cells are then transfected with the plasmids using Qiagen's SuperFect transfection reagent. HEK296 cells (1.4×10^5 in 2 mL of medium) are seeded onto 35-mm dishes coated with fibronectin (Sigma, F2006) and grown in DME H21 with 10% fetal bovine serum, 2 mM glutamine, and Pen/Strep (100 U/mg/mL).

13. *Assay for function.* For mutations that obviously disrupt the gene, this difficult and expensive step is unnecessary, but for missense mutations a functional assay is essential. Assays require knowledge of what the gene product does. CFTR does many things, but its best-documented role is as a protein kinase A (PKA)-dependent anion channel. A simple assay for this CFTR function is to measure the ability of cells transfected with CFTR to increase their conductance to ^{125}I (a convenient surrogate for Cl$^-$) after exposure to forskolin, which elevates cAMP via a direct action on adenylate cyclase *(48)*. HEK cells transfected with plasmid alone do not respond to forskolin, while cells transfected with wild-type CFTR show rapid increases in ^{125}I efflux. If mutations lead to diminished CFTR function, cells transfected with such mutations are predicted to show efflux responses that are significantly reduced relative to those from cells expressing wild-type CFTR. Cells are incubated at 37°C for 2 h in efflux buffer containing ~2 µCi of ^{125}I/mL, then washed 3× with 1-mL aliquots of 22°C buffer. Efflux samples are collected at 30-s intervals with total fluid replacement. Remaining counts are removed by lysing cells, scintillation fluid iss added, and samples are counted in a Beckman liquid scintillation counter. Efflux rate constants were estimated according to the formula given by Venglarik et al. *(48)*.

14. *Establish breeding groups.* Animals carrying mutations that lead to diminished CFTR function are selected for breeding to homozygosity. All animals used for this study are already maintained as part of breeding populations in NIH primate facilities. Thus breeding groups are established by housing the animals together in a facility separate from other animals.

15. *Screen offspring for homozygous individuals.* As offspring are born in the breeding groups, they are genotyped and then either maintained within the group or returned to the main colony. Homozygous animals are subjected to physiological and biochemical examinations as appropriate to assess possible phenotypic manifestations of the altered genes.

Acknowledgments

This work was supported by the Cystic Fibrosis Foundation, by NIH HL51776, and by RR00169 to the California Regional Primate Research Center. We thank the staffs of the Primate Research Centers in California, Louisiana, Oregon, and Washington, especially Jenny Short, Phil Allen, Ron Walgenbach, Margaret Clarke, Mark Murchison, Steve Kelley, and

Debra Glanister. S. Vuillaumier, INSERM, Paris, supplied the sequence of exon 1 and flanking segments from several primate species. We thank Ron Kopito and Cristi Ward for supplying 293 cells, the pRBG4 vector, CFTR-pRBG4, and help with transfection protocols. Numerous individuals assisted with SSCP and functional analysis, especially Gregory Hurlock, Eugene Kuo, Mauri Krouse, Clare Robinson, Margaret Lee, Uros Potocnik, and Metka Ravnik-Glavac.

References

1. Mitler, M. M., Soave, O., and Dement, W. C. (1976) Narcolepsy in seven dogs. *J. Am. Vet. Med. Assoc.* **168,** 1036–1038.
2. Knecht, C. D., Oliver, J. E., Redding, R., Selcer, R., and Johnson, G. (1973) Narcolepsy in a dog and a cat. *J. Am. Vet. Med. Assoc.* **162,** 1052,1053.
3. Green, E. L. (1966) The Jackson Laboratory: a center for mammalian genetics in the United States. *J. Hered.* **57,** 3–12.
4. Thomas, K. R. and Capecchi, M. R. (1987) Site-directed mutagenesis by gene targeting in mouse embryo-derived stem cells. *Cell* **51,** 503–512.
5. Capecchi, M. R. (1989) Altering the genome by homologous recombination. *Science* **244,** 1288–1292.
6. Clarke, A. R. (1994) Murine genetic models of human disease. *Curr. Opin. Genet. Dev.* **4,** 453–460.
7. O'Neal, W., P. Hasty, McCray, Jr., P. B., Casey, B., Rivera-Perez, J., Welsh, M. J., Beaudet, A. L., and Bradley, A. (1993) A severe phenotype in mice with a duplication of exon 3 in the cystic fibrosis locus. *Hum. Mol. Genet.* **2,** 1561–1569.
8. Brigman, K. K., Latour, A. M., Malouf, N. N., Boucher, R. C., Smithies, O., and Koller, B. H. (1992) An animal model for cystic fibrosis made by gene targeting. *Science* **257,** 1083–1088.
9. Kent, G., Iles, R., Bear, C. E., Huan, L. J., Griesenbach, U., McKerlie, C., et al. (1997) Lung disease in mice with cystic fibrosis. *J. Clin. Invest.* **100,** 3060–3069.
10. Cherny, R. A., Stokes, T. M., Merei, J., Lom, L., Brandon, M. R., and Williams, R. L. (1994) Strategies for the isolation and characterization of bovine embryonic stem cells. *Reprod. Fertil. Dev.* **6,** 569–575.
11. Thomson, J. A. and Marshall, V. S. (1998) Primate embryonic stem cells. *Curr. Top. Dev. Biol.* **38,** 133–165.
12. Shim, H., Gutierrez-Adan, A., Chen, L. R., BonDurant, R. H., Behboodi, E., and Anderson, G. B. (1997) Isolation of pluripotent stem cells from cultured porcine primordial germ cells. *Biol. Reprod.* **57,** 1089–1095.
13. Harris, A. (1997) Towards an ovine model of cystic fibrosis. *Hum. Mol. Genet.* **6,** 2191–2194.
14. Venter, J. C., Adams, M. D., Myers, E. W., Li, P. W., Mural, R. J., Sutton, G. G., et al. (2001) The Sequence of the human genome. *Science* **291,** 1304–1351.
15. Crow, J. F. (1995) Spontaneous mutation as a risk factor. *Exp. Clin. Immunogenet.* **12,** 121–128.

16. Keightley, P. D. and Caballero, A. (1997) Genomic mutation rates for lifetime reproductive output and lifespan in *Caenorhabditis elegans*. *Proc. Natl. Acad. Sci. USA* **94**, 3823–3827.

17. Imaizumi, Y. (1995) Incidence and mortality rates of cystic fibrosis in Japan, 1969–1992. *Am. J. Med. Genet.* **58**, 161–168.

18. Yamashiro, Y., Shimizu, T., Oguchi, S., Shioya, T., Nagata, S., and Ohtsuka, Y. (1997) The estimated incidence of cystic fibrosis in Japan. *J. Pediatr. Gastroenterol. Nutr.* **24**, 544–547.

19. Gregory, R. J., Rich, D. P., Cheng, S. H., Souza, D. W., Paul, S., Manavalan, P., et al. (1991) Maturation and function of cystic fibrosis transmembrane conductance regulator variants bearing mutations in putative nucleotide-binding domains 1 and 2. *Mol. Cell. Biol.* **11**, 3886–3893.

20. Cheng, S. H., Gregory, R. J., Marshall, J., Paul, S., Souza, D. W., White, G. A., et al. (1990) Defective intracellular transport and processing of CFTR is the molecular basis of most cystic fibrosis. *Cell* **63**, 827–834.

21. Ward, C. L., Omura, S., and Kopito, R. R. (1995) Degradation of CFTR by the ubiquitin-proteasome pathway. *Cell* **83**, 121–127.

22. Welsh, M. J. and Smith, A. E. (1993) Molecular mechanisms of CFTR chloride channel dysfunction in cystic fibrosis. *Cell* **73**, 1251–1254.

23. Choi, J. Y., Muallem, D., Kiselyov, K., Lee, M. G., Thomas, P. J., and Muallem. S. (2001) Aberrant CFTR-dependent HCO-3 transport in mutations associated with cystic fibrosis. *Nature* **410**, 94–97.

24. Tebbutt, S. J., Wardle, C. J., Hill, D. F., and Harris, A. (1995) Molecular analysis of the ovine cystic fibrosis transmembrane conductance regulator gene. *Proc. Natl. Acad. Sci. USA* **92**, 2293–2297.

25. Ballard, S. T., Trout, L., Bebok, Z., Sorscher, E. J., and Crews, A. (1999) CFTR involvement in chloride, bicarbonate, and liquid secretion by airway submucosal glands. *Am. J. Physiol.* **277**, L694–699.

26. Menotti-Raymond, M. and O'Brien, S. J. (1993) Dating the genetic bottleneck of the African cheetah. *Proc. Natl. Acad. Sci. USA* **90**, 3172–3176.

27. Zhang, Y. P. and Shi, L. M. (1993) Phylogenetic relationships of macaques as inferred from restriction endonuclease analysis of mitochondrial DNA. *Folia Primatol.* **60**, 7–17.

28. Zhang, Y.-P. and Shi, L.-P. (1993) Phylogeny of Rhesus Monkeys (Macaca mulatta) as revealed by mitochondrial DNA restriction analysis. *Int. J. Primatol.* **14**, 587–605.

29. Taylor, C. J., Baxter, P. S., Hardcastle, J., and Hardcastle, P. T. (1988) Failure to induce secretion in jejunal biopsies from children with cystic fibrosis. *Gut* **29**, 957–962.

30. Berschneider, H. M., Knowles, M. R., Azizkhan, R. G., Boucher, R. C., Tobey, N. A., Orlando, R. C., and Powell, D. W. (1988) Altered intestinal chloride transport in cystic fibrosis. *FASEB J.* **2**, 2625–2629.

31. Behm, J. K., Hagiwara, G., Lewiston, N. J., Quinton, P. M., and Wine, J. J. (1987) Hyposecretion of beta-adrenergically induced sweating in cystic fibrosis heterozygotes. *Pediatr. Res.* **22**, 271–276.

32. Gabriel, S. E., Brigman, K. N., Koller, B. H., Boucher, R. C., and Stutts, M. J. (1994) Cystic fibrosis heterozygote resistance to cholera toxin in the cystic fibrosis mouse model. *Science* **266,** 107–109.

33. Cuthbert, A. W., Halstead, J., Ratcliff, R., Colledge, W. H., and Evans, M. J. (1995) The genetic advantage hypothesis in cystic fibrosis heterozygotes: a murine study. *J. Physiol. (Lond)* **482,** 449–454.

34. George, J. W. and Lerche, N. W. (1990) Electrolyte abnormalities associated with diarrhea in rhesus monkeys: 100 cases (1986-1987). *J. Am. Vet. Med. Assoc.* **196,** 1654–1658.

35. Elmore, D. B., Anderson, J. H., Hird, D. W., Sanders, K. D., and Lerche, N. W. (1992) Diarrhea rates and risk factors for developing chronic diarrhea in infant and juvenile rhesus monkeys. *Lab. Anim. Sci.* **42,** 356–359.

36. Cotten, J. F., Ostedgaard, L. S., Carson, M. R., and Welsh, M. J. (1996) Effect of cystic fibrosis-associated mutations in the fourth intracellular loop of cystic fibrosis transmembrane conductance regulator. *J. Biol. Chem.* **271,** 21,279–21,284.

37. Seibert, F. S., Linsdell, P., Loo, T. W., Hanrahan, J. W., Riordan, J. R., and Clarke, D. M. (1996) Cytoplasmic loop three of cystic fibrosis transmembrane conductance regulator contributes to regulation of chloride channel activity. *J. Biol. Chem.* **271,** 27,493–27,499.

38. Anguiano, A., Oates, R. D., Amos, J. A., Dean, M., Gerrard, B., Stewart, C., et al. (1992) Congenital bilateral absence of the vas deferens. A primarily genital form of cystic fibrosis. *JAMA* **267,** 1794–1797.

39. Mak, V., Jarvi, K. A., Zielenski, J., Durie, P., and Tsui, L. C. (1997) Higher proportion of intact exon 9 CFTR mRNA in nasal epithelium compared with vas deferens. *Hum. Mol. Genet.* **6,** 2099–2107.

40. Snouwaert, J. N., Brigman, K. K., Latour, A. M., Malouf, N. N., Boucher, R. C., Smithies, O., and Koller, B. H. (1992) An animal model for cystic fibrosis made by gene targeting. *Science* **257,** 1083–1088.

41. Wine, J. J., Kuo, E., Hurlock, G., and Moss, R. B. (2001) Comprehensive mutation screening in a cystic fibrosis center. *Pediatrics* **107,** 280–286.

42. Wine, J. J., Glavac, D., Hurlock, G., Robinson, C., Lee, M., Potocnik, U., et al. (1998) Genomic DNA sequence of Rhesus (M. mulatta) cystic fibrosis (CFTR) gene. *Mamm. Genome.* **9,** 301–305.

43. Zielenski, J., Rozmahel, R., Bozon, D., Kerem, B., Grzelczak, Z., Riordan, J. R., et al. (1991) Genomic DNA sequence of the cystic fibrosis transmembrane conductance regulator (CFTR) gene. *Genomics* **10,** 214–228.

44. Orita, M., Iwahana, H., Kanazawa, H., Hayashi, K., and Sekiya, T. (1989) Detection of polymorphisms of human DNA by gel electrophoresis as single-strand conformation polymorphisms. *Proc. Natl. Acad. Sci. USA* **86,** 2766–2770.

45. Ravnik-Glavac, M., Glavac, D., and Dean, M. (1994) Sensitivity of single-strand conformation polymorphism and heteroduplex method for mutation detection in the cystic fibrosis gene. *Hum. Mol. Genet.* **3,** 801–807.

46. Ravnik-Glavac, M., Glavac, D., Chernick, M., di Sant'Agnese, P., and Dean, M. (1994) Screening for CF mutations in adult cystic fibrosis patients with a directed and optimized SSCP strategy. *Hum. Mutat.* **3,** 231–238.

47. Ravnik-Glavac, M., Glavac, D., Komel, R., and Dean, M. (1993) Single-stranded conformation polymorphism analysis of the CFTR gene in Slovenian cystic fibrosis patients: detection of mutations and sequence variations. *Hum. Mutat.* **2,** 286–292.
48. Venglarik, C. J., Bridges, R. J., and Frizzell, R. A. (1990) A simple assay for agonist-regulated Cl and K conductances in salt-secreting epithelial cells. *Am. J. Physiol.* **259,** C358–364.

II

CFTR STRUCTURE AND FUNCTION: *STRUCTURE, GATING, AND REGULATION*

4

Electrophysiological Approach to Studying CFTR

Horst Fischer

1. Introduction

Cystic fibrosis transmembrane conductance regulator (CFTR) is a phosphorylation- and ATP-dependent Cl^- channel. It is predominantly expressed in the apical membrane of epithelial cells. The presence and function of CFTR in a cell is sensitively measured using electrophysiological techniques. The patch clamp technique is the most frequently used method to measure CFTR in single cells or in isolated patches of cell membrane. A key step for the successful recording of CFTR is its identification and distinction from other Cl^- channels. In patch clamp recordings this is done by probing for physiological, pharmacological, or biophysical characteristics of the channel. This chapter describes, first, how to successfully record CFTR currents using the patch clamp technique. Second, it focuses on current noise analysis as a useful tool to investigate the regulation of CFTR activity.

1.1. Patch Clamp Recording Modes

The patch clamp recording technique allows one to record CFTR-mediated Cl currents from a single cell or from a small membrane patch ($\sim$1 μm^2) of a cell (1). To do this a glass micropipet that is filled with salt solution is placed onto a single cell on the stage of a microscope. A tight seal between the glass pipet and the cell membrane is achieved by applying negative pressure to the pipet interior. The seal electrically and mechanically isolates a small membrane patch inside the pipet. The sealing procedure is a critical step during patch clamping of CFTR. The quality of the seal is measured by its electrical resistance. In order to measure CFTR, single-channel currents that are <1 picoampere (pA = 10^{-12} A or $\sim$6 million Cl^- ions per second) seals >10 gigaohms (GΩ) are necessary. Once a gigaseal is established, CFTR currents

From: *Methods in Molecular Medicine, vol. 70: Cystic Fibrosis Methods and Protocols*
Edited by: W. R. Skach © Humana Press Inc., Totowa, NJ

can be recorded across the membrane patch. This initial manipulation establishes the "cell-attached" recording configuration. This configuration is primarily used to record the physiological behavior of CFTR. In the cell-attached configuration the intact cell provides the factors necessary to regulate CFTR. Disadvantages of the cell-attached configuration are that the concentration of intracellular factors, ion concentrations, and the membrane potential are not known.

The "excised inside-out" configuration is obtained from the cell-attached configuration by quickly removing the patch pipet from the cell. This procedure mechanically excises the small membrane patch that is enclosed by the pipet. The seal that has been formed between the pipet and the membrane is mechanically stable, so in most cases the seal does not rupture during excision. After patch excision the cellular face of the membrane is exposed to the bathing solution ("inside-out"). Excised inside-out patches of CFTR are used to record channel activity where control of intracellular factors, ion concentrations, and membrane potential is needed. For example, inside-out patches are used to determine the ion selectivity (e.g., Cl^- vs I^-) of CFTR by changing the ion composition in the bathing solution, or to investigate the regulation by factors such as ATP or kinases, which can be added directly to the bath. A limitation of excised inside-out patches is that cellular factors that are part of normal CFTR function may be lost during excision. For example, the fast, flickery gating of CFTR that is a normal part of CFTR activity is lost after patch excision *(2,3)*. In addition, patch excision frequently induces inactivation ("run-down") of CFTR, which is caused by membrane-bound phosphatases that dephosphorylate CFTR *(4,5)*.

The "whole cell" recording mode is obtained from cell-attached patches by rupturing the membrane patch inside the pipet. This is done by applying negative pressure to the pipet interior of cell-attached patches. Mechanical rupture of the membrane results in electrical contact between the pipet interior and the cell interior so that current across the total membrane area of the cell ("whole cell") is recorded. In the whole-cell mode the sum of all CFTR channels of a cell is recorded. For example, Calu-3 cells (a cell line with characteristics of airway gland serous cells *[2]*) show large CFTR-mediated currents and each cell expresses several thousand of CFTR channels in their plasma membrane. The whole-cell recording mode is used when the determination of single-channel parameters is not necessary. For example, it is a useful mode to test CFTR activators and blockers. In the whole-cell mode the cell interior is dialyzed with the pipet solution, which can lead to loss of regulatory factors from the cell. On the other hand, it can be used to dialyze factors into the cell interior, for example, ATP or a high Cl^- concentration.

1.2. Identification of CFTR Using Physiological Characteristics

The initial task during a recording is to identify CFTR as the current carrier. Conditions must be used that immediately identify the ion species that carries the measured current. This is most simply done by excluding most other small ions in the bath and pipet filling solution so that Cl⁻ is the major current-carrying ion. Commonly, small cations are exchanged for the large cation N-methyl-D-glucamine (NMDG), which does not support ion currents through most biological channels. Currents measured with symmetrical (i.e., bath and pipet) NMDG-Cl solutions are a good indication of Cl- currents.

The channel activity of CFTR is dependent on its phosphorylation status which is determined by intracellular protein kinases (PK) and protein phosphatases *(6)*. PKA is a prominent activator of CFTR which is the most commonly used criterion for the identification of a Cl⁻ current as being CFTR-mediated. This is readily tested in the cell-attached or whole-cell recording mode by addition of forskolin. Forskolin is a rapid and reversible activator of the ubiquitous adenylate cyclase, which causes increased intracellular cAMP concentrations and activation of cellular PKA. In excised inside-out patches PKA regulation is tested by adding the catalytic subunit of PKA (which is active without cAMP) directly to the bath.

The dependence of CFTR activity on ATP is another critical characteristic to distinguish CFTR currents from other Cl currents. When membrane patches are excised into ATP-free solution, CFTR channels inactivate quickly. In the absence of ATP, CFTR stays inactive. Addition of ATP to an excised patch that has been phosphorylated with PKA recovers CFTR activity *(7)*.

1.3. Identification of CFTR Using Pharmacological Characteristics

A small molecular probe that could be used to either block or activate CFTR with a high specificy would be extremely useful to identify CFTR in electrophysiological recordings. Unfortunately, currently there is no high-affinity probe for CFTR. That makes it necessary to use a pharmacological profile of several rather unspecific drugs to identify CFTR. CFTR is blocked by DPC (N-phenyl-antranylic acid) and glibenclamide, but not by DIDS (4,4'-diisothiocyanato-stilbene-2,2'-disulfonate), which blocks other Cl⁻ channel types. This CFTR blocker profile is readily tested in whole-cell recordings. However, conclusions from blocker studies are limited because glibenclamide also blocks the outwardly rectifying Cl channel ORCC *(8,9)* and DPC blocks various other Cl channels. On the other hand, DIDS (which does not block CFTR from the outside) induces a voltage-dependent flicker-block when applied to CFTR in excised patches *(10)*. In excised inside-out patches, CFTR is blocked by a number of compounds. Several negatively charged, chemically unrelated molecules have been shown to cause voltage-dependent block of the CFTR pore when applied from the intracellular side *(10–12)*. Genistein is a widely used CFTR activator. When added to cell-attached recordings, CFTR readily activates *(13)*. However, inactive CFTR in excised patches (or in whole-cell recordings when the basal level of cAMP is dialyzed to very low levels) are insensitive to genistein *(14–16)*. Although genistein is frequently used, its isomer apigenin is an approximately three times more potent CFTR activator *(14)*.

1.4. Identification of CFTR Using Biophysical Characteristics

The biophysical single-channel characteristics readily distinguish CFTR from other Cl^- channels. CFTR has a comparably small single channel conductance of $g = 6$–10 picosiemens (pS). Variations are largely explained by different recording conditions, such as temperature, Cl^- concentration, and low-pass filter setting *(17–19)*. Its conductance is linear in excised patches in the presence of symmetrical Cl^- concentrations. In cell-attached patches, CFTR rectifies outwardly (*see* **Note 1**). **Figure 1** shows the typical steady-state activity of CFTR in a cell-attached patch clamp recording. Active CFTR shows a distinct and characteristic open–close behavior, which is an explicit identifier of CFTR. The gating of CFTR is characterized by long openings broken by fast (millisecond) closures. This typical gating behavior is an important identifier of CFTR in cell-attached recordings. At the same time, the gating of CFTR contains information about its regulation.

The steady-state gating of CFTR has been modeled with at least three states *(2,3,19,20)* in a linear transition model of the form

$$\begin{array}{ccccc} & k_{10} & & k_{02} & \\ closed_1 & \leftrightarrow & open & \leftrightarrow & closed_2 \\ & k_{01} & & k_{20} & \end{array} \qquad \text{(Scheme 1)}$$

$$Pc_1 \qquad\qquad Po \qquad\qquad Pc_2$$

The open channel is in a steady-state equilibrium with a long-lasting closed state ($closed_1$) and a very brief closed state ($closed_2$). Each state is described by its respective probability of being in that state (P) which are related to the transition rates (k) between the states by

$$Po = k_{10} \cdot k_{20}/K \qquad Pc_1 = k_{01} \cdot k_{20}/K \qquad Pc_2 = k_{10} \cdot k_{02}/K \qquad \text{(1a–c)}$$

with $K = k_{01} \cdot k_{20} + k_{10} \cdot k_{02} + k_{10} \cdot k_{20}$. The left-hand $closed_1$–open transition expresses mean state lifetimes ranging from ~60 to 200 ms *(19–21)*. It has been shown that this transition is dependent on ATP *(20,22,23)*, and we will refer to this transition as the slow gate of CFTR.

The right-hand open–$closed_2$ transition in **Scheme 1** describes the rapid closings of CFTR. The lifetime of the $closed_2$ state was reported in the range of <1 to 5 ms and the transition rate k_{02} into the $closed_2$ state appears to be volt-

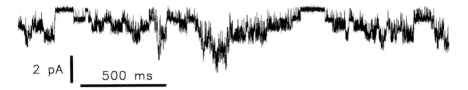

2 pA | 500 ms

Fig. 1. Typical appearance of CFTR in a cell-attached patch clamp recording. Pipet and bath contained NMDG-Cl solutions. Holding potential is –85 mV, filtered at 500 Hz. 3T3 cell stably expressing recombinant CFTR was stimulated with 10 μ*M* forskolin. Downward deflections are openings, uppermost level is the all-closed level, six open levels are apparent. Note the clearly discernible slow and fast gate.

age-dependent *(19)*. The closed$_2$ state is readily observed in cell-attached patches of CFTR but is greatly reduced after patch excision *(3,24)* , suggesting that it is caused by a diffusible intracellular factor *(25)*. Conversely, addition of various anionic compounds to excised patches mimicks the closed$_2$ state *(12)*. The open–closed$_2$ transition will be referred to as the fast gate of CFTR in this chapter.

The three-state model of **Scheme 1** describes the steady-state gating of phosphorylated (i.e., activated) CFTR. The steady-state open probability of CFTR is $Po \approx 0.5$, with reports ranging from 0.3 to almost 1.0 in different cell types, which is probably a reflection of different levels and kinds of phosphorylation obtained under different conditions *(2,19,26)*. Additional states outside of this gating scheme with longer time constants have been reported and likely reflect phosphorylation-dependent states *(19,27,28)*.

1.5. Noise Analysis of CFTR Recordings

Virtually all patch clamp recordings in the cell-attached or excised patch clamp mode contain multiple, in some cases hundreds, of CFTR channels. This makes it difficult to extract information about channel gating using classical single-channel analysis, which yields detailed gating kinetics only for single-channel recordings. Noise analysis is the appropriate analytical method for recordings that contain many channels. It describes gating kinetics in noise analytical terms and allows one to extract information about the channel open probability (*Po*) and the number of channels (*N*). The method is similarly applicable to recordings containing few or many channels, and it is useful to analyze CFTR-mediated currents in cell-attached, excised, or whole-cell patch clamp recordings.

For a population of channels the time-averaged current (*I*) is given by

$$I = N \cdot Po \cdot i \tag{2}$$

where *i* is the single-channel current that passes through the channel in its open state. The current fluctuations (current variance, σ^2) around *I* for channels gating between a conductive and a nonconductive state are described by *(29)*

$$\sigma^2 = i^2 \cdot N \cdot Po \cdot (1 - Po) \tag{3}$$

Equations 2 and **3** provide the basic relation between the measured I and σ^2 and the single channel parameters i, N, and Po. Because i can be estimated from g of CFTR and the known electrochemical driving forces in a patch clamp experiment, **Eqs. 2** and **3** are used to determine N and Po.

Fourier transformation (or its digital approximation, a fast fourier transform, FFT) of the channel-generated current noise results in a current noise spectrum. It displays the distribution of the spectral densities (S) of the frequencies (f) contained in the original current noise and it is used to determine rate constants and state probabilities in a kinetic gating scheme. Channel-generated currents show Lorentzian noise in the spectrum described by a distribution of frequencies according to

$$S(f) = S_0/[1 + (f/fc)^2] \tag{4}$$

Up to the corner frequency (fc) Lorentzian noise shows a constant amplitude (S_0) and then rolls off with a slope of -2 in a double-logarithmic plot (*see* **Note 2**). The number (n) of observed Lorentzians in the spectrum predicts $n + 1$ states in a steady-state gating scheme. Spectra recorded from CFTR-mediated currents contain two distinct Lorentzian noise components (**Fig. 2**), which is consistent with the gating model of **Scheme 1**. The total channel-generated noise is equal to the area under the Lorentzian function, that is,

$$\sigma^2 = S_0 \cdot fc \cdot \pi/2 \tag{5}$$

1.6. Technique for Acquiring Patch Clamp and Noise Data

Analog electrophysiological signals have to be appropriately digitized for subsequent analysis. Patch clamp analysis and noise analysis require significantly different methods of digitizing, although the analog signal for both analyses is initially the same. Single-channel patch clamp data are generally sampled at a sampling frequency (fs) that is five times the filter frequency (ff). In contrast, the digitized noise signal that is subsequently transformed by a FFT requires a ratio of $fs/ff = 2.5$ (for an ideal filter, $fs/ff = 2$, which is the Nyquist rate). In other words, in order to faithfully reconstruct the original current signal and the current spectrum, different sampling frequencies are required.

Multichannel recordings of CFTR frequently contain a large DC current component. When digitizing a DC-containing signal, the resolution of the analog-to-digital (A/D) converter is often unsuitable to reconstruct the original current noise. In particular, high frequencies (which show low intensities in the spectrum) are prone to be missampled and distorted during A/D conversion.

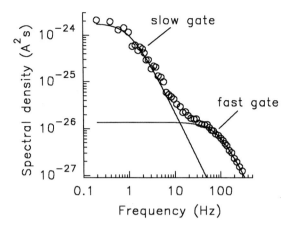

Fig. 2. Current noise spectrum of CFTR-mediated current. Spectrum was fitted with the sum of two Lorentzians (*lines*) according to **Eq. 4**. The low-frequency Lorentzian showed $fc_1 = 1.1$ Hz and $S_{01} = 1.8E{-}24$ A^2s and represents the slow gate of CFTR. The high-frequency Lorentzian showed $fc_2 = 90$ Hz and $S_{02} = 1.4E{-}26$ A^2s and is an expression of the fast gate of CFTR. Current was recorded in the cell-attached mode from a Calu-3 cell stimulated with forskolin, holding potential was -75 mV, frequency band was 0.2–330 Hz, and 12 consecutive spectra were averaged.

We find that the high-frequency Lorentzian of CFTR is largely distorted when noise analyzing standard patch clamp recordings.

To avoid sampling artifacts but still be able to perform simultaneous patch clamp and noise analyses successfully, we use selective signal conditioning and A/D conversion for the patch clamp current and the current noise, as shown schematically in **Fig. 3**. The signal for patch clamp analysis is low-pass-filtered and then digitized and sampled by a computer (*top branch* in **Fig. 3**). The same signal from the patch clamp amplifier is separately conditioned for noise analysis. First the DC current is removed with a high-pass filter (*see* **Note 3**), then the signal is low-pass-filtered (*see* **Notes 4** and **5**) and amplified to scale up the noise signal before A/D conversion. This setup allows for continuous, parallel, and independent recording of a patch clamp experiment and its current noise using optimal sampling conditions for either signal.

The FFT reads noise data in segments whose length and sampling frequency determine the bandwidth of the recording. The number of samples per segment (n) determines the total length (T) of one data segment by $T = n/fs$. The frequency bin-width (Δf), which also corresponds to the lowest frequency analyzed (f_{min}), is the reciprocal of T ($\Delta f = 1/T = f_{min}$) and the maximal frequency $f_{max} = fs/2.5$. Thus, the frequency band (ranging from f_{min} to f_{max}) available for noise analysis is predetermined by the selection of n and fs.

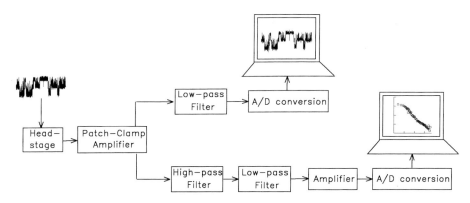

Fig. 3. Flow chart of the current signal for the simultaneous recording of both patch clamp current and current noise. The analog output signal from the patch clamp amplifier is conditioned selectively for either patch clamp analysis (*top branch*) or noise analysis (*bottom branch*), and both branches use independent A/D conversion steps.

2. Materials

1. Borosilicate glass patch pipets. Use thick-walled glass (PG52150-4, World Precision Instruments, Sarasota, FL) for cell-attached and inside-out excised recordings, and thin-walled glass for whole-cell recordings (PG52165-4). Wash pipets with methanol and let air dry.
2. Eppendorf Microloader tip for back-filling of the pipets.
3. Silver wire. Use to make a Ag/AgCl bath electrode by submersing the wire in bleach. A grayish-black AgCl layer forms within minutes.
4. Forskolin (Calbiochem, LaJolla, CA). Prepare 20 mM stock in dimethylsulfoxide, store at 4°C for up to 4 mo. Use at 10 μM (i.e., at a dilution of 1/2000).
5. Protein kinase A (PKA) catalytic subunit (Promega, Madison, WI) comes as 2500 U reconstituted in ~25 μL of 350 mM potassium phosphate/0.1 mM dithiothreitol (DTT). Prepare 5-μL aliquots (containing ~500 U). Store aliquotes at –70°C until use. Avoid freeze-thaw cycles; thaw and use up one aliquot per experimental day, do not refreeze. Keep leftovers refrigerated (4°C) for several days. Use at 50 U/mL.
6. NMDG-Cl buffers (concentrations in mM):

	I Standard extracellular solution	**II** Bath solution for excised recordings	**III** Pipet solution for whole cell recordings
NMDG	140	144	140
HCl	140	144	140
CaCl$_2$	2	—	—
MgCl$_2$	1	1	1
HEPES	10	10	2
Glucose	10	10	1
Manitol	10	2	—

EGTA	—	5	5
Mg-ATP	—	1	5
Li-GTP	—	—	0.1
pH	7.3	7.3	7.3

The standard extracellular solution **I** is used as bath solution in cell-attached and whole-cell recordings, and as pipet solution in cell-attached and excised recordings. The pipet solution for whole-cell recordings (**III**) is hypotonic with respect to the bath solution in order to prevent cell swelling in the whole-cell mode *(30)*. The pH of all solutions is adjusted with a 1 *M* NMDG solution to 7.3. Before use, filter all solutions (0.2 µm). Keep standard extracellular solution **I** refrigerated for ~1 mo. Freeze (–20°C) ATP/GTP-containing solutions. NMDG, *N*-methyl-D-glucamine; HEPES, N-[2-hydroxyethyl]piperazine-*N'*-[2-ethanesulfonic acid]; EGTA, ethyleneglycol-bis-(β-aminoethyl ether) *N,N,N',N'*-tetraacetic acid. All chemicals are available from Sigma.

3. Methods

3.1. Recording CFTR in the Cell-Attached Configuration

1. Place cells in chamber on an inverted microscope. Make sure that cells are firmly attached in the chamber. Add ~500 µL of solution **I** to chamber, heat to 37°C. Place bath electrode wire directly in solution (*see* **Note 6**).
2. Use thick-walled glass to pull patch pipets to ~10 MΩ (when filled with NMDG-Cl buffer) using a two-stage pull.
3. Tip-filling solution: sterile-filter 1.5 mL of solution **I** into an Eppendorf tube. Keep solution covered.
4. Back-filling solution: fill a 1-mL syringe with filtered solution **I**, attach microloader tip.
5. Dip pipet tip into tip-filling solution, apply suction to the back of the pipet, then back-fill pipette. Remove air bubbles by tapping pipet from the side. Insert pipet into the pipet holder of the headstage amplifier.
6. Contact recording pipet and bath solution. Keep amplifier in voltage-clamp mode. Adjust current offset to zero. Set amplification to 1 mV/pA.
7. Continuously apply 5-mV/500-µs voltage pulses, and observe current pulse. **Figure 4A** shows an example of a typical current pulse. Determine the pipet resistance from current deflection.
8. Select cell for recording, navigate pipette over cell, and carefully contact cell so that a slight indentation forms in the cell membrane. Observe the current pulses, which drop to ~50% of original size .
9. Use a 20-mL glass syringe with the barrel pulled back halfway to apply slight suction to the pipet until a seal forms. Application of a negative holding potential (–40 mV) supports seal formation. Seal should be >10 GΩ. **Figure 4B** shows a typical current pulse after seal formation.
10. Cancel the current transient caused by the pipet capacitance with the controls of the amplifier. **Figure 4C** shows the curent pulse response after cancelation of the transient. Then turn pulses off.

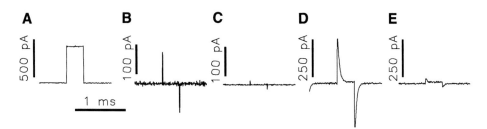

Fig. 4. Shapes of current pulses during patch clamping. The current pulse measured when the pipet contacts the bath solution (**A**) is used to determine the pipet resistance. After seal formation (**B**) current pulse disappears. The capacitance of the pipet causes large transients, which are canceled (**C**) with the amplifier controls. After break-in into the whole-cell mode a large current transient appears (**D**), which is canceled (**E**) using the amplifier whole cell controls.

11. Set amplification to 200 mV/pA, clamp voltage to +80 mV, continuously record current. Basal CFTR activity is frequently present.
12. Add forskolin (10 μ*M*) to the bath to stimulate CFTR activity. Effects are seen after ~30 s. In order to determine the current–voltage relation, clamp potential from –100 mV to +100 mV in 20-mV increments.

3.2. Recording CFTR in the Excised Inside-Out Configuration

1. Keep ATP-containing solution **II** and PKA preparation on ice.
2. Establish the cell-attached recording condition as described above and start recording at a holding potential of +80 mV and an amplification of 200 mV/pA.
3. Quickly move the pipet away from the cell to obtain an excised inside-out patch.
4. Observe current recording. Add ATP-containing solution **II** to the bath to maintain CFTR activity.
5. Add 50 U (i.e., 0.5 μL) of PKA preparation directly to bath. Effects on CFTR activity are seen within seconds.

3.3. Recording CFTR in the Whole-Cell Configuration

1. Keep ATP/GTP-containing pipet filling solution **III** on ice.
2. Use thin-walled glass to pull patch pipets to 2–3 MΩ using a two-stage pull. Fill pipet with solution **III** and establish the cell-attached configuration as described above.
3. Break into the whole-cell mode: set amplification to 5 mV/pA and continuously apply 5-mV/ 500-μs pulses. Observe current pulse, which looks as shown in **Fig. 4C**. Steadily apply increasing suction to the pipet interior until a large current transient appears (as shown in **Fig. 4D**). This transient is caused by the *Ra/Cm* element formed by the access resistance (*Ra*, which includes the pipet resistance) and the cell membrane capacitance (*Cm*) once the membrane patch ruptures.
4. Use the whole-cell controls of the amplifier to determine *Ra* and *Cm* and cancel the capacitative transient (as shown in **Fig. 4E**). Try to decrease *Ra* to values as

low as possible by further applying light suction to the pipet. *Ra* values <20 MΩ are good. Make a note of *Ra* and *Cm*.

5. Clamp holding potential to –60 mV, record current at 5-mV/pA amplification. Add forskolin (10 μ*M*) to the bath. Within ~30 s, current activation can be observed. During a continuous recording, test *Ra* frequently as described in **step 4**. *Ra* tends to increase over time.

6. Apply current–voltage step protocols from –100 mV to +100 mV, step 20 mV, 1-s duration for each potential. CFTR currents typically show no voltage-dependent activation or inactivation and currents change linear with voltage.

3.4. Noise Analysis of CFTR

3.4.1. Current and Noise Recording in the Cell-Attached Mode

1. Establish the cell-attached recording condition as described above and start recording at a holding potential of +80 mV and an amplification of 200 mV/pA.

2. Stimulate cell in the cell-attached mode with 10 μ*M* forskolin.

3. Continuously record patch clamp currents at an amplification of 200 mV/pA, filtered at 500 Hz, and sampled at 2 kHz.

4. Continuously record current noise high-pass-filtered at 0.1 Hz, low-pass-filtered at 330 Hz and additionally amplified 10-fold. Record noise signal continuously and perform FFTs after the experiment, off-line. Alternatively, calculate spectra on-line when currents are in a steady state.

5. To calculate spectra, use $n = 4096$ samples/segment and $fs = 820$ Hz (which results in a frequency band from $f_{min} = 0.2$ Hz to $f_{max} = 330$ Hz; *see* **Note 7**). Average at least 10 spectra calculated from consecutive segments to smooth the data sufficiently. Fifty seconds of steady-state current are needed (*see* **Note 8**).

3.4.2. Analysis of Activating or Inactivating (Nonstationary) Currents

This analysis allows the calculation of *N* and *Po* of multichannel recordings. An example of this analysis is shown in **Fig. 5.**

1. Visually inspect the current and noise signals. Recordings frequently contain additional noise from sources such as mechanical disturbances by solution changes. Eliminate segments with excessive noise.

2. Calculate *I* and σ^2 pairs from consecutive single segments of a continuous recording. Select a segment length of 5–10 s (*see* **Note 9**). *I* and σ^2 are readily calculated as the arithmetic mean and the statistical variance ($\sigma^2 = \Sigma[(I(t) - I)^2/(n - 1)]$; n, number of samples) from digitized data for each segment (*see* **Note 10**).

3. Plot the resulting data in a current variance-to-mean current plot. Fit plot with Sigworth's parabola *(31)*,

$$\sigma^2 = I \cdot i - I^2/N \qquad (6)$$

which is derived by combining **Eqs. 2** and **3** (through elimination of P_o). The fit estimates the parameters *i* and *N* (*see* **Note 11**).

4. Use the fitted *i* and *N* values to calculate P_o for every *I* using **Eq. 2.**

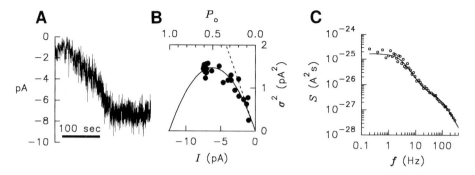

Fig. 5. **(A)** Cell-attached recording from a 3T3 cell stably expressing recombinant CFTR. Current was activated by stimulation with 10 μM forskolin. Holding potential was –75 mV. For display in this figure, data were sampled at 25 Hz. **(B)** Current variance-to-mean current plot. Data points represent σ^2 and *I* pairs calculated from successive 10-s sweeps filtered at 500 Hz from the recording in (A). Fit of data to **Eq. 6** (*solid line*) resulted in estimates for $i = -0.47 \pm 0.03$ pA (corresponding to $g = 6.3$ pS at –75 mV) and $N = 26 \pm 4$. *Dashed line* shows the initial slope, which is $i = -0.47$ pA. *Po* values are displayed as *top axis*. Maximal $Po = 0.59$. **(C)** Current noise spectrum calculated from steady-state current after forskolin stimulation. Frequency range is 0.2–330 Hz. Spectrum was fitted with the sum of two Lorentzians (*line*) which resulted in $fc_1 = 3.1$ Hz, $fc_2 = 90$ Hz, $S_{01} = 1.6 \times 10^{-25}$ A²s, $S_{02} = 4.1 \times 10^{-27}$ A²s. When assuming $k_{01} = 6$ s⁻¹, then $k_{10} = 13.5$ s⁻¹, $k_{02} = 112$ s⁻¹, $k_{20} = 452$ s⁻¹, and the probabilities for the two closed states are $Pc_1 = 0.26$ and $Pc_2 = 0.15$.

3.4.3. Analysis of Steady-State Currents

The analysis of current noise spectra yields information about channel gating kinetics, the minimal number of states in a gating model, rate constants, and state probabilities.

1. Inspect noise spectra. If the spectrum contains extraneous line frequency (50 or 60 Hz), eliminate this frequency point and its harmonics (i.e., multiples).
2. Decide whether to fit spectra with one or with the sum of two Lorentzian functions (**Eq. 4**; *see* **Note 12**).
3. Fit Lorentzian function(s) to spectral data in order to estimate the parameters fc and S_0.
4. A two-state model is indicated when the spectrum shows one Lorentzian. As a test for accuracy of the spectral data, compare the Lorentzian noise (**Eq. 5**) with the corresponding σ^2 calculated in **Subheading 3.4.2., step 3** for this current segment.
5. The rate constants in a two-state model (k_{01}, k_{10}) are determined from the fitted f_c value and from the Po that has been determined in **Subheading 3.4.2., step 4**, with

$$2\pi fc = k_{01} + k_{10} \quad \text{and} \quad Po = k^{10} k^{01} + k^{10} \qquad (7a,b)$$

6. When the spectrum contains two Lorentzians (i.e., at negative holding potentials), a three-state model (**Scheme 1**) is indicated where the fitted parameters fc_1 and S_{01} describe the slow gate, and fc_2 and S_{02} describe the fast gate of CFTR. The reaction rates are related to the measured corner frequencies by (*see* **Note 13**)

$$2\pi fc_1 = k_{01} + k_{10} \quad \text{and} \quad 2\pi fc_2 = k_{02} + k_{20} \qquad (8a,b)$$

7. Additional information is needed to determine all four rate constants of a three-state model. One practical way is to estimate one (for example, k_{01}, which then determines k_{10} with **Eq. 8a**). Then,

$$k_{20} = 2\pi fc_2 \cdot k_{10}/[(k_{10}/Po) - k_{01}] \qquad (9)$$

(where Po is used from **Subheading 3.2., step 4**) and k_{02} is determined from **Eq. 8b**. The probabilities of the two closed states (Pc_1, Pc_2) are determined with **Eqs. 1b,c**. **Figure 4** shows an example for the analysis.

4. Notes

1. Outward currents are defined as positive charge moving out of the cell and are given as positive currents. Outward rectification means that currents measured at positive potentials are larger than currents measured at negative potentials. For the negatively charged Cl^- ion, an outward current means Cl^- flux into the cell. Membrane potentials are given as intracellular potentials as if measured with an intracellular electrode. Since the patch pipet in the cell-attached and the excised mode represents an extracellular electrode, applied voltages and measured currents have to be inversed (multiplied by -1) in these recording modes.

2. The slope of -2 of a Lorentzian at frequencies larger than fc is a useful practical characteristic. For example, an observed fc that expresses a roll-off of intensities different from -2 is likely not channel-generated noise, but probably a time constant of the recording system. However, a simple RC element (as a low-pass) can generate Lorentzian-type noise. A spectrum that contains a linear background with a slope of -2 indicates that the fc of a Lorentzian noise component lies to the left of the recorded bandwidth.

3. High-pass filtering can be done most simply with an RC element. For example, a capacitor $C = 47$ μF in series with a resistor $R = 210$ kΩ results in an f_c for the current measured over the resistor of 0.1 Hz. Noise intensities near the f_c will be attenuated, and, if necessary, should be corrected numerically by multiplying with $1 + [1/(R \cdot C \cdot 2\pi f)^2]$.

4. Filtering of noise signals is frequently done with a Butterworth filter because of its excellent amplitude matching to the fc. In comparison, Bessel filters, which are mostly used to filter patch clamp data, show worse amplitude matching; however, they show no "ringing" at the corners of square-wave signals, which Butterworth filters do. Ringing is caused by the phase shift from high-frequency components around fc. Since square-wave-like single-channel steps are usually present in excised or cell-attached CFTR recordings, the ring-free Bessel filter has advantages for this application. Under no circumstance should a digital filter be used without prior analog filtering of the signal. Digitized data that have not

been appropriately analog-filtered will alias (*see* **Note 5**), no matter what the *fc* of the digital filter is.

5. Filtering of a signal has two purposes: (1) it reduces background noise; and (2) it prevents aliasing of high frequencies during A/D conversion. *Aliasing* is a misrepresentation of high frequencies as lower frequencies and occurs only in digital sampling systems because data samples are taken at brief time points and fixed time intervals.

6. Direct contact of the Ag/AgCl bath electrode with the bath solution can be done only when the bath and the pipet solutions have identical Cl⁻ concentrations. If the bath contains another Cl⁻ concentration (e.g., Cl⁻ free), then the bath electrode wire must be placed in pipet-filling solution and electrical contact to the bath is established through a 3% agar bridge.

7. The frequency range depends on the process under investigation and has to be adjusted for the experimental conditions. The given frequency window of 0.2 to 330 Hz will allow one to investigate both the slow and the fast gates of CFTR. For the investigation of a rapid blocker, for example, the frequency window has to be shifted to higher frequencies by (1) increasing *fs* and/or (2) increasing the number *n* of samples per data segment.

8. Increasing the recording time, and thus the number of analyzed segments, will further smooth the resulting spectrum. However, there are technical limits for keeping a patch clamp recording stable over a long time. Another way to smooth the spectral data is to overlap adjacent segments during the FFT. Up to 50% overlap doubles the number of analyzed segments and significantly smoothes the resulting spectrum.

9. Within the current segment, the I and σ^2 have to be stable. During an experiment where the current rises or falls, the selection of the segment length can be tricky. To include CFTR's slow gate, a length of 5–10 s is indicated. If within the segment the average current changes significantly, then the segment length has to be reduced.

10. σ^2 is ideally calculated from recordings that cover the full frequency range of CFTR. However, in any experimental situation the calculated values for σ^2 from the recorded data will be frequency-limited, whereas σ^2 in **Eq. 3** is not. The practical frequency limitation of the calculated σ^2 values tends to underestimate the true σ^2, which is a frequently found error during noise analysis. This problem can be minimized by selecting f_{max} and f_{min} of the analysis carefully, so that the frequency spectrum of CFTR's gating kinetics is largely included. To include 95% of the true σ^2 in the calculations, f_{min} should be ideally selected at ~1/20th of f_c and f_{max} ~35 times fc. f_{max} can be calculated with $f_{max} = f_c \cdot \tan[0.95 \cdot \pi \cdot 0.5 + \arctan(1/20)]$. CFTR's fc values lie far apart (2 Hz and 90 Hz). In order to include the noise of both Lorentzians in the calculation of σ^2, a bandwidth of 0.1–3 kHz is indicated to measure 95% of true σ^2. Dependent on the background noise situation in the recording, this wide frequency band may not be fully usable. When using a $T = 10$ s and $ff = 500$ Hz, then 97% of the slow gates, and 88% of the fast gate's noise will be included. A current noise spectrum helps to identify the usable frequency range and distinguishes CFTR-generated noise from contaminating noise.

11. The σ^2-to-*I* plot has interesting characteristics. (1) The initial slope is an estimate of the single-channel current. In fact, under conditions where *Po* is small (i.e., in unstimulated recordings), the ratio σ^2/I approximates *i*. (2) Maximal current noise is found at *Po* = 0.5 (where the curve peaks), and *Po* = 0 or *Po* = 1 results in zero channel-generated noise. (3) *N* is constant during this analysis, and any change in *I* is caused by a change of *Po* as long as the data adhere to **Eq. 7**. A systematic deviation of the data from the fitted equation is an indication for a change in *N* during the recording. For example, if both *N* and *Po* increase with *I*, then the data will be right-skewed (for negative currents), or if only *N* changes with *I* (and *Po* is constant), then the σ^2-to-*I* plot will be linear (with the slope *i*).

12. At negative potentials in the cell-attached mode, CFTR-mediated current noise spectra express two clear Lorentzians. When patches are excised or clamped to positive (depolarized) potentials, the fast gate is significantly reduced *(3,19)*, and fits to a single Lorentzian may suffice.

13. In a three-state model, both observed *fc* values are determined by all four rate constants (k_{01}, k_{10}, k_{02}, k_{20}) *(32)*. Since CFTR's two *fc* values lie far apart, f_{c1} is practically determined by **Eq. 8a** and the effects of k_{02} and k_{20} are small. Similarly, fc_2 is determined by **Eq. 8b** with very little effects of k_{01} and k_{10}. Thus, **Eq. 8** is for practical purposes a good estimator for CFTR's rate constants from *fc* values. However, if necessary, a correction factor that accounts for the effects of all *k* values can be calculated with

$$c = 0.5 \cdot [(k_{02} + k_{20} - k_{01} - k_{10}) - \sqrt{(k_{02} + k_{20} - k_{01} - k_{10})^2 + 4 \cdot k_{01} \cdot k_{02}}\,].$$

Then $2\pi fc_1 = k_{01} + k_{10} + c$ and $2\pi fc_2 = k_{02} + k_{20} - c$.

Acknowledgments

Work in the author's laboratory is supported by the National Institutes of Health (1P50HL60288-01) and the Cystic Fibrosis Foundation.

References

1. Penner, R. (1995) Pracical guide to patch clamping, in *Single Channel Recording* (Sakmann, B. and Neher, E., eds.), Plenum Press, New York, London, pp. 3–30.
2. Haws, C., Finkbeiner, W. E., Widdicombe, J. H., and Wine, J. J. (1994) CFTR in Calu-3 human airway cells: channel properties and role in cAMP-activated Cl conductance. *Am. J. Physiol. Cell Physiol.* **266 (10)** L502–L512.
3. Fischer, H. and Machen, T. E. (1996) The tyrosine kinase p60[c-src] regulates the fast gate of the cystic fibrosis transmembrane conductance regulator chloride channel. *Biophys. J.* **71**, 3073–3082.
4. Zhu, T., Dahan, D., Evagelidis, A., Zheng, S., Luo, J., and Hanrahan, J. W. (1999) Association of cystic fibrosis transmembrane conductance regulator and protein phosphatase 2C. *J. Biol. Chem.* **274**, 29,102–29,107.
5. Becq, F., Jensen, T. J., Chang, X. B., Savoia, A., Rommens, J. M., Tsui, L. C., Buchwald, M., Riordan, J. R., and Hanrahan, J. W. (1994) Phosphatase inhibitors activate normal and defective CFTR chloride channels. *Proc. Natl. Acad. Sci. USA* **91**, 9160–9164.

6. Hwang, T. C., Horie, M., and Gadsby, D. C. (1993) Functionally distinct phospho-forms underlie incremental activation of protein kinase-regulated Cl conductance in mammalian heart. *J. Gen. Physiol.* **101,** 629–651.

7. Anderson, M. P. and Welsh, M. J. (1992) Regulation by ATP and ADP of CFTR chloride channels that contain mutant nucleotide-binding domains. *Science* **257,** 1701–1704.

8. Julien, M., Verrier, B., Cerutti, M., Chappe, V., Gola, M., Devauchelle, G., and Becq, F. (1999) Cystic fibrosis transmembrane conductance regulator (CFTR) confers glibenclamide sensitivity to outwardly rectifying chloride channel (ORCC) in Hi-5 insect cells. *J. Membr. Biol.* **168,** 229–239.

9. Rabe, A., Disser, J., and Frömter, E. (1995) Cl⁻ channel inhibition by glibenclamide is not specific for the CFTR-type Cl⁻ channel. *Pflugers Arch.* **429,** 659–662.

10. Linsdell, P. and Hanrahan, J. W. (1996) Disulphonic stilbene block of cystic fibrosis transmembrane conductance regulator Cl⁻ channels expressed in a mammalian cell line and its regulation by a critical pore residue. *J. Physiol. (Lond.)* **496,** 687–693.

11. Linsdell, P. (2000) Inhibition of CFTR Cl channel currents by arachidonic acid. *Can. J. Physiol. Pharmacol.* **78,** 490–499.

12. Linsdell, P. and Hanrahan, J. W. (1996) Flickery block of single CFTR chloride channels by intracellular anions and osmolytes. *Am. J. Physiol. Cell Physiol.* **271,** C628–634.

13. Illek, B., Fischer, H., Santos, G. F., Widdicombe, J. H., Machen, T. E., and Reenstra, W. W. (1995) cAMP-independent activation of CFTR Cl channels by the tyrosine kinase inhibitor genistein. *Am. J. Physiol. Cell Physiol.* **268,** C886–C893.

14. Illek, B. and Fischer, H. (1998) Flavonoids stimulate Cl conductance of human airway epithelium in vitro and in vivo. *Am. J. Physiol. Lung Cell. Mol. Physiol.* **275,** L902–L910.

15. Illek, B., Lizarzaburu, M. E., Lee, V., Nantz, M. H., Kurth, M. J., and Fischer, H. (2000) Structural determinants for activation and block of CFTR-mediated chloride currents by apigenin. *Am. J. Physiol. Cell Physiol.* **279,** C1838–C1846.

16. Wang, F., Zeltwanger, S., Yang, I. C., Nairn, A. C., and Hwang, T. C. (1998) Actions of genistein on cystic fibrosis transmembrane conductance regulator channel gating. Evidence for two binding sites with opposite effects. *J. Gen. Physiol.* **111,** 477–490.

17. Berger, H. A., Anderson, M. P., Gregory, R. J., Thompson, S., Howard, P. W., Maurer, R. A., Mulligan, R., Smith, A. E., and Welsh, M. J. (1991) Identification and regulation of the cystic fibrosis transmembrane conductance regulator-generated chloride channel. *J. Clin. Invest.* **88,** 1422–1431.

18. Tabcharani, J. A., Low, W., Elie, D., and Hanrahan, J. W. (1990) Low conductance Cl channel activated by cAMP in the epithelial cell line T84. *FEBS Lett.* **270,** 157–163.

19. Fischer, H. and Machen, T. E. (1994) CFTR displays voltage dependence and two gating modes during stimulation. *J. Gen. Physiol.* **104,** 541–566.

20. Winter, M. C., Sheppard, D. N., Carson, M. R., and Welsh, M. J. (1994) Effect of ATP concentration on CFTR Cl⁻ channels: a kinetic analysis of channel regulation. *Biophys. J.* **66,** 1398–1403.

21. Carson, M. R., Travis, S. M., and Welsh, M. J. (1995) The two nucleotide-binding domains of cystic fibrosis transmembrane conductance regulator (CFTR) have distinct functions in controlling channel activity. *J. Biol. Chem.* **270,** 1711–1717.

22. Gunderson, K. L. and Kopito, R. R. (1995) Conformational states of CFTR associated with channel gating: the role ATP binding and hydrolysis. *Cell* **82,** 231–239.

23. Venglarik, C. J., Schultz, B. D., Frizzell, R. A., and Bridges, R. J. (1994) ATP alters current fluctuations of cystic fibrosis transmembrane conductance regulator: evidence for a three-state activation mechanism. *J. Gen. Physiol.* **104,** 123–146.

24. Haws, C., Krouse, M. E., Xia, Y., Gruenert, D. C., and Wine, J. J. (1992) CFTR channels in immortalized human airway cells. *Am. J. Physiol. Lung Cell. Mol. Physiol.* **263,** L692–707.

25. Fischer, H. (1997) CFTR's fast gate is caused by an intracellular non-diffusible factor (abstr.). *Ped. Pulmonol.* **suppl. 14,** 230.

26. Gray, M. A., Harris, A., Coleman, L., Greenwell, J. R., and Argent, B. E. (1989) Two types of chloride channel on duct cells cultured from human fetal pancreas. *Am. J. Physiol. Cell Physiol.* **257,** C240–251.

27. Baukrowitz, T., Hwang, T. C., Nairn, A. C., and Gadsby, D. C. (1994) Coupling of CFTR Cl⁻ channel gating to an ATP hydrolysis cycle. *Neuron* **12,** 473–482.

28. Gadsby, D. C. and Nairn, A. C. (1999) Control of CFTR channel gating by phosphorylation and nucleotide hydrolysis. *Physiol. Rev.* **79,** S77–S107.

29. Ehrenstein, G., Lecar, H., and Nossal, R. (1970) The nature of the negative resistance in bimolecular lipid membranes containing excitability-induced material. *J. Gen. Physiol.* **55,** 119–133.

30. Worrell, R. T., Butt, A. G., Cliff, W. H., and Frizzell, R. A. (1989) A volume-sensitive choride conductance in human colonic cell line T84. *Am. J. Physiol. Cell Physiol.* **256,** C1111–C1119.

31. Sigworth, F. J. (1980) The variance of sodium current fluctuations at the node of ranvier. *J. Physiol. (Lond.)* **307,** 97–129.

32. Colquhoun, D. and Hawkes, A. G. (1995) The principles of the stochastic interpretation of ion-channel mechanisms, in *Single-Channel Recording*, 2nd ed. (Sakmann, B. and Neher, E., eds.), Plenum Press, New York.

5

Quantitative Analysis of ATP-Dependent Gating of CFTR

Allan Powe, Zhen Zhou, Tzyh-Chang Hwang, and Georg Nagel

1. Introduction

CFTR, the chloride ion channel encoded by the gene mutated in cystic fibrosis patients, has been the subject of intense investigation since its discovery in 1989 *(1)*. A member of the ATP Binding Cassette (ABC) superfamily, the CFTR channel possesses two nucleotide-binding domains (NBDs) that hydrolyze ATP in vitro and are thought to use the resulting energy to drive the opening and closing of the channel. In addition to its NBDs and the putative pore-forming transmembrane regions, CFTR also contains a unique domain believed to regulate gating by modulating the activity of the two NBDs. This regulatory (R) domain is a substrate for phosphorylation by protein kinase A (PKA). PKA-dependent phosphorylation not only activates but also finely modulates ATP-dependent gating *(2)*.

There have been a few challenges in understanding how ATP hydrolysis drives CFTR gating: (1) obtaining good-quality recordings from stably phosphorylated, rundown-free channels, (2) distinguishing between ATP-dependent and ATP-independent gating, and (3) analyzing and interpreting data to determine the roles of each NBD in gating from experiments using various electrophysiological, biochemical and molecular biological approaches. Developing clear, consistent experimental protocols has been critical for overcoming some of these obstacles to understanding CFTR gating. This chapter outlines some of the procedures we use to examine how ATP controls opening and closing of the CFTR chloride channel.

From: *Methods in Molecular Medicine, vol. 70: Cystic Fibrosis Methods and Protocols*
Edited by: W. R. Skach © Humana Press Inc., Totowa, NJ

1.1. Issues in Understanding the Nature of ATP-Dependence in CFTR Gating

The role of ATP in CFTR gating is complex. The requirement for ATP in channel gating was first shown for recombinant CFTR by Anderson et al. *(3)* and for endogenous CFTR by Quinton and Reddy *(4)* and Nagel et al. *(5)*. Gamma phosphate-hydrolyzable nucleotides, such as ATP, GTP, ITP, UTP, CTP, and AMPCPP, can open PKA-phosphorylated CFTR channels, while nonhydrolyzable gamma-phosphate analogs, such as AMPPNP, AMPPCP, ATPγS, and nucleotides lacking a gamma phosphate, such as ADP and cAMP, cannot (**Figs. 1** and **2A**). This need for hydrolyzable ATP analogs, as well as the similarity between the rate of ATPase activity by purified CFTR in vitro and the rates of opening and closing *(6)*, strongly suggest that the channel uses ATP hydrolysis to power the opening of the gate.

Even though CFTR cannot use nonhydrolyzable analogs to open the channel, the addition of these analogs in the presence of hydrolyzable ATP greatly stabilizes the open state of the channel (**ref. 7**; **Fig. 1**). This effect suggests a second site for ATP action in controlling gating. Further evidence for two functional nucleotide-binding sites comes from kinetic studies of a hydrolysis-deficient NBD2 mutant, K1250A *(8)*. The presence of micromolar concentrations of ATP permits K1250A-CFTR channels to open briefly as in wild-type, whereas millimolar concentrations promote extremely prolonged openings, similar to those seen with nonhydrolyzable analogs. Such results suggest the presence of two functional sites for ATP. One hydrolyzes ATP to open the channel. Once open, the other site prolongs channel opening upon binding of a second ATP; ATP hydrolysis at that second site releases this stabilization of the open state (reviewed in **ref. 9**). This presence of two functional ATP sites certainly complicates attempts to understand how CFTR's nucleotide-driven gating occurs (*see* **Subheading 1.2.5.**).

This complexity is further compounded by the fact that ATP-driven gating is activated and quantitatively regulated by phosphorylation and dephosphorylation (for review, *see* **ref. 2**). The R domain possesses multiple, apparently redundant, sites for PKA-dependent phosphorylation, which contribute to regulating ATP-dependent gating. Moreover, several types of phosphatases, some membrane-bound, dephosphorylate CFTR *(10–12)*. Although this antagonism serves to regulate CFTR exquisitely in the intact cell, it creates difficulties in establishing stable, consistent experimental conditions for studying channel gating by ATP.

Finally, in addition to ATP-driven gating, CFTR shows a faster, ATP-independent form of gating. This "flickery" gating is thought to be the result of relatively brief blockade of the pore by intracellular anions and perhaps by a part of CFTR itself *(13,14)*. This "flickery" gating occurs on the order of tens of milliseconds *(14–18)*, whereas ATP-dependent gating happens on the scale

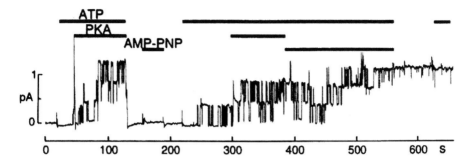

Fig. 1. Activation of CFTR by PKA and ATP but not AMPPNP and stabilization of the open state by ATP plus AMPPNP. Trace of an excised "giant" patch from a guinea-pig cardiac myocyte showing activation by both PKA and ATP. Upward deflections indicate channel openings. No channel activity is evident in the presence of ATP prior to introduction of PKA. After phosphorylation, introduction of AMPPNP alone does not elicit channel opening. Reintroduction of ATP reopens the channels, and a mixture of ATP and AMPPNP "locks" the channels in the open state. Reproduced from *Proceedings of the National Academy of Sciences, USA (7)* by permission of the National Academies of Sciences.

of hundreds of milliseconds to seconds *(8,19,20)* (**Fig. 3**). Thus, although these two forms of gating can be kinetically separated, care must be taken to identify ATP-dependent gating transitions.

1.2. Performing Kinetic Analyses on Recordings of Microscopic and Macroscopic CFTR Currents

1.2.1. Assessing Recording Quality for Quantitative Analysis of CFTR Gating

Before performing analyses on recorded data, some care must be taken to assure uniform conditions and behavior of channel activity throughout the recording interval to be analyzed. In excised inside-out patch experiments, one critical quality control factor is controlling channel rundown. Rundown takes two forms in recordings of CFTR channel activity: phosphorylation-dependent and phosphorylation-independent. Here, phosphorylation-dependent rundown is defined as reductions in channel activity that can be prevented by the presence of phosphatase inhibitors or restored by the addition of PKA (for example, *see* **ref. 12**). Phosphorylation-independent rundown is both unrecoverable loss in channel activity after patch excision from the cell and irreversible time-dependent changes in channel kinetics during the length of the experiment. Both phosphorylation-independent and phosphorylation-dependent rundown present significant hurdles in establishing stable experimental conditions.

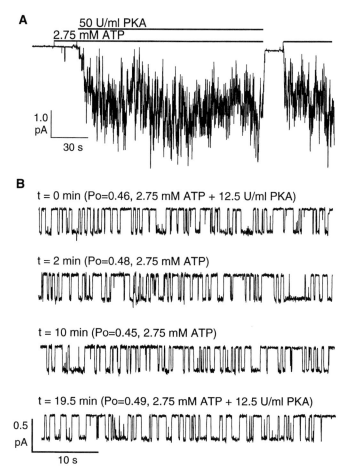

Fig. 2. PKA activation and ATP dependence of CFTR gating. **(A)** Representative trace from an excised inside-out patch from an NIH3T3 cell stably transfected with CFTR showing no channel activity in the presence of ATP prior to introduction of PKA. The presence of both PKA and ATP activates a multitude of CFTR channels. Downward deflections indicate channel openings. Upon withdrawal of kinase and nucleotide, channels shut completely. Reintroducing ATP alone rapidly opens channels to approximately the same level of steady-state activity. **(B)** Single-channel trace sweeps from the same experiment showing the consistency of channel activity over time. Reproduced from the *Journal of General Physiology (8)* by permission of the Rockefeller University Press.

As a result of membrane-bound phosphatases remaining after patch excision, the level of CFTR phosphorylation changes throughout the course of the experiment, consequently altering channel gating kinetics. For example, when examining macroscopic relaxations of CFTR currents in *Xenopus* oocytes, the time constants for opening and for closing changed significantly after PKA

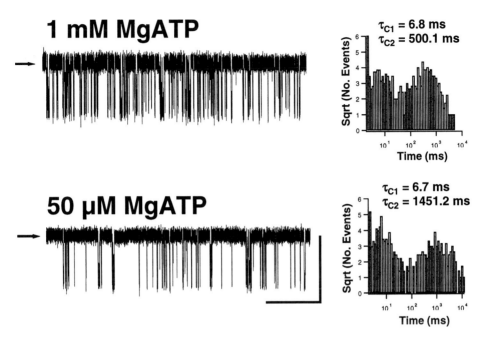

Fig. 3. ATP-dependent and -independent closed times for CFTR gating. On the left are single-channel traces from the same experiment showing channel activity at 50 μ*M* and 1 m*M* ATP. Arrows indicate the current baseline; downward deflections indicate channel openings. On the right are corresponding closed dwell-time histograms plotted using a log-scale binning method *(69)* to isolate more clearly the two components of CFTR gating. While the duration of the slow component (C2) demonstrably changes with ATP concentration, the fast component (C1) does not. This modulation is also apparent in the traces themselves: the interburst duration becomes longer when ATP concentration is reduced. The nadir in the distribution occurs at about 80 ms and is used to set a cutoff for discriminating between ATP-independent flickers and ATP-dependent closings. From Zhou and Hwang, unpublished observations.

had been applied and then washed out (**ref. *21*; Fig. 4**). The authors observed a gradually diminished ATP-dependent steady-state current and accelerating rates of opening and closing during the course of their experiment. In fact, after exposure to and removal of PKA at the beginning of the experiment, subsequent current activation relaxations by pulses of ATP could be fit, not with a single-, but with a double-exponential function (**Fig. 4**, insets). The time constant of one component was 1.7 s and that of the other several seconds. Furthermore, the relative contribution of the faster component increased over time, accounting for the acceleration of opening. This modulation of channel kinetics is at least in part due to the degree of phosphorylation of CFTR, as

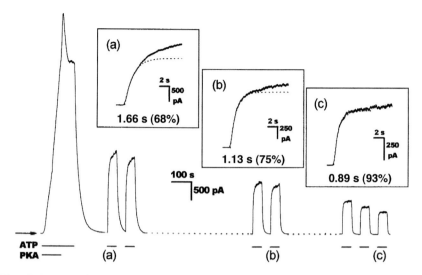

Fig. 4. Pre-steady-state macroscopic relaxations and rundown in excised "giant" patches. Representative trace of channel activity in a "giant" patch from a *Xenopus* oocyte heterologously expressing CFTR. Arrow indicates the current baseline; upward deflections indicate channel activation. Dashed regions indicate portions of the trace deleted for clarity. Initially, PKA and ATP activate a large number of channels. Upon withdrawal of PKA, activity markedly declines, most likely due to rapid dephosphorylation. Removal of ATP results in relaxation back to baseline. However, reintroduction of ATP alone restores channel activity to a reduced level. Subsequent pulses of ATP elicit progressively smaller responses. Insets show the change in kinetics of activation over time; indicated are time constants (and their relative weights) for fits to the fast relaxation component (dotted lines). Reproduced from the *Journal of General Physiology (21)* by permission of the Rockefeller University Press.

renewed application of PKA partially reversed these changes in opening and closing rates.

Although there is no way to control for phosphorylation-independent rundown, some measures can be taken to establish a steady-state condition for CFTR phosphorylation. One way to abate phosphorylation-dependent rundown would be to include phosphatase inhibitors throughout the course of the experiment. Although strong specific phosphatase inhibitors, such as calyculin A and okadaic acid, exist for phosphatase 2A (PP2A), one of the two main phosphatases shown to dephosphorylate CFTR *(10,11)*, none exist for phosphatase 2C (PP2C), another phosphatase shown to downregulate CFTR *(12,22)*. To complicate matters further, a recent study suggests that PP2C, through its close association with CFTR, is a strong candidate for the endogenous membrane-bound phosphatase responsible for dephosphorylating the channel in intact cells and excised patches *(23)*. Other means available to control PP2C-mediated dephosphorylation, that is, use of orthovanadate, a broad-spectrum phosphatase inhibitor, or reduction of free magnesium, a cofactor for PP2C activity, are extremely problematic because they drastically affect channel gating kinetics *(19,24,25)* (*see* **Subheading 1.2.5.**).

Alternatively, inclusion of protein kinase A (PKA) throughout the experiment can ameliorate phosphorylation-dependent rundown. Although the channel may not be maximally phosphorylated, the antagonism between kinase and phosphatase allows for stable, steady-state conditions during recording. As most of our patch experiments are performed with constant superfusion, continuous perfusion of kinase, phosphatase inhibitors, or both is an expensive proposition. Hence, having a static bath, except when changing solutions, would be advisable if using costly kinases and phosphatase inhibitors to control steady-state phosphorylation levels. Nevertheless, kinase/phosphatase-driven transitions between partially phosphorylated and dephosphorylated states become nested within transitions due solely to ATP-dependent gating, adding further variability to the extracted kinetic parameters.

Regardless of phosphorylation-dependent rundown, establishing stationarity in CFTR channel recordings before analysis is very important. For example, in Zeltwanger et al. *(8)*, care was taken to show that the open probability of a single CFTR channel did not change over a long period, as a way to ensure that gating behavior remained constant throughout the experiment (**Fig. 2B**). Also, the authors established a bracketing procedure in order to reduce the influence of rundown: applying a control condition, in this case, perfusion of 2.75 m*M* MgATP, before and after (i.e., bracketing) the test condition. If channel activity diminished by more than 20% upon the second application of the control condition, the experiment was discarded. Hence, bracketing allows pairing of the test condition with the control in the same experiment over a short period of time. Also, with the control condition as a standard for comparison, the variability among experiments can be assessed more reliably. Both bracketing during the experiment and establishing the stationarity of the recording are essential quality control measures to ensure reliability in estimates of gating kinetics.

1.2.2. Methods for Analyzing Single- and Few-Channel Data

The methods for analysis of CFTR single-channel recordings are the standard ones used by others in the ion channel field: (1) all-point histograms used to determine single-channel amplitude and open probability, (2) idealization of single channel traces, (3) detection of open and closed events and generation of an event list, (4) plots of open and closed dwell times as histograms or survivor functions, and finally (5) fitting those plots with exponential functions or a probability density function (pdf) to estimate mean dwell times. The theory and hazards associated with these techniques are thoroughly explained by Rudy and Iverson *(26)* and by Sakmann and Neher *(27)*. Gating analysis is most easily performed using single-channel recordings. Unfortunately, the occurrence of single CFTR channel patches is quite rare, necessitating the need for ways to analyze multiple-channel recordings.

One way to deal with multiple-channel recordings involves an approach originated by Fenwick et al. *(28)* and modified by Wang et al. *(29)* (**Fig. 5**; *see* also **Subheading 3.3.4.**). In Wang et al. *(29)*, a multiple-channel open event (with *N* channels opened simultaneously at most) is converted into *N* single-channel events, each with an open duration defined by the arithmetic mean of the duration of the multiple-channel event. The authors use this method to estimate the change in mean open time caused by applying genistein to excised inside-out patches with CFTR exposed to ATP. The open time estimates obtained by this conversion of a multiple-channel event to several single ones are not much different from the ones obtained via bona-fide single-channels recordings. For example, the estimated mean open time for CFTR in the presence of 0.5 m*M* ATP from Wang et al. *(29)* (**Fig. 5C**) is nearly identical to that derived from single-channel experiments in Zeltwanger et al. *(8)*. However, it should be mentioned that this technique has only been applied to recordings with five or fewer channels. With increasing numbers of channels and the accompanying open-channel noise created by flickers (*see* **Subheading 1.2.3.**), resolving step transitions between current levels becomes progressively difficult, therefore limiting the ability to use the modified Fenwick method.

In addition to the Fenwick method, other means for analyzing multichannel data are available. For example, Csanády *(30)* has developed a suite of programs designed to extract kinetic constants from multichannel patch data under the constraints of a simplified model. This methodology has been used in two recent studies examining the role of the R domain in CFTR gating *(31)* and delineating the functional boundaries of NBD1 *(32)*. Although this powerful

----

Fig. 5. *(facing page)* Modified Fenwick transformation of multichannel recordings. (**A**) Hypothetical trace of two channels gating. Arrows indicate the time spent open by either channel; upward deflections indicate channel openings. (**B**) Event list after detection by the Csanady program *(30)*. The dwell times from a multiple-channel open event are shaded. These events are averaged using the equation in Fenwick, et al. *(28)* (**Subheading 3.3.4.**). (**C**), Survivor plots of dwell times from multichannel recordings in the presence of 0.5 mM ATP and 0.5 mM ATP plus 50 µM genistein *(29)*. The resulting mean open time at 0.5 mM ATP alone obtained by Wang et al. *(29)* is virtually identical to the mean open time at the same concentration shown in Zeltwanger et al. (ref. *8*; cf. Fig. 4). Reproduced from the Journal of General Physiology *(29)* by permission of the Rockefeller University Press.

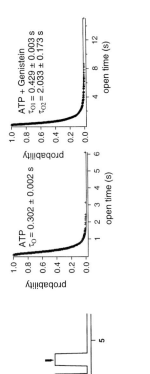

Fig. 5

75

method is extremely rapid and less computationally intensive than other analogous programs, there are a few limitations to the Csanády program. First, users must employ a simplified model, restricting the amount of kinetic information that can be immediately extracted. Second, the program cannot accomodate cyclic gating schemes, such as the ones proposed by Hwang et al. *(7)*, Weinreich et al. *(21)*, Zeltwanger et al. *(8)*, and Csanády et al. *(31)*, without simplifying portions of the proposed schemes. Verification of those composited steps might then require different experiments or other means of analysis to be performed. Nevertheless, using the Csanády program, in conjunction with the modified Fenwick method, may allow CFTR investigators to make better use of their multichannel data.

Once dwell-time information has been gathered, that information can be used to construct kinetic models for CFTR gating. One important piece of information that can be almost immediately garnered from open and closed time histograms is information on microscopic reversibility *(33)*. If a gating mechanism contains no irreversible steps, then the pdf fitted to dwell-time histograms will decrease monotonically, without a maximum or point of inflection. On the other hand, for schemes with irreversible steps, the fitted pdf will first go through a maximum, then monotonically decrease. Thus, having a negative exponential component in the pdf indicates the presence of microscopic irreversibility in the gating mechanism. Zeltwanger et al. *(8)* use the negative exponential component present in their closed-time pdf as evidence for an irreversible step in the opening of CFTR channels (**Fig. 6**). The presence of such a step would be consistent with the idea that ATP hydrolysis opens the channel.

1.2.3 Separating Slow ATP-Dependent and Fast ATP-Independent ("Flickery") CFTR Gating

CFTR channels tend to open in bursts that are separated by long closures in the range of hundreds of milliseconds to seconds, or the so-called slow gating of CFTR channels. Within each individual burst, brief closures with a time scale of several to tens of milliseconds are readily observed *(14–18)*. These brief closures, called flickers, represent the fast gating of CFTR channels. Accordingly, a closed-time histogram of CFTR channels contains two components with different time scales (**Fig. 3**). The slow component, corresponding to the mean time of the long closures between bursts, is ATP-dependent such that it becomes longer when ATP concentration is decreased. The other, faster component, corresponding to the mean time of the flicker, is ATP-independent (**Fig. 3**).

Fast flickers in CFTR have two defining characteristics. They are dramatically diminished after patch excision and are voltage-dependent, with more flickers observed at hyperpolarizing potentials *(14–18,34)*. This fast gating of CFTR is thought to result from transient block from the cytoplasmic side of the

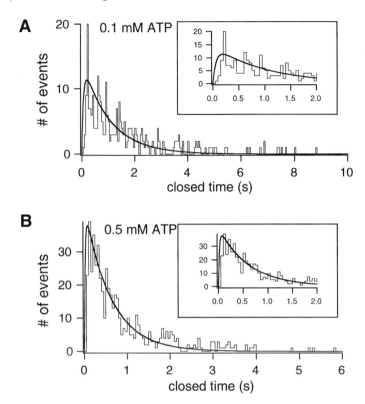

Fig. 6. Closed time histograms with fitted probability density functions (pdfs). Histograms show the distribution of closed times from single channels at two different concentrations of ATP (**A**, 0.1 m*M*; and **B**, 0.5 m*M* ATP) fitted with a pdf derived from the kinetic scheme outlined in Zeltwanger et al. *(8)*. The insets demonstrate more closely the presence of a negative exponential component in the dwell-time histogram, as highlighted by the fitted pdf. Reproduced from the *Journal of General Physiology (8)* by permission of the Rockefeller University Press.

channel, although the precise nature of the blocker is unknown. A recent study *(14)* examined the detailed kinetics of this flickery gating and its underlying voltage dependence. Within an ATP-dependent burst, the kinetics of the flickers can be described by a simple two-state model: open–closed. Moreover, the closed time, but not the open time, is voltage-dependent and sensitive to the concentration of external permeant anions. These results suggest that, within the pore, a permeant anion, entering from the extracellular side and occupying its binding site in a voltage-dependent manner, can electrostatically repel the blocker entering from the intracellular side, therefore accounting for the voltage dependence of the flickers.

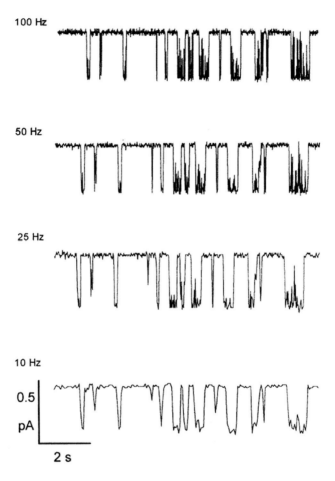

Fig. 7. Effect of filtering on CFTR gating events *(35)*. A 10-s sweep of a single CFTR channel recording filtered at different frequencies. Downward defelctions indicate channel openings. As the filter frequency decreases from 100 to 10 Hz, the flickery gating becomes less apparent, whereas the longer, ATP-dependent events remain relatively unadulterated. Reproduced from the doctoral dissertation of Shawn Zeltwanger *(35)* by permission of the author.

Given that the flickery gating of CFTR occurs on a millisecond time scale, these fast events can be removed through low-pass filtering before recording or analysis of single- or multiple-channel data. For example, Zeltwanger *(35)* shows that filtering data at 25 Hz during playback and digitization has little effect on ATP-dependent gating events, whereas flickers are virtually eliminated (**Fig. 7**). A number of studies have used filtering in their analyses of CFTR's ATP-dependent gating *(8,36)*. Flickers remaining after low-pass filtering can be removed by discarding events briefer than some cutoff value. For example, Zeltwanger et al. *(8)* use an 80-ms cutoff to exclude flickers from their kinetic analysis (*see* **Subheading 3.3.4.**). This choice of cutoff is justified by the fact that the nadir in the overlap between the flickers and ATP-dependent closed times occurs approximately at 80 ms (**Fig. 3**). At this nadir the probability of misclassifying an event as either a flicker or an ATP-dependent transition is at a minimum. Li et al. *(6)* also used this approach graphically to eliminate flickery gating from their analysis of ATP-dependent transitions, whereas Csanády et al. (31) solved for the optimum cutoff analytically.

1.2.4. Garnering Gating Information from Pre-Steady-State Current Relaxations

As discussed above, single-channel studies are one way to obtain kinetic constants for channel gating. These derived rate constants can then be used to construct different models of CFTR's gating mechanism. One major drawback of the single-channel approach is that long recordings of channel activity are required to collect enough events for accurate kinetic analyses of single channels, especially if the opening and closing rates (i.e., long bursts or interburst intervals) are extremely slow. For example, assuming a CFTR mutant has a mean burst duration of 180 s (similar to that for the K1250A mutant; *see* **ref.** *8*), tens of hours of single-channel recording on average would be required to collect about 1000 events! Another drawback is that results from many single-channel experiments have to be averaged in order for the results to be statistically significant. Given the difficulty of obtaining patches with only a single CFTR channel, other approaches to extract kinetic information from multichannel recordings are essential for fully characterizing CFTR gating.

An alternative approach to obtain kinetic constants is the simultaneous observation of many channels following a perturbation of steady-state conditions, such as a sudden change of temperature, voltage, or substrate concentration. Perturbation analysis allows rapid estimation of kinetic parameters when the responses of many channels (tens to hundreds) are tracked simultaneously. Examples of such investigations are studies of the Na^+,K^+-ATPase (e.g., *see* **refs.** *37–39*) and voltage-activated channels *(40,41)*.

In these types of experiments, kinetic constants for conformational changes of proteins are obtained by fast perturbation and measurement of the consequent relaxation to a new steady-state. This perturbation—for example, a change of nucleotide concentration—must be faster than the ensuing relaxation if rate-constant information is to be gained from the change. In the context of studying CFTR's gating *(21)* (**Fig. 8**), changes in ATP concentration can be achieved on the order of milliseconds, either through fast switching of the superfusing solution or by photolytic release of caged ATP *(42,43)*. For these experiments, one requires many channels in a membrane patch. After a rapid concentration jump, the resulting change in channel activity will produce

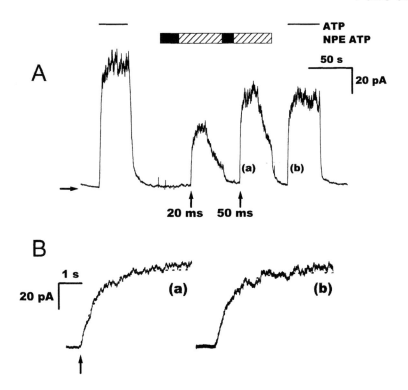

Fig. 8. Comparison of CFTR activation by rapid solution exchange and by caged ATP photolysis. (**A**) Trace shows activation of CFTR channels by rapid introduction of ATP, then by specific decaging of ATP-P3-[1-(2-nitrophenyl)ethyl]ester (NPE-ATP). NPE-ATP does not induce activity until photolyzed by UV irradiation. Upward deflections indicate channel openings. Thin bars indicate rapid perfusion of ATP, filled bars perfusion of NPE-ATP, and stippled bars interruption of continuous perfusion. UV-laser pulses decaging NPE-ATP indicated by arrows with the duration of the pulses shown beneath. Relaxations (a) and (b) expanded in **B**. (**B**) Activation relaxations by rapid exchange and caged ATP release have nearly identical time courses, as revealed by the superimposed exponential fits. Dashed curves are exponential fits to current relaxations; time constants for (a) and (b) are 1.3 s^{-1} and 1.4 s^{-1}, respectively. Reproduced from the *Journal of General Physiology (21)* by permission of the Rockefeller University Press.

a smooth relaxation of electrical current, as the channels reach a new level of steady-state behavior (**Fig. 8**). Such relaxations are subsequently fitted with exponential functions to extract rate-constant information. Because of the large numbers of channels required to produce smooth relaxations, channel recordings are preferentially made from "macro" or "giant" membrane patches *(44,45)*, which permits the presence of more channels per patch than found in conventionally sized excised membrane patches.

Alternatively, high levels of CFTR expression through use of viral vectors allow the recording of large numbers of channels per conventionally sized patch (e.g., *see* **refs. *3,46,47***). Furthermore, ensembles of quasi-macroscopic relaxations from conventionally sized patches with fewer channels ($5 \geq n \geq 20$) can be used to create a macroscopic one for the purposes of extracting kinetic information. For example, Zeltwanger et al. *(8)* used his approach to estimate the mean open time for the wild-type channel exposed to AMPPNP and the K1250A mutant.

1.2.5. Using Channel Mutants, Drugs, and Other Probes to Dissect CFTR Gating

Another powerful tool for dissecting CFTR gating is the use of nucleotide and phosphate analogs. As mentioned above, the use of the nonhydrolyzable ATP analog, AMPPNP, and the NBD2 mutant K1250A, implicated the involvement of ATP hydrolysis in channel opening and closing and established the presence of two functional sites for ATP (*see* above). These results from few channel patches were corroborated by macroscopic relaxation experiments using rapid solution changes. Switching from AMPPNP to ATP and then back to AMPPNP revealed that both opening and closing of CFTR are delayed *(21)* (**Fig. 9**). The delayed closing upon switching from ATP to AMPPNP is consistent with the above-mentioned binding of AMPPNP to a second binding site, where its binding inhibits channel closing. The delayed opening when changing from AMPPNP to ATP indicates the binding of AMPPNP to a nucleotide-binding site from which it must be released before ATP can open CFTR.

These experiments also used ADP to elucidate CFTR gating via NBDs. Macroscopic rate constants were determined from relaxation analysis in the presence of ADP *(21)*. When changing rapidly from ADP to ATP, the rate of opening deduced from current relaxations was decreased significantly. It was interpreted that the bound ADP had to be released before ATP can bind and open the channel. On the other hand, when changing from ATP to ADP, the rate of closing was increased significantly, perhaps due to binding of ADP to a second nucleotide-binding site that enhanced release of ATP or its hydrolysis products from the first binding site. Taken together, experiments using nucleotide analogs AMPPNP and ADP along with pre-steady-state relaxation analysis and steady-state single-channel kinetics have clearly demonstrated the presence of two functional ATP-binding sites in CFTR.

As alluded to earlier (*see* **Subheading 1.2.1.**), orthovanadate and beryllium fluoride, transition-state analogs of inorganic phosphate, can also prolong the open time of CFTR *(25)*. These authors argued that the ability of these analogs to "lock" CFTR open suggested a coupling of ATP hydrolysis to channel opening. In addition, other conventional means of manipulating the rate of ATP

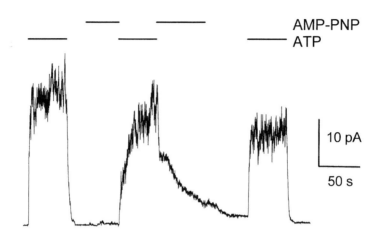

Fig. 9. The effect of AMPPNP on CFTR current relaxations. Trace shows rapid activation and deactivation of CFTR current by a pulse of ATP. Upward deflections indicate channel openings. Exposure to AMPPNP prior to and after an ATP application prolongs activation and deactivation of CFTR channels, respectively. Reproduced from the *Journal of General Physiology (21)* by permission of the Rockefeller University Press.

hydrolysis have been employed to examine their effects on CFTR gating. For example, two groups have used temperature-shift experiments to elucidate the thermodynamics for channel gating and correlate them to the energy of ATP binding and hydrolysis *(48,49)*.

Moreover, a number of groups have examined the role of magnesium, demonstrated to be a cofactor in certain ATPase reactions, in the opening and closing of the channel. Whereas Anderson et al. *(3)* and Dousmanis *(19)* reported that ATP failed to open CFTR in Mg^{2+}-free buffer, other studies demonstrated that micromolar amounts of free Mg^{2+} are sufficient for ATP-mediated opening of CFTR *(19,36,50)*. On the other hand, evidence from other studies *(46,51)* suggests that ATP is indeed able to open CFTR channels in the apparent absence of free Mg^{2+}. Harrington et al. *(52)* showed that substitution of Mg with certain other divalent cations greatly slowed channel closing but had little effect on channel opening. It is completely unclear what may account for the discrepancies in the literature. One possible explanation is that CFTR, like myosin *(53)* or elongation factor Tu *(54)*, may be able to use monovalent cations in lieu of divalents to ligand the phosphates of nucleotides during hydrolysis. Further experiments are needed to understand clearly how magnesium participates in CFTR function. Resolution of this controversy may prove key in supporting or refuting the argument that CFTR requires ATP hydrolysis for channel gating.

Finally, the introduction of mutations into CFTR's NBDs has been and currently serves as a powerful approach not only to understand how ATP gates the channel but also to provide insight into the structure of the ion channel. Several groups have also investigated the effects of mutating conserved lysines within each NBD thought to be intimately involved with ATP hydrolysis *(36,46,55–57)*, a notion supported by the finding that mutation of either lysine reduces CFTR-mediated ATP hydrolysis in vitro *(56)*. As with magnesium, it is difficult to reconcile the absolute requirement for ATP hydrolysis with the observed ATP-dependent opening of CFTR channels, where Walker A lysines in both nucleotide-binding sites are mutated to alanines (K464A/K1250A) *(56,57)*. Additionally, Gadsby and co-workers have used a "severed" domain approach to establish the functional boundaries for the N-terminal NBD *(32)* and to investigate the role of the R domain in regulating ATP-dependent gating *(31)*. With the resolution of the three-dimensional structures of NBDs from ABC transporters, HisP *(58)*, RbsA *(59)*, and MalK *(60)*, CFTR channel investigators have begun to use these structures as templates to test ideas about the structure–function relationships *(61,62)*. Such studies have begun to merge structural and functional data to provide an increasingly more complete picture of CFTR gating.

2. Materials

The materials and methods listed here are by no means the only ones that can be used for performing electrophysiological experiments examining CFTR gating. The following sections enumerate the materials we personally have used for our studies (*see* **refs.** *8* and *21*). Information on alternative hardware and software options can be found in Rudy and Iverson *(26)*, Sakmann and Neher *(27)*, or via the World Wide Web (e.g., http://www.axon.com/MR_Axon_Guide.html).

2.1. Patch Clamp Experiments Using Heterologous Expression of CFTR in NIH3T3 Cells

2.1.1. Culture of NIH3T3 Cells

1. Dulbecco's modified Eagle's medium (DMEM)/2 m*M* glutamine (Life Technologies, Rockville, MD).
2. Calf serum (Harlan Sera-Lab, Leicestershire, UK).
3. Phosphate-buffered saline (PBS) (Life Technologies, Rockville, MD).
4. 0.05% Trypsin, 1 m*M* ethylenediaminetetraacetic acid (EDTA) (Life Technologies).
5. Cover glass, 24 × 50 mm (Fisher Scientific, Pittsburgh, PA).
6. Falcon tissue culture dishes, polystyrene, 35 × 10 mm (Becton Dickinson, Franklin Lakes, NJ).

7. Cell culture flasks, polystyrene, 25 cm^2 (Corning, Corning, NY).

2.1.2. Electrophysiological Recording (Excised Inside-Out Patch Clamp) of Heterologously Expressed CFTR in NIH3T3 Cells

All chemicals are the purest grades available from Sigma Chemical (St. Louis, MO), unless otherwise indicated.

1. Pipet solution: 140 mM N-methyl-D-glucamine chloride (NMDG-Cl), 2 mM MgCl$_2$, 5 mM CaCl$_2$, 10 mM HEPES, pH 7.4 with NMDG (use either solid or 1 M stock). A 2 M stock solution of NMDG-Cl can be made by the addition of concentrated HCl to solution of NMDG to a final pH of 7.4; then this NMDG-Cl stock can be used to make the appropriate solutions.
2. Bath solution (prior to patch excision): 150 mM NaCl, 2 mM MgCl$_2$, 1 mM EGTA, 5 mM glucose, 5 mM HEPES, pH 7.4 with 1 N NaOH.
3. Superfusion solution (during and after patch excision): 150 mM NMDG-Cl, 10 mM EGTA, 10 mM HEPES, 8 mM Tris-HCl, and 2 mM MgCl$_2$, pH 7.4 with NMDG.
4. MgATP (Sigma). Stock concentration 250 mM. Upon addition of millimolar ATP to the superfusion solution, noticeable acidification occurred, so the pH of superfusion solution is readjusted to 7.4 with NMDG (1 M stock solution) after ATP addition.
5. Li$_4$AMPPNP (Roche Biochemicals, Indianapolis, IN). As a solid or in a 250-mM stock solution, both stored at –20°C, AMPPNP is quite labile and decomposes into ADP. The solid remains stable for approx 6–8 wk, the stock solution for about 2 wk.
6. PKA catalytic subunit (Promega Corp., Madison, WI). PKA catalytic subunit is shipped frozen on dry ice and stored at –70°C upon arrival; aliquots thawed for use are stored at 4°C and remain good for about a month. As the specific activity per lot varies, attention is paid to maintaining a consistent specific activity across multiple experiments rather than a constant concentration.
7. Glass capillary tubing (Corning 7056; Corning).

2.1.3. Data Acquisition, Storage, Analysis, and Display for Conventional Patch Clamp Experiments

1. EPC-9 patch clamp amplifier (Heka Elektronik, Lambrecht, Germany). The headstage and pipet holder are included with the amplifier. Different configurations of interfaces, acquisition software and analysis program suites can be selected and bundled with the amplifier upon purchase.
2. Microforge. Ours are home-made, but commercially manufactured ones are also available (e.g., Narishige, Tokyo, Japan).
3. Pipet puller (Narishige).
4. Microscope, inverted (Olympus America, Melville, NY).
5. Micromanipulator (Newport, Irvine, CA).
6. Air table (Technical Manufacturing, Peabody, MA).
7. Faraday cage. Ours are home-made, but commercially manufactured ones are also available (e.g., Heka Elektronik.).

 8. Perfusion chamber. Ours are home-made, but commercially manufactured ones are also available (e.g., Warner Instruments, Hamden, CT).
 9. Eight-Pole Bessel filter (Warner Instruments).
10. Pulse code modulator/VCR (Vetter/JVC). Although this pulse code modulator/ VCR fusion is quite useful for its ability to store broad-bandwidth analog data, other means of storing data (e.g., DAT) are adequate. For a more in-depth discussion of the relevant issues, see French and Wonderlin *(63)*.
11. Oscilloscope (Hewlett-Packard, Palo Alto, CA).
12. Chart recorder (Kipp & Zonen, Delft, Holland).
13. Macintosh Quadra 450 (Apple, Cupertino, CA). Windows-based PC versions of Heka's hardware and software are also available.
14. Igor Pro, v3.13 (Wavemetrics, Lake Oswego, CA). The most current update of this program at this writing is Version 4.01, which features much friendlier user interfaces for its analytical macros.

2.2. "Giant Patch" Experiments Using Heterologous Expression of CFTR in Xenopus Oocytes

2.2.1. Harvesting and Culture of Xenopus Oocytes

All chemicals are purchased from Sigma Chemical (St. Louis, MO), unless otherwise indicated.

1. 0.2% tricaine solution for anesthesia of the animals.
2. Collagenase. One can use collagenase from Worthington (Lakewood, NJ), Roche, or Sigma. Specific batches tested empirically for quality are more important than the particular supplier (*see* **Subheading 3.2.**). Accordingly, it is useful to track lot numbers for certain batches of collagenase to ensure consistent digestion.
3. mMessage mMachine kit (Ambion, Austin, TX).
4. RNase-free water (Promega, Madison, WI).
5. Injection pipets and injector (Drummond Scientific, Broomall, PA).
6. Pipet puller (David Kopf, Tujunga, CA). Pulled pipets are either broken with tweezers or beveled (with pipet grinding dishes from World Precision Instruments) to a diameter of 25 to 30 μm.
7. Penicillin/streptamycin.
8. Modified Ringer's solution (ORi): 110 mM NaCl, 5 mM KCl, 2 mM CaCl$_2$, 1 mM MgCl$_2$, 5 mM HEPES pH 7.6 with NaOH.
9. Ca^{2+}-free ORi: 110 mM NaCl, 5 mM KCl, 1 mM MgCl$_2$, 5 mM HEPES, pH 7.6 with NaOH.

2.2.2. Electrophysiological Recording (Excised Inside-Out Giant Patch) of Heterologously Expressed CFTR in Oocytes

1. Hypertonic shrink solution: 200 mM K-aspartate, 20 mM KCl, 2 mM MgCl$_2$, 5 mM EGTA, 10 mM HEPES, pH 7.4 with KOH.
2. Pipet solution: 150 mM NMDG, 2 mM BaCl$_2$, 2 mM MgCl$_2$, 0.5 mM CdCl$_2$, 10 mM HEPES, pH 7.4 with HCl.

3. Ca^{2+}-free bath solution: 140 mM NMDG, 20 mM TEA-OH, 5 mM reduced glutathione, 5 mM EGTA, 2 mM MgCl$_2$, 10 mM HEPES, pH 7.4 with aspartate.

4. Patch pipets are the type (N-51A from Drummond) originally used by Hilgemann *(45)*, with a diameter of more than 2 mm, which requires careful drilling of the provided pipet holders. Pipets can be pulled in two stages to a desired tip diameter of 20 µm by most conventional pipet pullers, such as PP-83 from Narishige.

2.2.3. Data Acquisition, Storage, and Analysis for "Giant Patch" Experiments

All other equipment necessary for completing a "giant patch" rig are similar or identical to ones listed above (*see* **Subheading 2.1.3.**). For some of our previous "giant patch" studies (e.g., *see* **ref. *21***) data acquisition was accomplished using two Windows-based PCs with digitizing hardware and PCLAMP software from Axon Instruments (Foster City, CA). One computer triggered solution changes and recorded resulting changes in current, while the other continuously acquired data at low frequency. For subsequent analysis, we used PCLAMP or ORIGIN (OriginLab Corp., Northampton, MA) software for fitting current relaxations.

3. Methods

3.1. Patch Clamp Experiments Using Heterlogous Expression of CFTR in NIH3T3 Cells

3.1.1. Culture and Preparation of NIH3T3 Cells for Patch Clamp

Both wild type- *(64)* and K1250A-CFTR *(8)* channels were stably expressed in NIH3T3 cells. NIH3T3- K1250A cells stably expressing K1250A-CFTR were established using the retroviral vector pLJ *(8)*. Typically, we maintain both cell lines at 37°C under 95% O$_2$/5% CO$_2$ in 5 mL DMEM supplemented with 2 mM glutamine and 10% calf serum in Corning T-25 flasks. When cell growth reaches 80–100% confluence, the adherent NIH3T3 cells are trypsinized and passaged into a new flask. For patch clamp recording, cells are trypsinized then plated onto small, sterile glass chips in 35-mm tissue culture dishes and allowed at least a 24-h recovery period before recording. Sterile conditions should be maintained throughout. Antibiotics can be used but are not critical if careful sterile technique is followed.

1. From a flask with 80–100% confluence, remove old medium via suction with a sterile glass Pasteur pipet under a sterile hood.
2. Wash 1X with sterile isotonic PBS to remove residual serum, which will inhibit trypsinization.
3. Remove PBS via suction; add 0.5 mL 0.1% trypsin/1 mM EDTA solution. Rock flask back and forth to ensure complete coverage of the cell layer.

4. After approx 1 min, tap the flask gently to release the cells from the flask surface.
5. Immediately add 4.5 mL DMEM with calf serum to stop trypsinization and dilute the enzyme.
6. Titurate thoroughly to break up clumps of cells.
7. For cell maintenance, remove 1 mL of the cell suspension and add to a new flask with 4 mL DMEM with calf serum. Place in incubator and allow cells to settle. Typically, healthy cells will become confluent within 2–3 d after passage.
8. For patch clamp recording, prepare 35-mm dishes by placing sterile glass chips inside and overlaying with about 1 mL DMEM/calf serum. Make sure chips are completely submerged, using a sterile glass pipet to push the chips beneath the fluid surface onto the bottom of the dish.
9. Put approx 2–3 drops of cell suspension into the dishes with chips; swirl gently to disperse cells, then place in incubator. Allow at least 24 h for recovery before performing the patch clamp experiment.

3.1.2. Recording Steady-State Currents in Excised Inside-Out Patches from NIH3T3 Cells

1. Patch clamp pipet electrodes were made using a two-stage vertical puller (Narishige) and their tips fire-polished with a home-made microforge to ~1 μm external diameter, resulting in a pipet resistance of 3–6 MΩ in the bath solution.
2. Cells expressing CFTR are placed in home-made perfusion chamber and superfused with bath solution at room temperature (25°C) before recording.
3. Pipet electrodes are briefly front-filled by carefully dipping the tips into 0.22 μm-filtered pipet solution for 10–20 s, back-filled with pipet solution via filtered syringe, then mounted into the pipet holder.
4. Using a Huxley-type micromanipulator, the pipet is lowered into the recording chamber while a small command potential is applied to produce a step current to assess pipet resistance. Once the pipet makes contact with the cell, the step will be slightly reduced; suction through the pipet is then applied and a gigaohm seal will begin to form. Pipet potential is held at 50 mV in reference to the bath throughout.
5. Once the seal has reached approximately 50–100 GΩ, the bath solution is exchanged with superfusion solution. Once exchange has occurred, the pipet is quickly and abruptly raised from the cell while remaining in the bath solution to excise the membrane patch.
6. Once excised, PKA and ATP in superfusion solution activate CFTR channels in the patch. CFTR channel currents are then recorded with an EPC-9 patch clamp amplifier, filtered at 100 Hz with a built-in three-pole Bessel filter, and stored on videotape. Current fluctuations can also be simultaneously monitored on a chart recorder.
7. Once channels are active, the patch can be exposed to various experimental solutions, such as AMPPNP, by superfusion. Care must be taken that the previous test solution has been completely washed away before beginning the next (*see* **Note 1**).

3.2. Electrophysiological Recording ("Giant Patch") of Heterologously Expressed CFTR in Xenopus Oocytes

3.2.1. Harvesting and Culture of Xenopus Oocytes

1. 10–20 female *Xenopus laevis* are kept in a 200-L tank, with filtered water continuously exchanging every 24 h.
2. Ovary lobes are removed from anesthetized animals (by immersion into a 0.2% tricaine solution for 5–10 min) through a small incision that is sutured afterwards. Ovary lobes can be removed from the same animal up to eight times.
3. Oocytes are prepared by digestion with collagenase in Ca^{2+}-free ORi for 2–4 h (or overnight with 1-mg/mL collagenase) at room temperature and afterwards washed extensively (10 times) before they are stored in normal ORi. As collagenase from the same supplier may vary considerably, it is advisable to test a sample of a new batch in parallel with an established one before ordering more of the newer enzyme.
4. Stage V oocytes (~1.1 mm in diameter) are injected with 20 ng CFTR-cRNA in 50 nL RNAase-free water and incubated at 18°C for at least 3 d in ORi with penicillin and streptamycin.

3.2.2. Electrophysiological Recording (Excised Inside-Out Giant Patch) of Heterologously Expressed CFTR in Oocytes

Recording from giant patches of plasma membrane of oocytes was described in detail by Hilgemann *(45)* and by Weinreich et al. *(21)* (*see* **Note 2**).

1. Oocytes are shrunk in a hypertonic solution and the vitelline layer is removed mechanically with sharpened forceps.
2. Patch pipets of ~20-μm tip diameter are pulled on conventional pipet pullers and are fire-polished until a small decrease of the tip diameter is observed.
3. Using a micromanipulator, the giant patch electrode, filled with pipet solution under a slight outward pressure (1–2 cm water column), is lowered carefully toward the oocyte. Upon contact between pipet and oocyte, a slight suction (1–2 cm water column) is applied to form the seal. After establishing an apparent seal resistance of 0.5–1 GΩ, the patch is carefully excised and the pipet is transferred to the solution exchange chamber (*see* **ref. 65**).
4. Inside-out configuration of the excised patch can be confirmed by applying a solution with several micromolar free Ca^{2+}, which will activate the endogenous Ca^{2+}-activated chloride conductance. Seal resistance in Ca^{2+}-free bath solution typically ranges between 2 and 20 GΩ.

3.2.3. Photolysis of Caged ATP

For most transporters or ligand-gated channels it is impossible to achieve a rapid enough concentration jump by fast solution exchange at the membrane. Therefore "caged substrates" were developed so that a flash of ultraviolet light will induce a rapid release of substrate from a "caged" (i.e., chemically modified and inert) precursor, for example, the release of ATP from its γ-phosphate

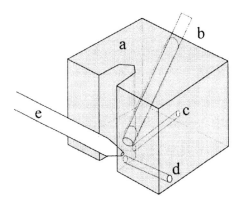

Fig. 10. Photolysis/perfusion chamber for "giant patch" experiment. Schematic of a temperature-controlled perfusion chamber used for photolysis of caged ATP. The brass cube (a) enclosed the inlets for the UV-laser (c), the perfusion solutions (c), and the temperature sensor (d). The pipet position (e) is also indicated. The brass cube is water-jacketed (not shown) for temperature control. The cube's dimensions are 10 mm³. Reproduced from the *Biophysical Journal (65)* by permission of the Biophysical Society.

nitro-phenyl-ethyl ester (caged ATP) *(42)*. UV-light-induced ATP release was shown to be accelerated at lower pH and to proceed with a time constant of about 10 ms at physiological pH *(43)*. For giant excised membrane patches a laser-photolysis system was developed to investigate the kinetics of the Na^+,K^+-ATPase *(65)*, which was also used to analyze the response of CFTR to a sudden increase of ATP concentration *(21)*. A typical protocol is shown in **Fig. 8**.

3.2.4. Rapid Solution Exchange Using Giant Patches of Excised Plasma Membrane

The measuring chamber for UV-laser flash-induced photolysis or fast solution exchange was built in the workshop of the Max-Planck-Institute (Frankfurt, Germany; **Fig. 10**). The original design *(65)*, with a volume of ~10 μL and a solution exchange time of ~1 s was improved further to obtain exchange time constants below 100 ms *(21)*. Eight solution-carrying lines were switched by computer-controlled electrical valves (General Valve, NJ) and were connected close to the solution inlet. Giant excised inside-out membrane patches (~ 20 μm diameter) are more sensitive to hydrostatic pressure but have a favorable shape in the patch pipet to allow rapid solution exchange at the membrane *(5,44)*. The time constant for exchange of the solution can easily be measured by changing the concentration gradient of a certain ion species with high conductance in the membrane and observing the change in electrical current. For CFTR, expressed in oocytes, we measured this time constant in every experiment by activating the endogenous Ca^{2+}-activated chloride conductance and changing the bath chloride concentration *(21)*. The solution exchange time constant typically ranged from 15 to 100 ms, and experiments were analyzed only when the CFTR-related time constants were at least five times longer (*see* **Fig. 8**).

3.3. Analysis of Recorded Data

3.3.1. Filtering and Sampling Data from Excised Patch Experiments

3.3.1.1. PROCEDURE FOR EXCISED PATCH/NIH3T3 EXPERIMENTS

As mentioned under **Subheading 1.1.**, CFTR exhibits fast ATP-independent (i.e., flickers) and slow ATP-dependent gating. To eliminate these flickers from our analysis of ATP-dependent gating, we filtered our signals at a relatively low cutoff frequency (–3 dB) of 25 Hz using an eight-pole Bessel filter. Our 25-Hz filter setting results in a 10–90% rise time of 12 ms; therefore, ATP-dependent gating transitions are likely to be unaffected by the filter, whereas flickers with durations of 10 ms or less are greatly attenuated (*see* **Note 3**). The played-back data are then sampled by computer using the Pulse software accompanying the EPC-9 patch clamp amplifier. The sampling rate should be at least five times the filtering frequency—in this case, 125 Hz. Once recorded data has been played back and adequately sampled by the computer, the resulting files are imported into the Igor program or some other software package for further analysis.

3.3.1.2. PROCEDURE FOR "GIANT PATCH"/*XENOPUS* OOCYTE EXPERIMENTS

Electrical current and solution switching pulses are recorded on a chart recorder. Current may also be filtered at 20 Hz and continuously recorded at 100 Hz on a PC using KAN1 software (MFK, Niedernhausen, Germany). For the analysis of relaxation time courses, current is filtered at 100 Hz and recorded at 500 Hz with PCLAMP software (Axon Instruments) on another computer, which also drives the laser, electrical shutter, and valves *(21)*. Digitized current traces were fitted with exponential functions using either PCLAMP or ORIGIN.

3.3.2. Determination of N, i, and P_o

From the stretch of recording to be analyzed, an all-point amplitude histogram is generated using the Histogram macro in the Igor software. From such a histogram, Gaussian functions can be used to determine the value at each peak using the Curve Fitting macro. The single-channel amplitude (*i*) is obtained by measuring the difference between the two adjacent peaks in the histogram. The number of channels (*N*) present is usually determined by the maximum number of channels seen under maximal stimulation conditions

(PKA 40 U/mL and 2.75 m*M* MgATP). However, one can also apply AMPPNP along with PKA and ATP to "lock" most of the channels open and more easily detect the maximum number of channels in the patch (*see* **Note 4**). The open probability (P_o) of the channels can then be calculated using the area under each peak (a_j) at each current level (j) in the histogram along with the number of channels (N) as follows:

$$P_o = \frac{\sum_{j=0} (j \times a_j)}{N \times \sum_{j=0}^{N} a_j}$$

The area under each peak can be calculated using the relevant Igor macro or from the parameters obtained from the fitted Gaussian function for each peak (*see* **Note 4**).

3.3.3. Idealization and Event Detection of Single-Channel Recordings

For idealization and event detection of single-channel recording, we use the PAT analysis software (http://www.strath.ac.uk/Departments/PhysPharm/ses.htm). For both single- and multiple-channel recordings, we use the relevant program in the suite of programs written by Dr. Lászlo Csanády *(30)*. Both programs generate lists of open and closing events that can be imported into the Igor program for further processing (*see* **Note 5**).

In addition to filtering during playback, the flickery, ATP-independent gating is also eliminated by defining open events as intervals separated by closings of 80 ms or greater. Such closed events are redefined as open and concatenated with adjacent open events (*see* **Subheading 1.2.3.**). The PAT program allows for this procedure within the program itself; with the Csanády program, the event list can be opened in Igor or any other spreadsheet program for editing.

For event discrimination using a predetermined cutoff, as in Zeltwanger et al. *(8)*, the investigator searches for closed events shorter than the cutoff duration, then reclassifies the event as open and concatenates it with the two flanking open events to generate one corrected open event. This procedure can be accomplished by computer algorithm or by manual inspection and recalculation. Determination of the cutoff can be done graphically by estimating the ordinate value at the nadir between the flicker and ATP-dependent components. Alternatively, an analytical method derived by Jackson et al. *(66)* can be used to calculate the optimum cutoff (t_c):

$$t_c = [(\tau_1 \cdot \tau_2)/(\tau_2 - \tau_1)] \cdot \ln [(\tau_2 \cdot a_1)/(\tau_1 \cdot a_2)]$$

where τ_1, τ_2, a_1, and a_2 are the time constants and fractional amplitudes for the two-exponential fit to the closed time histogram. Csanády et al. *(31)* used this method to justify a cutoff of 30–80 ms for wild-type and most of their mutant channels.

3.3.4. Dwell-Time Analysis

Once an event list has been generated and imported into Igor, a probability density function can be created by generating a frequency histogram from the event list using Igor's Histogram macro. The resulting histogram can be fitted with exponential functions to yield mean time constants for opening or closing or with pdfs derived from more complex kinetic schemes.

In situations where there are relatively few (<1000) events, survivor plots can be used to extract information about mean dwell time. To create a such plot, the open dwell times are ranked from longest to shortest. Then the ranks are divided by the total number of events and plotted as the abscissa against the corresponding duration on the ordinate. Thus, the plot indicates the probability that a particular opening event will last at least time t given that it was open at $t = 0$. Accordingly, the probability of an event lasting for the shortest defined duration in the event list is 1. This method is similar to that used by Baukrowitz et al. *(25)*. The resulting curve can be subsequently fitted with single, double, or multiple exponential functions using Igor's Curve Fitting macro. The resulting fits will yield time constants for each exponential fit (**Fig. 5C**).

3.3.5. Fenwick Method for Dwell-Time Analysis

For multiple-channel recordings, the durations of adjacent multiple channel open events bounded by closed events greater than 80 ms are summed and then divided by the number of events. The resulting average duration is entered into the event list as many times as the number of events averaged. As a result, the multiple-channel open event is transferred to several single-channel open events with average open time for each event. This procedure is based on that used by Fenwick et al. *(28)* to obtain a single mean open time for an entire event list from the following equation:

$$t_o = \frac{\displaystyle\sum_{j=0}^{N} (j \times t_j)}{\displaystyle\sum_{j=0}^{N} n_{j \rightarrow j+1}}$$

where t_o represents mean open time, j each current level, N the total number of channels, and $n_{j \rightarrow j+1}$ the number of transitions between the jth and $(j + 1)$th levels. Here, rather than applying the equation to an entire event list, each multiple channel event is converted to a series of single events, as in Wang et al. *(29)* (**Fig. 5A**). Then, the Fenwick-transformed event list can be treated by the same methods for the single channel event lists to determine mean dwell times. This modified procedure allows the detection of multiple exponential components (**Fig. 5C**).

3.3.6. Current Relaxation Analysis

Relaxation currents are fitted either with the PCLAMP simplex fitting algorithm or with the Levenberg-Marquardt fitting tool of ORIGIN *(21)*. In a first approach a monoexponential function is fitted to the data. If this is obviously unsatisfying, a biexponential function is fitted to the data and the relative amplitudes are recorded together with the two time constants.

4. Notes

1. For more extensive information on setting up and troubleshooting patch clamp experiments, we refer the reader to Rudy and Iverson *(26)* and Sakmann and Neher *(27)*. Both books contain extensive information on various patch clamp methodologies and the theoretical underpinnings necessary for obtaining good-quality recordings.
2. Before performing "giant patch" experiments, an investigator should test for functional CFTR expression using conventional two-electrode voltage clamping. However, because injection of 20 ng CFTR cRNA per oocyte may easily result in conductances of more than 1 mS, conventional two-electrode configuration may not be able to clamp membrane voltage reliably once CFTR channels are activated (*see* **ref. 67**).
3. A more extensive discussion of filtering and event detection can be found in Sakmann and Neher *(27)*.
4. Determining the open probability of CFTR channels can be somewhat problematic. The issue involves obtaining an accurate assessment of the number of channels, N, given the low P_o of certain CFTR mutants. Visual inspection of the experimental record alone as a way to determine N can be insufficient, especially when using submaximal stimulating conditions or working with mutant channels possessing very low P_o. When the ratio of mean open time to mean closed time is relatively small (< 0.01), then the probability of the actual number of channels present being greater than the observed maximum becomes frighteningly high (*see* **ref. 33**).
   A statistical test for determining the probability of possessing a given number of channels in the patch can be used to assess the confidence in one's estimate *(33)*. This test sets out to test the hypothesis that a recording with only single-channel openings evident actually contains two (or more) channels. Csanády et al. *(31)* have extended this method to test the hypothesis that the number of channels in the patch is greater than the observed maximum where the observed maximum number of channels is more than one.
   In conjunction with these statistical tests, CFTR investigators can use maneuvers that greatly enhance open probability to reveal the number of channels in the patch. For example, Csanády et al. *(31)* use AMPPNP or pyrophosphate to lock

open CFTR channels for counting at the end of their experiments. At a minimum, such an experimental maneuver should be used whenever evaluating CFTR or kinetics, as one might run the risk of grossly overestimating P_o in situations where the actual P_o is truly very low.

However, these statistical and experimental means for assessing N have limitations. For example, maneuvers to maximally open channels, such as exposure to AMPPNP or pyrophosphate, may prove less effective for some mutants, such as K464A, since their ability to stabilize the open state is somewhat impaired *(62,68)*. In fact, some mutants might not be able to be locked open by AMPPNP at all (e.g., G551D; Hwang, unpublished observations). Furthermore, the statistical approaches make the assumption that all the channels in a patch behave independently and identically, which may not hold during real experiments. Thus, the experimenter must take care to question and scrutinize empirically derived estimates for N and P_o and to use every means at their disposal to verify their measurements.

5. A number of other analysis programs are available that can be used to analyze single-channel recordings (*see* **ref.** *63* for a partial list).

References

1. Riordan, J. R., Rommens, J. M., Kerem, B.-S., Alon, N., Rozmahel, R., Grzelczak, Z., Zielenski, J., Lok, S., Plavsik, N., Chou, J.-L., Drumm, M. L., Iannuzzi, M. C., Collins, F. S. and Tsui, L.-C. (1989) Identification of the cystic fibrosis gene: cloning and characterization of complementary DNA. *Science* **245,** 1066–1073.
2. Gadsby, D. C. and Nairn, A., C. (1999) Control of CFTR channel gating by phosphorylation and nucleotide hydrolysis. *Physiol Rev.* **79,** S77–S107.
3. Anderson, M. P., Berger, H. A., Rich, D. P., Gregory, R. J., Smith, A. E., and Welsh, M. J. (1991) Nucleoside triphosphates are required to open the CFTR chloride channel. *Cell* **67,** 775–784.
4. Quinton, P. M. and Reddy, M. M. (1992) Control of CFTR chloride conductance by ATP levels through non-hydrolytic binding. *Nature* **360,** 79–81.
5. Nagel, G., Hwang, T. C., Nastiuk, K. L., Nairn, A. C., and Gadsby, D. C. (1992) The protein kinase A-regulated cardiac Cl⁻ channel resembles the cystic fibrosis transmembrane conductance regulator. *Nature* **360,** 81–84.
6. Li, C., Ramjeesingh, M., Wang, W., Garami, E., Hewryk, M., Lee, D., Rommens, J. M., Galley, K., and Bear, C. E. (1996) ATPase activity of the cystic fibrosis transmembrane conductance regulator. *J. Biol. Chem.* **271,** 28,463–28,468.
7. Hwang, T. C., Nagel, G., Nairn, A. C., and Gadsby, D. C. (1994) Regulation of the gating of cystic fibrosis transmembrane conductance regulator Cl channels by phosphorylation and ATP hydrolysis. *Proc. Natl. Acad. Sci., USA* **91,** 4698–4702.
8. Zeltwanger, S., Wang, F., Wang, G. T., Gillis, K. D., and Hwang, T. C. (1999) Gating of cystic fibrosis transmembrane conductance regulator chloride channels by adenosine triphosphate hydrolysis. Quantitative analysis of a cyclic gating scheme. *J. Gen Physiol.* **113,** 541–554.

9. Zou, X. and Hwang, T. C. (2001) ATP hydrolysis-coupled gating of CFTR chloride channels: structure and function. *Biochemistry* **40,** 5579–5586.

10. Hwang, T. C., Horie, M., and Gadsby, D. C. (1993) Functionally distinct phosphoforms underlie incremental activation of protein kinase-regulated Cl⁻ conductance in mammalian heart. *J. Gen. Physiol.* **101,** 629–650.

11. Berger, H. A., Travis, S. M., and Welsh M. J. (1993) Regulation of the cystic fibrosis transmembrane conductance regulator Cl⁻ channel by specific protein kinases and protein phosphatases. *J. Biol. Chem.* **268,** 2037–2047.

12. Luo, J., Pato, M. D., Riordan, J. R., and Hanrahan, J. W. Differential regulation of single CFTR channels by PP2C, PP2A, and other phosphatases. (1998) *Am. J. Physiol.* **274,** C1397–C1410.

13. Ishihara, H. and Welsh, M. J. (1997) Block by MOPS reveals a conformation change in the CFTR pore produced by ATP hydrolysis. *Am. J. Physiol.* **273,** C1278–C1289.

14. Zhou, Z., Hu, S., and Hwang, T. C. (2001) Voltage-dependent flickery block of an open CFTR channel pore. *J. Physiol.* **532,** 435–448.

15. Gray, M. A., Harris, A., Coleman, L., Greenwell, J. R., and Argent, B. E. (1989) Two types of chloride channel on duct cells cultured from human fetal pancreas. *Am. J. Physiol.* **257,** C240–C251.

16. Tabcharani, J. A., Chang, X. B., Riordan, J. R., and Hanrahan, J. W. (1991) Phosphorylation-regulated Cl⁻ channel in CHO cells stably expressing the cystic fibrosis gene. *Nature* **352,** 628–631.

17. Haws, C., Krouse, M. E., Xia, Y., Gruenert, D. C., and Wine, J. J. (1992) CFTR channels in immortalized human airway cells. *Am. J. Physiol.* **263,** L692–L707.

18. Fischer, H. and Machen, T. E. (1994) CFTR displays voltage dependence and two gating modes during stimulation. *J. Gen Physiol.* **104,** 541–566.

19. Dousmanis, A. G. (1996) The CFTR (cystic fibrosis transmembrane conductance regulator) channel: anion permeation and regulation by adenylyl cyclase and ATP hydrolysis. Thesis, Rockefeller University, New York,.

20. Bear, C. E., Li., C., Galley, K., Wang, Y., Garami, E., and Ramjeesingh, M. (1997) Coupling of ATP hydrolysis with channel gating by purified, reconstituted CFTR. *J. Bioenerg. Biomembr.* **29,** 465–473.

21. Weinreich, F., Riordan, J. R., and Nagel, G. (1999) Dual effects of ADP and adenylylimidodiphosphate on CFTR channel kinetics show binding to two different nucleotide binding sites. *J. Gen. Physiol.* **114,** 55–70.

22. Travis, S. M., Berger, H. A., and Welsh, M. J. (1997) Protein phosphatase 2C dephosphorylates and inactivates cystic fibrosis transmembrane conductance regulator. *Proc. Natl. Acad. Sci. USA* **94,** 11,055–11,060.

23. Zhu, T., Dahan, D., Evagelidis, A., Zheng, S., Luo, J., and Hanrahan, J. W. (1999) Association of cystic fibrosis transmembrane conductance regulator and protein phosphatase 2C. *J. Biol. Chem.* **274,** 29,102–29,107.

24. Cohen, P. (1990) The structure and regulation of protein phosphatases. *Adv. Second Messenger Phosphoprotein Res.* **24,** 230–235.

25. Baukrowitz, T., Hwang, T. C., Nairn, A. C., and Gadsby, D. C. (1994) Coupling of CFTR Cl⁻ channel gating to an ATP hydrolysis cycle. *Neuron* **12,** 473–482.

26. Rudy, B. and Iverson, L. E. (eds.) (1992) Ion channels, in *Methods in Enzymology*, vol. 207. Academic Press, San Diego, CA.
27. Sakmann, B. and Neher, E. (eds.) (1995) *Single-Channel Recording* 2nd ed., Plenum, New York.
28. Fenwick, E. M., Marty, A., and Neher, E. (1982) Sodium and calcium channels in bovine chromaffin cells. *J. Physiol.* **331,** 599–635.
29. Wang, F., Zeltwanger, S., Yang, I. C., Nairn, A. C., and Hwang, T. C. (1998) Actions of genistein on cystic fibrosis transmembrane conductance regulator channel gating. Evidence for two binding sites with opposite effects. *J. Gen Physiol.* **111,** 477–490.
30. Csanády, L. (2000) Rapid kinetic analysis of multichannel records by a simultaneous fit to all dwell-time histograms. *Biophys. J.* **78,** 785–799.
31. Csanády, L., Chan, K. W., Seto-Young, D., Kopsco, D. C., Nairn, A. C., and Gadsby, D. C. (2000) Severed channels probe regulation of gating of cystic fibrosis transmembrane conductance regulator by its cytoplasmic domains. *J. Gen Physiol.* **116,** 477–500.
32. Chan, K. W., Csanady, L., Seto-Young, D., Nairn, A. C., and Gadsby, D. C. (2000) Severed molecules functionally define the boundaries of the cystic fibrosis transmembrane conductance regulator's NH2-terminal nucleotide binding domain. *J. Gen. Physiol.* **116,** 163–180.
33. Colquhoun, D. and Hawkes, A. G. (1995) The principles of the stochastic interpretation of ion-channel mechanisms, in *Single Channel Recording* (2nd ed.), (Sakmann, B. and Neher, E., eds.), Plenum, New York, pp. 397–482.
34. Fischer, H. and Machen, T. E. (1996) The tyrosine kinase p60c-src regulates the fast gate of the cystic fibrosis transmembrane conductance regulator chloride channel. *Biophys. J.* **71,** 3073–3082.
35. Zeltwanger, S. (1998) Gating of cystic fibrosis transmembrane conductance regulator (CFTR) chloride channels by nucleoside triphosphates. Thesis, University of Missouri, Columbia, Missouri.
36. Gunderson, K. L. and Kopito, R. R. (1995) Conformational states of CFTR associated with channel gating: the role of ATP binding and hydrolysis. *Cell* **82,** 231–239.
37. Fendler, K., Grell, E., Haubs, M., and Bamberg, E. (1985) Pump currents generated by the purified Na+K+-ATPase from kidney on black lipid membranes. *EMBO J.* **4,** 3079–3085.
38. Fendler, K., Grell, E., and Bamberg, E. (1987) Kinetics of pump currents generated by the Na+K+-ATPase. *FEBS Lett.* **224,** 83–88.
39. Nakao, M. and Gadsby, D. C. (1986) Voltage dependence of Na translocation by the Na/K pump. *Nature* **323,** 628–630.
40. Hodgkin, A. L. and Huxley, A. F. (1952) A quantitative description of membrane current and its application to conduction and excitation in nerve. *J. Physiol.* **117,** 500–544.
41. Armstrong, C. M. and Bezanilla, F. (1974) Charge movement associated with the opening and closing of the activation gates of the Na. channels. *J. Gen. Physiol.* **63,** 533–552.

42. Kaplan, J. H., Forbush, B., and Hoffman, J. F. (1978) Rapid photolytic release of adenosine 5'-triphosphate from a protected analogue: utilization by the Na:K pump of human red blood cell ghosts. *Biochemistry* **17**, 1929-1935.

43. McCray, J. A., Herbette, L., Kihara, T., and Trentham, D. R. (1980) A new approach to time-resolved studies of ATP-requiring biological systems laser flash photolysis of caged ATP. *Proc. Natl. Acad. Sci. USA* **77**, 7237–7241.

44. Hilgemann, D. W. (1989) Giant excised cardiac sarcolemmal membrane patches: sodium and sodium-calcium exchange currents. *Pflugers Arch.* **415**, 247–249.

45. Hilgemann, D. W. (1995) The giant membrane patch, in *Single Channel Recording* (2nd ed.), (Sakmann, B. and Neher, E., eds.), Plenum, New York.

46. Ikuma, M. and Welsh, M. J. (2000) Regulation of CFTR Cl⁻ channel gating by ATP binding and hydrolysis. *Proc. Natl. Acad. Sci. USA* **97**, 8675–8680.

47. Linsdell, P., Tabcharani, J. A., and Hanrahan, J. W. (1997) Multi-ion mechanism for ion permeation and block in the cystic fibrosis transmembrane conductance regulator chloride channel. *J. Gen. Physiol.* **110**, 365–377.

48. Mathews, C. J., Tabcharani, J. A., and Hanrahan, J. W. (1998) The CFTR chloride channel: nucleotide interactions and temperature-dependent gating. *J. Membr. Biol.* **163**, 55–66.

49. Aleksandrov, A. A. and Riordan, J. R. (1998) Regulation of CFTR ion channel gating by MgATP. *FEBS Lett.* **431**, 97–101.

50. Schultz, B. D., Bridges, R. J., and Frizzell, R. A. (1996) Lack of conventional ATPase properties in CFTR chloride channel gating. *J. Membr. Biol.* **151**, 63–75.

51. Aleksandrov, A. A., Chang, X. B., Aleksandrov, L., and Riordan, J. R. (2000) The non-hydrolytic pathway of cystic fibrosis transmembrane conductance regulator ion channel gating. *J. Physiol.* **528**, 259–265.

52. Harrington, M. A., Gunderson, K. L., and Kopito, R. R. (1999) Redox reagents and divalent cations alter the kinetics of cystic fibrosis transmembrane conductance regulator channel gating. *J. Biol. Chem.* **274**, 27,536–27,544.

53. Connolly, B. A. and Eckstein, F. (1981) Structures of the mono- and divalent metal nucleotide complexes in the myosin ATPase. *J. Biol. Chem.* **256**, 9450–9456.

54. Fasano, O., De Vendittis, E., and Parmeggianni, A. (1982) Hydrolysis of GTP by elongation factor Tu can be induced by monovalent cations. *J. Biol. Chem.* **257**, 3145–3150.

55. Anderson, M. P. and Welsh, M. J. (1992) Regulation by ATP and ADP of CFTR chloride channels that contain mutant nucleotide-binding domains. *Science* **257**, 1701–1704.

56. Ramjeesingh, M., Li, C., Garami, E., Huan, L. J., Galley, K., Wang, Y., and Bear, C. E. (1999) Walker mutations reveal loose relationship between catalytic and channel-gating activities of purified CFTR (cystic fibrosis transmembrane conductance regulator). *Biochemistry* **38**, 1463–1468.

57. Carson, M. R., Travis, S. M., and Welsh, M. J. (1995) The two nucleotide-binding domains of cystic fibrosis transmembrane conductance regulator (CFTR) have distinct functions in controlling channel activity. *J. Biol. Chem.* **270**, 1711–1717.

58. Hung, L. W., Wang, I. X., Nikaido, K., Liu, P. Q., Ames, G. F., and Kim, S. H. (1998) Crystal structure of the ATP-binding subunit of an ABC transporter. *Nature* **396**, 703–707.

59. Armstrong, S., Tabernero, L., Zhang, H., Hermodson, M., and Stauffacher, C. (1998) The 2.5Å structure of the N-terminal ATP-binding cassette of the ribose ABC transporter. *Pediatr. Pulmonol.* **17,** 91,92.

60. Diederichs, K., Diez, J., Greller, G., Muller, C., Breed, J., Schnell, C., Vonrhein, C., Boos, W., and Welte, W. (2000) Crystal structure of MalK, the ATPase subunit of the trehalose/maltose ABC transporter of the archaeon thermococcus litoralis *EMBO J.* **19,** 5951–5961.

61. Berger, A. L., Thomas, P. J., Hunt, J. F., and Welsh, M. J. (2001) Testing the predicted contacts between CFTR and ATP. *Biophys. J.* **80,** 469a.

62. Vergani, P., Basso, C., Csanády, L., Kopsco, D., Sanchez, R., Sali, A., Nairn, A., C., and Gadbsy, D. C. (2001) Roles of ATP binding and hydrolysis in CFTR Cl⁻ channel gating. *Biophys. J.* **80,** 354a.

63. French, R. J. and Wonderlin, W. F. (1992) Software for acquisition and analysis of ion channel data: choices, tasks and strategies, in *Ion Channels*, Methods in Enzymology, vol. 207 (Rudy, B. and Iverson, L. E., eds.), Academic Press, San Diego, CA, pp. 711–728.

64. Berger, H. A., Anderson, M. P., Gregory, R. J., Thompson, S., Howard, P. W., Maurer, R. A., Mulligan, R., Smith, A. E., and Welsh, M. J. (1991) Identification and regulation of the cystic fibrosis transmembrane conductance regulator-generated chloride channel. *J. Clin Invest.* **88,** 1422–1431.

65. Friedrich, T., Bamberg, E., and Nagel, G. (1996), Na(+), K(+) - ATPase pump currents in giant excised patches activated by an ATP concentration jump. *Biophys, J.* **71,** 2486–2500.

66. Jackson, M. B., Wong, B. S., Morris, C. E., Lecar, H., and Christian, C. N. (1983) Successive openings of the same acetylcholine receptor channel are correlated in open time. *Biophys. J.* **42,** 109–114.

67. Nagel, G., Szellas, T., Riordan, J. R., Friedrich, T., and Hartung, K. (2001) Unspecific activation of the epithelial sodium channel by the CFTR chloride channel. *EMBO Reports* **2,** 249–254.

68. Powe, A. C., Al-Nakkash, L., and Hwang, T. C. (2001) The role of CFTR's Walker-A lysine 464 in ATP-dependent gating. *Biophys. J.* **80,** 470a.

69. Sigworth, F. and Sine, S. (1987) Data transformations for improved display and fitting of single channel dwell-time analysis. *Biophys. J.* **52,** 1047–1054.

6

CFTR Regulation by Phosphorylation

Tang Zhu, Deborah A. R. Hinkson, David Dahan, Alexandra Evagelidis, and John W. Hanrahan

1. Introduction

The cystic fibrosis transmembrane conductance regulator (CFTR) is a tightly regulated anion channel expressed in epithelial and other cells. It conducts chloride and bicarbonate ions through the plasma membrane and also influences the activity of other channels and transporters through unknown mechanisms. CFTR has two membrane domains (TM1, TM2), each comprised of six transmembrane segments, two nucleotide-binding folds (NBD1, NBD2) that bind and hydrolyze ATP, and a central regulatory or "R" domain (*1*). Phosphorylation of the R domain by protein kinases (**Table 1**) stimulates channel activity and may also enhance interactions of CFTR with other proteins. This chapter describes methods that we have found useful for studying the phosphorylation and dephosphorylation of CFTR. We emphasize simple approaches for the partial purification of CFTR and for assaying kinase and phosphatase activities using either CFTR or casein as substrate.

2. Materials

2.1. Equipment and Reagents

1. Disposable cell scrapers: Sarstedt, Inc., cat. no. 83.1830.
2. Homogenizer: 5 mL Safe-Grind plastic-coated tissue grinders with Teflon pestle from VWR Canlab, cat. no. 62400-314.
3. Rotators: Glas-Col tissue culture rotators: VWR Canlab, cat. no. 62404-006.
4. Protein G immobilized on Sepharose 4B: Sigma, cat. no. P-3296.
5. NiNTA Agarose beads: Qiagen, cat. no. 30230
6. Sepharose G-50: Pharmacia Biotech AB, cat. no. 17-0573-01.
7. Bio-Rad Protein Assay Kit: Bio-Rad, cat. no. 500-0006.

From: *Methods in Molecular Medicine, vol. 70: Cystic Fibrosis Methods and Protocols*
Edited by: W. R. Skach © Humana Press Inc., Totowa, NJ

Table 1
Predicted Phosphorylation Sites in the R Domain
for Protein Kinase A (PKA), Protein Kinase C (PKC),
and Casein Kinase 2 (CK2)

A

Pos	Context ↓	Score	Pred	Kinase
631	----SELQN	0.002	.	
641	QPDFSSKLM	0.390	.	
642	PDFSSKLMG	0.015	.	
649	MGCDSFDQF	0.007	.	
654	FDQF SAERR	0.590	*S*	
660	ERRNSILTE	0.981	*S*	PKA
670	LHRFSLEGD	0.997	*S*	PKA
678	DAPVSWTET	0.997	*S*	CK2
686	TKKQ SFKQT	0.986	*S*	PKA/PKC
700	KRKN SILNP	0.958	*S*	PKA
707	NPIN SIRKF	0.096	.	PKC
712	IRKF SIVQK	0.889	*S*	PKA
728	IEEDSDEPL	0.985	*S*	
737	ERRLSLVPD	0.988	*S*	PKA
742	LVPDSEQGE	0.783	*S*	
753	LPRISVIST	0.990	*S*	PKA
756	ISVISTGPT	0.927	*S*	
768	RRRQ SVLNL	0.990	*S*	PKA
776	LMTH SVNQG	0.009	.	
790	KTTA STRKV	0.892	*S*	PKC
795	TRKVSLAPQ	0.954	*S*	PKA
809	LDIYSRRLS	0.023	.	
813	SRRLSQETG	0.997	*S*	PKA

8. Bicinchoninic acid (BCA) protein assay kit: Pierce, cat. no. 23225
9. Protease inhibitor cocktail tablets: Roche, cat. no. 1873580.
10. M3A7 CFTR monoclonal antibody: Chemicon Intl., cat. no. MAB3480, or Research Diagnostics, cat. no. RDI-CFTRabm-A7.
11. H89: Calbiochem, cat. no. 371963.
12. Chelerythrine chloride: Calbiochem, cat. no. 220285.
13. Okadaic acid: Sigma, cat. no. O-1506.
14. Protein phosphatase inhibitor-2 (I-2): Calbiochem, cat. no. 539516.
15. Calmodulin: Sigma, cat. no. P1062.
16. Brij 35 solution: Sigma, cat. no. 430AG-6.
17. Bovine serum albumin (essentially fatty acid free): Sigma, cat. no. A 6003.

Table 1 (continued)

B

Pos	Context ↓	Threonines Score	Pred	
663	NSILTETLH	0.064	.	
665	ILTETLHRF	0.235	.	
680	PVSWTETKK	0.055	.	
682	SWTETKKQS	0.903	*T*	PKC
690	SFKQTGEFG	0.068	.	
717	IVQKTPLQM	0.122	.	
757	SVISTGPTL	0.023	.	
760	STGPTLQAR	0.033	.	
774	LNLMTHSVN	0.024	.	
787	IHRKTTAST	0.814	*T*	PKA
788	HRKTTASTR	0.498	.	
791	TTASTRKVS	0.760	*T*	PKC
803	QANLTELDI	0.021	.	
816	LSQETGLEI	0.050	.	

C

Pos	Context	Tyrosines Score	Pred
808	ELDIYSRRL	0.474	.

Score indicates probability the site would be phosphorylated according to NetPhos 2.0, a program that uses experimentally observed phosphorylations in a large protein database.

18. Filter paper: 3MM, cut into 2×2 cm squares.
19. Scintillation vials and BetaMax liquid scintillation cocktail: ICN, cat. no. 880020.
20. $[^{32}P]PO_4$-casein or $[^{32}P]PO_4$-GST-R prepared as described below.
21. $[\gamma^{-32}P]ATP$: Amersham Pharmacia Biotech, cat. no. PB10132.

2.2. Buffers

1. Phosphate-buffered saline (PBS): 140 mM NaCl, 2.7 mM KCl, 10 mM Na$_2$HPO$_4$, and 1.8 mM KH$_2$PO$_4$, pH7.4.
2. 50X protease inhibitor cocktail: one tablet is dissolved in 1 mL distilled water as 50X stock solution and kept at $-20°C$.
3. RIPA buffer: 1% v/v Triton X-100, 0.1% w/v deoxycholic acid, 0.1% w/v sodium dodecyl sulfate (SDS), 150 mM NaCl, 20 mM Tris-HCl, pH 8.0.
4. Sucrose buffer: 500 mM sucrose, 10 mM HEPES, pH 7.2.
5. Solution A: 50 mM Tris-HCl, pH 7.0, 0.1 mM EGTA, stored at 4°C.
6. Phosphorylation buffer: 140 mM NaCl, 4 mM KCl, 2 mM MgCl$_2$, 0.5 mM CaCl$_2$, 10 mM Tris-HCl, pH 7.4.

7. Solution A with 1% bovine serum albumin (BSA), stored at 4°C.
8. Calmodulin buffer: 0.01% Brij-35, 1 mg/mL BSA, 0.1 mM calmodulin in solution A, stored at –20°C.
9. 300 pM and 300 nM okadaic acid (OA) in solution A, stored at –20°C.
10. 30 ng/μL protein phosphatase inhibitor-2 (I-2) in solution A, stored at –20°C.
11. 60 mM and 120 mM magnesium acetate in solution A, stored at 4°C.
12. 2.4 mM $CaCl_2$ in solution A, stored at 4°C.
13. 20% TCA.

3. Methods

3.1. Preparing CFTR for Use in Phosphorylation Studies

3.1.1. Immunoprecipitations

1. A 10-cm-diameter dish of confluent BHK cell monolayer (79 cm^2 or about 3×10^6 cells expressing CFTR) is washed twice in cold phosphate-buffered saline (PBS: 8 g/L NaCl, 0.2 g/L KCl, 1.44 g/L Na_2HPO_4, 0.24 g/L KH_2PO_4, pH 7.4). Cells are harvested by scraping with a rubber policeman into a 15-mL screw-cap tube. Monolayers may be pretreated in culture for 30 min with kinase inhibitors (PKC inhibitor chelerythrine chloride 5 μM and PKA inhibitor H-89 [500 nM]) to reduce endogenous phosphorylation.
2. Cells are collected by centrifugation (500g, 5 min), then resuspended in RIPA buffer supplemented with EDTA-free protease inhibitor cocktail. The cells are left on ice for 30–60 min to lyse, then centrifuged at 21,000g for 15 min to remove cellular debris.
   Alternatively, detergent can be avoided during early lysis steps by: (a) incubating cells on ice for 10 min in 1.6 mL RIPA buffer without Triton X-100, (b) homogenizing 10X by hand in a 5-mL tissue grinder, (c) adding sucrose buffer (1.6 mL), (d) homogenizing the sample again 15X, (e) collecting the soluble fraction by centrifugation at 7500g for 10 min at 4°C, and (f) adjusting with 10% Triton X-100 to 1% final concentration (*see* **Note 1**).
3. After insoluble material has been removed from the lysate, an aliquot of the supernatant is used to determine total protein (typically about 5 mg/mL) using either the bicinchoninic acid or Bio-Rad protein assay kits. The amount of CFTR in the sample can be estimated by Western blotting by calibrating with a recombinant protein containing the appropriate epitope. For this we have used monoclonal R-domain antibody (previously sold by Genzyme, now available from Research Diagnostic, cat. no. RDI-CFTRRabm), and calibrated the luminescence signal in Western blots using known amounts of recombinant R-domain protein purified from bacteria or yeast.
4. Cell lysates are diluted with RIPA to a final concentration of 2 mg total protein/mL.
5. CFTR is immunoprecipitated from diluted lysates containing 1 mg protein by incubating them with 0.5–2.0 μg/mL M3A7 antibody and 20 μL protein G Sepharose 4B beads (preequilibrated in 1 mL RIPA buffer) in an Eppendorf tube at 4°C on a benchtop rotator (e.g., Glas-col, TerreHaute, IN) for 20–60 min.

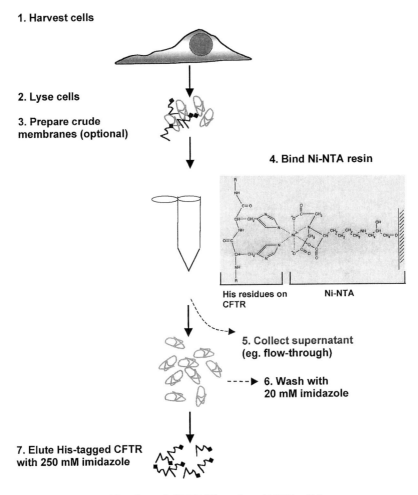

Fig. 1. Purification of CFTRHis$_{10}$ from BHK cell lysates.

Alternatively, lysates are incubated overnight with Ab at 4°C, and protein G Sepharose 4B beads are added at a concentration of 25 μL beads/mL lysate during the last hour of incubation.

6. The lysate/M3A7/protein G Sepharose 4B bead mixture is washed with ice cold RIPA 6–8 times by centrifugation (21,000g, 30 s) to remove unbound proteins. The washed beads with immunoprecipitates attached can be stored in 50 μL RIPA at –20°C.

3.1.2. Nickel-Chelate Affinity Purification

An alternative approach for obtaining semipurified CFTR uses Ni-NTA beads (**Fig. 1**). For this we added 10 histidine codons to the 3' end of the CFTR cDNA, subcloned it into the pNUT expression plasmid, and transfected pNUT-

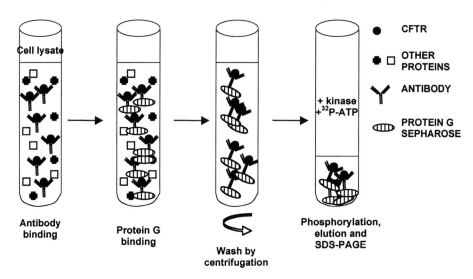

Fig. 2. Immunoprecipitation and in vitro phosphorylation of CFTR.

CFTR$_{His10}$ into BHK cells by calcium phosphate coprecipitation *(2,3)*. Colonies in which integrated sequences are highly amplified were selected using 500 μ*M* methotrexate, and CFTR$_{His10}$ expression confirmed by immunoblotting.

1. 10 medium (i.e., 10-cm-diameter) culture plates of confluent monolayer BHK cells expressing CFTR$_{His10}$ (about 790 cm^2) are washed with ice cold PBS, harvested by scraping, and centrifuged at 1500g for 5 min at room temperature.
2. The cell pellet is washed and centrifuged twice with ice-cold PBS, resuspended in 4 mL RIPA buffer, and stirred for 1 h at 4°C.
3. Insoluble material is removed by centrifugation at 3000g for 5 min.
4. Protein concentration of the supernatant (i.e., cell lysate, typically 11–12 mg/mL) is determined and adjusted to 4.5 mg/mL by adding lysis buffer.
5. Ni-NTA agarose is added at a final dilution of 20 μL (packed volume)/mL.
6. The slurry is allowed to equilibrate on a benchtop rotator overnight at 4°C.
7. Aliquots (1 mL) are placed in Eppendorf tubes and subjected to the phosphoryation protocol described above for immunoprecipitates.

3.2. In Vitro Phosphorylation

3.2.1. General

For phosphorylation experiments such as those illustrated in **Fig. 2**, we use Type II bovine cardiac protein kinase A (PKA catalytic subunit: 0.418 casein units/ng) from the laboratory of Dr. M. P. Walsh. Comparable preparations are available commercially from Promega and Upstate Biochemical. One unit (U) of activity corresponds to 1 pmol phosphate incorporated per min at 30°C using casein as the substrate. Activity is stable for more than 1 yr at –70°C, although it should be checked periodically (e.g., using the SigmaTECT PKA assay kit from Promega, Madison, WI). Rat brain protein kinase C II (a mixture of PKC isotypes:1.84 neurogranin units/ng, assayed using the SignaTECT PKC assay kit) is also available from UBI and Promega. Once thawed, PKA and PKC are kept for 1–2 wk at 4°C and are not refrozen. For immunoprecipitations and Western blotting we use the anti-CFTR antibody M3A7 or L12B4 (epitope between aa 386-412; available from the same companies, see above and *(4)*.

1. Beads (protein G Sepharose 4B or NiNTA agarose) are rinsed three times with phosphorylation buffer to remove remaining traces of detergent. The beads are resuspended in 100 μL of the same buffer supplemented with 20 mM MgATP, 10 μCi $\gamma[^{32}P]$ATP and 10 μg BSA at 30°C. PKA, PKC, or both kinases, are added to the mix and allowed to react for 2–8 h. The reaction is stopped by adding ice-cold RIPA buffer. When PKC is used, it is activated by adding the lipid activator DiC8 (5 μM from DMSO stock).
2. Beads are then rinsed five times in RIPA and twice in phosphorylation buffer as described above.
3. Radiolabeled protein is released from the beads by incubation in 30 μL of 2X SDS-PAGE sample buffer for 10 min at 20°C.
4. After centrifugation (21,000g, 2 min), the supernatant is resolved using SDS-PAGE, transferred to a PVDF membrane, and exposed to a storage phosphor screen.
5. Phosphorylation is analyzed using a PhosphorImager and Image QuaNT™ software (Molecular Dynamics). Counts are normalized to the amount of CFTR protein estimated by Western blotting the same PVDF membrane.

3.2.2. Modifications for Tyrosine Phosphorylation

1. CFTR is immunoprecipitated from RIPA lysates using M3A7 antibody as described (*see* above and **ref. 2**).
2. Protein G Sepharose 4B beads (25 μL; with the CFTR from one 6-cm-diameter plate of BHK cells bound to them) are washed in 100 mM Tris-HCl, pH 7.2, 25 mM MnCl$_2$, 2.0 mM EGTA, 0.25 mM Na$_3$VO$_4$, and 125 mM Mg·acetate and incubated with 10 μCi [γ-^{32}P]ATP (Amersham) and recombinant p60$^{c\text{-}Src}$ (15–30 U, UBI) for 15 min.
3. After extensive washing, CFTR is released by adding sample buffer, electrophoresed in SDS/7% polyacrylamide gels, dried, and exposed on X-ray film using standard methods.

3.3. In Vitro Dephosphorylation of CFTR

3.3.1. Preparation of GST-R Domain for Phosphatase Studies

Construct design: cDNA corresponding to amino acids M645-M837 (expected *Mr* 53,000) was amplified using Vent® polymerase and polymerase chain reaction (PCR) primers that contained BamHI sites for subcloning into the pGEX-2T vector (a Kozak consensus sequence was also included in the upstream primer sequence for future studies requiring expression in mammalian cells). The PCR product was ligated into pGEX-2T and transformed into *Escherichia coli* Top 10 cells. Plasmids were isolated and confirmed by DNA sequencing.

3.3.2. Expression of GST-R Domain Fusion Protein

1. *E. Coli* HB101 cells are transformed and grown to late log phase in LB broth, collected by centrifugation (10 min/5000), resuspended in minimal medicine (M9) at 30°C. Expression of GST-R domain protein is induced for 15 min with 0.1 mM isopropyl β-D-thiogalectopyranoside (IPTG).
2. Fusion protein is bound to glutathione Sepharose 4B beads and eluted by addition of 20 mM glutathione in 100 mM Tris-HCl/pH8.0, 120 mM NaCl, and 0.1% Triton X-100 at 4°C according to the manufacturer's instructions.
3. GST-R has been useful as a phosphatase substrate, when characterizing protein phosphatase activities in different cellular compartments *(3)*, and for pharmacological studies of the protein phosphatases, particularly their sensitivity to activators of the CFTR channel (*see* **Note 2**).

3.3.3. [^{32}P]PO$_4$ Labeling of Casein and GST-R Domain

1. Casein (10 mg, Sigma) or GST-R domain fusion protein (200 µg prepared as described above) are labeled by incubation with PKA (600 U) and [γ-^{32}P]ATP (50 µCi) in 1-mL reaction buffer containing 50 mM Tris-HCl, 0.1 mM EGTA, 10 mM magnesium acetate, 0.1% β-mecaptoethanol (pH = 7.0) for 5–12 h at 30°C (*see* **Note 2**).
2. The phosphorylation reaction is stopped by adding 100 µL of solution containing 100 mM EDTA and 100 mM sodium pyrophosphate, pH 7.0.
3. Free [γ-^{32}P]ATP is removed by passing the reaction mix through Sepharose G-50 after pre-equilibration of the column with 50 mM Tris-HCl, 0.1 mM EGTA, 5% glycerol, and 0.1% β-mercaptoethanol (pH = 7.0).
4. Free [γ-^{32}P]ATP remaining in the mixture is then determined by precipitating the protein with 100 µL trichloroacetic acid (TCA; 20% w/v), spinning down the precipitate at 15,000 rpm for 1 min at 4°C, and taking a sample of the supernatant for liquid scintillation counting. The amount of free [γ-^{32}P]ATP in the supernatant is normally less than 1% of the total radioactivity.

3.3.4. Assaying Phosphatase Activity as [^{32}P]PO$_4$ Release from Phospho-Casein and Phospho-GST-R Domain

All procedures are performed in a space dedicated to radioisotope work. Reaction tubes are prewarmed for 10 min in a water bath at 30°C.

1. Water bath and oven are prewarmed to 30 and 80°C, respectively. Filter paper squares are used for each test sample and two additional squares are used for the blank and a control (i.e., undephosphorylated) sample. ^{32}P-phospho-casein or phospho-GST-R domain is diluted with solution A to a final concentration of 1 nmol/µL.

2. Cell lysates are diluted to 10–50 μg/mL for assays using solution A containing 1% BSA. Samples to be assayed for protein phosphatase 2B (PP2B) assay are diluted with calmodulin buffer. The reaction mixes are prepared in 1.5-mL Eppendorf tubes.

3. Assaying total vs individual phosphatase activities within cell lysates:

   a. For total protein phosphatase (PP) activity we mix 10 μL of sample with 5 μL magnesium acetate stock (60 mM in solution A) and 5 μL calcium chloride stock (2.4 mM in solution A).

   b. For PP1 activity, we mix 10 μL sample and 10 μL OA stock (300 pM).

   c. For PP2A activity, we mix 10 μL sample and 10 μL of the I-2 stock (30 ng/μL).

   d. For PP2B activity, we mix 10 μL sample diluted with calmodulin buffer, 5 μL 300 nM OA, and 5 μL 60 mM CaCl$_2$.

   e. For PP2C activity, we mix 10 μL sample, 5 μL 300 nM OA, and 5 μL 120 mM Mg·acetate.

   f. For the blank, we mix 10 μL solution A containing 1% BSA and 10 μL solution A.

4. 10 μL of the 1-nmol/μL ^{32}P[PO$_4$]-casein or –GST-R domain are added to each reaction tube, making a total reaction volume of 30 μL. The mix is incubated at 30°C for 10 min.

5. To estimate initial radioactivity of the substrate (i.e., at time = 0 min), 10 μL of the 1-nmol/μL ^{32}P[PO$_4$]-casein or –GST-R domain solution are spotted onto a 3MM paper square.

6. All reactions are stopped by adding 30 μL of 20% TCA to make a total volume of 60 μL, mixing, and centrifuging at 15,000g for 2 min.

7. 50 μL of supernatant (from the total volume of 60 μL) are spotted onto 2 × 2 cm squares of 3MM paper. Paper squares are dried in a vacuum oven at 80°C for 20 min, including the time = 0 sample from **step 5**.

8. Each paper square is placed in a scintillation vial containing 10 mL BetaMax liquid scintillation cocktail for counting.

9. One unit (U) is defined as the amount of enzyme catalyzing dephosphorylation of 1.0 mmol of ^{32}P-casein per minute under the assay conditions. To calculate protein phosphatase activity "A" in μU/mg protein with these reaction volumes, we use the formula $A = (S - B) \times 12 \times$ sample dilution/total [^{32}P]casein cpm · sample protein conc. (in mg/mL), where S and B are the counts per minute in sample and blank, respectively.

4. Notes

1. Fresh samples are recommended for immunoprecipitations, but if frozen lysates must be used, it is important to centrifuge them before use at 21,000g for 10 min, at 4°C. Otherwise, protein precipitates formed during storage of the samples may be spun down with the beads, greatly increasing contamination of immunoprecipitated CFTR. Also, during immunoprecipitations, beads with antibodies still bound should be washed very gently in **step 4**, and high vortex settings (i.e., > 2 on a Fisher-type Vortex-Genie) should be avoided when resuspending beads in wash buffer.

2. Protein phosphatase types 1, 2A, 2B, and 2C (PP1, PP2A, PP2B, and PP2C, respectively) dephosphorylate CFTR in vitro with potencies in rank order PP2C ≥ PP2A > PP1 > PP2B. Dephosphorylation of casein, recombinant R-domain protein, and full-length CFTR are grossly similar, but kinetic differences probably exist. PP2C strongly prefers phosphothreonine as substrate compared to phosphoserine, thus PP2C activity should be higher for substrates containing more phosphothreonines. Full-length CFTR is obviously the preferred substrate for phosphatase studies, but the small amount of full-length CFTR expressed in mammalian cells means that phosphatase activity has to be monitored as residual radioactivity after running a gel and phosphorimager analysis. GST-R domain is a convenient alternative since most phosphorylation occurs on CFTR's R domain and $[^{32}P]PO_4$ released from the fusion protein can be quantified directly by liquid scintillation counting. Although casein is not expected to be an ideal substrate for PKA, phospho-casein provides a useful irrelevant protein; for example, when testing potential phosphatase inhibitors *(5)*. In such experiments it is important to use the same dilutions, since optimal PP activity depends on test sample dilution. Best results are obtained when phosphatase in the sample dephosphorylates approx 10% of the phospho-substrate available. As with immunoprecipitations, 50-μL samples of supernatant should be removed carefully in **step 7** to avoid contamination by the TCA precipitate.

CFTR is part of a regulatory complex in which scaffolding proteins, kinases, phosphatases, and other regulatory proteins are closely associated. An important caveat of in-vitro phosphorylation studies is therefore that phosphorylation of CFTR in a test tube may differ qualitatively and quantitatively from that in the plasma membrane if kinase and phosphatase activities depend on their locations within the complex. Such differences are expected to be apparent only when phosphorylation is measured at individual sites. Mass spectrometry (MS) has become the method of choice for identifying posttranslational modification of proteins *(6)*, but it is rarely quantitative and so far has been used mainly to confirm results from phosphopeptide maps and mutagenesis *(7–9)*.

Acknowledgments

This work was supported by the National Institutes of Health (NIDDK; DK54075-03), Canadian Cystic Fibrosis Foundation (CCFF), and Canadian Institutes of Health and Research (CIHR).

References

1. Riordan, J. R., Rommens, J. M., Kerem, B.-S., Alon, N., Rozmahel, R., Grzelczak, Z., Zielenski, J., Lok, S., Plavsic, N., Chou, J.-L., Drumm, M. L., Iannuzzi, M. C., Collins, F. S., and Tsui, L.-C. (1989) Identification of the cystic fibrosis gene: cloning and characterization of complementary DNA. *Science* **245,** 1066–1073.
2. Chang, X.-B., Tabcharani, J. A., Hou, Y.-X., Jensen, T. J., Kartner, N., Alon, N., Hanrahan, J. W., and Riordan, J. R. (1993) Protein kinase A (PKA) still activates CFTR chloride channel after mutagenesis of all ten PKA consensus phosphorylation sites. *J. Biol. Chem.* **268,** 11,304–11,311.

3. Zhu, T., Dahan, D., Evaglelidis, A., Zheng, S.-X., Luo, J., and Hanrahan, J. W. (1999) Association of cystic fibrosis transmembrane conductance regulator and protein phosphatase 2C. *J. Biol. Chem.* **274,** 29,102–29,107.

4. Kartner, N. and Riordan, J. R. (1998) Characterization of polyclonal and mono-clonal antibodies to cystic fibrosis transmembrane conductance regulator. *Meth. Enzymol.* **292,** 629–652.

5. Luo, J., Zhu, T., Evagelidis, A., Pato, M., and Hanrahan, J. W. (2000) Role of protein phosphatases in the activation of CFTR (ABCC7) by genistein and bromotetramisole. *Am. J. Physiol. (Cell Physiol.)* **279,** C108–C119

6. Townsend, R. R., Lipniunas, P. H., Tulk, B. M., and Verkman, A. S. (1996) Iden-tification of protein kinase A phosphorylation sites on NBD1 and R domains of CFTR using electrospray mass spectrometry with selective phosphate ion moni-toring. *Protein Sci.* **5,** 1865–1873.

7. Cheng, S. H., Rich, D. P., Marshall, J., Gregory, R. J., Welsh, M. J., and Smith, A. E. (1991) Phosphorylation of the R domain by cAMP-dependent protein kinase regu-lates the CFTR chloride channel. *Cell* **66,** 1027–1036.

8. Cohn, J. A., Nairn, A. C., Marino, C. R., Melhus, O., and Kole, J. (1992) Charac-terization of the cystic fibrosis transmembrane conductance regulator in a colonocyte cell line. *Proc. Natl. Acad. Sci. USA* **89,** 2340–2344.

9. Seibert, F. S., Chang, X.-B., Aleksandrov, A. A., Clarke, D. M., Hanrahan, J. W., and Riordan, J. R. (2000) Influence of phosphorylation by protein kinase A on CFTR at the cell surface and endoplasmic reticulum. *Biochim. Biophys. Acta* **1461,** 275–283.

7

Transepithelial Measurements of Bicarbonate Secretion in Calu-3 Cells

Robert J. Bridges

1. Introduction

The importance of impaired HCO_3^- secretion in the pathophysiology of the pancreas of cystic fibrosis (CF) patients has been well documented and known for many years *(1)*. Studies in 1990s from the Welsh *(2)* and Boucher *(3)* laboratories suggested that HCO_3^- secretion may also be impaired in the airways of CF patients. Perhaps because Cl⁻ secretion has been assumed to be of higher importance and thus received the greater attention, the transcellular mechanisms of HCO_3^- secretion remain poorly understood and underinvestigated. Studies from our own laboratory *(4)* and the laboratories of Wine and Widdicombe *(5)* have now established that the human airway serous cell line, Calu-3 cells, secrete HCO_3^- and not Cl⁻, in response to a cAMP-mediated secretory agonist. Serous cells are the most abundant cell type of the submucosal glands *(6)* and are the predominate site of CFTR expression in the airways *(7,8)*. Thus, a better understanding of the transport mechanisms of serous cells is of critical importance in establishing how mutations in CFTR lead to submucosal gland and airways pathophysiology. The focus of this chapter is to provide a description of the methods used to study Calu-3 cell monolayers grown on permeable supports by the short-circuit current (I_{SC}) technique. In addition, methods for ion flux studies and ion substitution studies of short-circuited monolayers are described along with background information necessary to interpret the experimental results specifically as they relate to the net secretion of HCO_3^-. To introduce the subject of HCO_3^- secretion, we provide a brief description of the mechanisms of transepithelial HCO_3^- secretion as they are presently understood.

From: *Methods in Molecular Medicine, vol. 70: Cystic Fibrosis Methods and Protocols*
Edited by: W. R. Skach © Humana Press Inc., Totowa, NJ

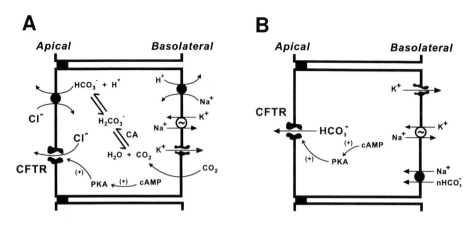

Fig. 1. Mechanisms of HCO_3 secretion.

Figure 1 illustrates two models of how HCO_3^- may be secreted by an epithelial cell. The model in **Fig. 1A** was proposed by Stenson et al. *(9)* for urinary bladder HCO_3^- secretion and by Novak and Gregor *(10)* for pancreatic HCO_3^- secretion. According to this model, extracellular CO_2 enters across the basolateral membrane and is hydrated by intracellular carbonic anhydrase to carbonic acid, which quickly dissociates to H^+ and HCO_3^-. Bicarbonate leaves the cell across the apical membrane in exchange for luminal Cl^-. Luminal Cl^- is provided by the secretion of Cl^- via an apical membrane Cl^- channel, namely, CFTR. Thus, according to this model, the absence of CFTR in CF cells would lead to diminished luminal Cl^- and thereby impair the secretion of HCO_3^-. However, this model does not explain how the exocrine pancreas achieves the secretion of an essentially Cl^--free, isotonic (140 m*M*) $NaHCO_3$ fluid. Indeed, Case and co-workers *(11,12)* have recently shown agonist-stimulated HCO_3^- secretion at low (less than 7 m*M*) luminal Cl^- concentrations in interlobular ducts of guinea pig pancreas. In our own studies on Calu-3 cells, forskolin-stimulated HCO_3^- secretion did not require Cl^- in the apical or basolateral membrane bathing solutions *(4)*. Thus, luminal Cl^- does not appear to be essential for the secretion of HCO_3^- (*see* **Note 1**).

The model shown in **Fig. 1B** emerged from our results on Calu-3 cells *(4)*. According to this model, HCO_3^- enters the cell across the basolateral membrane coupled to the movement of Na^+ on a Na^+:HCO_3^- cotransporter (NBC). Bicarbonate exits the cell via an apical membrane anion channel that we propose is CFTR. Studies from Case and co-workers *(11,12)* on pancreatic ducts and our own studies on Calu-3 cells have demonstrated the dependence of HCO_3^- secretion on serosal Na^+ and serosal HCO_3^- as well as an inhibition by the disulfonic stilbene, DNDS, a known inhibitor of NBCs. Molecular studies have recently shown the expression of an NBC isoform in the pancreas *(13)* and in Calu-3 cells *(14)*. Furthermore, immunofluorescence studies using NBC antibodies have revealed the basolateral membrane localization of the NBC in pancreatic ductal cells *(15)* and in Calu-3 cells *(14)*. Since the initial expression cloning of a renal NBC from the salamander kidney *(16)*, a number of NBC isoforms and splice variants have been cloned from different species and tissues. Indeed, it now appears that cells may express more than one type of NBC. Thus, further studies will be necessary to determine which NBC isoform(s) contributes to the transepithelial secretion of HCO_3^-. Calu-3 cells appear to be a good model cell line in which to perform such studies.

The second tenant of the model shown in **Fig. 1B** is the conductive exit of HCO_3^- from the cell via an apical membrane channel that we and others have proposed is CFTR. Because HCO_3^- secretion is stimulated by cAMP in both the pancreas and in Calu-3 cells, the anion channel mediating the secretion of HCO_3^- is likely to be activated by cAMP and protein kinase A, as is CFTR. As already noted, CFTR is highly expressed in pancreatic ductal cells, airway submucosal gland serous cells, and Calu-3 cells. Patch-clamp anion selectivity studies have shown that CFTR can conduct HCO_3^-, although at a fraction (0.15–0.25) of the Cl^- conductance *(17,18)*. Illek et al. *(19)* have shown, in α-toxin permeabilized monolayers of Calu-3 cells, the activation of an apical membrane anion conductance by cAMP with a similar HCO_3^- to Cl^- selectivity as observed in the patch-clamp studies of CFTR. Impedance analysis (*see* Chapter 8) as well as microelectrode studies on intact Calu-3 cell monolayers have also shown forskolin activates an apical membrane conductance *(20)*. Indeed, the apical membrane resistance of a forskolin-stimulated Calu-3 cells is remarkably low, $<20\ \Omega\ cm^2$, which translates into a conductance of >50 mS/cm^2. Thus, even at a HCO_3^- to Cl^- selectivity of 0.15, this high conductance requires an outwardly directed driving force of <7 mV across the apical membrane for the net secretion of HCO_3^-. Since Cl^- is not secreted in forskolin-stimulated Calu-3 cells *(4,5)*, Cl^- must be at its electrochemical equilibrium across the apical membrane. If one assumes a normal intracellular Cl^- concentration of 30 mM and an extracellular Cl^- concentration of 120 mM, the equilibrium potential for Cl (E_{Cl}) is approximately -35 mV. The difference between E_{Cl} and $E_{HCO_3^-}$ of -22 mV (-35 mV$-[-13$ mV$]$) would therefore be more than adequate to drive the secretion of HCO_3^- (*see* **Note 2**).

The above brief description of the mechanisms involved in the transepithelial secretion of HCO_3^- suggests that there is still much to be investigated before we fully understand how HCO_3^- is secreted. Several hypotheses predicated on these two models of HCO_3^- secretion are readily testable using the methods described in this chapter. The further use of Calu-3 cells is certain to aid in testing these hypotheses. Knowledge gained from the studies on Calu-3 cells may then reveal how better to study HCO_3^- secretion in intact airways, an experimental preparation that will be significantly more challenging to investigate.

2. Materials

2.1. Tissue Culture

1. Calu-3 cell American Type Culture Collection (cat. no. HTB55).
2. DMEM/F12 media (Sigma, cat. no. D-8900), prepared as described by manufacture.
3. Fetal bovine serum, FBS (Hyclone, cat. no. SH30070.03).
4. Calu-3 culture media: we typically add 353 mL FBS to 2000 mL of DMEM/F12.
5. T25-cm^2 flasks (Fisher, cat. no. 10-126-10).
6. Phosphate-buffered saline, PBS (Sigma, cat. no. P-4417).
7. Human placental collagen Type IV, HPC (Sigma, cat. no. C-7521).
8. A stock solution of HPC is prepared with 100 mg HPC plus 200 μL glacial acetic acid and 100 mL H_2O stored at 4°C.
9. Snapwell polycarbonate filters (Costar, cat. no. 3407).
10. Trypsin-ethylenediaminetetraacetic acid (EDTA) (Life Technologies, cat. no. 25200-056).

2.2. Ussing Chamber Setup

1. Ussing chambers. Snapwell vertical diffusion chambers (Costar, cat. no. 3430).
2. Silver chloride electrodes and electrode caps for Ussing chambers (Costar, cat. nos. 3433 and 3435).
3. Voltage clamp (Iowa Instruments model 558C-5).
4. Gas and heating manifold for Ussing chambers (Costar, cat. nos. 3431 and 3432).
5. Strip-chart recorder.
6. Ussing chamber buffers: 120 mM NaCl, 25 mM NaHCO$_3$, 3.3 mM KH$_2$PO$_4$, 0.8 mM K$_2$HPO$_4$, 1.2 mM MgCl$_2$, 1.2 mM CaCl$_2$, and 10 mM glucose. The pH of this solution is 7.4 when gassed with a mixture of 95% O_2, 5% CO_2 at 37°C. However, mannitol is substituted for glucose in the mucosal solution to eliminate the contribution of Na$^+$-glucose cotransport to the I_{SC}. We typically prepare 500 mL of the glucose and mannitol containing buffers in volumetric flasks from 20× stock solutions of the above salts. When not in use, the buffers are kept at 4°C and are gassed prior to each experiment. If the divalent salts have precipitated out of solution, usually because of the loss of CO_2 with storage, or if there is any growth in the solution, the buffer is discarded. Chloride-free solutions are prepared by equimolar replacement of the NaCl with Na-gluconate and MgCl$_2$ with Mg-gluconate. The 1 mM CaCl$_2$ is replaced with 4 mM Ca-gluconate to compensate for the Ca^{2+} buffing capacity of the gluconate. Bicarbonate-free solutions are prepared using 145 mM NaCl, 3.3 mM K$_2$HPO$_4$, 0.8 mM K$_2$HPO$_4$, 1.2 mM MgCl$_2$, and 1.2 mM CaCl$_2$, pH adjusted with NaOH, and this solution is gassed with air. A small pump for a fish tank is useful for this purpose. Sodium-free solution is prepared by the equimolar replacement of NaCl with

N-methyl-D-glucoamine (NMDG) Cl and chlorine-HCO_3. To avoid any cholinergic effects of the chlorine, 10 μM atropine is added to this solution. The NMDG-Cl is prepared from 23.42 g/L of NMDG and the addition of HCl until the pH of the solution is 7.0. As the pH of the solution approaches 7.0, the HCl should be added slowly to avoid overshooting the desired pH. Sodium-free and Cl^--free solutions are prepared by equimolar replacement of the NaCl with NMDG-gluconate, $NaHCO_3$ with choline-HCO_3, $MgCl_2$ with Mg-gluconate, and 4 mM Ca-gluconate for the $CaCl_2$. This solution should also contain 10 μM atropine. The NMDG-gluconate is prepared using 23.42 g/L of NMDG and approx 47 mL/L of gluconic (Sigma G1139) acid and the pH adjusted to 7.0 with either NMDG or gluconic acid. In general, gluconate-containing solutions should not be stored for more than a few days, and we generally prepare fresh solutions each day. Each of the above solutions should have an osmolarity of approx 290 mOsmol. It is a good practice to measure the osmolality each time a buffer is prepared, since this is a good check that it has been prepared correctly.
7. 1 M KCl.
8. 1 N HCl.

2.3. Chemicals

1. Forskolin (RBI, Cat. no. F-105).
2. DNDS (Pfaltz and Bauer, cat. no. D47973).
3. Acetozolamide (Sigma, cat. no. A6011).
4. Bumetanide (Sigma, cat. no. B3023).
5. ^{22}Na, ^{36}Cl, ^{86}Rb, and ^{42}K are purchased from NEN (Boston, MA).

3. Methods

3.1. Calu-3 Cell Cultures and Filter Preparation

Calu-3 cells are maintained in DMEM/F-12 plus 15% FBS culture media. Cells are kept in an incubator at 37°C in 5% CO_2 and passaged once per week. We have successfully passaged the cells for more than 1 yr without any loss in the transport phenotype. A confluent T25 flask is washed with PBS (5 mL) for 1 min. The PBS is removed and 1 mL of trypsin-EDTA is added, washed across the cells, and approx 0.5 mL is removed, leaving just enough to cover the cell surface. The cells are incubated at 37°C for 8–10 min, until the cells detach from the flask. Culture medium, 6.5 mL, is added to suspend the cells. An aliquot of 1.6 mL of the suspended cells are added to a T25 flask to passage the cells, equivalent to a 1:4 split. Eight drops of cells from a 10-mL pipet are seeded onto a collagen-coated Snapwell filter and 3 mL of culture medium are added to the basal side of the filter. To avoid any delay in plating the cells, we do not routinely take time to count the number of cells. Collagen-coated filters are prepared by overnight incubation at 37°C with 3 drops of HPC. Excess HPC is removed from the filter just before the addition of the cells. In our experience, it is essential to use polycarbonate filters and not poly-ester filters to obtain a consistent transport phenotype with the Calu-3 cells. On the second day, fluid is removed from the apical side of the filter and the cells are fed with fresh medium on the basolateral side. Thereafter, the cells are fed every other day on the basolateral side. Any fluid on the apical side is removed at each feeding. After approx 1 wk, the cells will hold back fluid and are then grown at an air–liquid interface for an additional 21 d. The monolayers will secrete mucus onto the apical surface, which will accumulate with time and appear as a shiny layer when viewed in bright light. However, there should not be any fluid on the apical surface. If fluid is observed, the filter should be discarded or cultured for an additional 7–10 d. The most consistent results are obtained with cells grown on filters for 28 d, but we have successfully used filters as old as 42 d. However, the forskolin responses are 30% reduced in older cells.

3.2. Ussing Chambers, Voltage-Clamp Setup, and Mounting Filters

The Costar vertical diffusion chambers were specifically designed to accommodate the Snapwell filters, and we strongly recommend the use of these chambers. In addition to the chambers, one must purchase the electrode caps and electrodes (*see* **Note 3**) to perform I_{SC} studies. Compared to the many different Ussing chamber designs available, the Costar chamber and electrodes are by far the most user-friendly chamber we have used. A more general discussion of I_{SC} methods can be found in the excellent volume edited by Wills, Reuss and Lewis *(21)*. The two halves of the chamber are held in place with retaining rings on the back and front sides of the chamber (*see* **Note 4**). Each half chamber is filled with 5 mL of buffer and when connected to the gas supply, the solution is circulated by a gas lift incorporated into the chamber design. The chambers are kept warm by a heating manifold, also available from Costar. The heating manifold is kept warm with a circulating water bath. The heating manifold also incorporates a gas supply manifold (*see* **Note 5**). Although the heating and gas manifold can accommodate six chambers, we recommend using fewer chambers or purchasing a second manifold. With six chambers in the manifold, the chambers are too close together and one can easily become confused when inserting the electrodes, making drug additions, or taking samples. Far fewer electrodes will be broken if there is some space between the chambers.

Before performing an experiment, the chambers are initially set up without a filter, filled with mannitol buffer and placed in the heating manifold. The four glass-barreled electrodes, two voltage-measuring, and two current-passing, are placed in the chamber and connected to the voltage clamp, care being taken to place the voltage-measuring and current-passing electrodes in their proper positions on each side of the chamber (*see* **Note 6**). We keep our elec-

trodes in 1 *M* KCl when not in use and connected to the voltage clamp to minimize any offset potential that could develop between the electrodes (*see* **Note 7**).
After a few minutes of equilibration, the offset potential, if any, is corrected for
using the offset circuit on the voltage clamp. In addition, the fluid resistance is
measured and corrected for using the clamp circuitry. The electrodes are left in
place for an additional few minutes to ensure that they remain stable. The Iowa
Instruments voltage clamp allows for the correction of a ±10-mV offset and a
solution resistance of 50 Ω. If the offset potential is greater than 10 mV, one must
replace the electrode or rechloride the existing electrodes. To rechloride the
electrodes, the electrodes are removed from the chamber and the plastic cap
and silver wire are removed. The silver wire is cleaned with fine steel wool and
connected to the positive pole of a DC power supply set at 1 V. The wire is
inserted into a vial of 1 *N* HCl. The circuit is completed by placing a silver wire
connected to the negative pole of the DC power supply, caring being taken not
to touch the two silver wires together in the vial of HCl. Within a minute or
two, a brown deposit of chloride will form on the electrode wire. The electrode
is then rinsed in distilled water and placed back into the 1 *M* KCl-filled glass
barrel of the electrode. This is repeated for each of the four electrodes required
for each chamber. Alternatively, one may have an extra set of electrodes already
prepared to replace any electrodes with a large offset potential or that are not
stable. With experience, the electrodes seldom require attention more than once
a month. When problems do develop, it is usually because the electrodes were
not properly positioned in the chamber and one has attempted to short-circuit
the epithelium. Another common mistake is to remove the electrodes at the end
of an experiment before switching the clamp to the standby position. In this
case, the clamp senses a large voltage difference and attempts to pass enough
current to short-circuit this voltage, causing the electrodes to become very
polarized. Therefore, it is best to train oneself always to place the clamp in the
standby mode before removing the electrodes from the chamber and to double-
check the placement of the electrodes in the chamber as well as all connections
before going to the clamp mode.

Once the offset and fluid resistance have been corrected, the electrodes are
removed and placed back into a holding vessel containing 1 *M* KCl. Fluid is
removed from each of the chambers, the gas supply is disconnected, and the
chambers are disassembled in preparation of mounting the filters. The opened
chambers should be left on top of the heating block to keep them warm. The cells
grown on filters—we usually do six filters at one time—are retrieved from the
incubator. Each filter is then dipped three times in warm gassed mannitol buffer
(37°C) and mounted into a chamber. Five milliliters of warm (37°C) gassed
mannitol buffer are added to the apical side and then 5 mL of warm gassed
glucose buffer are added to the basolateral side. It is critical to use warm

gassed buffer to both wash the filter and to add to the chamber. Solutions that are cold (< 37°C) will stimulate the cells, yielding an elevated I_{SC} that may require 15–30 min to return to baseline. It is also important to add the buffer to the apical side first to avoid subjecting the cells to a hydrostatic pressure gradient from the serosal side, since this can disrupt the integrity of the tight junctions and the monolayer. With practice, six filters can be mounted in less than 10 min.

After all the filters to be used are mounted, the gas supply to each chamber is reconnected. Each set of electrodes is then rinsed with distilled water to remove any 1 M KCl from the glass barrels, wiped gently with a Kimwipe, and placed in the chamber in its proper position. After all the electrodes are in place and after double-checking that they are in the proper position, one can then switch the voltage clamp from the standby position to the open-circuit mode. With the meter set on *Em* the displayed value is the transepithelial voltage (*VT*). This value is typically –5 to –10 mV in unstimulated Calu-3 cells. If the *VT* is much greater than –10 mV this usually indicates the electrodes are not in their proper positions, a wire is not properly connected, or there is an air bubble at the tip of one of the electrodes. In any case, one should not switch to the voltage clamp mode until the problem is corrected, because the voltage clamp will pass an artificially high current that can damage the cells. Therefore, one should switch back to the standby mode and then try to identify and rectify the problem. Once a satisfactory *VT* is achieved, the meter is switched to *IM* or the current-measuring mode and should read zero. The voltage clamp is then switched from the open-circuit mode to the short-circuit (voltage clamp) mode and the meter should read a value of 10–20 µAmp. One should be prepared to swtich quickly back to the open-circuit mode if a very high current (>100 µA) is displayed upon switching to the short-circuit (voltage clamp) mode. A very high current could mean that there is a problem with the position of the electrodes, a connection, or an air bubble. Once such potential problems have been eliminated, one must consider that the transepithelial resistance (*RT*) of the monolayer is low. The resistance of the monolayer can be estimated by dividing the *VT* measured in the open-circuit mode by the measured current in the short-circuit mode, which is the I_{SC}; $VT/I_{SC} = RT$ (*see* **Note 8**). Unstimulated Calu-3 cells grown under the above culture conditions have an *RT* of approx 300 Ωcm². Because the I_{SC} is inversely proportional to the *RT*, a high I_{SC} at a given *VT* indicates that the resistance of the monolayer is low, as discussed further below.

3.3. R$_T$ *Measurements*

An estimate of *RT* can be obtained from the *VT* measured in the open-circuit mode and the I_{SC} measured in the short-circuit/voltage clamp mode as described above. However, this requires switching the clamp between these two modes each time an estimate of the RT is desired. An alternative to this method is to pulse the monolayer intermittently to a new clamp potential (e.g., ±2 mV) and record the change in I_{SC}. RT is then calculated from the change in voltage divided by the change in current, where $RT = \Delta V/(\Delta I_{SC}/1.2)$ correcting for the 1.2-cm^2 surface area of a Snapwell. An external pulse generator can be connected to the voltage command input of the voltage clamp or one can purchase the voltage clamp with a pulse generator installed. In either case, both the amplitude and duration should be adjustable so that a stable measurable change in current is achieved. With Calu-3 cells, we find a 2-mV bipolar pulse of 3 s duration to be useful. We typically pulse the monolayer once every minute, and these pulses appear as vertical deflections in the current trace recorded on a strip-chart recorder. Under short-circuit conditions, the epithelium is usually voltage-clamped to 0 mV. When a bipolar pulse is used, the pulse generator gives a command to change the clamp potential to +2 mV and then –2 mV for 3 s at each new potential. The current-passing circuitry adjusts the I_{SC} to achieve these changes in the clamp potential. Thus, the ΔV is known, the ΔI_{SC} is measured, and from these values one can calculate RT.

Because the Calu-3 cells are a relatively leaky epithelium, a few words about solution resistance compensation are warranted. The VT and the resistance between the two voltage-measuring electrodes are what determines the amplitude of the I_{SC}. In most cases, one wishes to clamp the epithelium to 0 mV. However, the resistance between the electrodes is not just the resistance of the epithelium, but is also the resistance of the solution (and filter) between the two electrodes. In the Costar chamber, the latter is approx 30 Ω. In a tight epithelium (e.g., >1000 Ωcm^2), this solution resistance can essentially be ignored. However, in unstimulated Calu-3 cells the epithelial resistance is only 300 Ωcm^2 and this value falls further, to 200 Ωcm^2 in stimulated cells. If uncorrected, the 30-Ω solution resistance would cause an erroneous I_{SC} and, more important, the epithelium would not be clamped to 0 mV.

3.4. I_{SC} *Measurements*

The technique of short-circuit current measurements is technically rather simple once all the equipment is obtained and one becomes acquainted with the use of the equipment. The definition of the I_{SC} is the current required to clamp the epithelium at a defined voltage, usually 0 mV. The magnitude of the I_{SC} is given by Ohm's law, where $I_{SC} = VT/RT$. Many epithelia, but not all, display a spontaneous transepithelial potential difference (VT) indicative of the net active transport of an ion. When studied in solutions of equal ionic composition on both sides of the epithelium, the I_{SC} is a direct measure of net electrogenic ion transport. It is, however, important to appreciate the meaning of net ion transport and that significant net electroneutral active transport of ions goes unmeasured by I_{SC} studies alone. For example, in his initial studies, Ussing performed a careful series of experiments to show that the I_{SC} across frog skin was equivalent to the net absorption of Na^+ *(22)*. This required measuring the unidirectional fluxes of Na^+ (to be described later) and demonstrating the net movement of Na^+ was equal to the I_{SC}. Similar isotope flux studies have established that the I_{SC} is a measure of net Cl^- secretion in some tissues and cell lines. Thus, for certain tissues where unidirectional flux studies have established the ionic basis for the I_{SC}, the I_{SC} can be conveniently used as a routine measure of the net movement of the ion. However, there are examples of tissues and cell lines where the I_{SC} cannot be attributed to the net transport of a single ion species due to the simultaneous transport of two or more ion species. Stated differently, the I_{SC} is equal to the sum of the net fluxes of Na^+, K^+, Cl^-, and HCO_3^-. Because Mg^{+2}, Ca^{+2}, and PO_4^{-2} fluxes tend to be much smaller in magnitude, they can be ignored. For example, the rabbit colon both absorbs Na^+ and secretes Cl^- by electrogenic mechanisms, and the I_{SC} will be the sum of these two net fluxes. In addition, tissues such as the rat colon and the ileum of many species absorb Na^+ and Cl^- by an electroneutral mechanism and secrete HCO_3^- and Cl^- by electrogenic mechanisms, and the transport of each of these ions is subject to regulation by various mechanisms. Therefore, in tissues or cell lines where multiple ions are actively transported, the I_{SC} maybe difficult to interpret. In such tissues careful measurements of the unidirectional ion fluxes combined with ion substitution and pharmacological studies are required under each set of experimental conditions to establish the ionic basis of the I_{SC} (*see* **Note 9**). Unfortunately, airway surface epithelial cells and Calu-3 cells transport multiple ions and thus require careful analysis to determine the nature of the I_{SC}. Early studies on Calu-3 cells erroneously interpreted the spontaneous or cAMP-stimulated I_{SC} to be a measure of Cl^- secretion. Only after both the mucosal-to-serosal (J_{MS}) and serosal-to-mucosal (J_{SM}) unidirectional fluxes of Cl^- were measured was it realized that Calu-3 cells do not secrete Cl^- under these conditions *(4,5)*. Further studies revealed that the cAMP-stimulated I_{SC} in Calu-3 cells is actually the secretion of HCO_3^- (*see* **Note 10**).

3.5. Unidirectional Fluxes

Compared to I_{SC} measurements, unidirectional flux studies are tedious to perform, which probably accounts for why many laboratories do not perform these studies. When performing the flux studies, extra care should be taken to pipet exactly 5 mL into each half-chamber. In preparation for the flux studies, one must first weigh a series of vials with caps into which the radioactive samples will be pipetted. This is essential because the sample volume taken from the chamber is seldom the volume one assumes is pipeted. Given the nature of the calculations, small errors in the sample volume can lead to large differences in the calculated fluxes. We typical require 16 vials for each chamber and use only four chambers when performing flux studies. Two chambers are used for the mucosal-to-serosal flux (J_{MS}) and two chambers are used for the serosal-to-mucosal flux (J_{SM}). All samples are taken in duplicate. Once the filters have been mounted and the I_{SC} is stable, isotope (^{22}Na, ^{36}Cl, ^{86}Rb, or ^{42}K) is added to the serosal or mucosal side of the chamber. This side is referred to as the hot side and the opposite side as the cold side. A final concentration of 1 µCi/mL is usually adequate to obtain reliable flux measurements. If any drugs are to be added they should be added, at the same time as the isotope is added. After an additional equilibration period of 15–20 min, two samples of 100 µL are taken from the hot side of each chamber. Two samples of 200 µL are then taken from the cold side of the first chamber and a timer started. This is time zero (T_0) for the first chamber. Four hundred microliters of warm gassed solution are added to the cold side. If any drugs have been added to the buffer on the cold side, these too must be included in the buffer. The I_{SC} and ΔI_{SC} during a pulse are recorded. At an exact time 2, 200-µL samples are then taken from the cold side of the second chamber and this is time zero for chamber two. Four hundred microliters of buffer are added to the cold side of chamber 2. The I_{SC} and ΔI_{SC} are recorded, and this is repeated for each chamber. We usually use the pulses given at 1 min intervals to time when the samples are to be taken. With Calu-3 cells a flux period of 15 min has proven adequate. Therefore, at exactly T_{15} for chamber one, two, 200-µL samples are taken from the cold side, 400 µL of buffer are replaced, and the I_{SC} values are recorded. This is repeated for chambers 2, 3, and 4 at their respective T_{15} intervals. This sequence is repeated at T_{30}, T_{45}, T_{60}, and T_{75}. Typically, the first two flux periods, T_0 to T_{15} and T_{15} toT_{30}, are used as the control flux periods. At T_{30} various drugs are added (e.g., forskolin). The period from T_{30} to T_{45} is an equilibration period and if necessary can be extended to ensure that the I_{SC} has reached a new stable plateau. The periods from T_{45} to T_{60} and from T_{60} to T_{75} are used as the experimental flux periods. At the completion of the experiment, two 100-µL samples are taken from the hot side of each chamber.

The vials are then weighed a second time and the pipetted volumes are calculated. These values are then used in the flux calculations. The four samples from the hot side are averaged and used to calculate the specific activity of the hot side. For example, if ^{22}Na was used and the cpm of the hot side samples was 2900 cpm/µL, the specific activity would be 20,000 cpm/µmol given that the buffer contains 145 mM Na$^+$. At each time interval, the volume on the cold side is calculated using the initial volume of 5 mL minus the volume of the samples taken plus the addition of the 400 µL of buffer at each time interval.

For example, at T_0, the cold-side volume is 5000 µL minus the two samples (e.g., 190 and 195 µL), plus the 400 µL added, or 5015 µL. This volume is then the T_0 volume. However, because 385 µL were removed, the cpm (e.g., 6 cpm/µL) in this volume must be subtracted (6 · 385 = 2310 cpm) from the cpm in the cold side of the chamber. Therefore, the total cpm in the cold side at T_0 is 6 cpm/µL · 4615 µL = 27,690 cpm and these counts are now in a volume of 5015 µL. The cpm in the T_{15} samples (e.g., 9 cpm/µL) are then used together with the volume of 5015 to calculate the total cpm in the cold side at T_{15} (9 cpm/µL · 5015 µL = 45,135 cpm). The total cpm at T_0 is subtracted from the T_{15} value (45,135 cpm – 27,690 cpm = 17,445 cpm) and this value is divided by the specific activity of the hot side to yield the unidirectional flux over the T_0–T_{15} interval (17,445 cpm/20,000 cpm/µmol) = 0.87 µmol or 0.87 µEq/15 min. Since fluxes are conventionally stated in µEq cm^{-2} h^{-1}, this value is multiplied by 4 and divided by 1.2 to correct for the area of the Snapwell to yield a value of 2.9 µEq · cm^{-2} h^{-1}. The above calculations are then repeated for each of the four flux periods, T_0 to T_{15}, T_{15} to T_{30}, T_{45} to T_{60}, and T_{60} to T_{75}. The two initial periods are averaged, as are the two final periods. The average I_{SC} is also calculated from the recorded values over these same time intervals. The unidirectional fluxes from the two serosal-to-mucosal chambers are then compared to the two mucosal-to-serosal chambers and the net flux is calculated ($J_{MS} - J_{S-M}$ = J_{net}) and compared to the I_{SC} (*see* **Note 11**). We typically obtain values from six chambers for each unidirectional flux. The experiments are repeated for each of the isotopes (^{22}Na, ^{36}Cl, and ^{86}Rb).

In Calu-3 cells, we found a small net absorptive flux of Na$^+$ (0.46 µEq · cm^{-2} h^{-1}) that was not altered by forskolin. Although forskolin caused a fivefold increase in both unidirectional fluxes of Cl$^-$, there was no net secretion or absorption of Cl$^-$ (*see* **Note 12**). The ^{86}Rb fluxes, used as a measure of K$^+$ transport, revealed no net transport of K$^+$ in control or forskolin-stimulated cells. Thus, by the process of elimination, the I_{SC} across Calu-3 cells must be accounted for by the transport of some other ion besides Na$^+$, Cl$^-$, and K$^+$. The flux of this ion is often referred to as the net residual ion flux, or JR_{net} and is equal to the I_{SC} minus the net fluxes of Na$^+$, K$^+$, and Cl$^-$ (*see* **Note 13**). The ionic basis of JR_{net} has been shown in many tissues to correspond to the net secretion of HCO_3^-. Because HCO_3^- is in equilibrium with CO_2 and CO_2 has a high permeability, it is not possible to measure the HCO_3^- unidirectional fluxes directly in symmetric bathing solutions. However, pH measurements can be made across monolayers with an imposed HCO_3^- gradient, so called pH stat measurements *(23)*, and the results of such studies have helped establish that JR_{net} is equal to the net secretion of HCO_3^-. As with the flux of any ion, both unidirectional fluxes (J_{MS} and J_{SM}) of HCO_3^- must be measured to obtain an estimate of the net flux. The major shortcoming of the pH stat method is that one must impose a HCO_3^-

gradient. As with any ion substitution experiment, these changes in fluid composition can alter the transport properties of the epithelial cells and the results must therefore be interpreted with caution.

3.6. Ion Substitution and Pharmacology Studies

Based on the outcome of the unidirectional ion flux studies, one may perform ion substitution and pharmacological experiments to obtain supportive evidence for the net transport of a given ion as well as some insight into the mechanism involved in the transport of the ion. The utility of these types of studies is most easily illustrated by the following examples. The failure of bumetanide to inhibit the forskolin-stimulated I_{SC} in Calu-3 cells was the first piece of evidence that led us to suspect Cl^- secretion was not the ionic basis of the I_{SC}. Bumetanide is an inhibitor of the $Na:K:2Cl^-$ cotransporter that mediates the uptake of Cl^- across the basolateral membrane in Cl^- secreting epithelia. Bumetanide, 20 μM on the serosal side, did not inhibit the forskolin-stimulated I_{SC} in Calu-3 cells nor did it inhibit the J_{SM} of Cl^- suggesting that this cotransporter is inoperative in forskolin-stimulated Calu-3 cells. The symmetric substitution of Cl^- with gluconate also did not eliminate the forskolin-stimulated I_{SC}. This was an important observation since it demonstrated that HCO_3^- could be secreted without any need for Cl^-. Therefore, the secretion of HCO_3^- did not require a $Cl^-:HCO_3^-$ exchanger as proposed in earlier models of HCO_3^- secretion (**Fig. 1A**). This was further supported by the failure of mucosal DNDS to inhibit the forskolin-stimulated I_{SC}. DNDS is a noncolvalenty reactive disulfonic stilbene that inhibits $Cl^-:HCO_3^-$ exchangers and, at high concentrations, $Na^+:HCO_3^-$ cotransporters. The partial inhibition of the forskolin-stimulated I_{SC} by high concentrations of serosal DNDS was the first bit of evidence that a $Na^+:HCO_3^-$ cotransporter might be involved in the basolateral membrane entry of HCO_3^-. Ion substitution studies revealed that the forskolin-stimulated increase in I_{SC} required both Na^+ and HCO_3^- in the serosal solution, lending further support to a role for a basolateral membrane $Na^+:HCO_3^-$ cotransporter. Thus, through the use of I_{SC} measurements and isotope fluxes, we were able to ascertain that Calu-3 cells secrete HCO_3^- in response to forskolin. Ion substitution and pharmacology studies provided some insight into the underlying mechanisms involved in HCO_3^- secretion. The true power of these methods is in their combined use.

4. Notes

1. A number of studies suggest that HCO_3^- secretion does require luminal or extracellular Cl^-, and these results have been taken as evidence for a $Cl^-:HCO_3^-$ exchanger, which indeed they may accurately reflect. However, several studies have attempted to demonstrate the molecular identity of an apical membrane

anion exchanger in HCO_3^--secreting epithelia without success but have repeatedly shown the expression of an anion exchanger in the basolateral membrane. (The contribution of the latter to transepithelial anion secretion remains to be demonstrated.) When attempting to evaluate the Cl^- dependence of HCO_3^- secretion or efflux of HCO_3^- from a cell, it is important to distinguish between an electrochemical coupling of Cl^- and HCO_3^- movements from the obligatory exchange of Cl^- for HCO_3^- on an anion exchanger. Both would be electroneutral but the former could be mediated by an ion channel that allows for the entry of Cl^- and the exit of HCO_3^- and thus appears to behave like an anion exchanger. Since CFTR can conduct both Cl^- and HCO_3^-, it is important to distinguish these two different mechanisms experimentally. One means of doing so is to evaluate the voltage dependence of the HCO_3^- flux; a channel-mediated flux will show a clear voltage dependence, while the movement on an anion exchanger will be independent of the membrane voltage. However, this is not trivial with unpolarized cells grown on coverslips that express high levels of CFTR. Activation of CFTR is expected to dominate the conductance of the membrane, and attempts to alter the membrane potential with high extracellular K^+ and valinomycin may not lead to the expected changes in the membrane potential.

2. The actual driving force acting on HCO_3^- is the apical membrane potential (V_{ap}) minus $E_{HCO_3^-}$. Because the apical membrane conductance is dominated by the CFTR Cl^- conductance it will approach E_{Cl}, but must be corrected for the finite HCO_3^- permeability of CFTR. However, even at a HCO_3^--to-Cl^- permeability ratio of 0.25, this correction lowers V_{ap} by less than 2 mV as calculated using the Goldman, Hodgkin, Katz voltage equation.

3. The electrodes as provided by the manufacture have a small glass frit in the tip. We have found that this frit does not prevent the KCl inside the glass barrel from leaking into the chamber and thereby altering the KCl concentration of the buffer. In addition, the frit can become clogged with time and prevent the passage of current. Therefore, we recommend removing the frit and filling the tip of the glass barrel with 4% agar made with 1 *M* KCl. The frit can be removed by carefully rubbing the tip of the glass barrel against the smooth surface of a sharpening stone. Alternatively, one may purchase 200 µL glass pipets (Fisher, cat. no. 21-164-2J) and cut these to the correct length. One end of the shortened pipet is fire-polished to create a narrow tip and the other end is heated to create a flared end similar to that of the original glass barrel. The end with the narrow tip, is filled with agar, cooled, and then back-filled with 1 *M* KCl. With a little practice, one can prepare several dozen glass barrels in 1 h and store these in 1 *M* KCl for future use.

4. The tool provided by Costar to remove the retaining rings is difficult to use, and we recommend purchasing an alternative tool, one that has the tips at right angles. This tool can be purchased at a good hardware or automotive store along with additional retaining rings and O-rings, at a much lower price than available from Costar.

5. The gas supply manifold provided by Costar is not the best design we have experienced and requires some routine maintenance. When removing the gas supply

tube from the chamber, it is important not to pull on the tubing; rather, one must lift the connector with a small screwdriver or a fingernail. If there is no gas coming out of a given outlet, it is usually a problem with the valve and not the tubing. When gas flow stops at one of the outlets, it is necessary to take that outlet apart and repair it. This usually requires reattaching the rubber gasket on to the valve screw and reinserting the assembly into the value tube. The tube and gasket are actually parts of a 1-mL plastic syringe. While simple in design, the gas manifold is clearly the weakest portion of the Costar Ussing chamber system.

6. For the beginner and sometimes the expert, keeping track of which electrode goes where can be confusing. Costar provides four wires with the electrodes, two with white connectors and two with black connectors. We connect the two with white connectors to the voltage-measuring electrodes and the two with black connectors to the current-passing electrodes. In addition, a small piece of tape is placed on the wires of the electrodes, one voltage (E_1) and one current (I_1), that correspond to the serosal side of the chamber. The voltage across the epithelium is a differential measurement with the serosal side considered ground (0 mV) such that the absorption of a cation or the secretion of an anion will produce a negative membrane potential. Since one wants to measure the voltage across the epithelium, the voltage electrodes must be positioned as close to the epithelium as possible without touching. This is achieved by placing the voltage-measuring electrodes in the slanted inlets of the electrode caps. Likewise, to ensure an even current distribution over the entire monolayer, the current-passing electrodes are placed as far away from the cells as possible. In the Costar chamber, the current electrodes are placed in the vertical inlets of the electrode cap, which places the current-passing electrode at the most distal part of the chamber.

7. We usually keep our electrodes connected to the voltage clamp and stored in a vessel containing 1 M KCl. Only a few centimeters of the glass barrel need be immersed in the 1 M KCl, to ensure that the agar is kept hydrated. The glass barrel of the electrode should also be kept three-quarters full with 1 M KCl. It is usually best to fill the glass barrel of the electrodes after completing an experiment and then storing the electrodes overnight. We prefer to use 1 M KCl rather than the 3 M KCl used by many investigators. Because 3 M KCl is near the saturation concentration, the KCl will tend to crystallize and creep out of the vessel and up the shaft of the electrodes as water evaporates. This can quickly corrode the copper connectors of the electrodes and wires and thereby create many problems. The use of 1 M KCl avoids this problem and still provides an adequate solution for the AgCl electrodes. However, one must still be careful not to spill the 1 M KCl and to clean up any 1 M KCl that does spill. Many hours can be wasted trying to ascertain what is wrong with the electrodes, connections, or voltage clamp when the real source of the problem is actually a KCl salt bridge that has formed because of spillage or improper care of the equipment.

8. The resistance of the monolayer is obtained using Ohm's law where resistance (R) in ohms equals voltage in volts divided by current in amps ($R = V/A$). The use of the open circuit potential (VT) divided by the I_{SC} is one method of estimating

the *RT*. Because the Snapwell filter has a surface area of 1.2 cm^2 and because *RT* and I_{SC} are conventionally normalized per square centimeter, the I_{SC} or *RT* value must be corrected to obtain an *RT* value in Ω cm^2. Also, one must correct for the units of *VT* and I_{SC}. Most voltage clamps display the *VT* in microvolts and the I_{SC} in microamperes. Therefore, since R (Ω) = V/A, $RT = (VT \cdot 10^{-3})/[(I_{SC}/1.2) \cdot 10^{-6}]$. For example, with a Snapwell, if *VT* is 10 mV and I_{SC} is 100 μA, $RT = (10\ mV \times 10^{-3})/[(100\ \mu A/1.2) \cdot 10^{-6}] = 120\ \Omega cm^2$.

9. It is unfortunate, but many investigators in the CF community are guilty of concluding that any amiloride-insensitive I_{SC} is the result of net Cl$^-$ secretion, without a formal demonstration that this is the case. This erroneous conclusion has contributed to the underappreciation of the importance of HCO$_3^-$ secretion in CF-affected epithelia.

10. Calu-3 cells can be stimulated to secrete Cl$^-$ by the activation of basolateral membrane potassium channels. However, the secretion of Cl$^-$ by Calu-3 cells is not discussed in this chapter, and one is referred to the papers of Devor et al. *(4)* and Lee et al. *(5)* for further discussion of these results.

11. The units $\mu A\ cm^{-2}$ are converted to $\mu Eq\ cm^{-2}\ h^{-1}$ using the following constants and relationship: 1 A = 1 C/s; 1 C = 6.25 $\times$ 10^{18} electrons; 1 mole = 6.0221367 $\times$ 10^{23} atoms, so 1 μA = 1μC/s = 1.0378 $\times$ 10^{-5} μEq/s or 3.736 $\times$ 10^{-2} $\mu Eq\ h^{-1}$ and 1 $\mu Eq\ h^{-1}$ = 26.77 μA for a monovalent ion.

12. If one had only measured the serosal to mucosal flux of Cl$^-$ in response to cAMP, one might incorrectly conclude that the I_{SC} was the result of net Cl$^-$ secretion, as was reported in an earlier study on Calu-3 cells *(31)*. It is therefore necessary to measure both unidirectional fluxes to establish the net movement of an ion. This net transport can then be compared to the I_{SC} to establish its contribution to the I_{SC}.

13. One must take care to be consistent with the assignment of the sign designation and the valance of the ion. The net absorption of a cation or the secretion of an anion will by convention yield a positive current and when substracted from the I_{SC}, will yield the JR_{net}. Similarly, the net secretion of a cation or absorption of an anion will yield a negative current and, when added to the I_{SC}, will yield JR_{net}.

Acknowledgments

The author would like to thank Ms. Michele Dobransky for her excellent secretarial assistance in the preparation of this chapter, and Ms. Maitrayee Sahu and Mr. Matthew Green for their excellent technical assistance. The support given by the Cystic Fibrosis Foundation and the National Institutes of Health are also gratefully acknowledged.

References

1. Quinton, P. M. (1999) Physiological basis of cystic fibrosis: a historical perspective. *Physiol. Rev.* **79**, S3–S22.
2. Smith, J. J. and Welsh, M. J. (1992) cAMP stimulates bicarbonate secretion across normal, but not cystic fibrosis airway epithelia. *J. Clin. Invest.* **89**, 1148–1153.

3. Willumsen, N. J. and Boucher, R. C. (1992) Intracellular pH and its relationship to regulation of ion transport in normal and cystic fibrosis human nasal epithelia. *J. Physiol. (Lond)* **455,** 247–269.

4. Devor, D. C., Singh, A. K., Lambert, L. C., DeLuca, A., Frizzell, R. A., and Bridges, R. J. (1999) Bicarbonate and chloride secretion in Calu-3 human airway epithelial cells. *J. Gen. Physiol.* **113,** 743–760.

5. Lee, M. C., Penland, C. M., Widdicombe, J. H., and Wine, J. J. (1998) Evidence that Calu-3 human airway cells secrete bicarbonate. *Am. J. Physiol.* **274,** L450–L453.

6. Basbaum, C. B., Jany, B., and Finkbeiner, W. E. (1990) The serous cell. *Annu. Rev. Physiol.* **52,** 97–113.

7. Puchelle, E., Gaillard, D., Ploton, D., Hinnrasky, J., Fuchey, C., Boutterin, M. C., Jacquot, J., Dreyer, D., Pavirani, A., and Dalemans, W. (1992) Differential localization of the cystic fibrosis transmembrane conductance regulator in normal and cystic fibrosis airway epithelium. *Am. J. Respir. Cell Mol. Biol.* **7,** 485–491.

8. Engelhardt, J. F., Zepeda, M., Cohn, J. A., Yankaskas, J. R., and Wilson, J. M (1994) Expression of the cystic fibrosis gene in adult human lung. *J. Clin. Invest.* **93,** 737–749.

9. Stetson, D. L., Beauwens, R., Palmisano, J., Mitchell, P. P., and Steinmetz, P. R. (1985) A double-membrane model for urinary bicarbonate secretion. *Am. J. Physiol.* **249,** F546–F552.

10. Novak, I. and Greger, R. (1988). Properties of the luminal membrane of isolated perfused rat pancreatic ducts. *Pfluegers Arch Eur. J. Physiol.* **411,** 546–553.

11. Ishiguro, H., Steward, M. C., Wilson, R. W., and Case, R. M. (1996) Bicarbonate secretion in interlobular ducts from guinea-pig pancreas. *J. Physiol. (Lond)* **495,** 179–191.

12. Ishiguro, H., Steward, M. C., Lindsay, A. R., and Case, R. M. (1996) Accumulation of intracellular HCO3-by Na(+)-HCO3-cotransport in interlobular ducts from guinea-pig pancreas. *J. Physiol. (Lond)* **495,** 169–178.

13. Abuladze, N., Lee, I., Newman, D., Hwang, J., Boorer, K., Pushkin, A., and Kurtz, I. (1998) Molecular cloning, chromosomal localization, tissue distribution, and functional expression of the human pancreatic sodium bicarbonate cotransporter. *J. Biol. Chem.* **273,** 17,689–17,695.

14. Peters, K. W., Gangopadhyay, N. N., Devor, D. C., Watkins, S. C., Frizzell, R. A., and Bridges, R. J. (1999). *Ped. Pulmonol.* **S19,** 193.

15. Marino, C. R., Jeanes, V., Boron, W. F., and Schmitt, B. M. (1999) Expression and distribution of the Na(+)-HCO(-)(3) cotransporter in human pancreas. *Am. J. Physiol.* **277,** G487–G494.

16. Romero, M. F., Hediger, M. A., Boulpaep, E. L., and Boron, W. F. (1997) Expression cloning and characterization of a renal electrogenic Na+/HCO3-cotransporter. *Nature* **387,** 409–413.

17. Gray, M. A., Pollard, C. E., Harris, A., Coleman, L., Greenwell, J. R., and Argent, B. E. (1990) Anion selectivity and block of the small-conductance chloride channel on pancreatic duct cells. *Am. J. Physiol.* **259,** C752–C761.

18. Linsdell, P., Tabcharani, J. A., and Hanrahan, J. W. (1997) Multi-Ion mechanism for ion permeation and block in the cystic fibrosis transmembrane conductance regulator chloride channel. *J. Gen. Physiol.* **110,** 365–377.
19. Illek, B., Tam, A. W., Fischer, H., and Machen, T. E. (1999). Anion selectivity of apical membrane conductance of Calu 3 human airway epithelium. *Pflugers Arch.* **437,** 812–822.
20. Hug, M., Frizzell, R. A., and Bridges, R. J. (2000) Forskolin-stimulated Calu-3 cells have a very high apical membrane conductance with important implications for the mechanisms of anion secretion. *Pediatric Pulmonology* **S20,** 209.
21. Wills, N. K., Reuss, L., and Lewis, S. A. (eds.) (1996) *Epithelial Transport.* Chapman & Hall, London, 1996.
22. Ussing, H. H. and Zerahn, K. (1999) Active transport of sodium as the source of electric current in the short-circuited isolated frog skin. Reprinted from *Acta Physiol. Scand.* **23,** 110–127. *J. Am. Soc. Nephrol.* **20,** 2056–2065.
23. Guba, M., Kuhn, M., Forssmann, W. G., Classen, M., Gregor, M., and Seidler, U. (1996) Guanylin strongly stimulates rat duodenal HCO3- secretion: proposed mechanism and comparison with other secretagogues. *Gastroenterology* **111,** 1558–1568.

8

Transepithelial Impedance Analysis
of Chloride Secretion

**Ashvani K. Singh, Sangeeta Singh, Daniel C. Devor,
Raymond A. Frizzell, Willy van Driessche, and Robert J. Bridges**

1. Introduction

Transepithelial chloride secretion requires the activation of both apical membrane chloride channels and basolateral membrane potassium channels. Chloride channels are needed for the apical membrane exit of chloride and potassium channels are needed to repolarize the cell and thereby provide the driving force for chloride exit. Chloride entry on the basolateral membrane $Na:K:2Cl^-$ cotransporter must be carefully matched with the apical membrane exit of chloride to maintain cell volume integrity and to achieve a sustained level of chloride secretion. Endogenous secretory agonists acting via intracellular signal transduction cascades (e.g., cAMP, Ca^{2+}) coordinate the activities of the apical and basolateral membrane channels and transporters by mechanisms that are still poorly understood. Moreover, several different types of chloride and potassium channels are thought to contribute to the secretion of chloride. In an effort to better understand the mechanisms that regulate the coordinated activation of apical and basolateral membrane channels and to investigate the relative contribution of various candidate chloride and potassium channels in chloride secretion we have begun to utilize transepithelial impedance analysis.

Impedance analysis provides a noninvasive means of obtaining estimates of the apical and basolateral membrane resistances (Ra, Rb) and capacitances (Ca, Cb) under various experimental conditions (*see* **Note 1**). Impedance (Z) can be defined as the resistance of an electrical circuit of resistors and capacitors measured in response to a sinusoidal signal at a given frequency. The units of Z are ohms. In practice one measures Z at a number of sinusoidal frequencies to obtain an impedance spectrum (*see* **Note 2**). Thus, impedance analysis describes the

From: *Methods in Molecular Medicine, vol. 70: Cystic Fibrosis Methods and Protocols*
Edited by: W. R. Skach © Humana Press Inc., Totowa, NJ

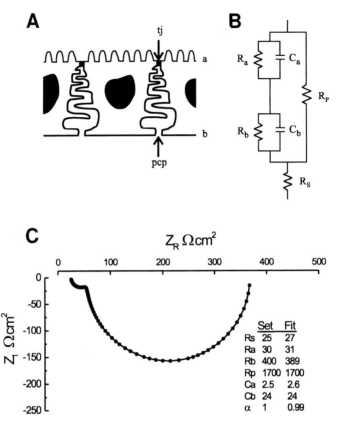

Fig. 1. Illustration of an epithelial monolayer, an equivalent electric circuit for an epithelial monolayer, and a Nyquist plot of an impedance spectrum. (**A**) The epithelial monolayer illustrates the apical and basolateral membrane domains separated at the tight junction (TJ) and the paracellular pathway (PCP). (**B**) The apical and basolateral membranes are shown as *RC* elements connected in series. These are connected to a parallel resistance (*RP*) and a series resistance (*RS*). *RP* is the resistance of the paracellular pathway and tight junction and *RS* is the solution resistance between the electrodes and the tissue. (**C**) The Nyquist plot shows the data points from an impedance spectrum taken with the analog circuit shown in B with known resistance and capacitance values (set) and the fitted values obtained by fitting the data using the BLIMP software. The solid line is the fit to the impedance spectrum.

properties of an epithelium in the frequency domain. A biological membrane can be modeled as a resistor (*R*) and capacitor (*C*) connected in parallel. An epithelium can be modeled as the equivalent electric circuit shown in **Fig. 1**. This model of an epithelial monolayer depicts two parallel *RC* elements connected in series, a parallel shunt resistance (*Rp*) and a series resistance (*Rs*). *Ra, Ca, Rb*, and *Cb* represent the resistances and capacitances of the apical and basolateral membranes, respectively. *Rp* is the resistance of the tight junction (TJ) and the paracellular pathway (PCP) and *Rs* is the solution resistance between the electrodes and the epithelium. This is the simplest model that can describe an epithelial monolayer and has been used by several laboratories to study transepithelial impedance *(1–6)* (*see* **Note 3**). In this chapter, we describe the methods we use to study chloride secretion in T84 monolayers by impedance analysis. Results from our studies will be presented to document the suitability of the equivalent electric circuit shown in **Fig. 1** to obtain estimates of the apical and basolateral electrical parameters in T84 monolayers. In addition, results will be presented to illustrate how one can use impedance analysis to define the site of action of some inhibitors of chloride secretion.

2. Materials

1. T84 cells (American Tissue Culture Collection, cat. no. CC1-248).
2. DMEM (Life Technologies, cat. no. 12100-046).
3. F-12 (Life Technologies, cat. no. 21700-075).
4. Fetal bovine serum, FBS (Hyclone, cat. no. SH30070.03).
5. Pen-Strep (Life Technologies, cat. no. 15140-122).
6. Trypsin (Life Technologies, cat. no. 15400-054).
7. Phosphate-buffered saline, PBS (Sigma, cat. no. P-4417).
8. T25-cm^2 flasks (Fisher, cat. no. 10-126-10).
9. Transwell filters (Costar, cat. no. 3470).
10. Ussing chambers, Snapwell vertical diffusion chambers (Costar, cat. no. 3430).
11. Silver chloride electrodes and electrode caps for Ussing chambers (Costar, cat. nos. 3433 and 3435).
12. Forskolin (RBI, cat. no., F-105).
13. Charybdotoxin, CTX (Sigma, cat. no. C7802).
14. 293B (Aventis, Germany).
15. Ussing chamber buffer: 120 mM NaCl, 25 mM NaHCO$_3$, 3.3 mM KH$_2$PO$_4$, 0.8 mM K$_2$HPO$_4$, 1.2 mM MgCl$_2$, 1.2 mM CaCl$_2$, and 10 mM glucose. The pH of this solution is 7.4 when gassed with a mixture of 95% O$_2$, 5% CO$_2$ at 37°C.
16. Heating manifold (Fisher, cat. no. 11-716-68; Thermolyne, cat. no. DB17615).
17. Voltage clamp aparatus.
18. 5,6-Dicholor-1-ethyl benzimidazolone (DCEBIO).

3. Methods
3.1. T84 Cell Cultures and Filter Preparation

1. T84 cells are maintained in DMEM/F12 (1/1) plus 5% FBS and 1% Pen-Strep culture medium. FBS is heat-inactivated at 56°C for 30 min. We typically add 100 mL FBS and 20 mL of Pen-Strep to 1900 mL DMEM and F12. The DMEM and F12 are prepared as described by the manufacturer. Cells are kept in an incubator at 37°C in 5% CO$_2$ and passaged once per week. We have successfully passaged the cells for more than 1 yr without any loss in transport phenotype. It is

important not to let the cells become overly confluent before passage and thus avoid the need for excessive exposure to the trypsin-ehtylenediaminetetraacetic acid (EDTA) solution.

2. To passage the cells, a 90%-confluent T_{25} flask of cells is washed with 5 mL of PBS for 1 min. The 10X trypsin-EDTA is diluted 1/1 with PBS to yield a 5X solution.
3. The PBS is removed and 1 mL of trypsin-EDTA is added, washed across the cells, and 0.5 mL is removed, leaving just enough to cover the cells.
4. The cells are incubated at 37°C for 8–10 min until the cells detach from the flask. Four milliliters of medium are added to the flask and the cells resuspended.
5. One milliliter of the resuspended cells is added to a T_{25} flask containing 4 mL of fresh media to passage the cells at a 1/4 split.
6. To prepare a Transwell filter, dilute 1 mL of the above cell suspension with 9 mL of fresh medium and mix well. Add 5 drops of the cell suspension to the top of a Transwell filter. Add 1.2 mL of fresh medium to the basolateral side. Feed both the flask and filters the day after seeding and every other day thereafter. The apical surface of the Transwell is fed with 3 drops of medium.
7. Filters are used 12–16 d after seeding, and we always feed the filters the night before using them. Grown in this manner, our T84 monolayers routinely have a transepithelial resistance of 1000–2000 Ω cm^2, a low basal I_{SC} of 1–3 µA/cm^2, and an I_{SC} response of 60–100 µA/cm^2 to maximal stimulatory concentrations of forskolin (2 µM).

3.2. Ussing Chamber Solutions

We typically prepare 500 mL of Ussing chamber buffer in a volumetric flask from 20X stock solutions of the above salts. When it is not in use the buffer is kept at 4°C, and it is gassed prior to each experiment. The solution is warmed to 37°C before use. This is important because cold solutions will stimulate chloride secretion in T84 cells. If the divalent salts have precipitated out of solution, usually because of the loss of CO_2 with storage, or if there is any growth in the solution, the buffer is discarded. The osmolarity of the buffer is checked each time a new flask is prepared and should be approx 290 mOsmol. It is good practice to measure the osmolarity each time a buffer is prepared since this is a good check that it has been prepared correctly.

3.3. Ussing Chamber Setup and Mounting Filters

1. The Costar vertical diffusion chamber modified to accept a Transwell filter is used to perform the impedance studies (*see* **Note 4**). In addition, one must purchase the electrode caps and electrodes to perform the impedance studies. A detailed description of how to set up the Costar chamber and the care and handling of the electrodes can be found in Chapter 7 of this volume. For technical reasons one must use the small surface area (0.33 cm^2) of the Transwell filters and not the larger surface area (1.1 cm^2) of the Snapwell filters.
2. Voltage-measuring electrodes must be fashioned so that they are as close to, but not touching, the filter as possible. In order to achieve this the mucosal electrode

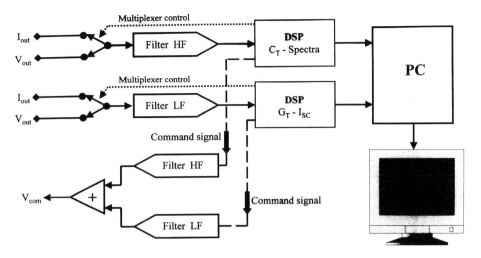

Fig. 2. Schematic of the impedance hardware. Two digital signal processing (DSP) boards (model 310B, Dalanco Spry, Rochester, NY) equipped with two high-speed (300 kHz) analog-to-digital converters (14-bit) and two digital-to-analog converters (12-bit) are connected to a personal computer (PC). The interface between the DSP boards and the high-speed voltage clamp consists of anti-aliasing filters, programmable gain amplifiers, and digital control circuits that are controlled by the DSP boards. One DSP board is used to record GT and I_{SC}. GT is measured by applying a 1-Hz sine wave voltage of 5 mV to the monolayer and calculated from the change in I_{SC}. The second DSP board is used to measure CT at five selectable frequencies via the high-pass filter. Impedance spectra were obtained by the same DSP board while I_{SC}, GT, and CT signals are interrupted.

    must have a small bend near the tip, so that it fits into the cup of the Transwell insert and thus can be placed close to the apical surface of the epithelium (*see* **Note 5**).

3. Once all the electrodes are in place, the chamber is placed in a heating manifold and the electrodes are connected to the voltage clamp. The heating manifold we use for the impedance studies is a custom aluminum jacket that surrounds the chamber and is mounted to an aluminum block that sets in a dri-bath-type heater The voltage clamp is a custom low-noise, high-bandwidth voltage clamp designed for the impedance studies by Dr. van Driessche's laboratory (*1,2*).

4. The voltage clamp is connected to two digital signal processing (DSP) boards mounted in a personal computer, as shown in **Fig. 2**. The impedance hardware and software were also developed by Dr. van Driessche and are available for purchase.

5. The software is run in a LabView environment and is very user friendly. The display is divided into three panels, one for the I_{SC}, one for GT, and one showing the capacitance at five different selectable frequencies. The I_{SC}, GT, and capacitance values at the five frequencies are all saved as an output file for further analysis. The display also has buttons to obtain an impedance spectrum as well as view previously obtained spectra. Thus, a spectrum can be obtained at any time during an I_{SC} experiment.

6. Each spectrum requires approx 35 s to acquire and calculate and is displayed as a Nyquist plot. Spectra can be acquired at fundamental frequencies of 1 or 4 Hz, and this too can be selected in the display window. Spectra are numbered consecutively and saved as an output file for further analysis. Details of the voltage clamp specifications and the impedance hardware and software have been published previously *(1,2)* (*see* **Note 6**).

3.4. Data Acquisition and Analysis

1. Impedance spectra can be acquired at any time during the experiment. In practice we wait for the I_{SC} to become stable and then acquire a set of three spectra. An experimental addition is then made (e.g., forskolin is added) and the I_{SC} allowed to change until a new stable value is achieved. At this time three additional spectra are acquired.
2. We have not found it necessary to discontinue gassing the chamber during the acquisition of the impedance spectra, nor has a Faraday cage been necessary.
3. Once the experiment is completed, the spectra are analyzed using a custom MatLab program called BLIMP, which was designed by the Bridges' laboratory and is available upon request. BLIMP uses a nonlinear least squares fitting routine to fit the impedance data to a one- or two-membrane model (*see* **Note 7**). The program requires an estimate of *RP*, which is obtained from the *y* intercept of a plot of *GT* vs I_{SC} as described by Wills et al. *(7)*.
4. We typically use the first 15–30 s of the initial *GT* vs I_{SC} response to forskolin and fit this by linear regression. Over a large number of experiments (>300), we have found that *RP* equals the reciprocal of 0.91 times the *GT* (*RP* = 1/0.91 *GT*) of a control unstimulated T84 monolayer. We assume R_P is constant under the different experimental conditions. We have validated this assumption using permeabilized monolayers. In addition, range analysis has shown that the value assigned to *RP* has little influence (<10%) on the estimates of *Ra*, *Ca*, and *Cb* but a larger influence on *Rb* (*see* **Note 8**).

3.5. Sample Results

1. As a test of the impedance hardware and software we prepared an analog circuit with resistors and capacitors with known measured values. This circuit was connected to the equipment and an impedance spectrum was obtained. The impedance values were then fitted using BLIMP to obtain estimates of the resistances and capacitances. As shown in **Fig. 1**, the equipment and software gave excellent estimates of the known values and an excellent fit (solid line) of the impedance spectrum. From this Nyquist plot one can see that each *RC* element appears as a semicircle (locus) and that the *RC* element of lower resistance and capacitance is seen at the left at the higher frequencies, while that of the higher resistance and capacitance is seen at the right at the lower frequencies.
2. Impedance results with T84 monolayers are shown in **Fig. 3**. The upper left panel is the I_{SC} response to forskolin, DCEBIO (*see* **Note 9**), CTX (charybdotoxin), and 293B. **Figures 3B–F** are the corresponding Nyquist plots from each of these experimental conditions. Under control, unstimulated conditions the transepithelial

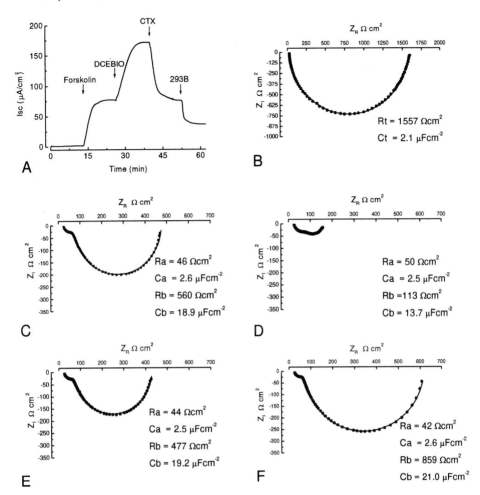

Fig. 3. Short circuit current trace and Nyquist plots from a T84 monolayer stimulated with forskolin and DCEBIO and inhibited with CTX and 293B: (**A**) I_{SC} trace; (**B**) Nyquist plot from control period; (**C**) After the addition of forskolin (2 µ*M*); (**D**) After DCEBIO (60 µ*M*), (**E**) After CTX (50 n*M*); (**F**) After 293B (10 µ*M*). Forskolin, DCEBIO, and 293B were added to both sides. CTX was added to the serosal side only. Spectra were fitted using BLIMP. Shown are the impedance values at 100 frequencies and the fit (solid line) to a one-membrane (A) or a two-membrane model (B–F).

impedance across T84 monolayers appears as a single impedance locus (semi-circle) in the Nyquist plot (*see* **Note 10**). Stimulation with forskolin causes a dramatic decrease in the total impedance and the resolution of two semicircles with distinctly separate loci. Addition of DCEBIO further reduces the total impedance due to a decrease in the right, low-frequency locus. Because DCEBIO under these experimental conditions affects the basolateral membrane potassium conductance, and based on morphological considerations, we suspected that the right locus corresponded to the basolateral membrane RC element. We confirmed this suspicion by showing that serosal CTX, a potent blocker of the DCEBIO-activated potassium channels (hIK1), decreased the DECBIO stimulated I_{SC}, increased the total impedance, and nearly restored the right locus to the pre-DCEBIO stimulated values. In addition, 293B, a blocker of cAMP-activated potassium channels, further decreased the I_{SC}, increased the impedance and caused a further shift of the right locus toward the pre-forskolin-stimulated values. Thus, the results of these pharmacological studies identify the right locus as the basolateral membrane and the left locus as the apical membrane in the Nyquist plot. The results also reveal that the apical membrane of forskolin-stimulated T84 cells has a remarkably low resistance of 40 Ω cm^2 and that DCEBIO does not further decrease the apical membrane resistance despite the substantial increase in I_{SC}. Therefore, in the presence of maximal stimulatory concentrations of forskolin, repolarization of the cell, mediated by the activation of basolateral membrane potassium channels, is rate-limiting to chloride secretion. Moreover, at this low apical membrane resistance (high conductance, 25 mS/cm^2), a driving force of only 4 mV is required to achieve a chloride secretory current of 100 μA/cm^2. Blockade of basolateral membrane potassium channels by CTX or 293B while decreasing the I_{SC} did not influence the apical membrane resistance, suggesting that there is little feedback regulation between the apical and basolateral membrane conductances. However, DCEBIO did cause Cb to decrease, and this was reversed by CTX. We speculate that this effect on Cb is due to the greater loss of intracellular KCl, which would cause the cell to shrink and thus decrease the surface area of the basolateral membrane. CTX, by blocking the DCEBIO activated potassium channels, reverses this effect.

3. The arylaminobenzoates such as DPC and NPPB and sulfonylureas such as glibenclamide have been shown by patch clamp methods to block CFTR *(8)*. There is in fact little doubt that under patch clamp conditions these compounds can block CFTR. Because of these patch clamp results, several studies have used these compounds as pharmacological tools to document the contribution of CFTR to a measured I_{SC}. Somewhat to our surprise, when DPC, NPPB, and glibenclamide were studied by impedance analysis, we observed a blockade of the basolateral membrane and only small changes on the apical membrane resistance (**Figs. 4–6**). Thus, the inhibitory effects of these compounds on I_{SC} cannot be attributed to a blockade of apical membrane CFTR. Rather, the effects of these compounds on I_{SC} must be attributed to a blockade of cAMP-activated potassium channels. Glibenclamide's blockade of K$_{ATP}$ channels is well documented *(8)*. Less studied are the effects of the arylaminobenzoates on potassium channels, although Greger and co-workers did warn against their blockade of basolateral membrane conductances in their original publication on this class of compounds *(9)*.

3.6. Summary

The above brief examples illustrate how one can use impedance analysis to study chloride secretion in T84 monolayers. Both the mechanisms regulating chloride secretion and the site of action of various pharmacological agents can

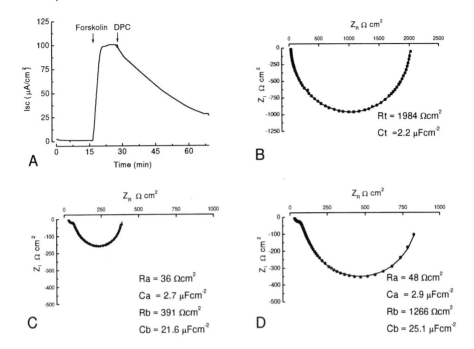

Fig. 4. Effects of forskolin and DPC on T84 cells. (**A**) I_{SC} trace; (**B**) Nyquist plot from the control period; (**C**) After the addition of forskolin (2 μM); (**D**) After the addition of DPC (1 mM). Forskolin and DPC were added to both sides. Other details are as given in **Fig. 3**.

be investigated. The methods for collecting impedance spectra can now easily be incorporated into an I_{SC} experiment to provide much more information than is made available from I_{SC} and RT measurements alone. The availability of the hardware and software to perform impedance studies should enable a larger number of laboratories to perform these studies and thus make impedance analysis a more commonly used method for transepithelial ion transport studies.

4. Notes

1. Recall that resistance (R) is equal to the reciprocal of conductance (G), so that $R = 1/G$. Therefore, estimates of the resistances provide a measure of the activation of the apical and basolateral membrane conductances that result from the opening of ion channels. Biological membranes also have a capacitance (C) such that 1 μF = 1 cm². Thus, estimates of C provide a measure of membrane surface area and are routinely used to study the insertion and retrieval of plasma membrane (but see **ref. 10** for an interesting discussion).

2. In principle, one does not have to use a sinusoidal signal, but this is a commonly used approach. A more detailed description of the use of impedance analysis for transepithelial studies, including additional theoretical background information, can be found in the excellent chapter by Lewis, Clausen, and Wills (*11*).

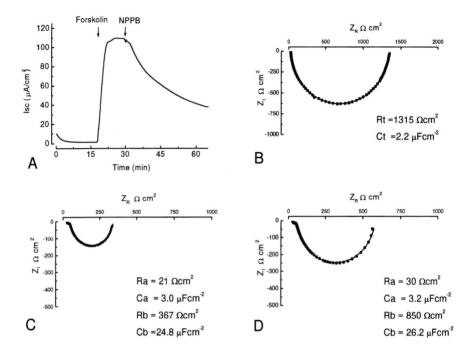

Fig. 5. Effects of forskolin and NPPB on T84 cells. (**A**) I_{SC} trace; (**B**) Nyquist plot from the control period; (**C**) After the addition of forskolin (2 μ*M*); (**D**) After the addition of NPPB (30 μ*M*). Forskolin and NPPB were added to both sides. Other details as given in **Fig. 3**.

3. Equivalent electric circuits of greater complexity have also been used to investi-gate transepithelial impedance, and the details of these models can be found in several references *(2,11–18)*. Several investigators have argued for the incorpo-ration of additional *RC* elements along the basolateral membrane, the so-called distributed model. As will be shown, the simpler model shown in **Fig. 1** appears to provide a good description of chloride secretion in T84 monolayers. Other cell types or the use of tissues of greater morphological complexity may require the use of more complex equivalent electric circuits to model the impedance results.

4. In their original design, the Costar chambers are made to accept a Snapwell filter. In order to accept a Transwell filter, the original Snapwell insert must be removed from the serosal side of the chamber and a new insert that accommodates the Transwell filter must be made and inserted. In addition, the mucosal side of the chamber must be milled out to accommodate the Transwell filter. Our machine shop would be happy to modify the chamber for a modest fee. Please contact Robert J. Bridges for further information.

5. It can be tricky to prepare the mucosal voltage-measuring electrode. As described for the preparation of the other electrodes (*see* Chapter 7), one may use a 200-μL glass pipet (Fisher, cat. no. 21-164-2J) cut to the proper length. The tip of this electrode (pipet) is bent under a flame so that it can slide into the Transwell filter

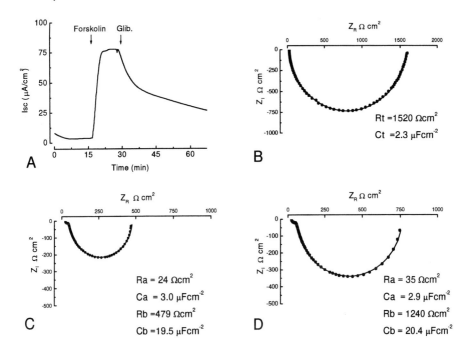

Fig. 6. Effects of forskolin and glibenclamide on T84 cells. (**A**) I_{SC} trace; (**B**) Nyquist plot from the control; (**C**) After the addition of forskolin (2 μM); (**D**) After the addition of glibenclamide (100 μM). Forskolin and NPPB were added to both sides. Other details as given in **Fig. 3**.

when attached to the electrode cap. The filter is first mounted in the chamber and then one must angle the electrode into the Transwell filter before securing the electrode cap. The current -passing electrode can then be inserted and the serosal electrode cap and electrodes placed in the chamber.

6. Impedance measurements are performed essentially as described by Margineanu and Van Driessche *(1)* and van Driessche et al. *(2)*. Briefly, the transepithelial electrical impedance is recorded with a computerized sine-wave method while the mean voltage across the epithelium is clamped to zero. A voltage signal composed of 99 sine waves is imposed on the tissue via the command input of the voltage clamp. The frequency range of the sine waves is 1–kHz and are equally spaced on a logarithmic scale. The transepithelial current (*It*) and voltage (*Vt*) signals are recorded consecutively. A synchronization pulse from the signal generator is used to initiate the sampling of a sweep of data points after first passing three training sweeps. The impedance (*Z*) is calculated as the ratio of the Fourier-transformed voltage and current signals. The calculations are done with data collected from a single sweep of sine waves. The impedance spectra are plotted as Nyquist plots.

7. The equivalent electric circuit shown in **Fig. 1** is used to calculate the apical and basolateral resistances (*Ra* and *Rb*) and capacitances (*Ca* and *Cb*). Each membrane is considered a simple *RC* network. Moreover, we assume a complex dielectric constant

(é–jé), which is generally found in biological membranes and results in the depression of the center of the semicircle into the region of the positive reactance. With this assumption, the impedance of one cell membrane can be described by the Cole-Cole equation *(19)*:

$$Z(f) = R_m/[1 + (jwR_mC_m)^\alpha \quad (1)$$

where $j = \sqrt{-1}$, and R_m and C_m represent the membrane resistance and capacitance respectively, $w = 2\pi f$ is the circular frequency and $\alpha = 1 - \theta$. θ is the angle in radians equal to $2\,\phi/\pi$, where ϕ is the angle (in degrees) between the real axis and the line that connects the center of the semicircle with its intersections with the real axis. Using **Eq. 1** to describe the impedance of apical and basolateral membranes and assuming an ohmic resistance for the impedance of the paracellular shunt path (*Rp*), the transepithelial impedance is given by **Eq. 2**:

$$Zt = Rs + [(As^\alpha + B)/(Cs^{2\alpha} + Ds^\alpha + 1)] \quad (2)$$

where *Rs* represents the resistance between the voltage electrodes in series with the epithelium and $s = jw$. *A*, *B*, *C*, and *D* are related to the resistances and capacitances of the apical and basolateral membrane:

$$A = Rp[Ra(RbCb)^2 + Rb(RaCa)^\alpha]/N \quad (3a)$$

$$B = Rp(Ra + Rb)/N \quad (3b)$$

$$C = Rp(RaCaRbCb)^\alpha/N \quad (3c)$$

$$D = \{Rb(RaCa)^a + Ra(RbCb)^\alpha + Rp[(RaCa)^\alpha + (RbCb)^\alpha]\} \quad (3d)$$

with $N = Ra + Rb + Rp$. *A*, *B*, *C*, and *D* are determined by the nonlinear curve fitting of **Eq. 2** to the impedance data. The real as well as imaginary parts are utilized in the fitting procedure. Weight factors, equal to the absolute value of the recorded data, are attributed to the data points and in this way all impedance data points deliver a comparable contribution to the sum of squares of differences. *Ra*, *Rb*, *Ca*, and *Cb* are calculated by solving **Eq. 3A–D**. *Rp* is determined independently by the method of Wills et al. *(18)* from the *y* intercept of a plot of the initial increase of I_{SC} vs *GT* in response to an agonist.

8. The lower limit for *RP* would be $RP = RT$ and this would be the case only when *Ra* and/or *Rb* approach an infinite resistance. An upper limit for *RP* cannot be stated with certainty. At low levels of stimulation, estimates of *Ra* and *Rb* are approx 3000 and 4000 Ω cm^2 respectively, suggesting that *RT* is dominated by *RP* in control unstimulated monolayers, results that are in good agreement with the estimate of *RP* obtained from the *GT* vs I_{SC} plots.

9. DCEBIO (5,6-dichloro-1-ethyl benzimidazolone) is a newly synthesized benzimidazolone derivative with improved potency compared to 1-EBIO for the activation of hIK-1 potassium channels *(20)*.

10. Although one might expect to see two impedance loci, given the presence of an apical and basolateral membrane, only one locus is observed in the Nyquist plot

from unstimulated T84 monolayers. Control experiments have shown that this spectrum is derived from the apical membrane capacitance and the paracellular resistance. Submaximal stimulation with forskolin (30 nM) to produce only a few microampers per square centimeter of chloride current is sufficient to reveal both apical and basolateral membranes in the Nyquist plot (data not shown).

Acknowledgments

The authors thank Mr. Matt Green and Ms. Maitrayee Sahu for their excellent technical assistances, and Ms. Michele Dobransky for her secretarial assistance. Robert J. Bridges would also like to thank Drs. Sandy Helman and Carol Bertrand for their many helpful discussions. This work was supported by a National Institutes of Health grant (no. 1P50DK56490) to Robert J. Bridges.

References

1. Margineanu, D. G. and Van Driessche, W. (1990) Effects of millimolar concentrations of glutaraldehyde on the electrical properties of frog skin. *J. Physiol.* **427,** 567–581.
2. Van Driessche, W., De Vos, R., Jans, D., Simaels, J., De Smet, P., and Raskin, G. (1999) Transepithelial capacitance decrease reveals closure of lateral interspace in A6 epithelia. *Eur. J. Physiol.* **437,** 680–690.
3. Kottra, G. (1995) Calcium is not involved in the cAMP-mediated stimulation of Cl-conductance in the apical membrane of Necturus gallbladder epithelium. *Pflugers Arch.* **429,** 647–658.
4. Bertrand, C. A., Durand, D. M., Saidel, G. M., Laboisse, C., and Hopfer, U. (1998) System for dynamic measurements of membrane capacitance in intact epithelial monolayers. *Biophys. J.* **75,** 2743–2756.
5. Bertrand, C. A., Laboisse, C. L., and Hopfer, U. (1999) Purinergic and cholinergic agonists induce exocytosis from the same granule pool in HT29-Cl. 16E monolayers. *Am. J. Physiol.* **276,** C907–C914.
6. Schifferdecker, E. and Fromter, E. (1978) The AC impedance of Necturus gallbladder epithelium. *Pflugers Arch.* **377,** 125–133.
7. Wills, N. K., Lewis, S. A., and Eaton, D. C. (1979) Active and passive properties of rabbit descending colon: a microelectrode and nystatin study. *J. Membr. Biol.* **45,** 81–108.
8. Schultz, B. D., Singh, A. K., Devor, D. C., and Bridges, R. J. (1999) Pharmacology of CFTR chloride channel activity. *Physiol. Rev.* **79,** S109–S144.
9. Wangemann, P., Wittner, M., Distefano, A., Englert, H. C., Lang, H. J., Schlatter, E., and Gregger, R. (1986) Cl$^-$ channel blockers in the thick ascending limb of the loop of Henle. Structure activity relationship. *Pflugers Arch.* **407,** S128–S141.
10. Awayda, M. S., Van Driessche, W., and Helman, S. I. (1999) Frequency-dependent capacitance of the apical membrane of frog skin: dielectric relaxation processes. *Biophys. J.* **76,** 219–232.
11. Lewis, S. A., Clausen, C. and Wills, N. K. (1996) Impedance analysis of epithelia, in *Epithelial Transport* (Wills, N. K., Reuss, L., and Lewis, S. A., eds.), pp. 118–145.

12. Clausen, C. (1989) Impedance analysis in tight epithelia. *Meth. Enzymol.* **171,** 628–663.
13. Kottra, G. and Fromter, E. (1984) Rapid determination of intraepithelial resistance barriers by alternating current spectroscopy. I. Experimental procedures. *Pflugers Arch.* **402,** 409–420.
14. Kottra, G. and Fromter, E. (1984) Rapid determination of intraepithelial resistance barriers by alternating current spectroscopy. II. Test of model circuits and quantification of results. *Pflugers Arch.* **402,** 421–432.
15. Gordon, L. G. M., Kottra, G., and Fromter, E. (1989) Electrical impedance analysis of leaky epithelia: Theory, techniques, and leak artifact problems. *Methods Enzymol.* **171,** 642-663.
16. Clausen, C., Machen, T. E., and Diamond, J. M. (1983) Use of AC impedance analysis to study membrane changes related to acid secretion in amphibian gastric mucosal. *Biophys. J.* **41,** 167–178.
17. Clausen, C., Lewis, S. A., and Diamond, J. M. (1979) Impedance analysis of a tight epithelium using a distributed resistance model. *Biophys. J.* **26,** 291–317.
18. Wills, N. K., Purcell, R. K., and Clausen, C. (1992) Na$^+$ transport and impedance properties of cultured renal (A6 and 2F3) epithelia. *J. Membr. Biol.* **125,** 273–285.
19. Cole, K. S. and Cole, R. H. (1941) Dispersion and absorption in dielectrics. I. Alternating current characteristics. *J. Chem. Phys.* **9,** 341–351.
20. Singh, S., Syme, C. A., Singh, A. K., Devor, D. C., and Bridges, R. J. (2001) Benzimidazolone activators of chloride secretion: potential therapeutics for cystic fibrosis and chronic obstructive pulmonary disease. *J. Pharmacol. Exp. Ther.* **296,** 605–616.

9

Studies of the Molecular Basis for Cystic Fibrosis Using Purified Reconstituted CFTR Protein

Ilana Kogan, Mohabir Ramjeesingh, Canhui Li, and Christine E. Bear

1. Introduction

Studies of purified, reconstituted cystic fibrosis transmembrane conductance regulator (CFTR) protein have proven invaluable in defining those functions that are intrinsic to the CFTR molecule. Reconstitution of purified CFTR protein in planar lipid bilayers provided direct evidence that CFTR possesses intrinsic activity as a protein kinase A (PKA)-regulated chloride channel *(1)*. Further, it appears that the regulation of the CFTR channel gate (the structure essential for opening and closing of the channel pore) reported in biological membranes has been recapitulated with fidelity in studies of reconstituted purified protein. For example, patch clamp studies on biological membranes revealed that ATP binding and/or hydrolysis by the PKA-phosphorylated CFTR channel caused channel opening and closing *(2–6)*. This unique requirement for ATP in channel gating was also reported in reconstitution studies of the purified protein *(7,8)*, indicating that the CFTR protein itself can mediate regulated chloride flux without the requirement for accessory proteins. These results also justify the use of purified protein in detailed biochemical and structural studies of mechanisms underlying the function of this protein. The CFTR molecule is known to be comprised of two membrane-spanning domains (TMDs), two nucleotide-binding domains (NBDs), and the phosphorylation-dependent regulatory or R domain *(9)*. However, to date, our understanding of the structure of these domains and the coordination of their activities is limited.

The apparent requirement for ATP hydrolysis in channel gating suggested that CFTR possesses intrinsic activity as an ATPase. Peter Pedersen and his colleagues were the first to demonstrate that the first NBD of CFTR exhibits

From: *Methods in Molecular Medicine, vol. 70: Cystic Fibrosis Methods and Protocols*
Edited by: W. R. Skach © Humana Press Inc., Totowa, NJ

ATPase activity *(10)*. We showed that the two nucleotide-binding folds function in a coordinated manner to mediate ATPase actvity in the intact CFTR protein *(11)*. Assessments of the catalytic activity by the intact CFTR protein revealed that ATP turnover is very slow, at 0.2 molecules ATP hydrolyzed per second. This slow hydrolysis rate is comparable to the slow rate of channel gating between the open and the closed state consistent with the model wherein ATPase activity is required for channel gating *(3–5,12–14)*. Future studies are required to investigate the mechanism for coupling between these functions of CFTR. Due to the low catalytic activity of CFTR and its relatively low expression in biological membranes, direct biochemical and biophysical studies of the coupling between the catalytic and conduction properties of this protein should ideally be performed using purified, reconstituted CFTR protein.

In the following paragraphs, we describe the current methods that we use for the purification, reconstitution, and functional assessment of the CFTR protein. Finally, we provide evidence of the utility of this reconstitution system for studying the molecular basis for disease associated with common mutations in the cystic fibrosis (CF) gene.

1.1. Expression of CFTR Protein in Sf9 Insect Cells

The availability of large quantities of biologically active protein is fundamental for studying the structure and function of membrane proteins. One method of producing high levels of recombinant CFTR protein is to use the *Spodoptera frugiperda* fall armyworm ovary (Sf9)-baculovirus expression system *(15,16)*. The yield of the recombinant protein produced by this method is high, i.e., approx 1% of total cellular proteins *(1)*. Due to high-level species specificity, infection of insect cells by the baculovirus is exclusive, thereby making this expression method a safe one to use. Moreover, insect cells can generate recombinant proteins that functionally resemble their native counterparts, due to the cells' ability to carry out many posttranslational modifications *(17)*. However, CFTR produced by Sf9 cells possesses only core glycosylation, as compared to the complex glycosylation pattern observed with CFTR produced in mammalian cells. To date, however, there is no evidence to suggest that differences in glycosylation patterns affect the structure or function of CFTR *(18)*. Sf9 insect cells also appear to have relatively permissive quality control mechanisms with respect to protein processing. As a result, CFTR variants such as CFTR-ΔF508, which are misprocessed and cannot reach the cell membrane in mammalian cells can be relatively well expressed at the cell surface of Sf9 cells *(19)*. Therefore, we use Sf9-baculovirus expression system for large-scale purification of wild-type and mutant CFTR proteins. The methods necessary for infection of the Sf9 cells with baculovirus containing the open reading frame (ORF) of CFTR have been described in detail in another recent publication *(18)*.

1.2. Solubilization and Purification of CFTR Protein Using Pentadecafluorooctanoic Acid (PFO)

Purification of membrane proteins requires their dissociation from interacting cellular proteins and membrane phospholipids using compatible detergents. The membrane protein of interest can then be purified from the mixed protein-detergent micelles by virtue of distinctive physicochemical properties or specific affinity with an immobilized ligand. CFTR is a very hydrophobic membrane protein and is poorly soluble in most detergents except the strong ionic detergent sodium dodecyl sulfate (SDS) and the salts of PFO *(1,20)*. In the original method we published with J. R. Riordan, CFTR solubilized in SDS was purified primarily by affinity to hydroxyapatite. Unfortunately, this purification procedure is quite complex and time-consuming *(1)*. Several membrane proteins have been purified by an easier method, using nickel-affinity chromatography. This method relies on the affinity of a polyhistidine tail (His), engineered onto the amino or carboxyl terminus of the protein, to nickle resin *(21,22)*. CFTR solubilized in SDS could not be purified by this method, as SDS prevented the binding of His-tagged proteins to the nickel resin *(20)*. On the other hand, purification of His-tagged CFTR, solubilized in PFO, by nickel-affinity chromatography is relatively rapid and simple, since PFO does not interrupt interaction of His-tagged proteins with the nickel column. PFO is a fluorinated surfactant with a hydrophobic fluorocarbon chain and a carboxyl group, making it much more surface-active than ordinary surfactants. Due to these characteristics, PFO is a more effective detergent for the solubilization of hydrophobic membrane proteins when compared to other detergents such as CHAPS or Triton *(20,23)*. This novel purification method has already had a major positive impact on our ability to produce purified wild-type and mutant CFTR protein.

2. Materials

2.1. CFTR Solubilization

1. Solubilization solution A (for Sf9 cell pellet): 150 mL phosphate-buffered saline (PBS) containing 2% Triton X-100, 5 mM MgCl$_2$, 20 U/mL DNase I, and a cocktail of the following protease inhibitors: 10 µg/mL, 10 µg/mL leupeptin, 10 µM aprotinin, 10 µM E64, 1 mM benzamidine, and 2 mM, dithiothreitol (DTT).
2. Solubilization solution B (for isolated membranes): 8% PFO (Oakwood Products, West Colombia, SC) in 25 mM phosphate, pH 8.0.
3. Buffer A: 4% PFO in 25 mM phosphate and 100 mM NaCl, pH 8.0 (filtered through Steritop-GP 0.22-µM filter, Millipore, Bedford, MA).
4. Buffer B: 4% PFO in 25 mM phosphate and 100 mM NaCl, pH 6.0 (filtered).
5. Buffer C: 8 mM HEPES, 0.5 mM EGTA, pH 7.2.

2.2. CFTR Reconstitution in Proteoliposomes

1. Phosphatidylethanolamine (PE; from egg; Avanti Polar Lipids, Birmingham, AL).
2. Phosphatidylserine (PS; from brain; Avanti Polar Lipids)
3. Phosphatidylcholine (PC; from egg yolk; Avanti Polar Lipids).
4. Ergosterol (Sigma, St. Louis, MO). Ergosterol is recrystallized from ethanol, dried under vaccum, and stored at –20°C.
5. Buffer C: 8 mM HEPES, 0.5 mM EGTA, pH 7.2.

2.3. Phosphorylation of CFTR by Protein Kinase A (PKA)

1. 10× PKA buffer: 2.5 μM catalytic subunit of PKA (Promega, Madison, WI), 5 μL 50 mM ATP, 0.5 μL 1 M MgCl$_2$, 42 μL 50 mM Tris-HCl/50 mM NaCl, pH 7.5.
2. 10× phosphorylation solution: 500 mM Tris-HCl, 500 mM NaCl, pH 7.5.
3. Buffer D: 8 mM HEPES, 0.5 mM EGTA, 0.025% NaN$_3$, pH 7.2
4. Buffer C: 8 mM HEPES, 0.5 mM EGTA, pH 7.2.

2.4. Analysis of CFTR Activity

1. Buffer E: 100 mM Tris base, 200 mM NaCl, 20 mM MgCl$_2$, pH 7.5.
2. [α-^{32}P]ATP, 10 μCi/μL (Amesham, Oakville, ON).
3. PEI cellulose TLC plastic plates, 20 × 20 cm (VWR, Mississauga, ON).
4. ADP/ATP separation solution: 1 M formic acid, 0.5 M LiCl.
5. Stop solution: 10% SDS, 88% formic acid (v/v).

3. Methods
3.1. Solubilization of Sf9 Cell Pellet in PFO

1. Sf9 cell pellet (from 1 L of Sf9 cell culture) expressing recombinant CFTR-His protein is thawed, resuspended in solubilization solution A, and mutated 2 h at room temperature.
2. The solubilized cell pellet is centrifuged at 100,000g for 2 h at 4°C and the supernatant is discarded.
3. The pellet, containing crude plasma membranes, is resuspended in 100 mL of solubilization solution B, stirred overnight at room temperature, and filtered through a 0.22-μM filteration unit before its application to the nickel column.

3.2. Purification of CFTR-His Using Nickel-Affinity Chromatography and Identification of Immunopositive Fractions

Purification of proteins using a column attached to an FPLC allows one to efficiently control the elution conditions—e.g., establish an accurate pH gradient—as compared to standard batch purification. Therefore, in these experiments we use an FPLC attached to a fraction collector to elute and collect the purified CFTR protein.

1. The filtered sample is applied to a freshly regenerated nickel column containing 25 mL of packed nickel chelating resin (Qiagen, Mississauga, ON), which is attached to an FPLC (Pharmacia Biotech, Piscataway, NJ) or any other liquid

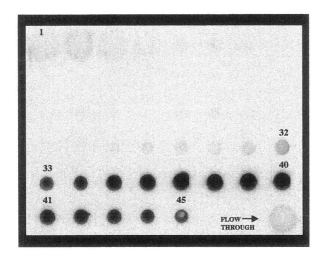

Fig. 1. A dot-blot showing the elution profile of CFTR with a pH gradient ranging from 8.0 (fraction 1) to 6.0. The immunopositive fractions (fractions 33–45) were eluted at pH 6.7, and identified by an anti-CFTR polyclonal antibody. This antibody was raised against the polyhistidine-tagged portion of the protein, corresponding to the predicted NBD2 and C-terminus domains of CFTR, amino acids N1197-L1480 (Kartner, N. and Riordan, J. R. [1998] *Meth. Enzymol.* **292,** 629–652). The flow-through did not display immunoreactivity.

    chromatography system that can generate a "linear" pH gradient. The CFTR-His sample is applied to the column at a 2 mL/min rate. The column is then washed with 100 mL of buffer A (*see* **Note 1**).

2. A pH gradient is applied to the column: buffer A is titered with buffer B, from 100% buffer A to 100% buffer B over 100 mL. The column is further washed with 50 mL buffer B.

3. Five-mililiter fractions are collected and analyzed by dot-blot for the presence of CFTR protein (**Fig. 1**) (*see* **Note 2**).

4. Immunopositive fractions are chosen to be concentrated. To maximize the stability and the catalytic activity of the purified CFTR protein, it is important to concentrate and reconstitute the selected fractions as soon as possible. Therefore, each immunopositive fraction is concentrated *separately* in a Centricon YM-100 concentrator (molecular cutoff 100 kDa; Millipore) to a final volume of approx 100 µL.

5. Concentrated samples in 4% PFO, 25 m*M* phosphate, and 100 m*M* NaCl are diluted 1:10 with buffer C and further concentrated to a final volume of 100 µL to reduce the PFO concentration to 0.4%.

6. Three microliters from each concentrated fraction are used to analyze the quantity and purity of CFTR protein by Western blot and silver-stained protein gel (**Fig. 2**). Best fractions are later combined, reconstituted into proteoliposomes, and phosphorylated (*see* **Subheading 3.4.**).

A

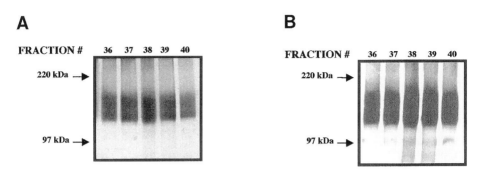

B

Fig. 2. A silver-stained gel (**A**) and Western blot (**B**) of a purified wild-type CFTR protein. The silver-stained gel shows the presence of a protein with the expected molecular weight in selected fractions eluted from the nickel column. The Western blot shows a major immunopositive band when a polyclonal anti-CFTR antibody is used. The minor immunopositive band represents a small fraction of degraded CFTR protein.

3.3. Reconstitution of CFTR Protein into Liposomes from PFO

To study the structure and function of a purified membrane protein, it is essential that the detergent in which the protein is purified be exchanged for phospholipids. This exchange is a time- and concentration-dependent process. Typically, phospholipids are added to detergent-solubilized proteins and then the detergent is removed by dialysis or detergent adsorption resins (24,25). Only when the detergent concentration decreases below a critical value (critical micelle concentration or CMC) can detergent monomers dissociate from the micelles and proteoliposomes be formed (26). Detergents with high CMC values, such as PFO, are easily removed by the dialysis method (20,27).

The choice of lipid composition used for the reconstitution procedure is essential for obtaining functionally active as well as correctly folded reconstituted protein. These phospholipids must give rise to well-sealed proteoliposomes and allow formation of biologically active proteins (26). Since PE and PS are likely important for enhancing the catalytic activity of other members of the ATP-binding-cassette (ABC) transporters such as P-glycoprotein, these lipids are also used for CFTR reconstitution (28). Further, PS (a negatively charged phospholipid) and PC are good bilayer-forming lipids, with the former helping maintain liposome integrity by decreasing the tendency of liposomes to aggregate (29). Although PE alone cannot form liposomes in physiological conditions, when used in combination with other lipids, it allows liposomes to be more fusogenic (29,30). This parameter is important for investigating the single-channel activity of CFTR in planar lipid bilayers. Ergosterol is also added to CFTR-containing liposomes, because it promotes their fusion with planar bilayers, once they are spiked with nystatin (1,31).

3.3.1. Liposome Preparation

1. A 2 mL lipid mixture containing PE/PS/PC in chloroform (ratio of 5/2/1 by weight; 10 mg/mL) is mixed with 250 μL of ergosterol (10 mg/mL in chloroform) in a 20-mL Pyrex test tube. The final PE/PS/PC/ergosterol ratio of the lipid mixture is 5/2/1/1 by weight.
2. The lipid mixture is dried first by nitrogen gas and then by argon gas to produce a layer of lipids on the bottom of the test tube. An even lipid layer is achieved by rotating the tube during the drying procedure.
3. Two milliliters of buffer C are added to the dry lipid mixture and the lipid/buffer combination is then sonicated in a bath sonicator (model G112SP1G, Laboratory Supplies, Hicksville, NY) until the solution becomes translucent. To prevent overheating of lipids and test tube, it is important to add ice to the sonicator during the sonication procedure. Aliquots of liposomes are kept frozen at –80°C and are sonicated before use.

3.3.2. Reconstitution of CFTR Protein into Liposomes by the Dialysis Procedure

Following elution of CFTR-His from the nickel column, the purified protein is first present in mixed micelles containing 4% PFO. After dilution of the micelles in buffer, pure CFTR in 0.4% PFO is mixed with excess of a sonicated lipid mixture containing PE/PS/PC/ergosterol. Next, the protein/lipid mixture is dialyzed, allowing slow removal of the remaining PFO and gradual formation of bilayer vesicles containing the purified protein.

1. Approximately 100 μL of each concentrated fraction (*see* **Subheading 3.2.**) is combined with 1 mg of the lipid mixture containing PE/PS/PC/ergosterol (5/2/1/1 by weight).
2. A lipid control is generated by diluting 1 mg of lipid mixture containing PE/PS/PC/ergosterol into 100 μL of buffer C. This control is essential for determining the amount of spontaneous ATP hydrolysis during the ATPase assay (*see* **Subheading 3.5.**).
3. The above concentrated CFTR fractions and the lipid control are dialyzed in a Spectra/Por dialysis membrane (Spectrum Laboratories, Rancho Dominguez, CA; molecular weight cutoff 50 kDa) overnight at 4°C against 4 L of buffer C.

3.4. Phosphorylation of CFTR Protein by the Catalytic Subunit of Protein Kinase A (PKA)

As mentioned previously, in addition to the two TMDs and NBDs, CFTR contains the unique R domain. This highly charged hydrophilic regulatory domain contains a number of potential phosphorylation sites for both protein kinase C and the cAMP-dependent protein kinase A (PKA) *(9,32–34)*. In CFTR, there are 10 dibasic consensus sites for recognition by PKA [(R/K)(R/K)X(S*/T*); asterisk represents potential phosphorylation sites], nine of which are found on the R domain *(35)*. Phosphorylation of the R domain by PKA plays an important role in CFTR regulation. Evidence to date suggests that phosphorylation of serine residues in the R domain by PKA is the primary mechanism controlling CFTR chloride channel activity *(36,37)*. However, phosphorylation of CFTR protein by PKA is not sufficient to activate chloride channel function. Electrophysiological studies suggest that ATP binding and/ or hydrolysis at each NBD is essential for normal opening and closing of the channel pore *(2–6)*. Further, studies with intact, purified CFTR protein show that PKA phosphorylation modulates the ATPase activity of CFTR by increasing CFTR's affinity to ATP *(7)*. In summary, since PKA phosphorylation is a prerequisite for both the channel function and the catalytic activity of the CFTR protein, it is important to phosphorylate the purified CFTR protein to study the complex structure and function of this molecule.

1. After the quantity and purity of CFTR protein in the different fractions eluted from the column are determined (*see* **Subheading 3.2.**), best fractions are removed from the dialysis bag and combined into one tube.
2. Half of the reconstituted CFTR protein and the lipid control are phosphorylated by the catalytic subunit of PKA. Reconstituted CFTR (200–500 μg of total purified CFTR) is phosphorylated for 1 h at room temperature in a reaction mixture containing 10× phosphorylation solution and 10× PKA buffer to yield the following final concentrations: 250 nM catalytic subunit of PKA, 1 mM MgCl$_2$, and 500 μM ATP. The other half of the CFTR sample and the lipid control are mock-phosphorylated (i.e., same reaction mixture as with the phosphorylated samples except that no PKA is added to the reaction).
3. Removal of PKA after the phosphorylation reaction is required to avoid interference of the kinase with the intrinsic ATPase activity of the pure CFTR protein *(18)*. Thus, to remove PKA, all samples are dialyzed in a Spectra/Por dialysis membrane (molecular weight cutoff 50 kDa) overnight at 4°C, against 4 L of buffer D. The next day, buffer D is changed to buffer C and the samples are further dialyzed at 4°C overnight.

3.5. Analysis of the Activity of Purified CFTR Protein

As we have published, a PKA activated 10 pS chloride channel is consistently observed in our planar bilayer studies of purified, reconstituted CFTR *(1,7,20)*. Further, we determined that the purified and phosphorylated channel recapitulates the unique dependence on ATP binding and hydrolysis observed for CFTR in biological membranes *(7,8)*. In conclusion, our biochemical studies documenting the ATPase activity of purified, reconstituted CFTR protein reinforce previous models wherein ATP binding and hydrolysis is necessary for normal CFTR channel function *(2,3,5,7,8,12)*. Furthermore, these findings support the application of this experimental system for detailed biochemical, biophysical, and structural studies of the mechanisms underlying function in the wild-type CFTR molecule, and investigations of how these mechanisms may be perturbed by mutations known to cause human disease.

In the following paragraphs we discuss our current biochemical methods for the measurement of CFTR ATPase activity as these methods have undergone revisions since the original protocols were published *(1,18,20)*. For example, one major change in the protocol is the requirement of the purified protein to be used fresh (i.e., immediately after the dialysis and without freezing). We observed that the catalytic activity of the purified and reconstituted CFTR protein markedly decreased after freezing and thawing cycles. Another revision of the previous protocol is the shorter time required for the ATPase assay, that is, 2 h rather than 4 h. On the other hand, our assays of CFTR channel have not been substantially revised since our description in *Methods in Enzymology (18)* and therefore will not be revisited in this chapter.

1. The ATPase assay is carried out in a 40-µL reaction mixture containing the following components: 30 µL of the freshly dialyzed proteoliposomes, 8 µL of 5 mM ATP in buffer E, and 2 µL [α-^{32}P]ATP (2 µCi/reaction). The ATPase mixture is sonicated for approx 3 s to distribute the different components equally inside and outside the proteoliposomes (*see* **Note 4**).
2. The ATPase reaction mixture is then incubated at 33°C for 2 h.
3. The reaction is stopped by the addition of 14 µL of stop solution. Reactions can be then stored at –80°C.
4. TLC plates are prespotted with 1 µL of 5 mM nonradioactive ADP/ATP mixture and allowed to air-dry. One-microliter samples from the ATPase reaction are then spotted onto the TLC plates and allowed to dry. Spotted plates are placed into a chamber containing ADP/ATP separation solution, and samples are allowed to run until the solution reaches the top of the plates. Plates are removed from the chamber and allowed to air dry.
5. STORM840 Molecular Dynamics PhosphorImager is used to visualize ADP production by phosphorylated and nonphosphorylated CFTR samples (**Fig. 3**). The quantity of ATP hydrolyzed is then determined using the ImageQuant software package (Molecular Dynamics, Sunnyvale, CA).

3.6. Methods for Analyzing the Molecular Basis for Disease Caused by CFTR Mutations

At last count, there were upwards of 900 putative disease-causing mutations identified in the CFTR gene, which are essentially scattered throughout the molecule (CF Genetic Analysis Consortium; accessible electronically at www.genet.sickkids.on.ca). Classification schemes have been proposed with which to categorize the molecular consequences for these mutations and to attempt to correlate these various categories with disease severity *(38,39)*. Many of the disease-causing mutations appear to belong to one or two of these categories and are described as "processing" and/or "regulation" mutants. The most common mutation, accounting for 70% of mutations in all alleles, is due to a deletion of phenylalanine in the first putative NBD at position 508 (ΔF508) and is described as a "processing" mutant. This variant exhibits a defect either

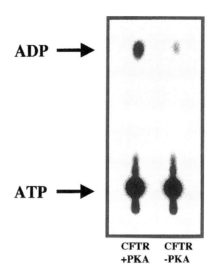

Fig. 3. ATPase activity of phosphorylated and nonphosphorylated wild-type CFTR protein. Separation of $[\alpha\text{-}^{32}P]ATP$ and $[\alpha\text{-}^{32}P]ADP$ by thin-layer chromatography. The phosphorylated CFTR sample displays significantly greater catalytic activity, that is, more ATP hydrolysis or ADP production, as compared to the nonphosphorylated sample.

in folding or conformation, which excludes it from the normal processing pathway and stable localization at the cell surface (40–43). Hence, the mislocalization of this mutant in epithelial cells likely accounts for disease severity (44). Furthermore, the relative lack of surface expression of the CFTR-ΔF508 channel on the plasma membrane is problematic for studying the channel activity using conventional patch clamp techniques. Compared to CFTR-ΔF508, all of the other mutations within the CFTR gene occur with far less frequency. Of these infrequent mutations, CFTR-G551D is relatively common, accounting for roughly 5% of mutations in all alleles. In contrast to CFTR-ΔF508, CFTR-G551D is stably expressed on the cell surface but functions abnormally as a channel (38,45,46).

In 1993, we reported that purified CFTR-ΔF508 protein exhibited near-normal channel function following reconstitution into planar lipid bilayers. These studies, along with findings in other experimental systems reporting chloride channel function of CFTR-ΔF508 (47,48), provided a rationale for developing pharmacological means to overcome the "processing" problem in affected cells. However, other studies of CFTR-ΔF508 in mammalian cell expression systems showed that the few molecules that escaped quality control and reached the cell surface exhibited abnormal gating kinetics, with a marked reduced rate of channel opening (49,50). A possible explanation for the differences in the

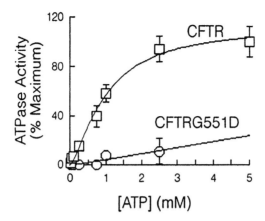

Fig. 4. CFTR-G551D displays defective ATPase activity compared to wild-type CFTR. The graph displays the relationship between the ATP concentration and the catalytic activity of purified and reconstituted wild-type ($n = 3$) and mutant ($n = 3$) CFTR proteins. The data were fitted by nonlinear regression analysis using the Hill equation. The mean ± standard deviation is shown for each point. With permission from ref. *(7)*.

channel kinetics reported in these studies, as compared to purified CFTR-ΔF508, was recently offered in a study reported by Wang et al. *(49)*. These authors found that ΔF508 channel function exhibited a defect in phosphorylation-dependent activation. However, once fully phosphorylated, CFTR-ΔF508 channels behaved like wild-type channels. It is possible that in our studies of purified, reconstituted CFTR-ΔF508 we observed activity close to that of the wild-type protein due to (1) the complete phosphorylation of the mutant by exogenous PKA and (2) lack of phosphatases in the reconstitution system. Thus, the studies of Wang et al., together with our findings regarding the regulation of CFTR ATPase activity, suggest a novel mechanism wherein the ΔF508 mutation could cause disease. We suggest that both the structural and functional coupling between the phosphorylated R domain and NBDs may be disrupted by the mutation. This hypothesis predicts that the catalytic activity of CFTR-ΔF508 may exhibit altered phosphorylation dependence, and this prediction is currently being tested in our laboratory.

In contrast to our findings with purified CFTR-ΔF508, we found that both the channel gating and the ATPase functions of CFTR-G551D were severely impaired, suggesting that the molecular bases for disease associated with CFTR-ΔF508 and CFTR-G551D are very different (**Fig. 4**). Further, our findings for CFTR-G551D provided direct evidence that the channel activity and the ATPase activity of CFTR are coupled *(7)*. Our current studies focus on understanding how mutation of the glycine residue in position 551 can have such a profound effect on both functions of CFTR. Alignment of the CFTR

sequence with the crystal structure of histidine permease *(51)* places this residue (aa 551) of CFTR in a location that is far removed from the ATP-binding
site of the first NBD. Hence, it is likely that mutation of glycine to aspartic acid
prevents domain–domain interactions, essential for both the catalytic and conduction functions of CFTR.

Recent data by Linsdell and Hanrhan suggest that CFTR may mediate not
only chloride conductance, but also the energy-dependent flux of organic
anions such as glutathione *(52,53)*. Future studies of the ability of purified
CFTR to mediate active transport are necessary to address these hypotheses
and correlate CFTR mutations to possible defects in transport functions.

In summary, studies with purified, reconstituted CFTR protein have informed
us and will continue to provide further knowledge about the intrinsic functional
properties of this protein. This reconstitution system will also help to identify the
specific functions, targetted by disease-causing mutations. Moreover, in the
future, studies with pure CFTR will yield the structural information required to
reveal how CFTR functions and how its regulation is perturbed in cystic fibrosis.

4. Notes

1. Buffers A and B and the nickel column should be all kept at a temperature higher
   than 25°C to avoid precipitation of PFO.
2. If not used immediately, eluted fractions should be kept at 4°C and warmed in
   lukewarm water prior to concentration of the immunopositive fractions.
3. The rotor and centrifuge should be kept at room temperature during the concentration procedure to prevent clogging of the filters by precipitated PFO.
4. After sonication, it is necessary to quick-spin the Eppendorf tubes to collect all
   the components of the ATPase reaction.

References

1. Bear, C. E. et al. (1992) Purification and functional reconstitution of the cystic
   fibrosis transmembrane conductance regulator (CFTR). *Cell* **68,** 809–818.
2. Hwang, T.-C., Nagel, G., Nairn, A., and Gadsby, D. C. (1994) Regulation of the
   gating of cystic fibrosis transmembrane conductance regulator Cl channels by
   phosphorylation and ATP hydrolysis. *Proc. Natl. Acad. Sci. USA* **91,** 4698–4702.
3. Gunderson, K. L. and Kopito, R. R. (1994) Effects fo pyrophosphate and nucleotide analogs suggest a role for ATP hydrolysis in cystic fibrosis transmembrane
   conductance regulator channel gating. *J. Biol. Chem.* **269,** 19,349–19,353.
4. Gunderson, K. L. and Kopito, R. R. (1995) Conformational states of CFTR
   associated with channel gating: the role of ATP binding and hydrolysis. *Cell* **82,**
   231–239.
5. Carson, M. R., Travis, S. M., and Welsh, M. J. (1995) The two nucleotide-binding
   domains of cystic fibrosis transmembrane conductance regulator (CFTR) have
   distinct functions in controlling channel activity. *J. Biol. Chem.* **270,** 1711–1717.

6. Zeltwanger, S., Wang, F., Wang, G. T., Gillis, K. D., and Hwang, T. C. (1999) Gating of cystic fibrosis transmembrane conductance regulator chloride channels by adenosine triphosphate hydrolysis. Quantitative analysis of a cyclic gating scheme. *J Gen Physiol* **113,** 541–554.

7. Li, C., et al. (1996) ATPase activity of the Cystic Fibrosis Transmembrane Conductance Regulator. *J. Biol. Chem.* **271,** 28,463–28,468.

8. Bear, C. E., et al. (1997) Coupling of ATP hydrolysis with channel gating by purified, reconstituted CFTR. *J. Bioenerg. Biomembr.* **29,** 465–473.

9. Riordan, J., et al. (1989) Identification of the cystic fibrosis gene: cloning and characterization of complementary DNA. *Science* **245,** 1066–1073.

10. Ko, Y. H. and Pedersen, P. L. (1995) The first nucleotide binding fold of the cystic fibrosis transmembrane conductance regulator can function as an active ATPase. *J. Biol. Chem.* **270,** 22,093–22,096.

11. Ramjeesingh, M., et al. (1999) Walker mutations reveal loose relationship between catalytic and channel-gating activities of purified CFTR (cystic fibrosis transmembrane conductance regulator). *Biochemistry* **38,** 1463–1468.

12. Anderson, M. P., et al. (1991) Nucleotide triphosphates are required to open the CFTR chloride channel. *Cell* **67,** 775–784.

13. Hwang, T. C., Horie, M., and Gadsby, D. C. (1993) Functionally distinct phospho-forms underlie incremental activation of protein kinase-regulated Cl- conductance in mammalian heart. *J. Gen. Physiol.* **101,** 629–650.

14. Baukrowitz, T., Hwang, T.-C., Nairn, A., and Gadsby, D. (1994) Coupling of CFTR Cl channel gating to an ATP hydrolysis cycle. *Neuron* **12,** 473–482.

15. George, S. T., Arbabian, M. A., Ruoho, A. E., Kiely, J., and Malbon, C. C. High-efficiency expression of mammalian beta-adrenergic receptors in baculovirus-infected insect cells. *Biochem. Biophys. Res. Commun.* **163,** 1265–1269.

16. Keinanen, K., Kohr, G., Seeburg, P. H., Laukkanen, M. L., and Oker-Blom, C. High-level expression of functional glutamate receptor channels in insect cells. *Biotechnology (NY)* **12,** 802–806.

17. Germann, U. A. (1998) Baculovirus-mediated expression of human multidrug resistance cDNA in insect cells and functional analysis of recombinant P-glycoprotein. *Meth. Enzymol.* **292,** 427–441.

18. Ramjeesingh, M., et al. (1999) Purification and reconstitution of epithelial chloride channel cystic fibrosis transmembrane conductance regulator. *Meth. Enzymol.* **294,** 227–246.

19. Li, C., et al. (1993) The cystic fibrosis mutation (delta F508) does not influence the chloride channel activity of CFTR. *Nat. Genet.* **3,** 311–316.

20. Ramjeesingh, M., et al. (1997) A novel procedure for the efficient purification of the cystic fibrosis transmembrane conductance regulator (CFTR). *Biochem. J.* **327,** 17–21.

21. Maduke, M., Pheasant, D. J.. and Miller, C. (1999) High-level expression, functional reconstitution, and quaternary structure of a prokaryotic ClC-type chloride channel. *J. Gen. Physiol.* **114,** 713–722.

22. Loo, T. W. and Clarke, D. M. (1995) Rapid purification of human P-glycoprotein mutants expressed transiently in HEK 293 cells by nickel-chelate chromatogra-

phy and characterization of their drug-stimulated ATPase activities. *J. Biol. Chem.* **270,** 21,449–21,452.

23. Shepherd, F. H. H. A. (1995) The potential of fluorinated surfactants in membrane biochemistry. *Analy. Biochem.* **224,** 21–27.
24. Cerione, R. A., et al. (1984) The mammalian beta 2-adrenergic receptor: reconstitution of functional interactions between pure receptor and pure stimulatory nucleotide binding protein of the adenylate cyclase system. *Biochemistry* **23,** 4519–4525.
25. Noel, H., Goswami, T., and Pande, S. V. (1985) Solubilization and reconstitution of rat liver mitochondrial carnitine acylcarnitine translocase. *Biochemistry* **24,** 4504–4509.
26. Rigaud, J. L., Pitard, B., and Levy, D. (1995) Reconstitution of membrane proteins into liposomes: application to energy-transducing membrane proteins. *Biochim. Biophys. Acta* **1231,** 223–246.
27. Egan, R. W. (1976) Hydrophile-lipophile balance and critical micelle concentration as key factors influencing surfactant disruption of mitochondrial membranes. *J. Biol. Chem.* **251,** 4442–4447.
28. Doige, C. A., Yu, X. Y., and Sharom, F. J. (1993) The effects of lipids and detergents on the ATP-ase active P-glycoprotein. *Biochim. Biophys. Acta* **1146,** 65–72.
29. Ramjeesingh, M., Huan, L.-J., Garami, E., and Bear, C. E. (1999) Novel method for evaluation of the oligomeric structure of membrane proteins. *Biochem. J.* **342,** 119–123.
30. Papahadjopoulos, D. and Watkins, J. C. (1967) Phospholipid model membranes. II. Permeability properties of hydrated liquid crystals. *Biochim. Biophys. Acta* **135,** 639–652.
31. Woodbury, D. and Miller, C. (1990) Nystatin-induced liposome fusion. A versatile approach to ion channel reconstitution into planar bilayers. *Biophys. J.* **58,** 833–839.
32. Cheng, S. H., et al. (1991) Phosphorylation of the R domain by cAMP-dependent protein kinase regulates the CFTR chloride channel. *Cell* **66,** 1027–1036.
33. Picciotto, M. R., Cohn, J. A., Bertuzzi, G., Greengard, P., and Nairn, A. C. *J. Biol. Chem.* **267,** 12,742–12,752.
34. Seibert, F. S., et al. (1995) cAMP-dependent protein kinase-mediated phosphorylation of cystic fibrosis transmembrane conductance regulator residue Ser-753 and its role in channel activation. *J. Biol. Chem.* **270,** 2158–2162.
35. Jia, Y., Mathews, C. J., and Hanrahan, J. W. (1997) Phosphorylation by protein kinase C is required for acute activation of cystic fibrosis transmembrane conductance regulator by protein kinase A. *J. Biol. Chem.* **272,** 4978–4984.
36. Anderson, M., Rich, D., Gregory, R., Smith, A., and Welsh, M. (1991) Generation of cAMP-activated chloride currents by expression of CFTR. *Science* **251,** 679–682.
37. Tabcharani, J. A., Chang, X. B., Riordan, J. R., and Hanrahan, J. W. (1991) Phosphorylation-regulated Cl- channel in CHO cells stably expressing the cystic fibrosis gene. *Nature* **352,** 628–631.
38. Welsh, M. J. and Smith, A. E. (1993) Molecular mechanisms of CFTR chloride channel dysfunction in cystic fibrosis. *Cell* **73,** 1251–1254.

39. Zielenski, J. and Tsui, L. C. (1995) Cystic fibrosis: genotypic and phenotypic variations. *Annu. Rev. Genet.* **29,** 777–807.

40. Cheng, S. H., et al. (1990) Defective intracellular transport and processing of CFTR is the molecular basis of most cystic fibrosis. *Cell* **63,** 827–834.

41. Denning, G. M., et al. (1992) Processing of mutant cystic fibrosis transmembrane conductance regulator is temperature-sensitive [see comments]. *Nature* **358,** 761–764.

42. Haardt, M., Benharouga, M., Lechardeur, D., Kartner, N., and Lukacs, G. L. (1999) C-terminal truncations destabilize the cystic fibrosis transmembrane conductance regulator without impairing its biogenesis. A novel class of mutation. *J. Biol. Chem.* **274,** 21,873–21,877.

43. Massiah, M. A., Ko, Y. H., Pedersen, P. L., and Mildvan, A. S. (1999) Cystic fibrosis transmembrane conductance regulator: solution structures of peptides based on the Phe508 region, the most common site of disease-causing DeltaF508 mutation. *Biochemistry* **38,** 7453–7461.

44. Kartner, N., Augustinas, O., Jensen, T. J., Naismith, A. L., and Riordan, J. R. (1992) Mislocalization of delta F508 CFTR in cystic fibrosis sweat gland. *Nat. Genet.* **1,** 321–327.

45. Gregory, R. J., et al. (1991) Maturation and function of cystic fibrosis transmembrane conductance regulator variants bearing mutations in putative nucleotide-binding domains 1 and 2. *Mol. Cell. Biol.* **11,** 3886–3893.

46. Yang, Y., et al. (1993) Molecular basis of defective anion transport in L cells expressing recombinant forms of CFTR. *Hum. Mol. Genet.* **2,** 1253–1261.

47. Drumm, M. L., et al. (1991) Chloride conductance expressed by delta F508 and other mutant CFTRs in Xenopus oocytes. *Science* **254,** 1797–1799.

48. Dalemans, W., et al. (1991) Altered chloride ion channel kinetics associated with the delta F508 cystic fibrosis mutation [see comments]. *Nature* **354,** 526–528.

49. Wang, F., Zeltwanger, S., Hu, S., and Hwang, T. C. (2000) Deletion of phenylalanine 508 causes attenuated phosphorylation- dependent activation of CFTR chloride channels. *J. Physiol. (Lond.)* **524 Pt 3,** 637–648.

50. Haws, C. M., et al. (1996) Delta F508-CFTR channels: kinetics, activation by forskolin, and potentiation by xanthines. *Am. J. Physiol.* **270,** C1544–1555.

51. Hung, L.-W., et al. (1998) Crystal structure of the ATP-binding subunit of an ABC transporter. *Nature* **396,** 703–707.

52. Linsdell, P. and Hanrahan, J. (1998) Adenosine triphosphate-dependent asymmetry of anion permeation in the cystic fibrosis transmembrane conductance regulator chloride channel. *J. Gen. Physiol.* **111,** 601–614.

53. Linsdell, P. and Hanrahan, J. (1998) Glutathione permeability of CFTR. *Am. J. Physiol.* **275,** C323–326.

10

Probing CFTR Channel Structure and Function Using the Substituted-Cysteine-Accessibility Method

Myles H. Akabas

1. Introduction

The cystic fibrosis transmembrane conductance regulator (CFTR) forms a chloride channel whose activation is regulated by phosphorylation and by ATP binding and hydrolysis *(1–4)*. The functional properties of the channel have been extensively studied using electrophysiological techniques *(4)*. Less is known about the structural bases for the functional properties. The cloning of CFTR in 1989 provided the primary amino acid sequence and a putative transmembrane topology of the protein *(5)*. In order to understand the structural bases for the functional properties of the channel, we sought to identify the residues lining the ion channel because they are likely to be the major determinants of the channel's functional properties. Although the channel-lining residues lie within membrane-spanning segments, they are part of the water-accessible surface of the protein. The substituted-cysteine-accessibility method (SCAM), which we developed, provides an approach to identify systematically the channel-lining residues *(6–9)*. We have applied SCAM to three of CFTR's 12 putative membrane-spanning segments *(9–11)*.

There are approx 240 residues in the 12 membrane-spanning segments. There is little *a priori* information as to which segments might contribute to the channel lining. Multiple membrane-spanning segments from an individual CFTR molecule are likely to contribute to the channel lining because CFTR is at most a dimer *(12,13)*. This situation is in marked contrast to the voltage-gated and neurotransmitter-gated channels that are formed by the assembly of four or five homologous subunits in a symmetrical or pseudosymmetrical pattern around the central pore axis *(14)*. In these channels, a similar region from

From: *Methods in Molecular Medicine, vol. 70: Cystic Fibrosis Methods and Protocols*
Edited by: W. R. Skach © Humana Press Inc., Totowa, NJ

each subunit contributes to the channel lining. Thus, for example, in the crystal structure of the bacterial K$^+$ channel, Kcsa, each of the four subunits contributes two membrane-spanning segments and a membrane reentrant P-loop to the channel lining *(15)*. This lack of homologous subunits increases the complexity of identifying CFTR's channel-lining residues.

In addition to identifying the channel-lining residues among the putative membrane-spanning segments of CFTR variations of SCAM facilitate the localization of functional domains of the channel, such as the size and charge selectivity filters and the gate, relative to identified channel-lining residues. SCAM has also been used to identify residues in receptor binding sites and in transporters *(16–18)*.

1.1. SCAM: An Overview

The basic experimental approach is to substitute systematically cysteine (Cys), one at a time, for each residue in a membrane-spanning segment. The Cys-substitution mutants are expressed heterologously in either *Xenopus* oocytes or transfected cells. If the functional properties of a mutant are near-normal, then the susceptibility of the engineered cysteine to covalent chemical modification by sulfhydryl-specific reagents is determined. For CFTR, the reagents that we have used are derivatives of methanethiosulfonate (MTS). The properties of these reagents are discussed below. Reaction of the MTS reagents with engineered Cys mutants was assayed functionally as a change in macroscopic currents recorded from oocytes maintained under two-electrode voltage clamp *(9–11)*. Alternatively, as has been done in other proteins, reaction could be assayed at the single-channel level *(19)* or biochemically *(20)*. It is important to note that for the purposes of assaying reaction for accessibility studies, an effect on currents is the critical issue. Whether the effect of modification causes inhibition or potentiation of subsequent currents is a secondary issue that requires single-channel studies to determine whether it arises from alterations in single-channel conductance or gating kinetics. Issues relating to performing SCAM experiments and interpretation of results will be discussed below.

1.2. Why Cysteine Substitution?

The ease and specificity with which Cys can be modified forms the basis for SCAM. The ability to substitute Cys and still obtain functional CFTR is essential for the method. In my experience with Cys substitutions at ~150 residues in three proteins (72 residues in CFTR, 36 in the acetylcholine receptor, and 43 in the GABA$_A$ receptor), Cys could be substituted for hydrophobic residues (alanine, glycine, isoleucine, leucine, methionine, phenylalanine, tyrosine, proline, and valine), polar residues (glutamine, asparagine, serine, and threonine), and charged residues (glutamic acid, arginine, and lysine), and all but one of these mutants displayed robust expression with near-normal function. One mutant in the acetylcholine receptor (αP221C) failed to express.

There are many reasons why Cys substitution may be so well tolerated. Cys is a relatively small amino acid; its volume is 108 Å^3 making it smaller than all other amino acids except glycine, alanine, and serine *(21)*. Cys occurs in proteins with a frequency of about 3% *(21)*. In globular proteins, about half of non-disulfide-linked Cys are buried in the interior of the protein and half are exposed on the water-accessible protein surface; this is similar to the percentage of buried residues for other non-polar amino acids *(22)*. Several groups have studied the frequency of occurrence of amino acids in regions of defined secondary structure. Relatively weak preferences have been identified for Cys, and the preferences vary with the study *(23,24)*. In addition, the data for secondary structural preferences is based on globular proteins, not integral membrane proteins. Recent studies suggest that the helical propensity of amino acids is different in the hydrophobic membrane environment *(25)*. This may be particularly true for Cys, which when it occurs in α helices has been shown to satisfy its hydrogen-bonding requirements by forming intrahelical hydrogen bonds to backbone carbonyls *(26)*: These bonds are entropically favorable due to the liberation of bound water. In sum, Cys tolerates both hydrophilic and hydrophobic environments, with little preference for any particular secondary structure.

1.3. Endogenous Cysteine Residues

Although ideally one might want to remove all endogenous Cys residues before beginning SCAM experiments, the more mutations introduced into a protein the less likely it will be in a conformation close to its native state. Thus, before substituting Cys residues into a protein one must demonstrate that the endogenous Cys residues are not accessible to the sulfhydryl reagents. CFTR contains 18 endogenous Cys, 4 in membrane-spanning segments (M2, M4, M6, and M7), and 14 in putative cytoplasmic domains. Application of the MTS reagents from the extracellular bath had no effect on the currents induced by wild-type CFTR *(9)*. This implies either that the endogenous Cys residues are inaccessible to react with extracellularly applied reagents or that modification of one or more of the endogenous Cys residues has no effect on CFTR channel function. In contrast, application of N-ethylmaleimide from the cytoplasmic bath to excised inside-out patches resulted in modification of Cys832 in the R domain; reaction at this position stimulated channel activity *(27)*. Thus, in order to conduct SCAM experiments using application of the reagents from the cytoplasmic side, Cys 832 would first have to be mutated.

1.4. The MTS Reagents and Other Sulfhydryl-Specific Reagents

For CFTR, the sulfhydryl reagents that we used were derivatives of methanethiosulfonate (MTS), one negatively charged, methanethiosulfonate-ethylsulfonate (MTSES$^-$; $CH_3SO_2SCH_2CH_2SO_3^-$) and two positively charged, methanethiosulfonate-ethylammonium (MTSEA$^+$; CH$_3$SO$_2$SCH$_2$CH$_2$NH$_3$$^+$) and methanethiosulfonate-ethyltrimethylammonium (MTSET$^+$; CH$_3$SO$_2$SCH$_2$CH$_2$N(CH$_3$)$_3$$^+$) (6,28). These reagents would all fit into a right cylinder 6 Å in diameter and 10 Å in length. MTSEA$^+$ is slightly smaller than the other two. The MTS reagents were synthesized as described (28,29) or can be obtained from Biotium, Inc. (Hayward, CA), Toronto Research Chemicals (North York, Ontario, Canada) or Anatrace (Maumee, OH). Other sulfhydryl reagents that have been used in studies of other proteins include mercurial derivatives, maleimides, and Ag$^+$ (20,30,31).

The reaction between free sulfhydryls and the MTS reagents involves an SN2 nucleophilic attack of the thiolate anion (RS$^-$) on the -S-S- bond in the MTS reagent. This leads to the high specificity of these reagents: they do not react with disulfide bonds. Reaction with a free sulfhydryl results in the addition of -SCH$_2$CH$_2$X to the sulfhydryl to form a mixed disulfide, where X is SO$_3$$^-$ for MTSES$^-$, NH$_3$$^+$ for MTSEA$^+$, and N(CH$_3$)$_3$$^+$ for MTSET$^+$. The rates of reaction of the MTS reagents with 2-mercaptoethanol, a model sulfhydryl compound, at 20°C and pH 7.0 are 1.7×10^4 L/mol/s, MTSES$^-$; 7.6×10^4 L/mol/s, MTSEA$^+$; and 21.2×10^4 L/mol/s, MTSET$^+$ (32). The differences in the rates of reaction are due in part to electrostatic interactions between the charge on the reagent and the thiolate anion. The reaction rates are pH-dependent due to effects of pH on the ionization state of the sulfhydryl. For Cys the thiol pKa is ~8.5 (21), thus, at pH 7.5 water-exposed Cys will be ionized about 10% of the time. The electrostatic environment at each substituted Cys residue may affect the thiol pKa and thus the relative reactivity toward the MTS reagents. Local protein environment has been shown to cause marked shifts in the pKa's of ionizable groups (33).

The MTS reagents undergo hydrolysis in aqueous solution. The hydrolysis reaction occurs in two steps and is pH-dependent. In the first step, OH$^-$ reacts to form a sulfinic acid (CH$_3$SO$_2$H) and a sulfenic acid (RSOH), which is sulfhydryl-reactive. In the second step, two sulfenic acids disproportionate to form a thiol (RSH) and a sulfinic acid. At pH 7.0 and 20°C the $T_{1/2}$ for hydrolysis is 12 min for MTSEA$^+$, 11 min for MTSET$^+$, and 370 min for MTSES$^-$ (32). The hydrolysis rates are about 5–10 times slower at pH 6.0.

Some of the MTS reagents, such as MTSES$^-$ and MTSET$^+$, are essentially membrane impermeant (17,34) whereas others, such as MTSEA$^+$, are membrane-permeant, probably in the deprotonated, uncharged form (34). The membrane permeability of MTSEA$^+$ and of uncharged MTS derivatives limits their utility for determining the sidedness of substituted Cys residues. In intact cells the reducing environment of the cytoplasm, may scavenge MTS reagents that cross the membrane into the cytoplasm but Cys residues in the cytoplasmic domains of integral membrane proteins may be exposed to higher reagent concentrations since they are in closer contact with the membrane than soluble cytoplasmic proteins whose labeling is often used as a control for membrane permeability of reagents. As with other biotin derivatives, MTS-biotin is slowly membrane-permeant and may react with intracellular Cys residues. Care must be exercised in using it for determination of membrane topology. In patch clamp experiments the inclusion of 10 m*M* cysteine or glutathione on the opposite side of the membrane as the MTS reagent has been used to scavenge reagent that permeates across the membrane *(34)*.

1.5. Interpretation of Results and Locating Functional Domains Within the Channel

1.5.1. Interpretation of Reactive Residues

Reactive Cys are inferred to be on the water-accessible surface of the protein, at least transiently, for several reasons. First, the MTS reagents react more than 10^9 times faster with the ionized thiolate form of Cys (RS^-) than with the uncharged thiol form (RSH) *(35)*. Only Cys on the water-accessible surface will ionize to a significant extent. Second, at pH 7.5, $MTSES^-$ and $MTSET^+$ are permanently charged and membrane impermeant *(17,34)*. Therefore, they are unlikely to enter hydrophobic regions in the lipid bilayer or in the interior of proteins. This implies that these reagents traverse an aqueous pathway to the reactive Cys. Third, in a protein of known crystal structure, the aspartate chemotaxis receptor, Falke and colleagues showed that cysteine reactivity was well correlated with calculated solvent accessibility measured from the high-resolution structure *(36)*. Thus, we infer that reactive Cys residues are on the water-accessible surface of the protein, at least part of the time. Based on the assumption that if the function of a Cys-substitution mutant is similar to wild-type then its structure is also similar, we infer that the side chain of the corresponding wild-type residue is also, at least transiently, on the water-accessible protein surface and, thus, may line the channel. Localization on the water-accessible surface, however, is not sufficient to prove that the residues are in the channel; additional evidence, as described below, such as voltage dependence of reaction rates or protection by channel blockers, is necessary.

Interpretations for Cys mutants where the currents are not statistically significantly affected by the reagents include: (1) they are not on the water-accessible surface; (2) the rate of reaction is below our detection threshold; (3) they are on the water-accessible surface but access to them is sterically hindered; or (4) they have reacted but reaction has no functional effect or the maximal effect of modification is less than 25%, our statistical detection threshold. We cannot distinguish between these possibilities and thus the negatives must be interpreted with caution. Furthermore, water-accessible residues are not necessarily always on the water-accessible surface but may move between the accessible and inaccessible parts of the protein due to thermal fluctuations in the protein structure. The percentage of time spent on the water-accessible surface will be one of the variables that affects the reaction rate.

1.5.2. Secondary Structure of Channel-Lining, Membrane-Spanning Segments

If a channel-lining segment has a regular secondary structure, then the pattern formed by the water-accessible residues identified by SCAM may provide insight into the secondary structure of that segment. If, when plotted on an α-helical wheel plot, the water-accessible residues lie on one face of the helix; this suggests that the secondary structure of the segment is α-helical. It is important to recognize that an ideal α helix oriented perpendicular to the membrane has 3.6 residues per turn; however, in proteins with multiple α helices the helices often form coiled-coil structures that alter the periodicity. Thus, in left-handed coiled-coils with a crossing angle of –20° there are 3.5 residues per turn and in right-handed coiled-coils with a 40° crossing angle there are ~4.0 residues per turn, (37). If the membrane-spanning segment is bent or crosses another segment, then the pattern of accessible residues may not form a perfect stripe on a helical wheel plot. Also, if the segment exists in different conformations in different states of the channel (i.e., open vs closed), both conformations may be sampled during the time scale of a SCAM experiment (seconds to minutes).

Alternatively, the secondary structure might be β strand, in which case one would expect that every other residue would be accessible, or there may be no regular secondary structure resulting in a pattern of accessible residues that is not consistent with either α helix or β strand as was reported for the P-loop in K^+ channels (30,38).

In the CFTR M1 segment the channel-lining residues lie within an arc of 80° on one side of an α-helical wheel plot. This strongly suggests that the segment has an α-helical secondary structure (9). In the M3 and M6 segments the pattern formed by the accessible residues was not as clear-cut, raising the possibility that they are not straight α helices (10,11).

1.5.3. Location of the Charge-Selectivity Filter

Ion channels are generally selectively permeant to either anions or cations. As a first step toward understanding the structural basis of charge selectivity it is important to determine the location of the charge-selectivity filter relative to identified channel-lining residues. Subsequently, one can determine the role of residues in that region of the channel in the process of charge selectivity.

The location of the charge-selectivity filter can be determined by comparing the relative rates of reaction of anionic and cationic MTS reagents, such as $MTSES^-$ and $MTSET^+$, with identified channel-lining Cys mutants (39). If the charge-selectivity filter is located at a more cytoplasmic position than an engineered Cys residue, then the ratio of the reaction rates of MTSES$^-$ and MTSET$^+$ applied extracellularly will be similar to the ratio of their reaction rates with sulfhydryls in free solution. In contrast, in an anion-selective channel, such as CFTR, if the Cys mutant is at or more cytoplasmic than the charge-selectivity filter, then the ratio of the reaction rates of MTSES$^-$ and MTSET$^+$ will be much greater than the ratio of their reaction rates with sulfhydryls in free solution. We used this approach to show that both anions and cations could enter the extracellular end of the CFTR channel and that charge selectivity occurred near the cytoplasmic end of the channel *(39)*. We subsequently showed that mutations that changed the charge at the position of Arg352 near the cytoplasmic end of the M6 segment altered the Cl$^-$-to-Na$^+$ permeability ratio. This suggested that Arg352 was a major determinant of charge selectivity in the CFTR channel *(40)*.

1.5.4. Voltage Dependence of Reaction Rates

The reaction of an MTS reagent with a channel-lining, substituted Cys occurs in two steps. In the first step, the MTS reagent moves from bulk solution through the channel to the level of the Cys. In the second step, the MTS reagent reacts with the thiolate of the Cys. For charged MTS reagents, the first step, movement through the channel, will be dependent on the membrane potential. If the first step is rate-limiting, then, the second-order rate constant for the overall reaction will be voltage-dependent. (These assumptions are similar to those used to analyze proton block of sodium currents *[41]*.) Assuming that the reagent is impermeable through the channel, the magnitude of the voltage dependence will be determined by the fraction of the electrical potential through which the charge on the MTS reagent moves in order to reach the Cys. The electrical distance, δ, can be calculated by fitting the rate constants as a function of membrane potential with the Boltzmann relationship (**Eq. 1**). Thus, the second-order rate constant $k_{(\psi)}$ determined at a membrane potential, ψ, should be

$$k_{(\psi)} = k_{(\psi = 0)} \exp(-zF\delta\psi/RT) \tag{1}$$

where $k_{(\psi = 0)}$ is the rate constant at a membrane potential of 0 mV, z is the charge on the MTS reagent, F is Faraday's constant, ψ is the electrical distance (i.e., the fraction of the electrical potential traversed by the charge on the MTS reagent), ψ is the membrane potential, R is the gas constant, and T is the temperature in kelvin. It should be noted that the influence of the electrostatic potential arising from fixed charges, dipoles, and so on, in the protein enters into $k_{(\psi = 0)}$, the rate constant at 0 mV. It is these forces that determine the anion selectivity of the access pathway. The influence of the applied transmembrane potential on the rate constant enters into the exponent of the Boltzmann equation (**Eq. 1**). Thus, the effects of these two potentials on the rates of reaction can be separated.

1.5.5. State-Dependent Conformational Changes and the Location of the Channel Gate

Channel gating from the closed to the open state involves conformational changes in the channel protein. These changes may alter the reaction rate of MTS reagents with substituted Cys residues. This may occur either by changes in the access pathway to the residue if access of the reagent involves movement through the channel lumen, or due to local conformational changes at the site of the Cys. Thus, reaction rates with extracellularly applied MTS reagents would be expected to change significantly for channel-lining Cys mutants at or more cytoplasmic to the level of the channel gate. This approach has been used to identify the position of the channel gate in the nicotinic acetylcholine receptor channel *(8,42)*.

1.5.6. Location of Channel Blocker Binding Sites

The reaction rate of MTS reagents with Cys substituted for residues that form a ligand-binding site should be slowed by the presence of the ligand. Thus, the ligand will protect the Cys residues from covalent modification. In a channel, if the ligand obstructs the channel lumen, that is, it is an open channel blocker, then more cytoplasmically located Cys residues will also be protected by the presence of the ligand. This approach has been used in other channels to identify channel-blocker binding sites *(31,43)* and in G-protein coupled receptors to identify residues forming the ligand-binding site *(18)*.

2. Materials
2.1. Mutagenesis
1. Cysteine-substitution mutants in pBluescript II KS(–) plasmid.

2.2. Preparation and Maintenance of Oocytes
1. 0.2% Tricaine solution (3-aminobenzoic acid ethyl ester) (Sigma).
2. ND-96 buffer: 96 mM NaCl, 2 mM KCl, 1 mM MgCl$_2$, 5 mM HEPES, pH 7.5 with NaOH, 2.5 mM NaPyruvate, 100 U/mL penicillin, 1 mg/mL streptomycin (Specialty Media, Phillipsburg, NJ).
3. Collagenase Type IA (Sigma, St. Louis, MO).
4. OR3 medium: 100 mL Lebovitz L-15 medium (Gibco-BRL, Grand Island, NY), 1 mL 200 mM glutamine, 3 mL 1 M HEPES, 400 µL 50 mg/mL gentamicin (Sigma). Adjust pH to 7.6 with 1 M NaOH. Add distilled H$_2$O to final volume of 200 mL. Sterile filter through 0.45-µm filters into autoclaved glass bottles. Store at 4°C.

2.3. Preparation of mRNA
All solutions and materials used in the preparation of mRNA must be RNase free (see **Notes 1** and **2**).

2.3.1. Preparation of RNase-Free cDNA Template

1. CFTR pBS plasmid DNA (~50 mg) linearized with *Sma*I.
2. 1 mg/mL proteinase K, store at –20°C.
3. Phenol/chloroform/isoamyl alcohol (25/24/1) (Sigma).
4. Isoamyl alcohol/chloroform (1/24).
5. 3 *M* NaAcetate, pH 5.2.
6. Ethanol.
7. TE pH 8.0: 10 m*M* Tris-HCl, 1 m*M* ethylenediaminetetraacetic acid (EDTA), pH adjusted to 8.0 with HCl.

2.3.2. mRNA Synthesis by In Vitro Transcription

1. RNase-free cDNA template linearized with *Sma*I restriction enzyme.
2. 5× transcription buffer (Promega, Madison, WI).
3. 0.1 *M* dithiothreitol (DTT) (Promega).
4. RNasin (Promega).
5. 10 m*M* m^{7}G(5')ppp(5')G RNA Cap Structure Analog (New England Biolabs, Beverly, MA).
6. 10 m*M* rATP, 10 m*M* rCTP, 10 m*M* rUTP, 1 m*M* rGTP (Promega).
7. [^{3}H]-UTP (New England Nuclear, Boston, MA).
8. T7 RNA Polymerase (Promega).
9. Phenol/chloroform/isoamyl alcohol (25/24/1) (Sigma).
10. Chloroform/isoamyl alcohol (24/1).
11. 3 *M* NaAcetate.
12. Ethanol.

2.4. Electrophysiology

1. Ca^{2+}-free frog Ringer's solution (CFFR): 115 m*M* NaCl, 2.5 m*M* KCl, 1.8 m*M* MgCl$_2$, 10 m*M* HEPES, pH 7.5 with NaOH (*see* **Note 3**).
2. MTS reagents (MTSES$^-$, MTSEA$^+$, MTSET$^+$) (*see* **Note 4**).
3. Two-electrode voltage clamp setup (TEV-200 amplifier [Dagan, Minneapolis, MN]; Digidata 1200 A/D interface running either Axobasic or pClamp software [Axon Instruments, Foster City, CA]; a PC computer and printer; analog oscilloscope; dissecting microscope; 2 micromanipulators and stands; oocyte perfusion chamber; Faraday cage).
4. 3 *M* KCl solution and agar bridges with 3 *M* KCl + 3% agar.
5. 20 m*M* 8-(4-chlorophenylthio) adenosine cyclic monophosphate (cpt-cAMP) (Sigma) in H$_2$O. Store at –20°C.
6. 500 m*M* 3-isobutyl-1-methylxanthine (IBMX) (Sigma) in DMSO. Store at –20°C.
7. 20 m*M* forskolin (Sigma) in DMSO. Store at –20°C.

3. Methods

3.1. Mutagenesis

Cysteine-substitution mutants should be prepared using your favorite site-directed mutagenesis technique. The mutants should be subcloned into an appropriate expression vector. We have used CFTR cloned into the pBluescript II KS(–) vector (CFTR-pBS) (Stratagene, La Jolla, CA).

3.2. Preparation and Maintenance of Oocytes

1. Anesthetize toad by placing it in a tank containing 0.2% tricaine solution until it loses its withdrawal response to toe pinch.
2. Place toad on her back on a bed of ice. With forceps, lift up skin over lower, lateral abdomen and make a 1–2 cm long incision with a pair of fine scissors (*see* **Note 5**).
3. Using forceps, pull a portion of the ovary out through the incision.
4. Using scissors, cut off a suitable-sized piece of ovary.
5. Push ovary back into abdomen and close incision with two or three 3-0 silk sutures. Be careful not to catch any loops of intestine in the sutures. Allow toad to recover from anesthesia.
6. Place the pieces of ovary in a 60-mm sterile Petri dish. Tease the membrane off the pieces of ovary and rinse in 20 mL of ND-96 buffer.
7. Incubate ovary pieces in 20 mL of solution containing 3 mg/mL collagenase Type 1A in ND-96 in the 60-mm Petri dish for 1 h at 18°C with gentle swirling on a Belly Dancer Agitator.
8. Wash the oocytes three times for 15 min each in 20 mL OR3 medium at 18°C with gentle swirling on a Belly Dancer Agitator.
9. Sort the oocytes under a dissecting microscope to remove small and damaged oocytes.
10. Maintain oocytes in OR3 medium at 18°C. Change medium daily to avoid bacterial or fungal growth in the medium.
11. Inject oocytes with 50 nL of mRNA solution (*see* **Note 6**).

3.3. Preparation of mRNA

Gloves should be worn throughout the procedure (*see* **Note 1**).

3.3.1. Preparation of RNase-Free cDNA Template

1. Linearize ~50 µg of Cys mutant CFTR-pBS plasmid DNA with *Sma*I restriction enzyme.
2. Add 1 µL of 1 mg/mL proteinase K per 50 µL of restriction digest.
3. Incubate 30 min at 37°C.
4. Add DEPC treated water to bring volume to 300 µL.
5. Extract two times with 300 µL of phenol/chloroform/isoamyl alcohol (25/24/1).
6. Extract once with 300 µL of chloroform/isoamyl alcohol (24/1).
7. Ethanol precipitate the DNA by adding 1/10 vol 3 *M* NaAcetate, pH 5.2, and 2 vol ethanol. Incubate 15 min at 4°C. Pellet the precipitated DNA in a microcentrifuge 30 min at 4°C. Aspirate off supernatant. Wash pellet with 70% ethanol in DEPC-treated H_2O (–20°C). Pellet DNA in microcentrifuge. Aspirate off supernatant. Allow ethanol to evaporate (*see* **Note 7**).
8. Dissolve DNA in TE, pH 8.0 buffer (*see* **Note 8**).
9. Measure the DNA concentration. Take 1 µL of DNA solution and mix it with 499 µL of H_2O. In a UV/visible spectrophotometer, measure the absorbance at 260 nm. Use a blank containing an equal volume of TE in H_2O. 1 OD_{260} = 50 µg/mL solution of double stranded DNA.
10. If the DNA concentration is greater than 1 µg/µL, adjust the concentration to 1 µg/µL.

3.3.2. mRNA Synthesis by In Vitro Transcription

1. Make a master mix of reaction components. Make an extra volume of master mix for scintillation counting to quantify mRNA yield. Thus, to make mRNA for *n* mutants, make (n + 1) volumes of master mix. For one volume (40 μL) of master mix add 7.25 μL DEPC-treated H_2O, 10 μL 5× transcription buffer, 5 μL 0.1 *M* DTT, 1.25 μL 40 U/μL RNasin, 2.5 μL 10 m*M* m^{7}G(5')ppp(5')G RNA Cap Structure Analog, 2.5 μL 10 m*M* rATP, 2.5 μL 10 m*M* rCTP, 2.5 μL 10 m*M* rUTP, 2.5 μL 1 m*M* rGTP, 1 μL 1 μCi/μL [^{3}H]-UTP, 3 μL 15 U/μL T7 RNA polymerase (*see* **Note 9**).
2. Mix 10 μL of 0.5 μg/μL plasmid DNA template and 40 μL of master mix.
3. Incubate 1 h at 37°C.
4. Add 2.5 μL of 1 m*M* rGTP and 2 μL of T7 RNA polymerase.
5. Incubate 1 h at 37°C.
6. Add DEPC-treated H_2O to make total volume 300 μL in order to minimize losses in subsequent extraction steps.
7. Extract two times with 300 μL phenol/chloroform/isoamyl alcohol (25/24/1).
8. Extract once with 300 μL chloroform/isoamyl alcohol (24/1).
9. Ethanol precipitate the RNA by adding 1/10 vol 3 *M* NaAcetate, pH 5.2, and 2.5 vol ethanol. Incubate at least 30 min at –70°C. Pellet the precipitated RNA in a microcentrifuge for 30 min at 4°C. Aspirate off supernatant. Wash pellet with 80% ethanol in DEPC-treated H_2O (–20°C). Pellet DNA in microcentrifuge. Aspirate off supernatant (*see* **Notes 7** and **10**).
10. Dissolve RNA in 100 μL DEPC-treated H_2O.
11. Repeat ethanol precipitation as in **step 9**. Allow all ethanol to evaporate.
12. Dissolve RNA pellet in 10 μL DEPC-treated H_2O (*see* **Note 8**).
13. Scintillation count 1 μL of each RNA solution and 5 μL of the initial master mix. Calculate the fractional incorporation of [^{3}H]-UTP into the RNA and thus the yield of RNA (*see* **Note 11**).
14. Adjust the mRNA concentration to 200 ng/μL with DEPC-treated H_2O.

3.4. Electrophysiology, Screening for MTS Reactive Residues, Measurement of Reaction Rates

1. Prepare two glass microelectrodes filled with 3 *M* KCl and a resistance of 0.5–2 MΩ.
2. Prepare a ground electrode containing a 3 *M* KCl/3% agar bridge to connect to the bath.
3. Place an oocyte in the perfusion chamber (volume ~250 μL) in Ca^{2+}-free frog Ringer (CFFR) solution at room temperature.
4. Impale the oocyte with both microelectrodes.
5. Maintain the oocyte under voltage clamp at a holding potential of –10 mV.
6. Determine the membrane conductance by periodically ramping the potential from –120 mV to +50 mV over 1.7 s and record the induced current (*see* **Note 12**).
7. Perfuse oocyte with 2 mL of solution containing 200 μ*M* cpt-cAMP, 20 μ*M* forskolin, 1 m*M* IBMX in CFFR buffer (subsequently referred to as "cAMP-activating solution") to activate CFTR.

8. Determine membrane conductance as described above at 5-min intervals after applying the cAMP-activating solution until CFTR-induced conductance approaches a plateau (*see* **Note 13**).
9. After the CFTR-induced conductance approaches a plateau, the membrane conductance is determined and the oocyte is immediately perfused with 2 mL of solution containing an MTS reagent + the cAMP-activating solution (*see* **Notes 14** and **15**).
10. Immediately following perfusion with the MTS reagent-containing solution, the membrane conductance is repeatedly determined for 5–8 min (*see* **Note 16**).
11. The pseudo-first-order reaction rate constant may be determined by fitting the conductance as a function of exposure time to the MTS reagent with a single exponential function. The second-order rate constant is then calculated by dividing the pseudo-first-order reaction rate constant by the MTS reagent concentration.
12. To determine whether the effects of the MTS reagents are irreversible, the oocyte is perfused with CFFR containing the cAMP-activating solution to remove the MTS reagent. If the effect persists after removal of the MTS reagent, it is deemed to be irreversible and therefore likely to be due to a covalent reaction between the reagent and a Cys residue.

4. Notes

1. RNase is a ubiquitous enzyme that is very hard to destroy. It is very efficient at degrading RNA. Gloves should be worn at all stages of the process of mRNA synthesis. Glassware should be baked at 180°C for 6 h. Plastic ware should be untouched by human hands. Autoclaving does not destroy RNase, it refolds very efficiently (that's how Christian Anfinsen won the Nobel Prize). To avoid RNase contamination of solutions and materials used for in vitro transcription, a separate area of the laboratory should be designated for RNA work and all solutions should be used only for RNA work.
2. All water used in the preparation of solutions for mRNA preparation should be treated with diethyl pyrocarbonate (DEPC) (0.2 mL DEPC per 100 mL of H_2O). Following vigorous mixing to dissolve DEPC the solution should be autoclaved to inactivate and remove unreacted DEPC. DEPC is a suspected carcinogen, so gloves should be worn when handling DEPC solutions. Before autoclaving it should be handled in a fume hood.
3. Ca^{2+}-free frog Ringer's solution (CFFR) is used in the oocyte perfusion bath to reduce the possibility of activating the endogenous Ca^{2+}-activated Cl^- current in *Xenopus* oocytes.
4. There are three sources of MTS reagents; check the prices, the quality appears similar. (a) Anatrace, 434 West Dussel Drive, Maumee, OH 43537. Tel: 800-252-1280; www.anatrace.com. (b) Toronto Research Chemicals, Inc., 2 Brisbane Road, North York, Ontario, Canada M3J 2J8. Tel: 416-665-9696; e-mail: torresh@interlog.com; www.trc-canada.com. (c) Biotium, Inc., 3423 Investment Blvd. Suite 8, Hayward, CA 94545. Tel: 510-265-1027; www.biotium.com
5. All surgical instruments should be sterilized by immersion in 70% ethanol solution and allowed to air-dry before use.

6. Oocytes may be injected the same day they are isolated, but allowing them a day to recover seems to result in fewer dead oocytes. Generally, CFTR expresses 2–5 d, following mRNA injection.

7. The DNA pellet does not always remain firmly stuck to the wall of the microcentrifuge. Be sure that you can see the DNA pellet before aspirating off the last drops of supernatant.

8. Assume that about half of the DNA will be lost during the preceding steps. Add a volume of TE that will make the DNA concentration ~1 μg/μL. DNA that is dried too much will go back into solution very slowly. Thus, allow sufficient time for the DNA to rehydrate. Incubation at 37°C speeds the rehydration time. Similar considerations regarding rehydration following drying apply to mRNA.

9. mRNA is more stable and better translated if the 5' end contains the $m^7G(5')ppp(5')G$ RNA Cap Structure. RNA polymerase will only incorporate the $m^7G(5')ppp(5')G$ RNA Cap Structure Analog at the initial position, but it does so in strict competition with GTP. Therefore, the $m^7G(5')ppp(5')G$ RNA Cap Structure Analog concentration is 10 mM along with the other NTPs, whereas the GTP concentration is only 1 mM. Thus, the molar ratio of $m^7G(5')ppp(5')G$ RNA Cap Structure Analog to GTP is 10/1. As long as the GTP concentration is sufficient to maintain processivity of the RNA polymerase, the lower GTP concentration will not affect the final mRNA yield. In order to avoid depleting the GTP, an additional aliquot of GTP is added for the second hour of incubation. Be sure to use ribonucleotides for RNA synthesis.

10. The goal of the two ethanol precipitation steps is to remove the unincorporated [^{3}H]-UTP from the reaction so that the amount of [^{3}H]-UTP incorporated into the mRNA can be determined, thereby allowing quantitation of the mRNA concentration. Alternatively the mRNA concentration can be estimated by comparison with standards following agarose gel electrophoresis. Agarose gel electrophoresis also allows one to assess whether full-length mRNA transcripts are being synthesized. If the expression level in *Xenopus* oocytes is poor, the size of the mRNA should be assessed.

11. The mRNA yield is typically between 5 and 20 μg per reaction.

12. The CFTR-induced conductance is determined from the current induced by the voltage ramp. The conductance is measured in this manner to avoid changing the intracellular Cl$^-$ concentration during the course of the experiments because Cl$^-$ is passively distributed in *Xenopus* oocytes. The initial membrane conductance before cAMP activation should be stable and less than 2.5 μS.

13. The time required for the CFTR-induced conductance to approach a plateau, that is, when the rate of increase of the current was less than 2%/min over a 5-min period, varies considerably between Cys-substitution mutants. For wild type it takes 15–20 min, but some of the mutants require as much as 60 min. In general, the time to approach the plateau current was inversely proportional to the magnitude of the mean plateau current for a mutant. This may be due to the extensive insertion of new membrane that accompanied CFTR activation in oocytes (*44*).

14. The concentration of the MTS reagents used for screening purposes to identify reactive mutants would be 10 mM MTSES$^-$, 2.5 mM MTSEA$^+$, and 1 mM

MTSET$^+$. These concentrations are roughly equireactive with 2-mercaptoethanol in free solution *(6,28,32)*. At these concentrations. residues with second-order reaction rate constants greater than 1 L/mol/s would be detected as reactive within 5 min. If the reaction rates for specific mutants are significantly faster, it may be necessary to use lower concentrations of the reagents in order to measure the rates.

15. In aqueous solution the MTS reagents hydrolyze in a pH- and temperature-dependent manner due to reaction with hydroxide anions (*see* **Subheading 1.4.**). Thus, care must be taken with solutions of the MTS reagents. A stock solution can be made in water, stored on ice, and used for a day. As hydrolysis begins, the pH of the stock solution will fall rapidly, stopping further hydrolysis. The stock solution should be diluted into pH 7.5 CFFR buffer immediately before use. Alternatively, weighed aliquots of the dried powder can be dissolved in CFFR buffer immediately before perfusion of the oocyte.

16. Reactive residues are identified as those where the effect of application of the MTS reagents is statistically significantly different from the effect on wild-type CFTR by a one-way ANOVA using the SPSS-PC statistics package (SPSS, Chicago, IL).

References

1. Riordan, J. R. (1993) The cystic fibrosis transmembrane conductance regulator. *Annu. Rev. Physiol.* **55,** 609–630.
2. Gadsby, D. C. and Nairn, A. C. (1999) Control of CFTR channel gating by phosphorylation and nucleotide hydrolysis. *Physiol. Rev.* **79,** S77–S107.
3. Sheppard, D. N. and Welsh, M. J. (1999) Structure and function of the CFTR chloride channel. *Physiol. Rev.* **79,** S23–45.
4. Akabas, M. H. (2000) Cystic fibrosis transmembrane conductance regulator. Structure and function of an epithelial chloride channel. *J. Biol. Chem.* **275,** 3729–3732.
5. Riordan, J. R., Rommens, J. M., Kerem, B. S., Alon, N., Rozmahel, R., Grzelczak, Z., Zielenski, J., Lok, S., Plavsic, N., Chou, J. L., Drumm, M. T., Iannuzzi, M. C., Collins, F. S., and Tsui, L. C. (1989) Identification of the cystic fibrosis gene: cloning and characterization of complementary DNA. *Science* **254,** 1066–1073.
6. Akabas, M. H., Stauffer, D. A., Xu, M., and Karlin, A. (1992) Acetylcholine receptor channel structure probed in cysteine-substitution mutants. *Science* **258,** 307–310.
7. Xu, M. and Akabas, M. H. (1993) Amino acids lining the channel of the γ-aminobutyric acid type A receptor identified by cysteine substitution. *J. Biol. Chem.* **268,** 21,505–21,508.
8. Akabas, M. H., Kaufmann, C., Archdeacon, P., and Karlin, A. (1994) Identification of acetylcholine receptor channel-lining residues in the entire M2 segment of the α subunit. *Neuron* **13,** 919–927.
9. Akabas, M. H., Kaufmann, C., Cook, T. A., and Archdeacon, P. (1994) Amino acid residues lining the chloride channel of the cystic fibrosis transmembrane conductance regulator. *J. Biol. Chem.* **269,** 14,865–14,868.
10. Cheung, M. and Akabas, M. H. (1996) Identification of CFTR channel-lining residues in and flanking the M6 membrane-spanning segment. *Biophys. J.* **70,** 2688–2695.

11. Akabas, M. H. (1998) Channel-lining residues in the M3 membrane-spanning segment of the cystic fibrosis transmembrane conductance regulator. *Biochemistry* **37,** 12,233–12,240.

12. Eskandari, S., Wright, E. M., Kreman, M., Starace, D. M., and Zampighi, G. A. (1998) Structural analysis of cloned plasma membrane proteins by freeze-fracture electron microscopy. *Proc. Natl. Acad. Sci. USA* **95,** 11,235–11,240.

13. Zerhusen, B., Zhao, J., Xie, J., Davis, P. B., and Ma, J. (1999) A single conductance pore for chloride ions formed by two cystic fibrosis transmembrane conductance regulator molecules. *J. Biol. Chem.* **274,** 7627–7630.

14. Karlin, A. and Akabas, M. H. (1995) Towards a structural basis for the function of nicotinic acetylcholine receptors and their cousins. *Neuron* **15,** 1231–1244.

15. Doyle, D. A., Cabral, J. M., Pfuetzner, R. A., Kuo, A., Gulbis, J. M., Cohen, S. L., Chait, B. T., and MacKinnon, R. (1998) The structure of the potassium channel: molecular basis of K^+ conduction and selectivity. *Science* **280,** 69–77.

16. Frillingos, S., Gonzalez, A., and Kaback, H. R. (1997) Cysteine-scanning mutagenesis of helix IV and the adjoining loops in the lactose permease of *Escherichia coli*: Glu126 and Arg144 are essential. *Biochemistry* **36,** 14,284–14,290.

17. Olami, Y., Rimon, A., Gerchman, Y., Rothman, A., and Padan, E. (1997) Histidine 225, a residue of the NhaA-Na^+/H^+ antiporter of *Escherichia coli* is exposed and faces the cell exterior. *J. Biol. Chem.* **272,** 1761–1768.

18. Javitch, J. A. (1998) Mapping the binding-site crevice of the D2 receptor. *Adv. Pharmacol.* **42,** 412–415.

19. Mindell, J. A., Zhan, H., Huynh, P. D., Collier, R. J., and Finkelstein, A. (1994) Reaction of diphtheria toxin channels with sulfhydryl-specific reagents: observation of chemical reactions at the single molecule level. *Proc. Natl. Acad. Sci. USA* **91,** 5272–5276.

20. Loo, T. W. and Clarke, D. M. (1995) Membrane topology of a cysteine-less human P-glycoprotein. *J. Biol. Chem.* **270,** 843–848.

21. Creighton, T. E. (1993) Proteins: structures and molecular properties, Freeman, New York

22. Chothia, C. (1976) The nature of the accessible and buried surfaces in proteins. *J. Mol. Biol.* **105,** 1–14.

23. Chou, P. Y. and Fasman, G. D. (1977) β-turns in proteins. *J. Mol. Biol.* **115,** 135–175.

24. Levitt, M. (1978) Conformational preferences of amino acids in globular proteins. *Biochemistry* **17,** 4277–4285.

25. Li, S. C. and Deber, C. M. (1994) A measure of helical propensity for amino acids in membrane environments. *Nat. Struct. Biol.* **1,** 368–373.

26. Gray, T. M. and Matthews, B. W. (1984) Intrahelical hydrogen bonding of serine, threonine and cysteine residues within α-helices and its relevance to membrane-bound proteins. *J. Mol. Biol.* **175,** 75–81.

27. Cotten, J. F. and Welsh, M. J. (1997) Covalent modification of the regulatory domain irreversibly stimulates cystic fibrosis transmembrane conductance regulator. *J. Biol. Chem.* **272,** 25,617–25,622.

28. Stauffer, D. A. and Karlin, A. (1994) Electrostatic potential of the acetylcholine binding sites in the nicotinic receptor probed by reactions of binding-site cysteines with charged methanethiosulfonates. *Biochemistry* **33,** 6840–6849.
29. Kenyon, G. L. and Bruice, T. W. (1977) Novel sulfhydryl reagents. *Meth. Enzymol.* **47,** 407–430.
30. Lu, Q. and Miller, C. (1995) Silver as a probe of pore-forming residues in a potassium channel. *Science* **268,** 304–307.
31. Xu, M., Covey, D. F., and Akabas, M. H. (1995) Interaction of picrotoxin with GABA$_A$ receptor channel-lining residues probed in cysteine mutants. *Biophys. J.* **69,** 1858–1867.
32. Karlin, A. and Akabas, M. H. (1998) Substituted-cysteine accessibility method. *Meth. Enzymol.* **293,** 123–145.
33. Yang, A.-S., Gunner, M. R., Sampogna, R., Sharp, K., and Honig, B. (1993) On the calculation of pKa's in proteins. *Proteins* **15,** 252–265.
34. Holmgren, M., Liu, Y., Xu, Y., and Yellen, G. (1996) On the use of thiol-modifying agents to determine channel topology. *Neuropharmacology* **35,** 797–804.
35. Roberts, D. D., Lewis, S. D., Ballou, D. P., Olson, S. T., and Shafer, J. A. (1986) Reactivity of small thiolate anions and cysteine-25 in papain towards methylmethanethiosulfonate. *Biochemistry* **25,** 5595–5601.
36. Danielson, M. A., Bass, R. B., and Falke, J. J. (1997) Cysteine and disulfide scanning reveals a regulatory alpha-helix in the cytoplasmic domain of the aspartate receptor. *J. Biol. Chem.* **272,** 32,878–32,888.
37. Lemmon, M. A. and Engelman, D. M. (1994) Specificity and promiscuity in membrane helix interactions. *Q. Rev. Biophys.* **27,** 157–218.
38. Pascual, J. M., Shieh, C. C., Kirsch, G. E., and Brown, A. M. (1995) K$^+$ pore structure revealed by reporter cysteines at inner and outer surfaces. *Neuron* **14,** 1055–1063.
39. Cheung, M. and Akabas, M. H. (1997) Locating the anion-selectivity filter of the cystic fibrosis transmembrane conductance regulator (CFTR) chloride channel. *J. Gen. Physiol.* **109,** 289–300.
40. Guinamard, R. and Akabas, M. H. (1999) Arg352 is a major determinant of charge selectivity in the cystic fibrosis transmembrane conductance regulator chloride channel. *Biochemistry* **38,** 5528–5537.
41. Woodhull, A. M. (1973) Ionic blockage of sodium channels in nerve. *J. Gen. Physiol.* **61,** 687–708.
42. Wilson, G. G. and Karlin, A. (1998) The location of the gate in the acetylcholine receptor channel. *Neuron* **20,** 1269–1281.
43. Pascual, J. M. and Karlin, A. (1998) Delimiting the binding site for quaternary ammonium lidocaine derivatives in the acetylcholine receptor channel. *J. Gen. Physiol.* **112,** 611–621.
44. Howard, M., DuVall, M. D., Devor, D. C., Dong, J. Y., Henze, K., and Frizzell, R. A. (1995) Epitope tagging permits cell surface detection of functional CFTR. *Am. J. Physiol.* **269,** C1565–1576.

11

Methods for the Study of Intermolecular and Intramolecular Interactions Regulating CFTR Function

Anjaparavanda P. Naren

1. Introduction

CFTR (Cystic Fibrosis Transmembrane Conductance Regulator) is a cAMP-activated chloride channel present on the apical surfaces of epithelial cells. This protein has been shown to be responsible for salt and water transport across epithelia (1). CFTR has been implicated in two major diseases, namely, cystic fibrosis (CF) and secretory diarrhea. In CF, the synthesis and or functional activity of the CFTR Cl⁻ channel is reduced. This autosomal recessive disorder affects approx 1 in 2500 Caucasians in the United States (1). Excessive CFTR activity is implicated in cases of toxin-induced secretory diarrhea (e.g., by cholera toxin and heat stable *Escherichia coli* enterotoxin) that stimulate cAMP or cGMP production in the gut (2). The protein encoded by the CF gene (CFTR) is a 1480-amino acid membrane-bound protein containing five major cytosolic domains, the N- and C-terminal tails, two nucleotide-binding domains (NBD 1 and 2), and a regulatory domain (R-domain). CFTR also has two sets of six transmembrane spanning domains. Physical interactions have been reported for various domains of CFTR with different proteins. The two opposing tails (N and C) of this Cl⁻ channel connect to different regulatory networks by interacting with distinct proteins. The amino-terminal tail interacts directly with syntaxin 1A and in part is responsible for inhibiting CFTR Cl⁻ current activity. Syntaxin 1A is highly expressed in the brain (3) and to a lesser extent in the lung and colon (4). Members of the syntaxin family of proteins have been implicated in membrane fusion (3,5). In the synapse, N-type calcium channels bind to syntaxin 1A (6–8), which negatively modulates the gating of these channels (9–11). The carboxy terminal tail interacts with PDZ

From: *Methods in Molecular Medicine, vol. 70: Cystic Fibrosis Methods and Protocols*
Edited by: W. R. Skach © Humana Press Inc., Totowa, NJ

(PSD-95, disc large, ZO-1) domain-containing proteins, and this interaction has been implicated in CFTR targeting to the apical (luminal) surface of polarized epithelial cells *(12)*. A recent review summarizes some of these interactions *(13)*. In this chapter, detailed methods will be presented and discussed that aid in the study of these interactions, with special emphasis on pulldown assays and pairwise binding assays.

1.1. Syntaxin 1A Binds Directly to the N Tail of CFTR and Modulates Cl⁻ Channel Function

We have observed that syntaxin 1A is expressed in native airway epithelial cells, where it localizes in part to the apical cell pole *(4)*. In addition, we have shown that syntaxin 1A interacts physically and functionally with CFTR *(14,15)* in an isoform-specific manner (i.e., syntaxins 2–4 do not bind to CFTR). The interacting sites have been mapped to the N-terminal tail of CFTR (1–79 a.a.) and the third helical domain (H3) of syntaxin 1A (194–266 a.a.) *(15)*. N-tail of CFTR syntaxin 1A binding has a 1:1 stoichiometry and is inhibited by a soluble syntaxin-binding protein, Munc 18 *(15)*. This physical interaction (between syntaxin 1A and CFTR) is essential for the modulation of CFTR activity by syntaxin 1A *(14)*. Evidence for this comes from functional studies conducted in two different systems. First, syntaxin 1A inhibits CFTR Cl⁻ currents when these proteins are co-expressed in *Xenopus* oocytes *(14)*. Syntaxin 1A must be membrane anchored to regulate CFTR currents and the inhibition can be completely blocked by reagents that disrupt the syntaxin-CFTR interaction (e.g., N tail of CFTR, cytosolic domain of syntaxin 1A, and munc 18 *(4,14,15)*. This inhibition is transporter specific to CFTR, in that it is not observed for other transporter proteins (e.g., the nicotinic acetylcholine receptor). This regulation of CFTR currents is also specific to syntaxin 1A (i.e., syntaxin 3 has no such effect; *see also* **ref. *14***). In a second series of experiments, whole-cell patch clamp studies were conducted on colonic epithelial cell lines *(14)* and primary airway epithelial cells *(4)* that normally express syntaxin 1A, CFTR, and Munc-18. Importantly, CFTR activity in these cells was augmented upon introducing agents that could disrupt the syntaxin 1A-CFTR interaction *(4,14,15)*. These studies clearly indicate that the intermolecular interaction between syntaxin 1A and the N tail of CFTR is essential for the downregulation of the channel.

1.2. Interdomain Interactions Between N Tail and R Domain Regulates CFTR Activity

We have also demonstrated that the N-terminal tail of CFTR is a positive regulator of Cl⁻ channel activity *(16)*. This regulation occurs via a direct domain–domain interaction between the N tail and the R domain of CFTR. A patch of acidic amino acids along one face of a putative helix in the N tail is involved in binding to the R domain as well as in regulating channel activity. The interacting sites have been mapped to a cluster of acidic residues (D47, E51, E54, and D58) on the N tail and to a small region on the R domain comprising a.a. residues 595-740 (*see* **Note 1** on the boundaries of the R domain). These acidic residues are strictly conserved between species. We observed a graded loss in CFTR activity with successive mutation of these negatively charged residues. Single-channel analysis showed a decreased open probability (*Po*) of the channel, which is due to the reduction of mean burst duration. We hypothesize that this is due in part to the disruption of the N tail and R domain interaction. This discovery of the N tail conferring a positive regulatory role through its interaction with the R domain establishes a novel determinant for the gating behavior of CFTR *(16)*. The precise mechanism by which this is accomplished is under investigation.

1.3. Biochemical Assays Used to Study These Interactions

Syntaxin 1A binds directly to the amino-terminal tail of CFTR, which is a region that also modulates CFTR gating. To understand how these intermolecular (between CFTR and syntaxin 1A) and intramolecular (between the N tail and R domain of CFTR) interactions influence the channel function, a detailed biochemical analysis is required of the binding regions/domains, stoichiometry and the half-maximal effective concentration of binding (EC_{50}). To obtain this information, a combination of several biochemical assays was performed and is reviewed below. **Subheadings 3.3.** and **3.4.** deal only with two specific assays (i.e., the pull-down and pairwise binding assays), which is used extensively in our laboratory to study protein–protein or domain–domain interactions.

1.3.1. Co-Immunoprecipitation

Co-Immunoprecipitation consists of immunoprecipitating a specific protein from a cell lysate using a specific antibody, and probing for the binding of another protein, either directly or indirectly. For example, we immunoprecipitated CFTR from a colonic epithelial cell lysate (HT29-CL19A cells) *(14)* using a CFTR-specific antibody (anti NBD-1; residues 426–588) *(17)* and have demonstrated specific co-immunoprecipitation of syntaxin 1A with CFTR. This was an early method that provided us with key evidence suggesting the existence of a protein–protein interaction between CFTR and syntaxin 1A. To carry out these experiments cell lysates were passed through a hydrazide deravitized disc (Actidisc, FMC Corp.) to which anti-CFTR antibodies were covalently linked. Bound protein was eluted with high-salt (1 *M* NaCl) and low-pH buffers (100 m*M* glycine, pH 2.5). In analysis of these eluted proteins, syntaxin 1A was detected. Non-immune antibodies were used as controls to rule out nonspecific interactions. It is to be noted, however, that the efficiency of co-immunoprecipitation was always low (<1% of input), which is consistent with the dynamic nature of the functional interaction between these two proteins *(14,15)*.

1.3.2. Pull-Down Assay

The pull-down assay utilizes a GST fusion protein that is incubated with a cell lysate. The complex is then "pulled down" with glutathione Sepharose beads and is probed by immunoblotting. In our case, syntaxin 1AΔC (where ΔC refers to deletion of the C-terminal membrane anchor) was expressed as a GST fusion protein and was allowed to bind CFTR in lysates of either colonic epithelial cells (HT29-CL19A) or in COS-7 cells expressing recombinant CFTR *(14,15)*. The protein complex was probed by immunoblotting for CFTR *(14,15)*. Using this assay we have shown intermolecular interactions between syntaxin 1A and CFTR *(14,15)*, shown in **Fig. 1**. We have also used this assay to detect intramolecular interactions between the N tail and the R domain of CFTR *(16)*, as is shown in **Fig. 2**. A limitation of this assay is that the fusion proteins (expressed in *E. coli*) used for binding studies has to be folded properly. We have both functional and structural information suggesting that the proteins described in this assay are folded properly. Although the evidence for protein–protein interactions between CFTR and syntaxin 1A was quite compelling using co-immunoprecipitation and pull-down assays, we could not rule out the possibility of an intermediary protein that could facilitate these interactions (i.e., cell lysate COS 7 or HT 29-CL19A was used as a source of CFTR and it contains several other proteins as well). We therefore utilized a pairwise binding assay.

1.3.3. Pairwise Binding Assay

Although it is very similar to the pull-down assay, the pairwise binging assay detects binding between two individually purified proteins. For this purpose, we purified these proteins as GST fusion proteins (e.g., GST-syntaxin 1AΔC, a.a. 1–266; and GST-N-tail of CFTR, a.a.1–75; or a.a. 1–79; *see* **Note 2**) and for one of these proteins the GST portion was clipped off (e.g., GST-syntaxin 1AΔC cleaved with thrombin to remove GST). Binding assays were performed using two purified proteins, and excess glutathione Sepharose beads were used to "pull down" the bound complex. An example of such an interaction is shown in **Fig. 3**. This assay has several advantages. First, we can determine if the interaction is direct. Second, the stoichiometry of interacting proteins can be determined (e.g., in our case we mixed a known amount of syntaxin 1AΔC with approx 100 molar excess GST-N-tail and the amount of syntaxin 1AΔC bound was estimated by immunoblotting using known amounts of syntaxin 1AΔC as standard *[15]*). Using such an assay we were able to show convincingly that the interaction between the N tail of CFTR (1–79 a.a.) and the H3 domain of syntaxin 1A (194–266 a.a.) was direct, with a stoichiometry of 1:1 *(15)*.

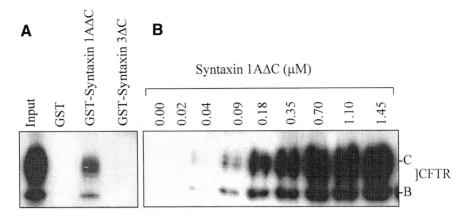

Fig. 1. CFTR interacts physically with syntaxin 1A. (A) GST-syntaxin 1AΔC (0.35 μM) can physically "pull down" recombinant CFTR from COS-7 cell lysates but not GST (0.76 μM) or GST-syntaxin 3ΔC (0.35 μM). (B) CFTR binding to syntaxin 1A saturates at submicromolar concentration (EC_{50} of ~350 nM). Immunoblots were probed with Genzyme-C-CFTR monoclonal antibody. Reprinted by permission from *Nature* **390,** 302–305, copyright 1997, MacMillan Magazine, Ltd.

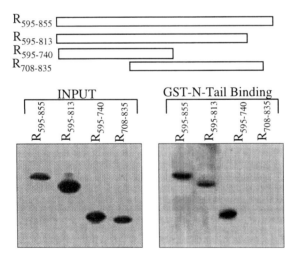

Fig. 2. The N tail interacts physically with the R domain of CFTR as detected by pull-down assay. Binding of GST-N-tail (2.85 μM) to various R-domain fragments expressed in COS-7 cells. Input corresponds to 20% of total lysate. Immunoblots were probed with Genzyme R-CFTR monoclonal antibody. Reprinted by permission from *Science* **286,** 544–548, copyright 1999, American Association for the Advancement of Science.

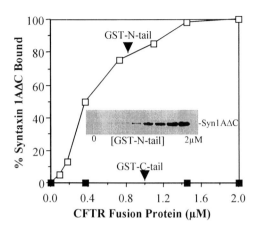

Fig. 3. Direct binding of GST-N-tail of CFTR to syntaxin 1AΔC as detected by pair wise binding assay. Cytosolic domain of syntaxin 1A (0.35 nM) binds saturally to increasing amounts of GST-N-tail of CFTR (0–2 μM) but does not bind to GST-C-tail (a.a. 1387–1480). Reprinted by permission from *Proc Natl. Acad. Sci. USA* **95,** 10,972–10,977, copyright 1998, The National Academy of Sciences.

1.3.4. Colorimetric Pairwise Binding Assay

We have also used a colorimetric pairwise binding assay to show a direct interaction between the R domain of CFTR and the N-tail peptide *(16)*. In this assay we used a small synthetic peptide (34 a.a. long). GST-R domain (a.a. 595–740) was immobilized on glutathione Sepharose beads and a biotinylated N-tail peptide (biotin-p30-63) was added to the mix. The amount of biotinylated peptide bound to the beads was detected by treating the bound complex with Streptavidin-HRP. After extensive washes, an HRP assay was performed (ABTS method, Pierce Chem. Co.) to detect the amount of the bound protein. Using this assay we have shown that there is a direct physical interaction between the N tail and R domain of CFTR. Although we did not quantitate the amount of peptide bound, running a standard curve for biotin p30-63 and estimating the amount bound from it can do this. One of the major disadvantages of using biotinylated synthetic peptide is lack of specificity. One way to control this is to utilize a large number of negative controls, as discussed earlier. For example, we have used GST and GST-R$_{740-813}$ as described earlier *(16)*. Competing with the unbiotinylated peptide is the method of choice to eliminate nonspecific interactions (e.g., p30-63 competes for the binding of biotin p30-63 but not the outer-loop CFTR peptide p107-117 *[16]*). Extensive washing of the bound complex on beads with buffer helps, but signals become weak due to the washing steps.

2. Materials

2.1. General Reagents

1. pGEX vectors (Amersham Pharmacia Biotech, Piscataway, NJ).
2. Glutathione Sepharose beads (Amersham).
3. Restriction enzymes (Promega, Madison, WI).
4. pCDNA3 (Invitrogen, Carlsbad, CA).
5. PCR reagents (Stratagene, La Jolla, CA).
6. Oligonucleotide primers (Genmed Synthesis, San Francisco, CA).
7. ECL reagents (NEN, Boston, MA).

All other reagents were purchased from Sigma (St. Louis, MO) unless otherwise stated.

2.2. Media and Buffers

1. Luria-Bertani containing Ampicillin (LB-Amp) medium (pH 7.0): 10 g Bacto-tryptone, 5 g Bacto yeast extract, and 10 g NaCl per liter. Autoclave, cool, and add filter-sterilized ampicillin (50 mg/L).
2. Sucrose buffer: 50 mM Tris-HCl (pH 8.0), 1 mM ethylenediaminetetraacetic acid (EDTA), 1 mM PMSF, and 10% sucrose.
3. Elution buffer: 25 mM Tris-HCl (pH 8.0), 140 mM NaCl, and 20 mM reduced glutathione.
4. Phosphate-buffered saline (PBS) (pH 7.4): 140 mM Na$_2$HPO$_4$, 1.5 mM KH$_2$PO$_4$, 2.7 mM KCl, and 140 mM NaCl.
5. Lysis buffer: PBS (pH 7.4) –0.2% Triton X-100 containing protease inhibitors (PMSF 1 mM, leupeptin [1 µg/µL], aprotinin [1 µg/µL] and pepstatin [1 µg/µL]).
6. 5× sample buffer: 0.6 M Tris-HCl (pH 6.8), 50% glycerol, 2% sodium dodecyl sulfate (SDS), 5% β-mercaptoethanol, and 0.1% bromophenol blue.

2.3. Cell Culture

1. COS-7 cells (ATCC).
2. DMEM with 10% fetal bovine serum (FBS).
3. Opti-mem (Gibco-BRL).
4. Vaccine virus encoding T7 polymerase (VTF 7-3).
5. DOPE/DOTAP.
6. HT29-CL19A cells.

2.4. CFTR Binding and Visualization

1. CFTR-Cterm antibody (Genzyme).
2. Nylon PVDF membrane.
3. Thrombin (Pharmacia).

3. Methods

3.1. Expression and Purification of GST Fusion Protein

1. Synthesize defined regions of syntaxin 1A (a.a. 1–266) and CFTR (N-tail; a.a. 1–75) by polymerase chain reaction. Incorporate restriction sites (Bam H1 in forward

and Xho 1 in reverse) 5'overhangs (TATA) and a stop codon into the primers. Clone the PCR product into pGEX5X-1 vector (Pharmacia) and transform in a protease-deficient *E. coli* strain (BL21-DE3), as protein integrity is often an issue.

2. Grow the culture overnight (37°C) in LB-Amp. Dilute the overnight culture 1:10 (LB-Amp) and grow a further 2 h at 37°C. Induce with 1 m*M* IPTG for the next 4 h at 30°C. Pellet the cells by centrifugation at 8000*g* for 10 min at 4°C.

3. Lyse the cells in sucrose buffer (20 mL for cell pellet originating from 1 L of culture) containing lysozyme (1 mg/mL), 0.2% Triton X-100, and protease inhibitors (*see* **Subheading 2.2.5.**). Mix on a rotary shaker for 30 min at 4°C.

4. Spin at 20,000*g* for 30min at 4°C. Take the clear supernatant.

5. Add 1 mL of glutathione Sepharose beads (50% slurry in sucrose buffer) to the clear supernatant and mix for 4 h at 4°C on a rotary shaker. Wash the beads by resuspending in PBS (15 mL), mix for 2 min, spin (800*g* for 2 min), and decant. This procedure is repeated six times.

6. Elute the protein from the beads using elution buffer (2 mL/mL of beads; *see* **Note 3**) and dialyze against 2 L with PBS. Change dialysate 4 times every 4 h. Concentrate the protein using a Centricon filter (10,000 cutoff) and store as small aliquots at –80°C. Determine the protein concentration by the BCA method *(18)*. Access the protein quality by SDS-PAGE *(19)*. If the purity of the protein is not satisfactory, secondary purification procedures such as gel filtration or ion exchange may be employed. (e.g., we have used a G-75 Sepharose column to further purify GST-N-tail)

3.2. Expression of CFTR in COS-7 Cells

1. Grow COS-7 cells to ~50–70% confluence overnight in a 6-well plate (DMEM–10% FBS). Wash each well of the plate with 1 ml of opti-MEM (Gibco-BRL). Infect the cells with vaccinia virus encoding T7 polymerase (VTF 7-3) at a multiplicity of infection of 5 in 0.8 mL of opti-MEM. The vaccinia system used as a transient expression system in COS-7 cells has the advantage of consistent high levels of expression and also high efficiency of transfection (>80–90% of the cells express the protein of interest). Refer to the excellent article by Ramachandra et al. *(20)* regarding this transient transfection method for details.

2. After 40 min, add 5 µg of pTM-1 plasmid *(21)* or pCDNA-3 plasmid expressing WT-CFTR or various R-domain constructs under regulatory control of the T7 promoter. Mix with 20 µg of lipid N-[1-(2,3-dioleoyloxy)propyl]-N,N,N-trimethylammonium chloride/dioleoyl phosphatidylethanolamine (DOPE/DOTAP) at 1/1 wt/wt ratio in opti-MEM (200 µL) for 20 min, to virus infected cells.

3. After 24 h, remove the medium and the cells are ready to be lysed (*see below*). Alternatively, HT29-CL19A cell lysate can be used as a source of native CFTR, as these cell lines express a substantial amount of CFTR *(14)*.

3.3. Pull-Down Assay

The experiment described below is specifically to monitor the CFTR–syntaxin 1A interaction. A similar assay was also used to detect binding of N tail to R domain of CFTR.

1. Lyse COS-7 cells expressing WT-CFTR (or R domain) in lysis buffer (200 µL/ well). Pool lysates from 6-well plates and mix at 4°C for 15 min on a rotary mixer. Centrifuge at 15,000*g* for 10 min at 4°C. Transfer the clear supernatant into a clean microfuge tube. This supernatant is the source of CFTR.

2. Add eluted GST, (*see* **Subheading 3.1., step 6**) GST-syntaxin 1AΔC and GST-Syntaxin 3ΔC (0–100 µg) to the clear supernatant (200 µL) and increase the volume to 1 mL with lysis buffer (or GST-N-tail, depending on the interaction). Mix on a rotary mixer. (CFTR is immunoprecipitated at the same time from an equal amount of lysate [200 µL] using Genzyme C-terminal antibody, which gives an indication of input amounts [*see* **Note 4** for CFTR immunoprecipitation]).

3. After 30–60 min, add glutathione Sepharose beads (Pharmacia; 50 µL of 50% slurry in lysis buffer) and continue to mix at 4°C for 3 h.

4. At the end of 3 h, spin at 800*g* for 2 min and discard the supernatant. Wash the beads three times with lysis buffer.

5. Elute the protein with 20 µL of 5× sample buffer for 15 min at 37°C (*see* **Note 5**). Spin at 12,000*g* for 1 min, recover the supernatant, and analyze by SDS-PAGE (5%).

6. Western blotting is done by transferring the protein on the gel to a nylon membrane (PVDF) and probed using Genzyme C-CFTR monoclonal antibody (0.1 µg/mL). (For N-tail–R-domain interaction, the Genzyme R-CFTR antibody at 0.2 mg/mL is used.) Detection is by ECL following the manufacturer's instructions. A typical pull-down experiment to detect intermolecular interactions between CFTR and syntaxin 1A is shown in **Fig. 1**, and intramolecular interaction between the N tail and R domain of CFTR is shown in **Fig. 2**. It is important that multiple controls to rule out nonspecific interactions be included. For example, CFTR binds to syntaxin 1AΔC but not GST, GST syntaxin 2ΔC, GST–syntaxin 3ΔC, GST–syntaxin 4ΔC, or GST–syntaxin 5ΔC. Also, CFTR cannot bind to GST–syntaxin 1AΔH3 (a.a. 1–194). We have also examined six other epithelially expressed proteins including aminopeptidase (apical membrane protein) for their ability to bind GST–syntaxin 1AΔC. None of these proteins bound under the binding conditions we used.

3.4. Pairwise Binding Assay

1. Cleave GST–syntaxin 1AΔC using 1 U of thrombin (Pharmacia)/100 µg of protein at 37°C for 1 h. Stop the reaction by adding 1 m*M* PMSF, estimate the protein content (BCA method), and store the protein in small aliquots at –80°C (typically we cleave 1–2 mg of GST–syntaxin 1AΔC at a time).

2. Transfer eluted GST-N-tail (0–2 µ*M*) in lysis buffer to microfuge tubes (200 µL total volume). Add 0.35 n*M* of thrombin-cleaved syntaxin 1A. Mix at 4°C.

3. After 30–60 min, add 20 µL of glutathione Sepharose beads and mix for an additional 3 h.

4. Spin the mix at 800*g* for 2 min and discard the supernatant. Wash three times with lysis buffer and process for Western blotting as described above except: (a) use 10% acrylamide gels are used to resolve the bound syntaxin 1AΔC and (b) detect syntaxin 1A using syntaxin 1A monoclonal antibody (14D8; **ref. *22***) at 0.1 µg/mL. A typical pairwise binding assay is shown in **Fig. 3**.

3.5. Conclusion

These techniques provide convenient and reproducible assays to biochemically define some of these protein–protein and domain–domain interactions.
Most compelling results are obtained using multiple assays. It is also to be
noted that researchers must use discretion in choosing the most appropriate
assay for the particular experiment of interest. For example, "pull-downs" may
not be useful if interactions are highly dynamic with high off-rates, which can
be detected using alternative binding assays such as surface plasmon resonance
assay *(23)*.

4. Notes

1. The boundaries of CFTR are currently being reevaluated based on the crystal
   structure of the NBD of His-P *(24)*. Based on this structure there is reason to
   believe that the NBD-1 of CFTR may extend from 433 to 634 a.a. This would
   mean that the region we define as R domain (595–740), which binds to the N tail,
   may contain the distal portion of NBD-1.
2. The N tail in our previous work has been defined as 1–79 of CFTR *(14,15)*. More
   recently we have made an N-tail fusion protein corresponding to residues 1–75,
   which is much better behaved as a fusion protein (higher yield and less protease
   sensitive) and easier to purify. The biochemical and functional properties of this
   construct are similar to 1–79 CFTR.
3. It is important that the pH of the elution buffer be adjusted to 8.0 after the addition of reduced glutathione. The pH can be as low as 3.0 after the addition of
   reduced glutathione; if the pH is not adjusted before elution, the efficiency of
   elution is drastically reduced.
4. Immunoprecipitation of CFTR: Genzyme-C-CFTR monoclonal antibody (0.5 µg)
   is bound to 20 µmL of protein A/G agarose (Santa Cruz Biotech, Santa Cruz, CA)
   for at least 1 h at 4°C. The bound IgG is washed once with 1 mL of 0.1 M N-ethyl
   morpholin (NEM) buffer. The IgG is cross-linked to protein A/G agarose using
   10 mM dimethyl pimelimidate (DMP; Pierce Chem. Co.) in NEM buffer for 30
   min at 22°C. The reaction is stopped by washing the beads once with 100 mM tris
   base (pH 8.0). Immunoprecipitation is done by mixing the beads with cell lysate
   (e.g., HT29-CL19A in PBS–0.2% Triton X-100) overnight. The beads are washed
   extensively with lysis buffer and the protein eluted with 20 µL of 5× sample
   buffer and immunoblotted using either a monoclonal or polyclonal antibody
   raised against CFTR (no heavy or light chain contamination is observed using
   this antibody and method of coupling). It is to be noted, however, that cross-
   linking is most efficient when Genzyme C-CFTR antibody is used (probably due
   to it being IgG 2a isotype; all other antibodies we have used are of IgG 1 isotype).
   Other antibodies can be cross-linked as well (e.g., Genzyme- R-CFTR mab,
   MATG 1031mab [first outer loop], MATG 1104mab [R domain], GA1-C-CFTR
   mab [recognizes a.a 1440–1460], NBD1-R-CFTR polyclonal [raised against a.a.
   521–828], N-CFTR polyclonal [raised against a.a. 46–63 and GST-N-tail], and
   C-CFTR polyclonal [raised against a.a. 1466–1480]). However ,these are not as

efficiently cross-linked as Genzyme C-CFTR mab. An alternative would be to cross-link a monoclonal (e.g., Genzyme R-CFTR, MATG 1031, or MATG 1104) and use a polyclonal (NBD1-R-CFTR polyclonal, N-CFTR polyclonal, or C-CFTR polyclonal) to detect by blotting, or vice versa.

5. It is strongly recommended not to boil the CFTR samples prepared for Western blotting, as aggregation is a common problem. Instead, the samples should be heated at 37°C for 10–15 min before loading the gel.

6. We have also detected interactions between syntaxin 1AΔC and the N tail of CFTR by the yeast 2-hybrid method. It is to be noted that the interaction is low affinity (EC_{50} of ~350 nM as detected by pull down assay; **Fig. 1**; **ref. 6**) and is just above the negative control (syntaxin 1A and the C tail were tested as negative controls and syntaxin 1A–munc 18 as a positive control). Yeast 2-hybrid is probably not an appropriate method to study interactions with low affinities.

Acknowledgments

I am indebted to Drs. Kevin Kirk, Estelle Cormet-Boyaka, David Nelson, John Clancy, Eric Sorscher, Douglas Cyr, and Eric Schwiebert for their comments. This work is supported by a grant from the Cystic Fibrosis Foundation (NAREN 99GO).

References

1. Welsh, M. J., Tsui, L.-C., Boat, T. F., and Beaudet, A. L .(1995) Cystic fibrosis, in *The Metabolic and Molecular Basis of Inherited Diseases: Membrane Transport Systems*, vol. 3, (Scriver, C. R., Beaudet, A. L., Sly, W. S., and Valle, D., eds.), McGraw-Hill, New York, pp. 379–387.

2. Chao, A. C., de Sauvage, F. J., Dong, Y. J., Wagner, J. A., Goeddel, D. V., and Gardner, P. (1994) Activation of intestinal CFTR Cl- channel by heat-stable enterotoxin and guanylin via cAMP-dependent protein kinase. *EMBO J.* **13,** 1065–1072.

3. Bennett, M. K., Garcia-Arrraros J. E., Elferink, L. A., Peterson, K., Fleming, A. M., Hazuka, C. D., and Scheller, R. H. (1993) The syntaxin family of vesicular transport receptors. *Cell* **74,** 863--873.

4. Naren, A.P., Anke, D., Cormet-Boyaka, E., Boyaka, P. N., McGhee,J. R., Zhou,W., Akagawa, K., Fujiwara, T., Thome, U., Engelhardt, J. F., Nelson, D. J., and Kirk, K. L. (1999) Syntaxin 1A is Expressed in Airway Epithelial Cells Where it Modulates CFTR Cl- Currents. *J. Clin. Invest.* **105,** 377–386.

5. Rowe, T., Dascher, C., Bannykh, S., Plutner, H., and Balch, W. E. (1998) Role of vesicle-associated syntaxin 5 in the assembly of pre-Golgi intermediates. *Science* **279,** 696–700.

6. Bennett, M. K., Calakos, N., and Scheller, R. H. (1992) Syntaxin: a synaptic protein implicated in docking of synaptic vesicles at presynaptic active zones. *Science* **257,** 255–259.

7. Yoshida, A., Oho, C., Omori, A., Kuwahara, R., Ito, T., and Takahashi, M. (1992) HPC-1 is associated with synaptotagmin and omega-conotoxin receptor. *J. Biol. Chem.* **267,** 24,925–24,928.

8. Sheng, Z. H., Rettig, J., Takahashi, M., and Catterall, W. A. (1994) Identification of a syntaxin-binding site on N-type calcium channels. *Neuron* **13,** 1303–1313.

9. Bezprozvanny, I., Scheller, R. H., and Tsien, R. W. (1995) Functional impact of syntaxin on gating of N-type and Q-type calcium channels. *Nature* **378,** 623–626.

10. Wiser, O., Bennett, M. K., and Atlas, D. (1996) Functional interaction of syntaxin and SNAP-25 with voltage-sensitive L- and N-type Ca^{2+} channels. *EMBO J.* **15,** 4100–4110.

11. Stanley, E. F. and Mirotznik, R. R. (1997) Cleavage of syntaxin prevents G-protein regulation of presynaptic calcium channels. *Nature* **385,** 340–343.

12. Moyer, B. D., Duhaime, M., Shaw, C., Denton, J., Reynolds, D., Karlson, K. H., et al. (2000) The PDZ interacting domain of CFTR is required for functional expression in the apical plasma membrane. *J. Biol. Chem.* 275, 27,069–27,074.

13. Naren, A. P. and Kirk, K. L. (2000) CFTR Cl⁻ channels and regulatory networks. *News in Physiol. Sci.* **15,** 57–61.

14. Naren, A. P., Nelson, D. J., Xie, W., Jovov, B., Tousson, A., Pevsner, J., et al. (1997) Regulation of CFTR chloride channels by syntaxin and Munc 18 isoforms. *Nature* **390,** 302–305.

15. Naren, A. P., Quick, M. W., Collawn, J. F., Nelson, D. J., and Kirk, K. L. (1998) Syntaxin 1A directly inhibits CFTR chloride channel by means of domain-specific interactions. *Proc. Natl. Acad. Sci. USA* **95,** 10,972–10,977.

16. Naren, A. P., Cormet-Boyaka. E., Fu, J., Villain, M., Blalock, E., Quick M. W., and Kirk, K. L. (1999) CFTR Chloride channel regulation by an interdomain interaction. *Science* **286,** 544–548.

17. Jovov, B., Ismailov, I. I., Berdiev, B. K., Fuller, C. M., Sorscher, E. J., Dedman, J. R., Kaetzel, M. A., and Benos, D. J. (1995) Interaction between cystic fibrosis transmembrane conductance regulator and outwardly rectified chloride channels. *J. Biol. Chem.* **270,** 29,194–29,200.

18. Smith, P. K., Krohn, R. I., Hermanson, G. T., Mallia, A. K., Gartner, F. H., Provenzano, M. D., et al. (1985) Measurement of protein using bicinchoninic acid. *Anal. Biochem.* **150,** 76–85.

19. Laemmli, U. K. (1970) Cleavage of structural proteins during the assembly of the head of bacteriophage T4. *Nature* **227,** 680–685.

20. Ramachandra, M., Gottesman, M. M., and Pastan, I. (1998) Recombinant vaccinia virus vectors for functional expression of P-glycoprotein in mammalian cells. *Meth. Enzymol.* **292,** 441–455.

21. Cheng, S. H., Rich, D. P., Marshall, J., Gregory, R. J., Welsh, M. J., and Smith, A. E. (1991) Phosphorylation of the R domain by cAMP-dependent protein kinase regulates the CFTR chloride channel. *Cell* **66,** 1027–1036.

22. Kushima, Y., Fujiwara, T., Sanada, M., and Akagawa, K. (1997) Characterization of HPC-1 antigen, an isoform of syntaxin-1, with the isoform-specific monoclonal antibody, 14D8. *J. Mol. Neurosci.* **8,** 19–27.

23. Villain, M., Jackson, P. L., Manion, M. K., Dong, W. J., Su, Z., Fassina, G., et al. (2000) De novo design of peptides targeted to the EF hands of calmodulin. *J. Biol. Chem.* **275,** 2676–2685.

24. Hung, L. W., Wang, I.X., Nikaido, K., Liu, P. Q., Ames, G. F. and Kim, S. H. (1998) Crystal structure of the ATP-binding subunit of an ABC transporter. *Nature* **396,** 703–707.

12

Fluorescent Indicator Methods to Assay Functional CFTR Expression in Cells

Alan S. Verkman and Sujatha Jayaraman

1. Introduction

Halide-sensitive fluorescent indicators have been useful in cystic fibrosis (CF) research in assaying functional cystic fibrosis transmembrane conductance regulator (CFTR) expression in cells. Some applications (for review, *see* **refs.** *1* and *2*) have included measurements in native airway cells *(3)*, demonstration that CFTR is a chloride channel *(4,5)*, functional analysis of mutant CFTRs *(6–8)*, and analysis of the efficacy of CFTR gene replacement in human gene therapy trials *(9–11)*. A promising new application of halide indicators is in high-throughput screening to discover drugs that may correct defective cellular processing and/or function of disease-causing CFTR mutants. Another new application is the use of cell-impermeable chloride indicators to measure chloride concentration in the airway surface liquid in cell culture models and in the in vivo trachea *(12)*. The first biological application of a chloride indicator, SPQ, was reported in 1987 *(13)*. As described below, numerous advances in indicator technology have been made since the first report, including the development of cell-permeable *(14)*, cell-impermeable *(15,16)*, long-wavelength *(17,18)*, and dual-wavelength *(19)* indicators, as well as the development of a targetable green fluorescent protein-based halide indicator *(20)*. The major advantages of a fluorescence-based assay of CFTR function are sensitivity, technical simplicity, and the ability to assay function in single cells and heterogeneous cell mixtures. Fluorescence assays are rapid, quantitative, and technically simple, and can be performed using fluorescence microscopy, automated fluorescence plate readers, or cell cytometry. In contrast, assays using radioactive ^{36}Cl require relatively large amounts of materials, are techni-

From: *Methods in Molecular Medicine, vol. 70: Cystic Fibrosis Methods and Protocols*
Edited by: W. R. Skach © Humana Press Inc., Totowa, NJ

cally difficult, and cannot be used to study single cells or heterogeneous cell mixtures. Single-channel electrophysiological measurements of CFTR function are also technically challenging and generally not suitable for screening applications; however, it should be noted that data on single-channel properties (open probability, gating kinetics, current–voltage relationships) cannot be obtained by fluorescence methods. This chapter describes the available fluorescence-based assays of CFTR function. Technical details and useful practical hints are provided, and potential pitfalls are mentioned.

1.1. Fluorescent Indicator Strategy to Assay CFTR Function

Fluorescence measurement of functional CFTR in cells involves first the labeling of cell cytoplasm with a chloride- or iodide-sensitive fluorescent indicator. Iodide and/or chloride transport across the cell plasma membrane are determined from the time-course of cell fluorescence in response to imposed chloride/iodide gradients, and after cAMP stimulation. **Figure 1** shows the classical chloride/nitrate exchange protocol to measure cAMP-stimulated CFTR function using the indicator SPQ. After loading cells with SPQ, extracellular chloride is replaced by nitrate, an anion that is transported by CFTR but does not quench SPQ fluorescence. Before CFTR activation, cell anion permeability is low and there is a slow increase in cell fluorescence. After activation of CFTR by the cAMP-agonist forskolin, fluorescence promptly increases as chloride exits the cell primarily in exchange for nitrate. The rate of fluorescence increase provides a quantitative measure of the CFTR chloride-transporting function. As detailed by Mansoura et al. (*9*), determination of absolute chloride flux (in millimoles per second) from the rate of the forskolin-induced fluorescence increase requires knowledge of the intracellular fluorescence vs [Cl] relationship. In addition, a two-point calibration is required because absolute fluorescence varies from experiment to experiment. As shown in **Fig. 1**, fluorescence *Fo* corresponds to zero intracellular chloride and *Fb*, measured after addition of a strong fluorescence quencher such as thiocyanate, corresponds to infinite intracellular fluorescence (background). Finally, computation of the absolute plasma membrane chloride conductance from chloride flux requires knowledge of the electrochemical driving force for chloride exit.

Although determination of absolute chloride flux or conductance can be useful, the indicator assay is most often used in a comparative or semiquantitative manner to compare CFTR function or to deduce the presence of functional CFTR. When experiments are set up in an identical manner and fluorescence is correctly calibrated, the activities of CFTR mutants can be compared or the efficacy of CFTR inhibitors/activators determined. The reader is referred to Mansoura et al. (*9*) for a full discussion of issues related to experimental design and data interpretation.

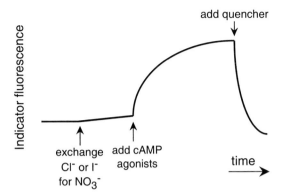

Fig. 1. Original SPQ assay protocol. SPQ-loaded cells were first perfused with Cl⁻ buffer, then with NO_3^- buffer and, where indicated, CFTR was stimulated by 20 μM forskolin (*see* **Subheading 3.** for buffer compositions).

1.2. Indicators

Figure 2 shows the structures of commonly used halide indicators for cellular measurements. The quinolinium indicator SPQ is a blue fluorescent zwitterionic compound whose fluorescence is quenched by halides by a collisional mechanism *(21)*. SPQ is loaded into cells by brief hypotonic shock or prolonged incubation, where it is well retained in cytoplasm because of its high polarity. The derivative diH-MEQ is a reduced (dihydro) quinolinium that rapidly enters cells, where it becomes oxidized to an indicator with similar properties to SPQ. Bis-DMXPQ is a chimeric, dual-wavelength indicator in which the blue fluorescent 6-methoxyquinolinium chromophore is linked to the chloride-insensitive yellow fluorescent 6-aminoquinolinium chromophore via a rigid, reducible 1,2-*trans*-bispyridylethylene spacer *(19)*. Also shown is a low-affinity, ratioable chloride-sensitive dextran that was used to measure chloride concentration in the ASL **(12)**. The recently introduced indicator LZQ is sensitive exclusively to iodide for assay of CFTR function using iodide/chloride or iodide/nitrate change protocols *(18)*. The fluorescence of LZQ is substantially brighter than that of SPQ or other quinolinium-based indicators, making it useful for plate-reader assays. Each of these compounds is nontoxic to cells, reasonably well retained in cytoplasm, and reports accurately changes in cytoplasmic chloride and/or iodide content. The choice of indicators depends on the system to be assayed in terms of loading requirements, detection sensitivity, and other factors.

Recently, a green fluorescent protein-based halide indicator was introduced, YFP-H148Q *(20)*. When cell transfection can be done to stain cytoplasm, we prefer this molecular indicator over exogenous chemical indicators because

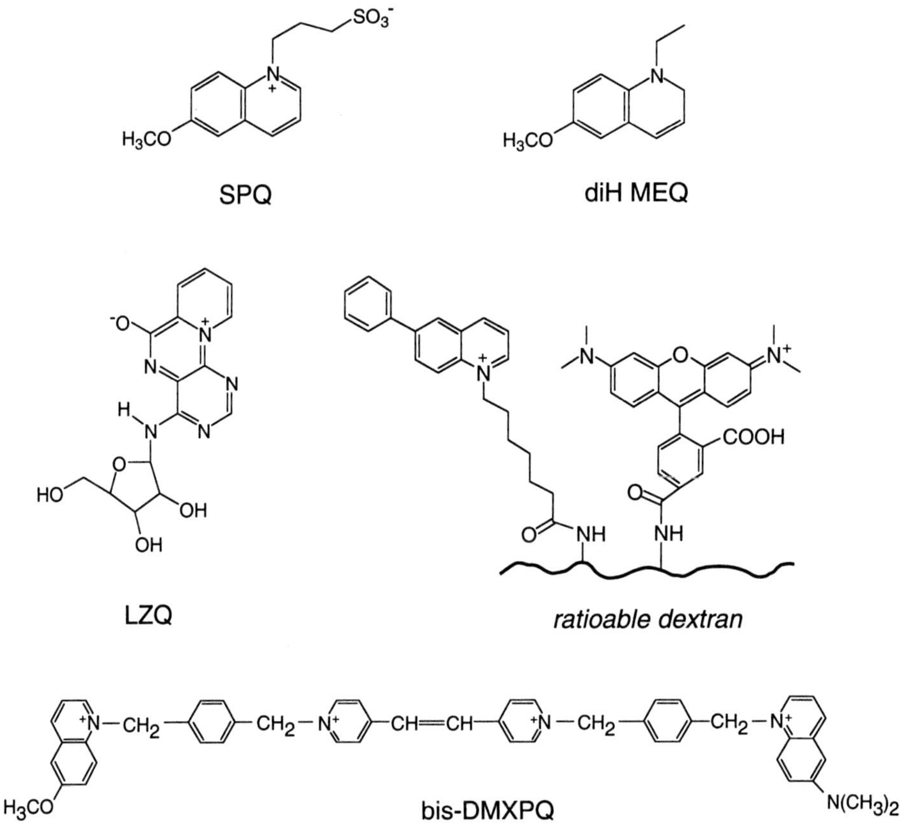

Fig. 2. Structures of widely used Cl⁻ sensitive blue quinolinium-based indicators SPQ and diHMEQ; the long-wavelength I⁻ sensitive indicator LZQ; and the dual-wavelength indicator bis-DMXPQ. Also shown is the low-affinity, ratioable Cl⁻ indicator conjugated to 40,000 MW dextran.

cell loading/washing is not necessary, cytoplasmic indicator retention is perfect, and the YFP chromophore has bright green/yellow fluorescence. **Figure 3** shows the application of YFP-H148Q fluorescence to detect functional CFTR using a Cl⁻/I⁻ exchange protocol. However, a potential concern is that the sensitivity of YFP fluorescence to halide concentration results from a shift in its pKa, so that YFP fluorescence depends on both iodide/chloride concentration and pH. By comparison, LZQ fluorescence is not pH-sensitive, and quinolinium fluorescence is mildly pH-sensitive because quinolinium fluorescence is quenched weakly by intracellular anions (such as proteins) whose charge is pH-dependent. A recent advance in green fluorescent protein-based halide indicators is the development of a dual-wavelength chimeric indicator

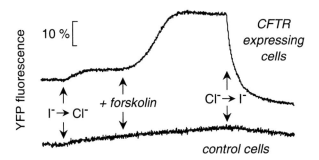

Fig. 3. CFTR-mediated Cl⁻/I⁻ transport detected using YFP-H148Q. Forskolin-stimulated Cl⁻/I⁻ transport is shown for Swiss 3T3 fibroblasts transiently transfected with YFP-H148Q. Cells (top, cells stably expressing CFTR; bottom, controls) were initially perfused with I⁻ buffer, followed by perfusion with Cl⁻ buffer and, where indicated, CFTR was stimulated by addition of 20 μ*M* forskolin (*see* **Subheading 3.** for buffer compositions).

consisting of YFP-H148Q in fusion with a halide- and pH-insensitive red fluorescent protein *(22)*. The chimeric indicator should be useful for applications involving ratio imaging or cell cytometry. In addition, random mutagenesis of YFP-H148Q has yielded mutants with improved chloride and iodide sensitivities *(23)*.

1.3. Instrumentation

For fluorescence microscopy, cells grown on transparent supports are mounted in a perfusion chamber in which solutions can be exchanged rapidly and cell fluorescence detected using a medium- or high-numerical-aperture objective lens. The supports may be glass or plastic for one-sided perfusion, or a transparent permeable substrate for two-sided perfusion *(3)*. Commercial or home-built perfusion chambers with temperature control, efficient mixing, and small chamber volume are recommended. Standard epifluorescence microscopes (upright or inverted) with appropriate filter sets and detector (charge-coupled device [CCD] camera, photomultiplier, or avalanche photodiode) are suitable. An important consideration is the use of low light and/or intermittent sample illumination to minimize photobleaching and light-induced cell injury. Illumination with a tungsten–halogen lamp powered by a stabilized direct current supply is preferred over arc lamp and laser sources because of superior stability. For plate-reader detection, we recommend a sensitive fluorescence plate reader equipped with high-quality bandpass filters, temperature regulation, bottom illumination/reading, and at least two software-controlled syringe pumps for solution additions. The choice of instrumentation depends on the cell system, fluorescent halide indicator, the need to resolve individual cells in a heterogeneous mixture, and the need to resolve small differences in CFTR activity. Some practical considerations are summarized in the Notes.

2. Materials

2.1. Indicators and Cells

1. High purity halide indicator (SPQ, LZQ, or diHMEQ).
2. Loading and experimental solutions (*see* below).
3. Cell line for loading with indicators, or cell line expressing YFP-H148Q. Cell lines that are generally used for the assays include Swiss 3T3 fibroblasts, Chinese hamster ovary (CHO) cells, MDCK cells, T84 cells, Calu-3 cells, HeLa cells, Fisher rat thyroid (FRT) cells, and C127 cells (*see* **Note 1** for considerations for suitable cell lines).

2.2. Solutions

1. Cl^- buffer: 137 mM NaCl, 2.7 mM KCl, 0.7 mM $CaCl_2$, 1.1 mM $MgCl_2$, 1.5 mM KH_2PO_4, 8.1 mM Na_2HPO_4, pH 7.4.
2. NO_3^- buffer: 137 mM $NaNO_3$, 2.7 mM KNO_3, 0.7 mM $CaNO_3$, 1.1 mM $MgNO_3$, 1.5 mM KH_2PO_4, 8.1 mM Na_2HPO_4, pH 7.4.
3. I^- buffer: 137 mM NaI, 2.7 mM KCl, 0.7 mM $CaCl_2$, 1.1 mM $MgCl_2$, 1.5 mM KH_2PO_4, 8.1 mM Na_2HPO_4, pH 7.4 (*see* **Note 2**).
4. KSCN buffer: 150 mM KSCN.
5. Forskolin: 50 mM stock in dimethyl sulfoxide (DMSO), or other activators and inhibitors for CFTR.

2.3. Instrumentation

1. Fluorescence measurements were carried out in a Nikon inverted epifluorescence microscope with appropriate filter sets and objective lens. SPQ filter set: excitation 365 ± 20 nm, dichroic 400 nm, emission 415 nm, barrier filter. LZQ filter set: excitation 420 ± 10 nm, dichroic 455 nm, emission 500 nm, barrier filter. YFP filter set: excitation 500 ± 10 nm, dichroic 515 nm, emission 535 ± 15 nm.
2. Perfusion chamber and water bath to maintain solution temperature at 37°C.
3. Solution reservoirs (50- or 60-mL tubes or syringes) and solenoid-driven valves (four- or eight-port D4/D8 valves, Hamilton Co., Reno, NV) or pinch-type valves with a 4 or 8 port manifold (ALA Scientific, Westbury, NY).
4. Photomultiplier (model R928S, Hamamatsu Corp., South Natick, MA) or CCD camera detector (e.g., AT 200; Photometrics, Tucson, AZ).
5. Computer interface consisting of 14-bit analog-to-digital converter and personal computer for data acquisition and storage.
6. For plate-reader assays: 96-well plates, plate reader (BMG LabTechnologies, Durham, NC) with appropriate filters (for LZQ, excitation 425 ± 15 nm; emission 530 ± 15 nm), equipped with heating block and two syringe pumps.

3. Methods

3.1. Preparing for Assay

3.1.1. For Fluorescence Microscopy

1. Set up the microscope with appropriate filter sets and objective lens (20–40× air or oil immersion objective). Excite fluorescence using a 100-W tungsten–halogen lamp powered by a stabilized DC supply in series with a OD 2 neutral density filter (*see* **Note 3** for more details). Use a concentric circular diaphragm to illuminate and measure ~50% of the field of illumination.
2. Check buffer osmolarities and adjust if needed to 295–300 mOsm using mannitol.
3. Set up the perfusion system by filling reservoirs with Cl$^-$ buffer; NO$_3^-$ buffer, NO$_3^-$ buffer with 20 μM forskolin and Cl$^-$ buffer with 20 μM forskolin for SPQ assay. For LZQ assay fill reservoirs with Cl$^-$ buffer, I$^-$ buffer, I$^-$ buffer with 20 μM forskolin, and Cl$^-$ buffer with 20 μM forskolin.
4. Load the cells with dye, either by hypotonic shock or by overnight incubation.
5. Set up the perfusion chamber by mounting the cover slip containing loaded cells in the chamber with the cells facing up, and close the chamber to make a watertight seal. Place the solution reservoirs in a water bath maintained at 37°C and perfuse through the chamber by gravity flow. The optimal flow rate for perfusion is 3–4 mL/min. Pass the solution leaving the perfusion chamber through a pinchcock to adjust the flow rate and drain into a reservoir placed below the stage.

3.1.2. For Plate Reader

1. Preheat platereader to 37°C.
2. Prime the pumps with I$^-$ buffers with and without 20 μM forskolin.

3.2. Indicator Loading/Cell Transfection

1. For loading cells by hypotonic shock method, incubate cells with 5–10 mM of SPQ or 0.2–0.5 mM of LZQ in a 1/1 Cl$^-$/I$^-$ hypotonic buffer (150 mOsm) for 5 min at room temperature, wash three times and allow to recover in isotonic Cl$^-$/I$^-$ buffer for 10 min.
2. For overnight loading, incubate cells overnight with the culture medium containing 10 mM of SPQ or 0.5 mM of LZQ at 37°C.
3. For loading with cell permeable reduced form of indicators such as diH-MEQ, incubate cells for 10 min with 20–50 mM of the dye in PBS at 37°C, followed by incubation in growth medium for 15 min to allow complete indicator reoxidation.
4. Cell transfection with YFP-H148Q. Cells are transfected 2 d after plating on solid supports (at 80% confluence) with 1 μL of plasmid DNA (containing the coding sequence for YFP-H148Q expression in a mammalian expression vector, pcDNA 3.1) and 8 μL of lipofectAMINE reagent (Life Technologies) in a 0.2-mL volume of Opti-MEM. The transfection medium is replaced at 5 h with 1 mL of culture medium. Cells are used 2–3 d after transfection.

3.3. Measurement Protocols

3.3.1. Fluorescence Microscopy

1. Indicator-loaded cells are washed, mounted in the perfusion chamber, and (for SPQ assay, for example) perfused for a specified time in succession with Cl^-/NO_3^-/NO_3^- + forskolin/Cl^- + forskolin buffers at a rate of 3–4 mL/min by selecting the buffers using a valve-perfusion system (*see* **Note 1** for choice of protocols).
2. Cell fluorescence is viewed using the filter sets for SPQ/LZQ/YFP and a 20× or 40× air or oil objective lens.
3. Integrated fluorescence intensity from a group of 20–30 cells is detected using a photomultiplier or the fluorescence is imaged using a cooled CCD camera. Fluorescence images are collected continuously.
4. Background fluorescence is measured in cells not loaded with dye.
5. Data analysis is carried out using standard data handling software such as Excel or Kaleidagraph. Data are usually presented as a plot of normalized background-subtracted fluorescence intensity vs time. To quantify the effect of agonists, the initial slope before and after activation of CFTR is measured from a linear or quadratic fit to the data acquired after switching to appropriate buffers (*see* **Note 4**).

3.3.2. Fluorescence Microplate Readers

1. The indicator loaded cells are bathed in 20 μL of isotonic Cl^-/I^- buffer.
2. 130–160 μL of I^-/Cl^- buffer is added from a stock solution to achieve a final [I^-/Cl^-] of 100–138 mM using the syringe pump.
3. CFTR is activated by addition of 50–80 μL of [I^-/Cl^-] buffer containing forskolin or other CFTR activators.
4. For CFTR mutants, cells are preincubated by adding specified concentrations (from nanomolar to millimolar) of test drugs to the culture medium and incubating at 37°C for minutes-to-hours as required.

4. Notes

1. The choice of a suitable assay protocol and indicator is important. For plate readers, LZQ or YFP-H148Q are recommended for their brightness. To avoid indicator loading and washing steps, YFP-H148Q is preferred when transfection is possible or stably expressing cell lines are available. If cell detachment during assay is a problem, consideration should be given to different cell lines, substrate coatings, and minimizing iodide concentration.
2. I^- buffers should be made freshly and kept out of the light to minimize oxidation to iodine.
3. Light intensity should be reduced by use of neutral-density filters to avoid photobleaching and photodynamic cell injury.
4. A significant halide transport rate in the absence of cAMP agonists suggests that CFTR or another halide transporter is activated. Approaches to minimize basal leak include cell line selection, addition of inhibitors (indomethacin, furosemide),

serum starvation, and increasing solution osmolality (to prevent activation of volume-sensitive channels).

References

1. Verkman, A. S. (1990) Development and biological applications of chloride-sensitive fluorescent indicators. *Am. J. Physiol.* **259,** C375–C388.
2. Verkman, A. S. and Biwersi, J. (1995) Chloride-sensitive fluorescent indicators, in *Methods in Neurosciences,* Vol. 27. (Kraicer, J. and Dixon, S. J., eds.), Academic Press, pp. 328–339.
3. Verkman, A. S., Chao, A. C.. and Hartmann, T. (1992) Hormonal regulation of chloride conductance in cultured polar airway cells measured by a fluorescent indicator. *Am. J. Physiol.* **262,** C23–C31.
4. Cheng, S. H., Rich, D. P., Marshall, J., Gregory, R. J., Welsh, M. J., and Smith, A. E. (1991) Phosphorylation of the R domain by cAMP-dependent protein kinase regulates the CFTR chloride channel. *Cell* **66,** 1027–1036.
5. Rommens, J. M., Dho, S., Bear, C. E., Kartner, N., Kennedy, D., Riordan, J. R., Tsui, L. C., and Foskett, J. K. (1991) cAMP-inducible chloride conductance in mouse fibroblast lines stably expressing the human cystic fibrosis transmembrane conductance regulator. *Proc. Natl. Acad. Sci. USA* **88,** 7500–7505.
6. Brown, R., Hong-Brown, L., Biwersi, J., Verkman, A. S., and Welch, W. (1996) Chemical chaperones correct the mutant phenotype of the DF508 cystic fibrosis transmembrane conductance regulator protein. *Cell Stress Chaperones* **1,** 117–125.
7. Cheng, S. H., Fang, S. L., Zabner, J., Marshall, J., Piraino, S., Schiavi, S. C., et al. (1995) Functional activation of the cystic fibrosis trafficking mutant DF508-CFTR by overexpression. *Am. J. Physiol.* **268,** L615–L624.
8. Rich, D. P., Anderson, M. P., Gregory, R. J., Cheng, S. H., Paul, S., Jefferson, D. M., et al. (1990) Expression of cystic fibrosis transmembrane conductance regulator corrects defective chloride channel regulation in cystic fibrosis airway epithelial cells. *Nature* **347,** 358–363.
9. Mansoura, M., Biwersi, J., Ashlock, M., and Verkman, A. S. (1999) Fluorescent chloride indicators to assess the efficacy of CFTR cDNA delivery. *Human Gene Therapy* **10,** 861–875.
10. Porteous, D. J., Dorin, J. R., McLachlan, G., Davidson-Smith, H., Davidson, H., Stevenson, B. J., et al. (1997) Evidence for safety and efficacy of DOTAP cationic liposome mediated CFTR gene transfer to the nasal epithelium of patients with cystic fibrosis. *Gene Ther.* **4,** 210–218.
11. Gill, D. R., Southern, K. W., Mofford, K. A., Seddon, T., Huang, L., Sorgi, F., et al. (1997) A placebo-controlled study of liposome-mediated gene transfer to the nasal epithelium of patients with cystic fibrosis. *Gene Ther.* **4,** 199–209.
12. Jayaraman, S., Song, Y., Vetrivel, L., Shankar, L., and Verkman, A. S. (2001) Non-invasive in vivo fluorescence measurement of airway surface liquid depth, salt concentration and pH. *J. Clin. Invest.* **107,** 317–324.
13. Illsley, N. P. and Verkman, A. S. (1987) Membrane chloride transport measured using a chloride-sensitive fluorescent indicator. *Biochemistry* **26,** 1215–1219.

14. Biwersi, J. and Verkman, A. S. (1991) Cell permeable fluorescent indicator for cytosolic chloride. *Biochemistry* **30,** 7879–7883.

15. Biwersi, J., Farah, N. Wang, Y. X. Ketchum, R., and Verkman, A. S. (1992) Synthesis of cell-impermeable Cl⁻ sensitive fluorescent indicators with improved sensitivity and optical properties. *Am. J. Physiol.* **262,** C243–C250.

16. Verkman, A. S., Sellers, M., Chao, A. C., Leung, T., and Ketcham, R. (1989) Synthesis and characterization of improved chloride-sensitive fluorescent indicators for biological applications. *Anal. Biochem.* **178,** 355–361.

17. Biwersi, J., Tulk, B., and Verkman, A. S. (1994) Long wavelength chloride-sensitive fluorescent indicators. *Anal. Biochem.* **219,** 139–143.

18. Jayaraman, S., Teitler, L., Skalski, B., and Verkman, A. S. (1999) Long-wavelength iodide-sensitive fluorescent indicators for measurement of functional CFTR expression in cells. *Am. J. Physiol.* **277,** C1008–C1018.

19. Jayaraman, S., Biwersi, J., and Verkman A. S. (1999) Synthesis and characterization of dual-wavelength chloride sensitive fluorescent indicators for ratio imaging. *Am. J. Physiol.* **276,** C747–C757.

20. Jayaraman, S., Haggie, P., Wachter, R., Remington, S. J., and Verkman, A. S. (2000) Mechanism and cellular applications of a green fluorescent protein-based halide sensor. *J. Biol. Chem.* **275,** 6047–6050.

21. Jayaraman, S. and Verkman, A. S. (2000) Charge transfer mechanism for quenching of quinolinium fluorescence by halides. *Biophys. Chem.* **85,** 49–57.

22. Haggie, P., Jayaraman, S., and Verkman, A. S. (2001) Ratioable GFP-based halide indicators utilizing a novel energy transfer strategy. *Biophys. J.* **80,** 654a.

23. Galietta, L. J. V., Haggie, P. M., and Verkman, A. S. (2001) Green fluorescent protein-based halide indicators with improved chloride and iodide affnities. *FEBS Lett.* **499,** 220–224.

II

CFTR Structure and Function:
Expression, Folding, and Degradation

13

Immunolocalization of CFTR in Intact Tissue and Cultured Cells

Christopher R. Marino

1. Introduction

Cloning of the cystic fibrosis (CF) gene provided, for the first time, the structural information needed to more precisely define the CF defect *(1–3)*. This genetic information was used to develop powerful molecular and antibody reagents that helped define cystic fibrosis transmembrane conductance regulator (CFTR) structure-function relationships and characterize CFTR expression throughout the body. This chapter focuses on how genetic information can be used to develop antipeptide antibodies and how these antibodies can be used to immunolocalize proteins in intact and cultured cells. By identifying which cells expressed CFTR, and correlating that information with existing knowledge of the physiology of those cells, the role of CFTR in normal cell function and the pathophysiology of CF was elucidated.

Successful immunolocalization, first reported in 1941 *(4)*, requires three basic elements: specific antibodies, well-preserved tissue, and a clear visualization method. This chapter discusses (a) antipeptide antibody production, (b) tissue preparation, (c) immunolocalization in intact tissues, and (d) immunolocalization in cultured cells. Because of the technical complexity associated with immunoelectron microscopy, this topic will be addressed only in general terms. The overall objective of the chapter is to provide investigators with a methodological framework from which the protein product of any newly cloned gene can be localized.

1.1. Overview

Gene expression in any tissue can be determined by measuring either transcription (mRNA production) or translation (protein production). Northern and

From: *Methods in Molecular Medicine, vol. 70: Cystic Fibrosis Methods and Protocols*
Edited by: W. R. Skach © Humana Press Inc., Totowa, NJ

Western blotting can be used to quantify total mRNA or protein expression, respectively, in tissue samples, but these techniques provide no information on which cells within that tissue express the protein of interest. *In situ* hybridization and immunocytochemistry identify which cells in a given tissue express the specific mRNA or protein of interest but are not particularly useful for quantifying gene expression. Thus, many investigators combine both blotting and localization techniques to fully characterize gene expression. Since *in situ* hybridization *(5)* is technically challenging and can only identify what cell type is expressing a given gene, protein localization using antibodies (i.e., immunolocalization) remains the most versatile approach to the study of gene product expression.

Immunolocalization involves the application of a specific (primary) antibody to a thin section of fixed and permeabilized tissue on a microscope slide (**Fig. 1**). After allowing the primary antibody to bind specifically to the protein of interest (CFTR in this case), the tissue is washed free of unbound antibody and reacted with a second antibody that is directed against some component of the primary antibody. This secondary antibody also contains a conjugate that allows for visualization of the entire antigen–antibody complex. These conjugates can be enzymes (e.g., horseradish peroxidase or alkaline phosphatase) that catalyze a specific colorimetric reaction, fluorescent tags (e.g., fluorescein or rhodamine) that can be visualized with a fluorescence microscope, or gold particles that can be detected by electron microscopy. In each case, the location of the original antibody–antigen complex is visualized under the microscope, thereby characterizing the cellular or subcellular distribution of the protein of interest. Since the signal being generated is associated with the secondary antibody, which is not interacting directly with the antigen itself, the technique is known as indirect immunomicroscopy.

1.2. Antibody Production

Although monoclonal and polyclonal antibodies can both be used for immunolocalization, this chapter focuses on the development of antipeptide polyclonal antibodies. This approach was used early on for the study of CFTR expression because it was not possible to produce enough full-length CFTR to raise antibodies against the entire protein. Using the published CF gene sequence *(3)*, a series of CFTR peptides of 13–15 amino acids in length were chosen as epitopes for polyclonal antibody production *(6)*. This size was selected because peptides of less than 12 amino acids may lack specificity and the synthesis of longer peptides can become quite costly. Since one cannot predict which sequence(s) will generate useful antibodies, multiple CFTR peptide sequences were chosen for immunization. Although the selection process is somewhat arbitrary, several principles should be adhered to. First, the peptides chosen should not have homology to peptides present in other proteins.

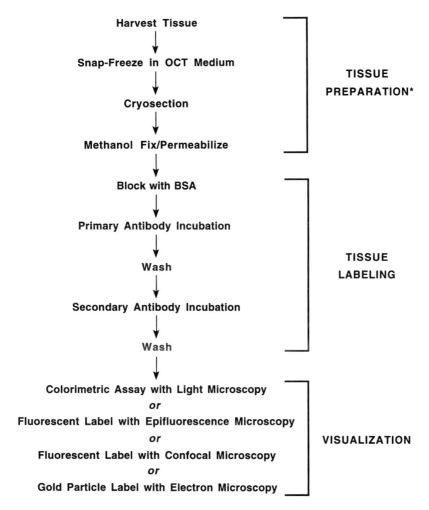

Fig. 1. Overview of the steps involved in the immunolocalization of cellular proteins. *Frozen tissue is highlighted in this figure, but gentle aldehyde fixation can also be used to prepare tissue for some labeling studies (see text for details).

Scanning of gene banks is necessary to avoid selecting sequences known to be present elsewhere. For CFTR, our greatest concern was avoiding homologous sequences present in P-glycoprotein or other members of the ATP-binding cassette family to which CFTR belongs. Second, the antigenic epitopes selected must have a reasonable likelihood of being accessible to antibody attack. Thus, sequences within putative transmembrane spanning domains (i.e., hydrophobic sequences) were avoided. Similarly, sequences containing putative glycosylation sites that could mask the antigenic epitope were avoided. Although one should also avoid epitopes hidden within the tertiary structure of a protein, genetic sequence information alone does not provide this information. However, some logical guesses can be made. For example, N-terminal and C-terminal peptides make good empiric choices since they are least likely to be completely buried within a protein's tertiary structure. Third, portions of the molecule containing so-called consensus sequences (for phosphorylation, glycosylation, and other posttranslational modifications) should be avoided, since these sequences are shared by many different proteins and can adversely affect the specificity of the antibody generated. And fourth, the addition of a lysine residue to the N-terminus of each peptide will allow for proper orientation of the peptide during preparation of affinity columns and is therefore a useful consideration when designing peptides for synthesis.

To convert these small peptides from haptens to antigens, they must be conjugated to larger proteins. Thyroglobulin, a large globular protein, is the protein we chose for CFTR antibody production *(7)*. In the presence of a large excess of peptide, glutaraldehye was used to bind the CFTR peptide nonspecifically to the exposed surface of the conjugate protein *(8)*. The rabbit's immune system, seeing a large foreign protein with only the CFTR peptide on its surface, generates antibodies against the CFTR sequence rather than thyroglobulin. The anti-CFTR antibodies produced are then purified from other serum components by affinity chromatography. This involves passing the antiserum through a Sepharose affinity column containing covalently linked CFTR peptide. Antibodies that recognize the CFTR peptide will bind to the column, while all other serum components pass through. Bound antibodies are then salt-eluted from the column, using increasing concentrations of salt to collect antibodies of increasing peptide affinity.

1.3. Tissue Processing

Since antigen–antibody reactions can be adversely affected by tissue fixation, immunolocalization studies are best performed on unfixed, frozen tissue *(9)*. To preserve morphology in the absence of fixation, it is important to minimize the effects of tissue hypoxia by snap-freezing the tissue as quickly as possible after procurement. Tissue pieces are frozen in standard laboratory cryosectioning medium (e.g., OCT compound) in plastic wells using isopentane cooled to a slurry with dry ice or using liquid nitrogen alone. The tissue is then cryosectioned (4–6 µm thick) onto coated glass slides for subsequent immunolocalization experiments.

Some antibodies, however, can function well in fixed tissue, particularly if the fixation is "gentle." Standard 10% neutral-buffered formalin used by pathology laboratories is rather harsh (~4% formaldehyde) and is associated with loss of antigenicity over time. Many antibodies will not work well on formalin-fixed tissue, including many CFTR antibodies *(10)*. Gentler fixation with 2% paraformaldehyde or PLP (periodate–lysine–paraformaldehyde *[11]*)

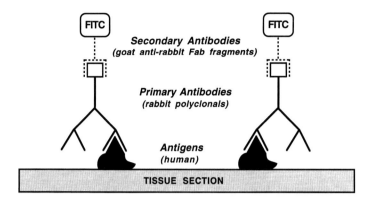

Fig. 2. Indirect immunolocalization technique. The protein antigen is recognized by a primary antibody directed against it. The conjugate carrying the visualization signal (in this case, the fluorescent tag FITC, also known as fluorescein) is linked to the secondary antibody. The secondary binds to the antigen–primary antibody complex via its affinity for the Fc portion of the primary antibody (*see* **Fig. 3**). Thus, visualization is an indirect process since the antibody containing the FITC signal is not directed against the protein antigen itself. Anti-rabbit secondaries will bind to any rabbit primary antibody, so they can be used in any immunolocalization study where the primary antibody is a rabbit polyclonal. The figure also illustrates the general concept that the antigen, primary antibody, and secondary antibody should all be from different species to avoid cross-reactivity and high background labeling.

causes less loss of antigenicity while providing good morphological preservation. Since individual antibodies behave differently, each must be tested against different fixatives to determine its efficacy.

1.4. Immunolocalization Techniques

Most immunolocalization experiments are performed using the indirect method. That is, the primary antibody reacting with the antigen does not generate the immunolocalization signal. The signal is indirectly generated by conjugates linked to a secondary antibody directed against the primary antibody (**Fig. 2**). This approach provides greater flexibility since it avoids the need to conjugate the primary antibody and allows the secondary antibodies (containing the conjugates) to be used with a variety of different primaries. For standard immunolocalization (i.e., at the light microscope level), visualization is achieved by either a colorimetric enzyme assay or by a fluorescent tag. For immunoelectron microscopy, an electron-dense gold particle or horseradish peroxidase (HRP) is linked to the secondary antibody for visualization.

Secondary antibodies with different conjugates are readily available from a variety of commercial sources. These antibodies are directed against an immunoglobin (Ig) component from the species that the primary antibody was

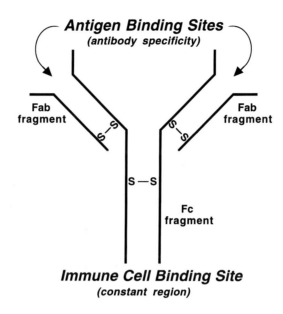

Fig. 3. Illustration of immunoglobulin G structure and components. The two main functional components of immunoglobulins are the Fab and the Fc fragments. The Fab fragments have variable sequences that bind to very specific antigens and represent the antibody specificity properties of the immunoglobulin molecule. The Fc fragment is more constant in structure and serves as the portion of the molecule that interacts with immune cells such as macrophages via Fc receptors on those cells. Thus, the Fab fragments are all that is needed to bind to antigens and for this reason they form good secondary "antibodies." Since the Fc fragments interact with immune cells, the use of whole Ig as a secondary can be associated with nonspecific labeling of immune cells in addition to the protein antigen of interest.

generated. Thus, if the primary antibody was raised in a rabbit, the secondary antibody is raised in a different species (e.g., goat or sheep) against either whole rabbit Ig or rabbit Fc fragments. Secondary antibodies themselves may be either whole Ig molecules or Fab fragments (**Fig. 3**). We routinely use Fab fragment secondaries since they lack the Fc fragment that can bind nonspecifically to receptors on immune cells and thereby increase background labeling. The conjugate is linked to a portion of the secondary Ig or Fab fragment that is distant from the antigen-binding site so as not to interfere with the antigen–antibody interaction.

Enzyme-linked secondaries have the advantage of requiring no special equipment for signal visualization. The most commonly used enzyme-linked secondary system utilizes HRP to peroxidize the exogenous substrate 3,3-diaminobenzidine (DAB) to a brown reaction by-product visualized by standard light microscopy. Alkaline phosphatase and glucose oxidase are alternatives with different proprietary substrates that produce red or blue reaction by-products. Unfortunately, colorimetric signals tend to be diffuse and the reaction must be watched continuously so that it can be terminated when the "right" signal-to-noise ratio is achieved. Although two different enzyme-linked conjugates can be used in double-label experiments, care must be take that the conditions of one reaction do not interfere with those of the other. Fluorescent-tagged secondaries, on the other hand, provide a sharper signal in my opinion and can be readily applied to double-labeling experiments. Visualization of the fluorescence signal, however, requires a fluorescence microscope, but this is worth the expense if more than occasional immunolocalization experiments are planned. Immunofluorescence localization can also be visualized on a confocal microscope. This laser-based detection system allows one to record fluorescence signals at defined micrometer depths within a cell or tissue section. Computer-based software allows these images to be digitally reconstructed into three-dimensional images for quantitation. It is important to note that the optical resolution of the confocal microscope is no better than that of a quality epifluorescence microscope. Thus, confocal microscopy does not improve resolution, but it expands one's ability to capture and reconstruct data for better signal interpretation. Accurate definition of protein expression at the subcellular level still requires immunoelectron microscopy.

Immunoelectron microscopy is a highly specialized technique that requires considerable experience for successful execution. Ideally, the labeling should be performed on fresh-frozen tissue that has been cryoprotected and ultrathinsectioned. Ultrathin cryosectioning is particularly challenging since very thin sections must be obtained from tissue that is not embedded in a supportive plastic matrix. Furthermore, it is more difficult to maintain good morphology with cryoprotected and crysectioned tissue than it is with fixed and plasticembedded tissue. Postembedding localization techniques are available, but they tend to be less reliable than immunolabeling of frozen tissue. The actual antibody labeling steps are similar to those used with standard immunolocalization except that a bridging antibody step is commonly used to amplify the gold signal. Since this technique is technically challenging and beyond the scope of this chapter, the interested reader should consult references dedicated to the subject *(12,13)*.

2. Materials
2.1. Stock Solutions
1. TBS (Tris-buffered saline): 100 mM NaCl, 10 mM Tris-HCl, pH to 7.4 .
2. 0.5 M PB, 7.4 (phosphate buffer): Place ~250 mL of 0.5 M Na$_2$HPO$_4$ in a 400-mL beaker. While stirring and measuring pH, slowly add 0.5 M NaH$_2$PO$_4$ to pH 7.4. Stable at 4°C.

3. 0.2 and 0.1 *M* PB, pH 7.4 (prepared from 0.5 *M* stock).
4. PBS (phosphate-buffered saline): Mix 100 mL of 1.5 *M* NaCl and 50 mL of 0.5 *M* PB,7.4. Bring the volume to1 L with water. Stable at 4°C.
5. 8% paraformaldehyde: Dissolve 8 g paraformaldehyde in ~95 mL water, then heat to 52–58°C with constant stirring (do not exceed 58°C). Add 1 *N* NaOH dropwise until solution clears (3–5 drops), then remove from heat and bring the volume to 100 mL with water. Pass through Whatman #1 filter paper and store at 4°C. Stable for ~1 wk at 4°C.

2.2. Antipeptide Antibody Production (For Each Immunization)

1. HPLC-purified peptide (~200 mg).
2. 0.5 *M* phosphate buffer, pH 7.4. Store at 4°C.
3. 0.1 *M* phosphate buffer, pH 7.4. Store at 4°C.
4. Bovine thyroglobulin (Sigma Chemical, St. Louis, MO), 33 mg in 2 mL of 0.1 *M* phosphate buffer. Prepare fresh.
5. 0.2% glutaraldehyde prepared in 0.1 *M* phosphate buffer. Prepare fresh.
6. Sodium borohydride, 12.5 mg/mL in water. Prepare immediately before use.
7. Dialysis tubing.
8. 0.2-μm sterile filters (Millipore, Burlington, MA) and a 5-mL sterile syringe.

2.3. Affinity Column Preparation

1. Epoxy-activated CH Sepharose 6B beads (Pharmacia, Vineland, NJ).
2. 1 *M* NaCO$_3$.
3. 0.1 *M* NaHCO$_3$. Bubble with CO$_2$ to pH 8.0.
4. 0.1 *M* sodium acetate, pH to 4.0 with acetic acid.
5. 1 *M* ethanolamine.

2.4. Affinity Purification of Rabbit Antiserum

1. Bovine serum albumin (BSA, Sigma).
2. Column wash buffer: TBS, 0.1% BSA, 5 m*M* benzamidine, 0.02% sodium azide.
3. BSA-free buffer: TBS, 0.5 m*M* benzamidine, 0.02% sodium azide.
4. High-salt buffer: 0.5 *M* NaCl, 10 m*M* Tris-HCl, 5 m*M* benzamidine, 0.02% Na azide.
5. Antibody elution buffer I: 4.9 *M* MgCl$_2$.
6. Antibody elution buffer II: 100 m*M* NaCl, 1 *M* acetic acid.
7. Dialysis buffer: 100 m*M* NaCl, 10 m*M* Tris-HCl, pH 7.4, 1 m*M* benzamidine. Make 4 L.
8. Dialysis tubing.
9. Aquacide II (Calbiochem, La Jolla, CA).

2.5. Tissue Proccessing for Cryoembedding Intact Tissue

1. Isopentane (2-methylbutane) cooled to a slurry with dry ice.
2. As a substitute for **item 1**, liquid nitrogen.
3. Disposable vinyl cryomolds, 15 mm × 15 mm × 15 mm.
4. OCT cryoembedding medium.
5. Coated glass slides.
6. Glass (not plastic) cover slips.

2.6. Processing Cultured Cells

1. Permeable membrane supports.
2. 2% paraformaldehyde: prepare 1/4 vol of 8% paraformaldehyde in 0.2 *M* PB, 7.4.

2.7. Immunolocalization in Frozen Tissue

1. Methanol, precooled to –20°C.
2. Stock protease inhibitor cocktail (PI) prepared in 25 m*M* HEPES, pH 7.5 (aliquot and store at –20°C): leupeptin, chymostatin, and pepstatin each at 0.2-mg/mL concentration; soybean trypsin inhibitor and aprotinin each at 0.5-mg/mL concentration.
3. Blocking buffer: PBS, 1.0% BSA, 1/200 dilution of stock PI.
4. PPD: 10 mg *p*-phenylenediamine, 1 mL 10× PBS, 2 mL water, 7 mL glycerol. For use in immunofluorescence labeling only. Prepare ~2 h before use. Protect from light. Stable for several days at –20°C. PPD is a poison: handle with care, wear gloves.
5. Colorimetric reagent kits for HRP, alkaline phosphatase, or glucose oxidase cytochemistry only—obtain commercially.
6. Crystal/Mount (Biomeda, Foster City, CA).

2.8. Cultured Cells

1. PBS.
2. 0.25% saponin in PBS.
3. 50 m*M* NH$_4$Cl (prepared in PBS). Prepare fresh and use immediately after preparation.
4. Blocking buffer: PBS, 1.0% BSA, 1/200 dilution of stock PI.

3. Methods

3.1. Overview

The following section provides detailed instructions on how to prepare affinity purified antipeptide antibodies from genetic sequence information and how to perform immunolocalization experiments with those antibodies. Notes provide additional insights into each protocol described, including helpful comments and troubleshooting suggestions.

3.2. Antipeptide Antibody Production (Modified from Czernik, et al. [8] and Used for Anti-CFTR Antibody Production in [6,7])

1. Peptide conjugation to thyroglobulin. Dissolve 33 mg (~50 nmol) of bovine thyroglobulin in 2 mL of 0.1 *M* phosphate buffer, pH 7.4. Filter through a 0.2-μm Millipore filter attached to a 5-mL sterile syringe.
2. Dissolve 1.25 μmol of peptide (assume each amino acid has a molecular mass of 110) in 100 μL of water. Check pH by applying a few microliters to pH paper. If necessary, bring pH to ~7.0 by adding microliter amounts of 0.5 *M* phosphate buffer, pH 7.4 (*see* **Note 1**).
3. Add the entire peptide solution to the thyroglobulin solution and mix at 4°C for 2 min.
4. To the peptide/thyroglobulin mixture, slowly add 1.5 mL of 0.2% glutaraldehyde in 0.1 *M* phosphate buffer at 4°C. The glutaraldehyde should be added drop by

drop over 20 min. Mix the entire solution for an additional 2 h at 4°C to complete the conjugation step.

5. Reduce the excess glutaraldehyde by adding 100 µL of freshly prepared sodium borohydride and mixing for 10 min at 4°C.
6. Dialyze the conjugate sample overnight against 2 L of PBS at 4°C.
7. Microfuge the conjugate sample to remove any particulate debris, filter the supernatant (0.2-µm Millipore), and aliquot the filtrate into sterile Eppendorf tubes (250 µL each). Store frozen at –70°C.
8. Use directly for rabbit immunization (*see* **Note 2**).

3.3. Affinity Column Preparation (For Use in Affinity Purification of Immune Antiserum) (see Note 3)

1. Swell 1 g of epoxy-activated Sepharose 6B beads in distilled water for 2 h.
2. Wash the beads 5 times with water using low-speed centrifugation to separate the beads from the water.
3. To the ~3 mL of bead slurry add an equal volume of water.
4. Dissolve 25 µmol (~40 mg) of peptide in 2 mL of 1 M NaCO$_3$, pH 11.5.
5. Add the peptide solution to the Sepharose bead suspension and mix overnight (16 h) at 37°C with gentle shaking to allow coupling to take place.
6. After removal of unbound peptide, wash the beads 3 times with water.
7. Wash the beads twice with 0.1 M NaHCO$_3$, pH 8.0.
8. Wash the beads twice with water.
9. Wash the beads twice with 0.1 M sodium acetate, pH 4.0.
10. Wash the beads twice with water.
11. Block unbound reactive groups overnight with 1 M ethanolamine.
12. Wash beads 3 times with TBS, pH 7.8 containing 1 mM benzamidine and 0.1% sodium azide. Store in a moist column at 4°C in the same.

3.4. Affinity Purification of Rabbit Antiserum (see Note 4)

1. Pool all high-titer serum samples together to obtain one large, uniform sample for purification.
2. Wash the peptide affinity column with ~30 mL of column wash buffer.
3. Apply several ml of antiserum to the column. Allow the antiserum to pass through the column (use a small volume of column wash buffer to complete the passage step). Collect the eluate and pass through the column 5 more times to assure adequate antibody–antigen interaction.
4. Wash the column with ~20 mL of BSA-free buffer (discard eluate).
5. Wash off low-affinity antibodies with ~40 mL of high-salt buffer (discard eluate).
6. Add 0.5 mL of antibody elution buffer I and mix well with the column matrix for 5 min. Collect the eluate in a tube labeled "bound antibody." Repeat this elution buffer **step 2** more times, adding each eluate into the "bound antibody" tube.
7. Wash the column with 30 mL of BSA-free buffer and store moist at 4°C in TBS containing 1 mM benzamidine and 0.1% sodium azide.
8. Prepare the dialysis tubing by boiling for 5 min in TBS containing EDTA and NaHCO$_3$ (to remove impurities) and then washing in water, and coating with 1 mg/mL

of BSA in water (to prevent nonspecific loss of antibody on the dialysis tubing). The "bound antibody" sample is then desalted by extensive dialysis over 36–48 h at 4°C against four changes of dialysis buffer.

9. Concentrate the antibody solution to a volume of ~0.5 mL by covering the dialysis tubing with Aquacide II.
10. Add an equal volume of glycerol to the concentrated antibody solution and store the final antibody sample in aliquots at –20°C (sample will not freeze).

3.5. Tissue Processing: Intact Tissue for Cryosectioning

1. Prepare the isopentane slurry over dry ice or bring a Dewar of liquid nitrogen in preparation for tissue procurement.
2. Place OCT embedding compound in plastic wells in preparation for tissue procurement.
3. Immediately after tissue procurement, submerge an ~2 × 2 mm tissue section in OCT in one of the plastic wells. Promptly submerge the underside of the well into the cooled isopentane or liquid nitrogen to snap-freeze the block from the bottom up.
4. Once frozen, keep the tissue blocks on dry ice until transferred to a –70°C freezer for storage. Dehydration occurs over weeks unless the blocks are stored in plastic bags with frozen saline (hydration can be maintained for up to a year).
5. Cryosection (4- to 6-μm thick) the frozen tissue onto coated glass slides.
6. Store the frozen sections on slides at –20°C in a nondefrosting freezer (*see* **Note 5**).

3.6. Processing Cultured Cells

1. Cut free the permeable support containing the cultured cells and place cell side up in a clean tissue culture well.
2. Wash the cells twice with PBS.
3. Wash once with 2% paraformaldehyde and then fix with fresh 2% paraformaldehyde for a minimum of 30 min (can keep in fixative for a day or so at 4°C if necessary) (*see* **Note 6**).

3.7. Immunolocalization Techniques: Intact Tissue

1. If labeling frozen, unfixed tissue sections, submerge the slides containing the cryosections in methanol cooled to –20°C (*see* **Note 7**). This will fix and permeabilize the frozen sections. After 20 min, remove the slides from the methanol and allow them to air-dry at –20°C for ~10 min. Proceed to **step 3**.
2. If labeling aldehyde-fixed tissue sections, do not methanol-fix. Instead, wash away excess fixative with PBS and then quench any free aldehyde residues by submerging the slides in freshly made 50 mM NH_4Cl (prepared in PBS) for 20 min at room temperature.
3. All subsequent labeling steps are performed at room temperature in a closed, moist chamber. As a moist chamber, I use a 100-slot slide box with moist tissue paper on the bottom and place the slides to be labeled flat on top of the slots with tissue sections up. This apparatus can easily hold 12 slides, and the top of the box can be closed to maintain a dark, moist environment.
4. Place a small drop of PBS over the tissue section to wash off excess methanol or NH_4Cl. Repeat 3 times (5 min per wash).

5. Block the tissue sections for 1 h with a drop of blocking buffer to reduce nonspecific labeling.

6. During **step 5**, prepare the desired primary antibody dilutions in blocking buffer. Microfuge the antibody dilutions at 10,000 rpm for 2 min to pellet any debris. Since <50 μL is needed to cover each tissue section, very little antibody is required for each experiment.

7. Apply the primary antibody to the blocked tissue sections for 1–2 h in the moist chamber.

8. Wash the tissue sections 5 times with blocking buffer (10–15 min per wash) to remove all unbound antibody.

9. Prepare secondary antibody dilutions in blocking buffer (the company from which they are purchased will suggest what dilution to use). Microfuge the antibody dilutions at 10,000 rpm for 2 min to pellet any debris. If the secondary antibodies are fluorescent conjugated, protect from the light by covering with aluminum foil.

10. Apply the secondary antibody to the washed tissue sections for 30–60 min.

11. Remove unbound secondary antibody by washing 3 times with blocking buffer, then 2 times with PBS (10–15 min per wash).

12. For immunofluorescent-labeled sections, blot the slide dry (without touching the tissue section) and place a small drop of PPD over the tissue section and cover with a glass coverslip. Apply nail polish to the edges of the coverslip to seal. Visualize the fluorescence labeling pattern with a fluorescence microscope.

13. For HRP or alkaline phosphatase cytochemistry, commercially available kits are used to produce the respective colorimetric reactions. These reactions must be observed under a quality light microscope and terminated manually when the optimal signal is achieved (if allowed to react for too long, the background signal will rise to levels that interfere with the specific signal). Place a small drop of Crystal/Mount over the tissue section and cover with a glass cover slip.

3.8. Immunolocalization in Cultured Cells (Aldehyde-fixed)

1. Wash cells with PBS twice to remove any residual fixative.

2. Permeabilize the cells by incubation in PBS containing 0.25% Saponin for 30 min.

3. Quench any remaining free aldehyde residues by reacting the cells on the permeable supports with freshly made 50 mM NH$_4$Cl in PBS for 20 min at room temperature.

4. Wash the cells twice with PBS.

5. Follow **steps 5–13** under **Subheading 3.7.**, keeping the cell side of the permeable support up (*see* **Note 8**).

4. Notes

1. The antibody production protocol has each peptide in a 25/1 molar ratio to assure that the thyroglobulin molecule is adequately coated with peptide. Use of significantly smaller amounts of peptide may lead to the development of antithyroglobulin antibodies. Although these will be removed during affinity purification, they can theoretically reduce the titer of the desired antipeptide antibody.

2. Since not all rabbits generate a good immune response, you should consider immunizing two rabbits with each antigen. The protocol as described prepares for the immunization of 2 rabbits, but if sufficient peptide is available, I suggest

preparing twice as much and immunizing each rabbit with a double dose. About half of the antigen is used for the first injection, with the remainder being divided up for 3 monthly boosts. You can do the rabbit immunizations yourself or you can have a commercial animal facility do it for you. In either case, obtain preimmune serum as well as antiserum samples before each boost for ELISA titer assays. Decisions re further boosts or a terminal bleed will be based on these titer assays. I suggest that a Western blot using tissue known to express the protein of interest be performed before deciding when to do a terminal bleed. If high-titer bleeds are confirmed by ELISA and antigen specificity is supported by Western blots, pool all desired immune sera samples to form a uniform serum sample for affinity purification.

Occasionally, no immune response will be detected after 3 boosts. This may mean that the peptide sequence chosen resembles a "self" protein to which the rabbit will not generate antibodies or that the peptide conjugate was insufficient to activate that particular animal's immune system. Conversely, an immune response may be stimulated but the antiserum recognizes too many different proteins by Western blot, failing to demonstrate specificity for your protein of interest. For these reasons, several different peptide sequences should be considered for antibody production.

3. Affinity column preparation is essentially a kit protocol with manufacturer's instructions (Pharmacia, Vineland, NJ). I have had no problems preparing peptide affinity columns when closely following the manufacturer's instructions.

4. Since the capacity of the column with regard to the particular antiserum being purified is not known, you have two options: either purifying only small amounts (2 mL) of antiserum at a time or performing experiments early on to assess the capacity of the column. To do the latter, I suggest starting with 2.5 mL of antiserum and doing an ELISA assay on the first 2.5 mL of eluate from **step 4**. If the titer is negative, the column capacity has not been exceeded and increasing amounts of serum (5, 7.5, 10 mL, etc.) can be tested on successive column runs. A positive titer in the eluate from **step 4** indicates that the capacity of the column has been exceeded and lesser amounts of antiserum should be used for each subsequent run.

Similarly, it is useful to test whether the high-salt wash (**step 5**) is advantageous. This step is intended to remove low-affinity antibodies so that the final antibody sample is as specific as possible. The high-salt wash may, however, remove specific antibodies. To test this, one can process the first 5 mL of eluate from **step 5** as one does for the final antibody sample and compare its Western blot profile to that of the final antibody sample. If the **step 5** sample produces a specific Western blot signal without significant background, this step may be eliminated in future purifications since it may only be removing specific antibodies. If the **step 5** sample generates a Western blot with many bands, the high-salt wash step must be maintained, since it is removing additional nonspecific antibodies.

The final concentrated affinity purified antibody sample is diluted with an equal volume of glycerol so that it can be stored at –20°C without freezing. This will better stabilize the protein than if it were stored at 4°C. If the antibody can tolerate a freeze–thaw cycle (test this first with a small aliquot), long-term storage should be at –70°C.

To determine the final antibody concentration, one needs to remember that some of the total protein concentration in the sample is BSA that was used to coat the dialysis tubing. The approximate contributions of antibody and BSA to the total protein concentration may be estimated by comparing the BSA and immunoglobulin Coomassie blue band densities on SDS-PAGE.

5. The major disadvantage of studying frozen (compared to fixed) tissue is that morphology is not as well preserved in frozen tissue. On the other hand, antigenicity is optimal with frozen tissue, hence it is advantageous for immunolocalization experiments. The morphology problem can be minimized by rapidly processing the tissue (hypoxia must be as short as possible), keeping the cryosection slides frozen at all times, and doing the cell labeling as soon as possible after cryosectioning. I routinely try to do my localization experiments the day of or shortly after cryosectioning. It is important to avoid storing the slides in self-defrosting freezers, which have automatic thawing cycles that will freeze–thaw the cryosections. In spite of all of the above, there are times when the tissue will simply have inadequate morphology. I routinely perform H&E staining of one of the cryosections of a set to determine whether morphology has been adequately preserved before proceeding with immunolabeling.

6. The cells should be labeled immediately after fixation. As mentioned in the introduction, other fixatives may be used but those containing glutaraldehyde or high concentrations of formaldehyde tend to reduce antigenicity and may completely destroy any chance of immunolabeling. Your antibody should be tested against other fixatives to determine its efficacy. Standard laboratory formalin is 4% formaldehyde, which explains why archival pathology specimens are frequently unsuitable for immunolocalization *(10)*.

   Although placing the permeable supports cell side down would help reduce the volume of antibody solution needed for labeling, we find that some cell types in this configuration dislodge from the filters during wash steps, so we prefer cell-side-up processing. If cells are dislodging in the upright position, consider culturing them on collagen-coated filters for greater tenacity.

7. For many reasons, I feel that immunofluorescent labeling of frozen tissue is the best way to do immunolocalization in intact tissue. Antigenicity is optimal, resolution is good, and double-labeling can be readily preformed to confirm one's interpretation of the labeling pattern obtained. If care is taken in tissue procurement and processing, the morphology of frozen tissue can be quite good.

   Double-labeling is a powerful tool that allows one to compare the distribution of two different proteins on the same tissue section simultaneously (**Fig. 4**). To perform a double-label experiment, the primary antibodies against the two antigens of interest must come from two different species (commonly a mouse monoclonal and a rabbit polyclonal). Anti-mouse and anti-rabbit secondaries, tagged with different fluorescent signals, can then be used to distinguish the labeling pattern of one protein from the other. The two primary antibodies are applied simultaneously, as are the two secondary antibodies, so the length of the experiment is unaffected. One simply changes the filter control on the fluorescence microscope to visualize the distribution of the two different proteins in the same visual field.

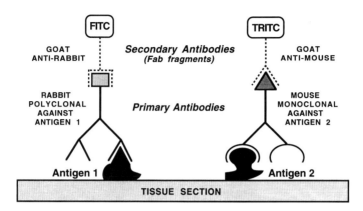

Fig. 4. Double-label immunolocalization. To perform double-labeling, two separate visualization signals are required to differentiate the two different antigens from one another. To accomplish this, two different secondary antibodies with different conjugates are required. In this figure, FITC and TRITC fluorescent tags represent two distinct signals (FITC or fluorescein generates a green fluorescence signal, while TRITC or rhodamine generates a red fluorescence signal). To prevent cross-reactivity of the secondaries, the primary antibodies must come from different species (this figure illustrates the common use of a rabbit polyclonal against one antigen and a mouse monoclonal against the other). Anti-rabbit and anti-mouse secondaries, each with their distinct fluorescent tag, are then targeted to the appropriate primary antibody for distinct antigen labeling.

If tissue morphology is good and the primary and secondary antibodies are of high specificity, indirect immunomicroscopy is a relatively straightforward and technically simple means of determining the cellular distribution of proteins. The major problems with immunolocalization have to do with demonstrating antibody specificity with proper controls. One should always process a slide without primary antibody to determine the degree of background labeling attributed to the secondary antibody and to tissue autofluorescence. This control, however, does not address the issue of primary antibody specificity. If you are using antiserum as your primary antibody preparation (i.e., immune serum that has not been affinity purified), preimmune serum must be used as control for nonspecific labeling. If one has an affinity-purified antibody, preincubation with excess peptide antigen to bind and inactivate the primary antibody before immunolabeling is the appropriate control. Loss of signal following peptide competition confirms that the signal is peptide-specific. Preimmune serum and peptide competition controls, however, still do not definitively prove that the immunolocalization pattern is specific for your protein of interest.

There are several ways to confirm that your labeling pattern is an accurate reflection of the true distribution of your protein. One way is to confirm your observations is with a second antibody, raised against a different epitope of the same protein *(7,14)*. Alternatively, one can demonstrate antibody specificity using

Marino

transgenic animal models or in vitro expression systems that demonstrate loss of signal in conjunction with targeted loss of gene expression. Lastly, antibody localization data can be supported by a clean Western blot identifying a protein of the appropriate molecular mass without significant background labeling. Without at least one of the above approaches to substantiate antibody specificity, one must interpret immunolocalization data with caution.

8. The same principles discussed in **Subheading 3.7.** apply to this section. The only difference one faces when working with cultured cells is the need to detergent permeabilize the cell membrane before quenching and labeling so that one's antibodies can access to the cell interior. If your primary antibody is directed against the extracellular epitope of a plasma membrane protein, this step is not essential.

The major technical problem with cultured cell work is not how to perform the labeling but how to visualize it. Ideally, one wants to examine the cells in cross section, but that cannot be done with the filter and cell monolayer lying flat on the microscope bridge. Filters can be perpendicularly oriented in OCT medium but they will not be sufficiently immobilized to permit cryosectioning. We have tried embedding prelabeled cell monolayers and their filters in Spurs (plastic) medium followed by routine plastic sectioning, but this was time-consuming and has not been uniformly successful in our hands. Others have reported success with folding the filters so that cells at the end of the fold could be examined in "cross section" *(15,16)*. It is difficult, however, to focus adequately on the cells using that approach.

The best way to examine immunolabeled cell monolayers is with the confocal microscope. Using this approach, the filters can be placed flat on the microscope bridge and successive images through the cells (from top to bottom) can be cleanly resolved and captured using confocal laser technology. Image software can then reconstruct the labeling pattern in a variety of ways to suit the goals of one's experiment. An added advantage of confocal image software is the ability to quantify signal intensity. Thus, if one is interested in immunolabeling cultured cells, access to a confocal microscope becomes almost a necessity.

References

1. Quinton, P. M. (1990) Cystic fibrosis: a disease in electrolyte transport. *FASEB J.* **4,** 2709–2717.
2. Welsh, M. J. (1990) Abnormal regulation of ion channels in cystic fibrosis epithelia. *FASEB J.* **4,** 2718–2725.
3. Riordan, J. R., Rommens, J. M., Kerem, B., et al (1989) Identification of the cystic fibrosis gene: Cloning and characterization of complementary DNA. *Science* **245,** 1066–1073.
4. Coons, A. H., Creech, H. J., and Jones, R. N. (1941) Immunological properties of an antibody containing a fluorescent group. *Proc. Soc. Exp. Biol. Med.* **47,** 200.
5. Chesselet, M.-F. (ed.) (1990) *In Situ Hybridization Histochemistry.* CRC Press, Boca Raton, FL.
6. Cohn, J. A., Melhus, O., Page, L. J., Dittrich, K., and Vigna, S. (1991) CFTR: Development of high-affinity antibodies and localization in sweat gland. *Biochem. Biophys. Res. Comm.* **181,** 36–43.

7. Marino, C. R., Matovcik, L. M., Gorelick, F. S., and Cohn, J. A. (1991) Localization of the cystic fibrosis transmembrane conductance regulator in pancreas. *J. Clin. Invest.* **88,** 712–716.

8. Czernik, A. J., Girault, J. A., Nairn, A. C., et al (1991) Production of phosphorylation state-specific antibodies. *Meth. Enzymol.* **201,** 264–283.

9. Taylor, C. R. and Cote, R. J. (ed.) (1994) *Immunomicroscopy: A Diagnostic Tool for the Surgical Pathologist*, 2nd ed., W. B. Saunders, Philadelphia, PA.

10. Claas, A., Sommer, M., de Jonge, H. R., Kalin, N., and Tummler, B. (2000) Applicability of different antibodies for immunohistochemical localization of CFTR in sweat glands from healthy controls and from patients with cystic fibrosis. *J. Histochem. Cytochem.* **48,** 831–837.

11. McLean, I. W. and Nakane, P. K. (1974) Periodate-lysine-parafromaldehyde fixative: a new fixation for immunoelectron microscopy. *J. Histochem. Cytochem.* **22,** 1077–1083.

12. Griffiths, G. (ed.) (1993) *Fine Structure Immunocytochemistry*. Springer Verlag, Heidelberg, Germany.

13. Cuello, A. C. (ed.) (1993) *Immunohistochemistry II*. John Wiley and Sons, West Sussex, UK.

14. Marino, C. R., Jeanes, V., Boron, W. F., and Schmitt, B. M. (1999) Expression and distribution of the Na^+-HCO_3^- cotransporter in human pancreas. *Am. J. Physiol.* **277,** G487–G494.

15. Prince, L. S., Tousson, A., and Marchase, R. B. (1993) Cell surface labeling of CFTR in T84 cells. *Am. J. Physiol.* **264,** C491–C498.

16. Tousson, A., Fuller, C. M., and Benos, D. J. (1996) Apical recruitment of CFTR in T-84 cells is dependent on cAMP and microtubules but not Ca2+ or microfilaments. *J. Cell Sci.* **109,** 1325–1334.

14

Analysis of CFTR Trafficking and Polarization Using Green Fluorescent Protein and Confocal Microscopy

Bryan D. Moyer and Bruce A. Stanton

1. Introduction

Expression of endogenous cystic fibrosis transmembrane conductance regulator (CFTR) in many epithelial cells is either low or difficult to detect or below the limit of detection using currently available microscopic techniques *(1,2)*. In addition, studies utilizing CFTR antibodies to detect CFTR frequently suffer from problems of antibody specificity *(3)*. Use of the green fluorescent protein (GFP) as a molecular marker for CFTR localization may circumvent the problems of low CFTR expression and poor antigenicity and facilitate research of CFTR in epithelial cells.

GFP, a 238-amino acid (27 kDa) protein from the jellyfish *Aequorea victoria*, has emerged as a reporter protein for studying complex biological processes such as organelle dynamics and protein trafficking *(4–7)*. GFP generates a green fluorescence when viewed with conventional fluorescein isothiocyanate (FITC) optics, is visible in both living and fixed specimens, and is resistant to photobleaching. In addition, GFP does not require any exogenous cofactors or substrates (besides molecular oxygen) to fluoresce, and, when ligated to other proteins, generally does not alter fusion protein function or localization *(8,9)*. Therefore, by using GFP fluorescence as a marker for CFTR localization, artifacts that may be introduced when studying CFTR in fixed cells stained with CFTR antibodies, such as the generation of false signals due to nonspecific antibody binding *(10)*, may be avoided.

We have used GFP as a marker to study cAMP-regulated CFTR trafficking and to identify the determinants that localize CFTR to the apical membrane in polarized epithelial cells. In this chapter we describe methods for using GFP fluorescence to quantitate CFTR subcellular localization and polarization by

From: *Methods in Molecular Medicine, vol. 70: Cystic Fibrosis Methods and Protocols*
Edited by: W. R. Skach © Humana Press Inc., Totowa, NJ

laser scanning confocal fluorescence microscopy and we provide details on the experimental approach we have optimized in our laboratory. The confocal microscope allows one to section rapidly through cell monolayers in the vertical dimension (i.e., along the *z* axis) and obtain *xz* vertical sections along the apical–basal axis, features that are not available with a conventional epifluorescence or wide-field microscope. Thus, the confocal microscope is ideally suited for determining the trafficking and polarization patterns of CFTR expressed in epithelial monolayers grown on permeable filter supports. We refer the reader to recent comprehensive overviews of GFP and confocal microscopy for additional references and further details concerning these subjects (*11–14*).

2. Materials
2.1. Cell Culture

1. MDCK type I or type II kidney epithelial cells stably transfected with GFP-CFTR (clone B7; GFP is ligated to the N terminus of CFTR and has no effect on CFTR function or localization [*15*]).
2. Minimal essential media (MEM) with Earle's salts (Life Technologies, Gaithersburg, MD).
3. Fetal bovine serum (FBS; Hyclone, Logan, UT).
4. Penicillin and streptomycin (Life Technologies).
5. Trypsin/EDTA solution: 0.05% trypsin, 0.53 mM ethylenediametetraacetic acid (EDTA) in Hanks' balanced salt solution; (Life Technologies).
6. Transwell filter bottom cups (Costar, Cambridge, MA).
7. G-418 (Life Technologies).
8. Sodium-*n*-butyrate (Sigma).
9. Cell culture incubator set to 33°C.

2.2. Cell Stimulation with cAMP and Staining with WGA–Texas Red

1. CPT-cAMP (monosodium salt; Boehringer Mannheim).
2. IBMX (Sigma).
3. Forskolin (Sigma).
4. Wheat germ agglutinin (WGA)–Texas Red (Molecular Probes).
5. Phosphate-buffered saline (PBS): 137 mM NaCl, 2.7 mM KCl, 1.5 mM KH$_2$PO$_4$, 9 mM Na$_2$HPO$_4$, pH 7.1.
6. *n*-Propyl gallate (Sigma; 10 mg/mL in 90% glycerol/10% PBS).
7. Coverslips (no. 1^1/$_2$ thickness; VWR Scientific, West Chester, PA).
8. Valap (1/1/1 mixture of <u>Va</u>soline, <u>la</u>nolin, and <u>p</u>araffin melted at 40–50°C).
9. Glass slides.

2.3. Cell Staining with ZO-1 Antibody

1. Acetone.
2. ZO-1 antibody (Zymed, South San Francisco, CA).
3. Goat anti-rabbit Texas Red secondary antibody (Molecular Probes).

4. PBS: 137 mM NaCl, 2.7 mM KCl, 1.5 mM KH$_2$PO$_4$, 9 mM Na$_2$HPO$_4$, pH 7.1.
5. 1% bovine serum albumin (BSA)/PBS.
6. *n*-Propyl gallate (Sigma): 10 mg/mL in 90% glycerol, 10% PBS.
7. Coverslips (no. 1^1/$_2$ thickness; VWR Scientific, West Chester, PA).
8. Valap.
9. Glass slides.

2.4. Laser Scanning Confocal Microscopic Analysis of GFP-CFTR Distribution Following cAMP Treatment and of GFP-CFTR Polarization

1. Confocal microscope (upright Zeiss Axioskop equipped with a laser scanning confocal unit model MRC-1024 (Bio-Rad, Hercules, CA) containing a 15-mW krypton-argon laser).
2. Objective lens (63× Plan Apochromat/1.4 NA oil immersion objective [Zeiss]).
3. National Institutes of Health (NIH) image software (Bethesda, MD Bethesda, MD; software can be downloaded at no cost at http://shareware.netscape.com/ computing/shareware/software_title.tmpl?p=MAC&category_id=60& subcategory_id=68&id=55652).

3. Methods
3.1. Cell Culture

1. Grow MDCK cells stably transfected with GFP-CFTR on tissue culture-treated polystyrene flasks in MEM with Earle's salts containing 10% FBS, 50 U/mL penicillin, 50 µg/mL streptomycin, 2 mM L-glutamine, and 150 µg/mL G-418 in 5% CO$_2$-balanced air at 37°C.
2. Replace ~80% of the media every 2 d.
3. When confluent (every 5–6 d), subculture cells by trypsinization (0.05% trypsin, 0.53 mM EDTA in Hanks' balanced salt solution) and seed at 200,000 cells/T75 flask to maintain the cells in culture (*see* **Note 1**).
4. For confocal microscopy experiments, seed cells at 50,000–75,000 cells/0.33 cm^2 Transwell filter bottom cup placed in an individual well of a 24-well plate and grow cells in 5% CO$_2$-balanced air at 33°C (*see* **Notes 2** and **3**).
5. Completely replace medium in apical and basolateral chambers daily for 5–7 d, at which point cells are fully polarized, and remove G-418 from medium 3–4 d prior to experimentation (*see* **Note 4**).
6. Treat monolayers with 5 mM sodium-*n*-butyrate for 15–18 h then remove sodium-*n*-butyrate 2 h prior to experimentation (*see* **Note 5**).

3.2. Cell Stimulation with cAMP and Staining with WGA–Texas Red

1. Quickly wash cells twice with PBS (wash apical and basolateral compartments).
2. Treat cells with 100 µM CPT-cAMP, 100 µM IBMX, and 20 µM forskolin (added to both apical and basolateral compartments) or vehicle for 10–60 min in MEM with Earle's salts lacking supplements in 5% CO$_2$-balanced air at 37°C (*see* **Note 6**).
3. Transfer cells to ice bucket in cold room.

4. Label apical and basolateral cell membranes with 10 μg/mL ice-cold WGA–Texas Red (added to both apical and basolateral compartments) in MEM with Earle's salts lacking supplements for 30 min (*see* **Note 7**).
5. Wash cells three times (2–3 min/wash) with MEM with Earle's salts lacking supplements (wash apical and basolateral compartments) to remove nonbound WGA–Texas Red.
6. Fix cells with 100% ice-cold MeOH (add fixative to both apical and basolateral compartments) for 10 min on ice.
7. Rinse cells twice with PBS (wash apical and basolateral compartments). Work can be performed at room temperature now.
8. Excise filters with a scalpel, place them apical side up on a glass slide, and overlay them with a drop (50 μL) of *n*-propyl gallate (to retard fading) followed by a coverslip (*see* **Note 8**).
9. Seal coverslips with liquid Valap heated to 40–50°C on a hot plate (*see* **Note 9**).

3.3. Cell Staining with ZO-1 Antibody

1. Quickly wash cells twice with PBS (wash apical and basolateral chambers).
2. Fix and permeabilize cells in 100% acetone (add fixative to both apical and basolateral chambers) for 2 min at –20°C.
3. Stain tight junctions with 10 μg/mL anti-ZO-1 rabbit polyclonal antibody in 1% BSA/PBS for 1 h at room temperature (*see* **Note 10**).
4. Wash cells three times with PBS (wash apical and basolateral chambers).
5. Stain with 1:100 goat anti-rabbit Texas Red secondary antibody in PBS (*see* **Note 10**).
6. Wash cells three times with PBS (wash apical and basolateral chambers).
7. Excise filters with a scalpel, place them apical side up on a glass slide, and overlay them with a drop (50 μL) of *n*-propyl gallate (to retard fading), followed by a coverslip.
8. Seal coverslips with liquid Valap heated to 40–50°C on a hot plate.

3.4. Laser Scanning Confocal Microscopic Analysis of GFP-CFTR Distribution Following cAMP Treatment

1. Acquire a complete z series beginning at the apical membrane and ending at the basal membrane (*see* **Note 11**).
2. Excite GFP fluorescence using the 488-nm laser line and collect GFP fluorescence using a FITC filter set (emission filter 530 ± 30 nm) (*see* **Note 12**).
3. Excite WGA–Texas Red using the 568-nm laser line and collect Texas Red fluorescence using a Texas Red filter set (emission filter 605 ± 32 nm) (*see* **Note 13**).
4. For each z series collected, acquire ~10 sections in 1.0-μm increments and average 3 scans (select Kalman method) per z section to filter out any pixel noise in the detector (*see* **Note 14**).
5. Quantitate the fraction of GFP-CFTR fluorescence located in each z section with NIH Image software.
6. Draw a box over the cell(s) to be measured and determine pixel counts within this area (click on "Analyze" menu and select "Measure;" then click on "Analyze" menu and select "Show Results" to see data). Keep box areas constant for all

sections of the same cell(s) and evaluate pixel intensity histograms (click on "Analyze" menu and select "Plot Profile") of boxed regions to ensure that GFP fluorescence is within the linear range (0–254) (*see* **Notes 15–17**). Draw a same-sized box over a region of the image where no GFP fluorescence is visible and determine the pixel counts within this area; this background fluorescence value is subtracted from each specific measurement.

7. Export measurements from NIH Image to Microsoft Excel or an equivalent software package (click on "Edit" menu, select "Copy Measurements," and paste into spreadsheet program) for assembly and analysis of data.
8. Quantitate GFP-CFTR localization along the apical to basal axis using the following formula: fraction GFP-CFTR fluorescence in section x = (GFP-CFTR pixel counts in section x – background fluorescence)/(sum of GFP-CFTR pixel counts in sections 1–10 – sum of background fluorescence), where x is a single confocal section of a 10 section z series. Evaluate 3–4 z series, each containing multiple cells per field, from each of 3–4 different monolayers to get a mean result. **Figure 1** illustrates the quantitation of GFP-CFTR distribution along the apical–basal axis as a function of cAMP treatment using this methodology.

3.5. Laser Scanning Confocal Microscopic Analysis of GFP-CFTR Polarization

1. Acquire a xz vertical section through a monolayer expressing GFP-CFTR fusion protein.
2. Excite GFP fluorescence using the 488-nm laser line and collect GFP fluorescence using a FITC filter set (530 ± 30 nm).
3. Excite Texas Red fluorescence associated with ZO-1 staining using the 568-nm laser line and collect Texas Red fluorescence using a Texas Red filter set (605 ± 32 nm).
4. Quantitate the fraction of GFP-CFTR fluorescence located in apical and basolateral membrane regions with NIH Image software.
5. Draw a box (~2 μm wide and encompassing the length of apical or lateral membranes) over the region to be measured (draw separate and similarly sized boxes over the apical membrane region, the right lateral membrane region, the left lateral membrane region, and the nuclear region) and determine pixel counts within the boxed regions (click on "Analyze" menu and select "Measure;" then click on "Analyze" menu and select "Show Results" to see data) (*see* **Note 18**). Evaluate pixel intensity histograms (click on "Analyze" menu and select "Plot Profile") of boxed regions to ensure that GFP fluorescence is within the linear range (0–254) (*see* **Note 15**).
6. Calculate an apical to basolateral polarity ratio (R) using the following formula: $R = (a - c)/[(b_l - c)/2 + (b_r - c)/2]$, where a corresponds to pixel counts in the boxed apical membrane region, b_l corresponds to pixel counts is the boxed left lateral membrane region, b_r corresponds to pixel counts in the boxed right lateral membrane region, and c corresponds to background pixel counts in the boxed nuclear region. Divide lateral membrane measurements by 2 when adjacent cells, with opposing lateral surfaces, display GFP fluorescence. GFP fluorescence is

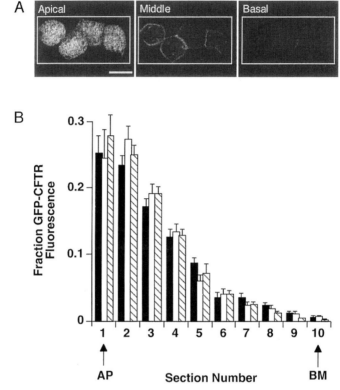

Fig. 1. Quantitative confocal microscopic analysis of GFP-CFTR localization along the apical to basal axis following cAMP treatment. **(A)** Selected *z* sections from the apical (section 2 in panel **B**), middle (section 6 in panel **B**) and basal (section 9 in panel **B**) regions of a monolayer of GFP-CFTR expressing cells not treated with cAMP. A box, used to quantitate GFP-CFTR fluorescence (shown in gray), is drawn around four cells. Scale bar is 10 µm. **(B)** Quantitative analysis. Cells were treated with 100 µ*M* CPT-cAMP, 100 µ*M* IBMX, and 20 µ*M* forskolin (added to both apical and basolateral compartments) for 10 min (black bars) or 60 min (white bars), or vehicle (60 min, hatched bars). GFP-CFTR fluorescence was measured in 1-µm confocal optical sections along the apical (section 1)-to-basal (section 10) axis. GFP-CFTR distribution did not change following cAMP treatment. For each treatment, three *z* series, each with 15–25 cells per field, were analyzed from each of four separate monolayers. Error bars display SEM. $P > 0.05$ for vehicle compared to 10-min or 60-min cAMP treatment for each section. AP, apical membrane; BM, basal membrane.

generally not observed in the basal membrane, which is excluded from analyses (*see* **Notes 16** and **17**). Evaluate multiple *xz* vertical sections from different cells from each of 3–4 different monolayers to get a mean result. **Figure 2** illustrates analysis of GFP-CFTR polarization along the apical–basal axis using this methodology.

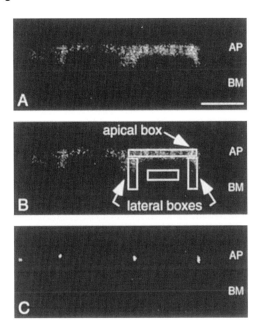

Fig. 2. Confocal micrographs (*xz* vertical sections) illustrating the apical polarization of GFP-CFTR. (**A**) GFP-CFTR fluorescence. (**B**) Same image as in (A) with boxes drawn around apical membrane (apical box), lateral membranes (lateral boxes), and nuclear region (unlabelled box between lateral boxes) for quantitation of GFP-CFTR apical to basolateral ratio. (**C**) ZO-1, a marker of tight junctions separating apical and basolateral membranes, immunoreactivity. GFP-CFTR is polarized to the apical membrane region and exhibits an apical to basolateral ratio ~10. AP, apical membrane; BM, basal membrane. Scale bar is 10 µm.

4. Notes

1. MDCK I cells are very adherent and difficult to trypsinize. To facilitate trypsinization, cells can be trypsinized in 10× trypsin (0.5% trypsin, 0.53 m*M* EDTA in Hanks' balanced salt solution; Life Technologies), which decreases trypsinization time from ~30 min (with 1× trypsin) to less than 5 min (with 10× trypsin). To facilitate removal of cells from culture plates, trypsinization can also be performed in 5% CO_2-balanced air at 37°C.

2. Transwell filters exhibit negligible green autofluorescence, and are optimal for viewing GFP-CFTR fluorescence. By contrast, other filters including Cellagen filters (ICN Biomedicals, Aurora, OH) exhibit high levels of green autofluorescence which preclude clear identification of GFP-CFTR-expressing cells.

3. Because correct folding of the GFP chromophore is temperature-sensitive (*9*), cells used for experiments are grown at 33°C to maximize GFP signal intensity. Culturing cells at reduced temperature does not affect cell growth or viability and does not alter GFP-CFTR localization compared to cells cultured at 37°C.

4. Aspirate media from basolateral chamber first and from apical chamber second; replace media in apical chamber first and in basolateral chamber second. This technique maintains constant positive pressure on cells and prevents cells from detaching from the filter. Add 2–3 drops (~100 μL) of medium to apical chamber and 0.4–0.5 mL of medium to basolateral chamber so that the heights of apical and basolateral solutions are equal.

5. GFP-CFTR fluorescence is dim and difficult to visualize in cells not induced with sodium-*n*-butyrate. Sodium-*n*-butyrate, which activates transcription from many viral promoters including the CMV promoter used to drive GFP-CFTR expression, increases GFP-CFTR expression levels ~30-fold, and facilitates identification of GFP-CFTR expressing cells without affecting CFTR localization or trafficking *(15)*. Five millimolar working solutions of sodium-*n*-butyrate are prepared in complete cell culture medium and filter-sterilized (0.2 μm) before use. Fresh solutions of butyrate are prepared immediately before use for each experiment.

6. CPT-cAMP stock solutions are prepared in sterile water at 10 mM and stored in single-use aliquots at –20°C. IBMX stock solutions are prepared in absolute EtOH at 40 mM and stored in single-use aliquots at –20°C. Forskolin stock solutions are prepared in dimethylsulfoxide (DMSO) at 20 mM and stored in single-use aliquots at –20°C. New stock solutions of CPT-cAMP, IBMX, and forskolin should be prepared every 3 mo.

7. WGA–Texas Red, a lectin that selectively binds N-acetylglucosamine and sialic acid carbohydrate residues present in glycoproteins at the plasma membrane in nonfixed cells, is prepared as a 2-mg/mL stock solution in PBS and stored at –20°C in single-use aliquots. Stock solutions are heated to 37°C for 10 min in a water bath and vortexed for 1 min to facilitate solubilization. Before use, WGA–Texas Red should be centrifuged for 2–3 min at 14,000g to pelletize insoluble material; only the supernatant is used for cell staining.

8. Retain a small amount of liquid on top of the filters (in the apical chamber) during excision. This decreases the tendency of the filters to wrinkle and roll up onto themselves. Because the filter and monolayer are each approx 10 μm tall, cells will be compressed and cellular morphology will be altered if no spacing is incorporated between the glass slide and coverslip. Therefore, two strips of scotch tape (~1 cm wide) should be placed along the long edges of the glass slides to create a small chamber for the excised filter to sit in. This small chamber minimizes compression of filter-grown cells when overlaid with the glass cover slip.

9. We do not recommend sealing cover slips with nailpolish, since nailpolish has been reported to quench GFP fluorescence *(4)*. Valap, by contrast, has not been reported to affect GFP fluorescence. As an alternative to *n*-propyl gallate, cells can be mounted in ProLong Antifade reagent (Molecular Probes). ProLong-mounted samples do not require Valap but should be allowed to dry/harden for at least several hours before the samples are visualized by confocal microscopy. Samples sealed with Valap can be viewed immediately.

10. To minimize the amount of antibody used for staining, add a sufficient volume to just cover the entire surface area (30–50 μL) of the apical membrane. It is not necessary to add antibody to the basolateral chamber, which can remain empty

during primary, and secondary antibody incubations. All antibody incubations (and washes) can be performed in the same 24-well plate in which cells were cultured. Keep filters covered with lid of 24-well plate to prevent antibody evaporation.

11. Apical and basal membranes are identified by WGA–Texas Red staining. All images from the same z series should be collected using the same values for laser power (range 3–10%), photomultiplier gain (range 1200–1500), iris (range 2.0–3.5), and black level (range –10 to –5). Using these values, the theoretical limits of resolution for the confocal microscope (~0.2 μm in the xy plane and ~0.8 μm in the xz plane at 488-nm excitation) can be approached *(14)*.

12. Alternatively, a Piston GFP filter (Chroma Optical, Brattleboro, VT; emission filter HQ 515 ± 30 nm) can be used to collect GFP fluorescence. Whereas the FITC filter (530 ± 30 nm) allows more long-wavelength background fluorescence to pass to the detector, the Piston GFP filter reduces background autofluorescence at wavelengths longer than 530 nm.

13. Using these filter sets, all fluorescent signals are spectrally isolated and negligible signal bleedthrough occurs between channels. To determine signal bleedthrough in a double-labeling experiment, the signal from the green channel (in cells not expressing GFP-CFTR) is first acquired in a specimen labeled only with ZO-1 (Texas Red fluorophore); then the signal from the red channel is acquired in a specimen expressing GFP-CFTR but labeled with Texas Red-coupled secondary antibody only (i.e., exclusion of the specific ZO-1 antibody during staining). If Texas Red fluorescence bleeds into the green channel, then green fluorescence will be visible in the first specimen; similarly, if GFP fluorescence bleeds into the red channel, then red fluorescence will be visible in the second sample. Signal bleedthrough can be avoided by proper selection of filter sets.

14. Since MDCK type I cells are ~10 μm tall when grown on filters, and the minimal resolution of the confocal microscope in the xz plane is 0.8 μm, stepping through the monolayer in 1.0-μm increments maximizes the amount of data collected in each section without duplicating information contained in neighboring sections. If sections are collected at intervals less than 1.0 μm, duplicate information present in multiple overlapping sections is generated without improving resolution. Minimal photobleaching of GFP-CFTR occurs during the ~30 scans (10 sections collected with a Kalman average of 3) required to collect a complete z series.

15. NIH Image may invert the data such that bright regions exhibit low pixel intensities (closer to 0) and dim regions exhibit high pixel intensities (closer to 254). If this is observed, merely subtract each pixel intensity measurement from 254 to obtain the correct value.

16. The confocal microscope can assess the relative levels of CFTR along the apical–basal axis; however, because the limit of resolution of the confocal microscope is ~0.2 μm in the xy plane and ~0.8 μm in the xz plane *(14)*, and cellular membranes are ~10 nm thick, it cannot accurately differentiate between CFTR localized in the plasma membrane and CFTR localized directly beneath the plasma membrane in endosomal vesicles. Thus, confocal microscopy cannot specifically be used to determine whether CFTR is localized in the plasma membrane and if a particular reagent, such as cAMP, stimulates insertion of CFTR-containing

vesicles into the plasma membrane. Therefore, we stress the need to compare semiquantitative measurements obtained by confocal microscopy with values obtained using a second, independent technique such as surface biotinylation. Using domain-selective cell surface biotinylation, we have validated pixel intensity counts as a measure of CFTR localization following cAMP treatment and of CFTR polarization (i.e., apical to basolateral polarity ratio) *(15,16)*.

17. Similar quantitative microscopic techniques have been used by other investigators to analyze both ion channel polarization and CFTR distribution following cAMP treatment, thereby independently verifying the utility of these approaches *(17,18)*.

18. The transition between apical and lateral membranes is identified by ZO-1 staining. Because the lengths of the apical and lateral membrane regions are not always equal, it may not be possible to draw boxes of the exact same size. If the apical and lateral membranes are not easily contained in a box, the outline of membranes can be traced using the kidney-shaped freehand drawing tool.

References

1. Crawford, I., Maloney, P. C., Zeitlin, P. L., Guggino, W. B., Hyde,S. C., Turley, H., Gatter, K. C., Harris, A., and Higgins, C. F. (1991) Immunocytochemical localization of the cystic fibrosis gene product CFTR. *Proc. Natl. Acad. Sci. USA* **88,** 9262–9266.

2. Engelhardt, J. F., Yankaskas, J. R., Ernst, S. A., Yang, Y., Marino, C. R., Boucher, R. C., Cohn, J. A., and Wilson, J. M. (1992) Submucosal glands are the predominant site of CFTR expression in the human bronchus. *Nature Gen.* **2,** 240–248.

3. Walker, J., Watson, J., Holmes, C., Edelman, A., and Banting, G. (1995) Production and characterization of monoclonal and polyclonal antibodies to different regions of the cystic fibrosis transmembrane conductance regulator (CFTR): detection of immunologically related proteins. *J. Cell Sci.* **108,** 2433–2444.

4. Chalfie, M., Tu, Y., Erskirchen, G., Ward, W. W., and Prasher, D. C. (1994) Green fluorescent protein as a marker for gene expression. *Science* **263,** 802–805.

5. Gerdes, H.-H. and Kaether, C. (1996) Green fluorescent protein: applications in cell biology. *FEBS Lett,* **389,** 44–47.

6. Lippincott-Schwartz, J., Cole, N., and Presley, J. (1998) Unravelling Golgi membrane traffic with green fluroescent protein chimeras. *Trends Cell Biol.* **8,** 16–20.

7. Lippincott-Schwartz, J. and Smith, C. L. (1997) Insights into secretory and endocytic membrane traffic using green fluorescent protein chimeras. *Curr. Biol.* **7,** 631–639.

8. Cubitt, A. B., Heim, R., Adams, S. R., Boyd, A. E., Gross, L. A., and Tsien, R. Y. (1995) Understanding, improving, and using green fluorescent proteins. *Trends Biochem. Sci.* **20,** 448–455.

9. Tsien, R. Y. (1998) The green fluorescent protein. *Annu. Rev. Biochem.* **67,** 509–544.

10. Griffiths, G., Parton, R. G., Lucocq, J., van Deurs, B., Brown, D., Slot, J. W., and Geuze, H. J. (1993) The immunofluorescent era of membrane traffic. *Trends Cell Biol.* **3,** 214–219.

11. Chalfie, M. and Kain, S. (eds.) (1998) *Green Flourescent Protein: Properties, Applications and Protocols*, Wiley-Liss & Sons, Inc., New York, NY.

12. Conn, P. M. (ed.) (1999) *Methods In Enzymology: Green Fluorescent Protein*, Academic Press, San Diego, CA.

13. Sullivan, K. F. and Kay, S. A. (eds.) (1999) *Methods In Cell Biology: Green Fluorescent Proteins*, Academic Press, San Diego, CA.

14. Sandison, D. R., Williams, R. M., Wells, K. S., Strickler, J., and Webb, W. W. (1995) Quantitive fluorescence confocal laser scanning microscopy (CLSM) in *Handbook of Biological Confocal Microscopy* (Pawley, J. B., ed.), Plenum Press, NY, pp. 39–53.

15. Moyer, B. D., Loffing, J., Schwiebert, E. M., Loffing-Cueni, D., Halpin, P. A., Karlson, K. H., et al. (1998) Membrane trafficking of the cystic fibrosis gene product, cystic fibrosis transmembrane conductance regulator, tagged with green fluorescent protein in Madin-Darby canine kidney cells. *J. Biol. Chem.* **273,** 21,759–21,768.

16. Moyer, B. D., Denton, J., Karlson, K. H., Reynolds, D., Wang, S., Mickle, J. E., et al. (1999) A PDZ-interacting domain in CFTR is an apical membrane polarization signal. *J. Clin. Invest.* **104,** 1353–1361.

17. Gottardi, C. J. and Caplan, M. J. (1993) An ion-transporting ATPase encodes multiple apical localization signals. *J. Cell Biol.* **121,** 283–293.

18. Lehrich, R. W., Aller, S. G., Webster, P., Marino, C. R., and Forrest, J. N., Jr. (1998) Vasoactive intestinal peptide, forskolin, and genistein increase apical CFTR trafficking in the rectal gland of the spiny dogfish, *Squalus acanthias*: acute regulation of CFTR trafficking in an intact epithelium. *J. Clin. Invest.* **101,** 737–745.

15

CFTR Folding and Maturation in Cells

Mohamed Benharouga, Manu Sharma, and Gergely L. Lukacs

1. Introduction

Structural predictions suggest that cystic fibrosis transmembrane conductance regulator (CFTR), a member of the ABC transporter family, consists of two homologous halves, each comprised of six transmembrane (TM) helices and a nucleotide-binding domain (NBD1 and NBD2), which are covalently connected by the regulatory (R) domain *(1)*. This complex, multidomain structure, conceivably renders the posttranslational folding of wild-type (wt) CFTR inefficient and sensitive to point mutations. Depending on the expression system examined, 50–80% of the newly synthesized wt CFTR degrades at the endoplasmic reticulum (ER), as core-glycosylated folding intermediate *(2–4)*. The remaining 20–50% of the CFTR undergoes an ATP-dependent conformational maturation *(3,4)* and attains an export competent, folded conformation, which is incorporated into transport vesicles at the endoplasmic reticulum. While traversing the cis/medial Golgi, the high-mannose-type N-linked oligosaccharides of CFTR (core-glycosylated form) are converted to complex-type oligosaccharides *(2)*.

More than 900 mutations have been identified in the cystic fibrosis (CF) gene, leading to impaired biosynthesis, processing, activation, and stability of CFTR or a combination of these *(5)*. Most of the missense mutations, including the most frequent one, deletion of phenylalanine at position 508 (ΔF508) in the NBD1 *(6,7)*, are believed to interrupt the posttranslational folding of CFTR *(2–4,8,9)* and to target the core-glycosylated intermediate for degradation, predominantly via the ubiquitin–proteasome pathway at the ER *(10,11)*. Exposure of ER-retention signals, however, may contribute to the inability of folding intermediate(s) to exit the ER *(12)*.

From: *Methods in Molecular Medicine, vol. 70: Cystic Fibrosis Methods and Protocols*
Edited by: W. R. Skach © Humana Press Inc., Totowa, NJ

The quality control mechanism prevents the exit of incompletely folded or misfolded polypeptides and unassembled oligomers from the ER *(13)*. It was demonstrated that the ATP-dependent conformational maturation of the nascent, core-glycosylated CFTR in the ER is a prerequisite for entering the distal stages of the secretory pathway *(3)*. Thus, appearance of the complex-type N-linked oligosaccharides can be taken as an indication that CFTR has undergone a conformational maturation, which enabled it to traverse the cis-medial Golgi. This conclusion was verified by examining the in vivo and in vitro protease susceptibility of the early folding intermediates and the fully mature CFTR either in its core- or complex-glycosylated form *(3,4,9)*.

While it is important to keep in mind that the processing of the N-linked-oligosaccharides is an indirect indicator of the folding competence of CFTR, it provides a relatively straightforward method to monitor the processing along the biosynthetic pathway. The sharp banding pattern of the core-glycosylated form (apparent molecular mass ~150 kDa, band B *[2]*) and the less mobile, diffusely migrating complex-glycosylated CFTR (apparent molecular mass ~170 kDs, band C *[2]*) can be separated by sodium dodecyl sulfate-polyacryla-mide gel electrophoresis (SDS-PAGE) and visualized with immunoblotting or fluorography as described under **Subheading 3.2.1.** Furthermore, distinction between the core- and complex-glycosylated CFTR could be confirmed with glycosidase digestion, a method described under **Subheading 3.2.2.**

Low-resolution structural information of the wt and mutant CFTR have been obtained by examining the protease susceptibility of the cytosolic domains, representing ~70% of the polypeptide mass of CFTR in its native environment (**Subheading 3.4.2.**). While this assay could only compare the protease suscepti-bility of those conformers that dominate the folding pathway, when the method is combined with metabolic pulse labeling and immunoprecipitation, the post-translational conformational transition between the folding intermediate(s) and the native form could be evaluated as well (**Subheading 3.4.3.**).

2. Materials

2.1. Expression of CFTR in Cultured Cells

1. Green monkey kidney epithelia (COS-1), baby hamster kidney (BHK-21), and Chi-nese hamster ovary (CHO-K1) cells (American Type Culture Collection, Rockville, MD, accession numbers CRL 1650, CCL10, and CRL9618 respectively).
2. Dulbecco's modified Eagle medium with high glucose (DMEM; Gibco-BRL, Gaithersburg, MD).
3. Fetal bovine serum (FBS; Gibco-BRL).
4. Transfection–quality plasmid DNA, i.e., pcDNA3 (CFTR) and pNUT (CFTR).
5. 2.5 M CaCl$_2$.
6. 0.1× TE: 10 mM Tris-HCl, 1 mM EDTA, pH 7.05.
7. 2× BES: 230 mM NaCl, 50 mM BES, 1.5 mM Na$_2$HPO$_4$, pH 6.96.

8. Phosphate-buffered saline (PBS): 2.7 mM KCl, 1 mM KH$_2$PO$_4$, 8.0 mM Na$_2$HPO$_4$, 137 mM NaCl.
9. Methotrexate (25 mg/mL, Faulding Inc., Quebec, Canada).
10. LipofectAMINE™ (Gibco-BRL).

2.2. Detection of Complex- and Core-Glycosylated CFTR by Western Blotting and Glycosidase Digestion

1. PBS *see* **Subheading 2.1.**
2. PBST: PBS supplemented with 0.1% Tween-20.
3. RIPA buffer: 150 mM NaCl, 20 mM Tris-HCl, pH 8.0, 0.1% (w/v) sodium dodecyl sulfate (SDS), 0.5% (w/v) sodium deoxycholate, 1% (v/v) Triton X-100. When indicated, protease inhibitors are added immediately before use: 5 μg/mL leupeptin, 5 μg/mL pepstatin A, 1 mM phenylmethylsulfonyl fluoride (PMSF), and 2 mg/mL idoacetamide (*see* **Note 1**).
4. Bicinchoninic acid (BCA) protein assay kit (Pierce, Rockford, IL).
5. 10× Laemmli sample buffer (LSB): 300 mM Tris-HCl, 40 mM EDTA, 20% SDS, 0.5 M dithiothreitol (DTT), 17.5% glycerol, 0.03% Bromophenol blue, pH 6.8.
6. Endoglycosidase H (New England Biolabs, Beverly, MA).
7. Peptide N-glycosidase F (New England Biolabs, Beverly, MA).
8. Standard components for SDS-PAGE, (e.g., acrylamide/bis-acrylamide mix, SDS, TEMED, vertical slab gel apparatus for running 1.5-mm thick gels).
9. Nitrocellulose (Trans-Blot, Bio-Rad, Hercules, CA).
10. Ponceau S stain: 0.1% (w/v) in 1% (w/v) trichloroacetic acid.
11. Protein blotting equipment: Trans-Blot cell from Bio-Rad (Hercules, CA).
12. Transfer buffer: 25 mM Tris-HCl, 192 mM glycine, 20% methanol, pH 8.1–8.4.
13. Blocking buffer: PBST containing 5% nonfat dry milk.
14. Affinity-purified mouse monoclonal M3A7, L12B4, or 24-1 anti-CFTR antibodies (Ab). The M3A7 and L12B4 antibodies were developed and provided by Drs. N. Kartner and J. Riordan *(14,15)*. The 24-1 Ab is commercially available from R & D Systems (Minneapolis, MN).
15. Horseradish peroxidase (HRP)-conjugated goat anti-mouse IgG (Amersham Pharmacia Biotech, Uppsala, Sweden).
16. Enhanced chemiluminescence detection kit (Amersham Pharmacia Biotech, Uppsala, Sweden).

2.3. Determination of the Processing Efficiency of CFTR by Metabolic Pulse Chase Labeling

1. Methionine- and cysteine-free αModified Eagel's Medium (αMEM-Cys/Met, Gibco-BRL).
2. ^{35}S-Methionine and ^{35}S-cysteine Pro-mix (>7.5 mCi/mL, >1000 Ci/mmoL, Amersham Pharmacia Biotech, Uppsala, Sweden).
3. Affinity-purified mouse monoclonal M3A7, L12B4, and 24-1 anti-CFTR antibodies (*see* **Subheading 2.2.**).
4. Protein G Sepharose (Sigma-Aldrich, St. Louis, MO).
5. Gel fixing solution (10% acetic acid, 40% methanol).

6. Amplify (Amersham Pharmacia Biotech).
7. End-over-end mixer.
8. Gel-dryer (Speed Gel, Savant, Farmingdale, NY).
9. Phosphorimager equipped with ImageQuant software (e.g., Molecular Dynamics, Sunnyvale, CA).

2.4. Monitoring the Conformation of the Cytosolic Domains of CFTR by Limited Proteolytic Digestion

1. PBS: *see* **Subheading 2.1.**
2. Homogenization buffer (HB): 0.25 M sucrose, 10 mM HEPES, 1 mM EDTA, pH 6.8. Protease inhibitors (10 μg/mL leupeptin and 10 μg/mL pepstatin) and 1 mM DTT added freshly.
3. Microsome resuspension buffer (RB): 0.25 M sucrose, 10 mM HEPES, 1 mM EDTA, pH 7.6.
4. Nitrogen-disrupting bomb (Park Instrument, Moline, IL).
5. Digestion buffer (DB): resuspension buffer (RB), with 4 mM CaCl$_2$ in the case of thermolysin.
6. Proteases: trypsin, proteinase K, thermolysine, and chymotrypsin (Sigma-Aldrich).

3. Methods

3.1. Expression of CFTR in Cultured Cells

While the transient expression system has the convenience of rapidity to screen the impact of a large number of mutations on the biosynthetic processing of CFTR, the more laborious stable mammalian expression system has the advantage of better reproducibility and larger yield for biochemical studies. Since a comprehensive review has recently been published about the requirements of vectors and hosts cells for CFTR expression *(12)*, in this section we will focus on the technical aspects of the most frequently used expression systems in our laboratory.

3.1.1. Transient Expression of CFTR in COS-1 Cells with Modified Calcium Phosphate Method

Transient expression of COS-1 and HEK-293 cells has been widely used to monitor the processing of wt and mutant CFTR by immunoblotting and metabolic pulse chase experiments *(2,8)*. The complementary DNA encoding CFTR has been inserted into pcDNA3 (Invitrogen, Carlsbad, CA) expression plasmid. Uptake of plasmid DNA into the target cell is based on the internalization of calcium phosphate co-precipitated DNA.

1. The day before transfection, seed COS-1 cells at 30% confluence on 60- or 100-mm-diameter tissue-culture dish in 4 or 12 mL DMEM with 10% (v/v) FBS.
2. Mix 25 μg DNA in 15-mL polystyrene test tube for each 100-mm plate and add H$_2$O to 450 μL by swirling the tube.

3. Add 50 μL 2.5 M CaCl$_2$ and mix it. Then combine the DNA with 500 μL 2× BES and leave it at room temperature for 30 min.
4. Supplement the DNA solution with 10 mL tissue culture medium (DMEM + 10% FBS).
5. Aspirate the medium from the cells and rinse them with PBS.
6. Add the precipitated DNA solution gently to the cell, while swirling the plates carefully to ensure an even distribution of DNA over the entire plate.
7. Harvest the cells after 48–72 h incubation at 37°C.

3.1.2. Transient Expression of CFTR in COS-1 Cells with LipofectAMINE™

LipofectAMINE can be used as an alternative complex-forming agent to shield the negative charges of the polyanionic DNA. This method appears to ensure higher transfection efficiency than the calcium phosphate precipitation and is recommended for the detection of mutant CFTR with attenuated level of expression.

1. Prepare cells as described above.
2. For each 100-mm plate, dilute 16 μg plasmid DNA into 800 μL serum-free medium (*see* **Note 2**).
3. Dilute 80 μL of LipofectAMINE into 800 μL of serum-free medium.
4. Combine the DNA and LipofectAMINE solutions slowly in a 10-mL polypropylene tube and leave them at room temperature for 30–45 min.
5. Wash the cells with serum-free medium twice to remove traces of serum.
6. Add 5 mL serum-free medium to the LipofectAMINE-DNA, mix gently, and overlay the entire plate evenly.
7. Incubate the cells for 6 hours to overnight at 37°C, 5% CO_2.
8. Replace the LipofectAMINE-DNA-containing medium with 10 mL of growth medium and incubate for an additional 24–48 h before harvesting.

3.1.3. Stable Expression of CFTR in Heterologous Systems

The complementary DNA-encoding CFTR has been inserted into pNUT expression plasmid for stable transfection. This expression vector harbors a dihydrofolate reductase (DHFR) gene, which allows the amplification of the copy number of the expression plasmid at increasing concentration of methotrexate, an inhibitor of the DHFR.

1. Day 1: transfect BHK-21 or CHO-K1 cells, grown on a 100-mm tissue culture dish, with the calcium phosphate precipitation method as described under **Subheading 3.1.1.**
2. Day 2: split the cells into four 100-mm culture dish.
3. Day 3: start the selection of clones with low concentration (10 μM) of Methotrexate-containing growth medium and increase the concentration of the drug progressively by 50–100 μM to achieve gene amplification. Medium has to be changed every 2 d.
4. Colonies are isolated and expanded from one of the two dishes after 12–16 d of selection (*see* **Note 3**). One of the dishes is expanded and saved as a mixture.

5. Verification of the transgene expression in individual clones is achieved by immunoblotting, as described under **Subheading 3.2.1.**

3.2. Detection of Complex- and Core-Glycosylated CFTR by Western Blotting and Glycosidase Digestion

Two consensus N-linked glycosylation sites have been identified in the predicted fourth extracellular loop of CFTR *(1)*. Addition of each mannose core-oligosaccharide results in an increase of 2–3 kDa in the apparent molecular mass of the polypeptide, determined by SDS-PAGE. N-linked glycosylation of both the ER-retained mutant and the fully mature wt CFTR can be confirmed by pepetide N-glycosidase F (PNGase F) digestion, which cleaves between the innermost N,N'-diacetylchitobiose and the asparagine and produces the nonglycosylated CFTR, with an apparent molecular mass of ~135 kDa (designated as band A, *[2]*). While the corc-glycosylated CFTR (band B), bearing high-mannose-type oligosaccharides, is sensitive to endoglycosidase H (endo-H) digestion, the complex-glycosylated form (band C) is endo H-resistant. Since the nonglycosylated, core- and complex-glycosylated CFTRs have distinct electrophoretic mobilities, immunoblotting analysis in conjuction with glycosidase treatment can reveal the processing state of CFTR variants along the biosynthetic pathway (*see* **Fig. 1**).

3.2.1. Detection of CFTR Expression by Western Blotting

Immunological detection of CFTR is an invaluable tool to identify the impact of various mutations on the processing and conformation of CFTR. Detailed comparative analysis of the specificity and affinity of previously used anti-CFTR antibodies for immunochemistry have been published and recommended as useful resources *(15–17)*. In this section the immunoblotting technique of CFTR is described as a general tool to monitor both the biosynthetic processing and the protease susceptibility of CFTR variants.

1. Grow CFTR expressing BHK-21 or CHO cells to 90% confluence on100-mm culture dish.
2. Place the dish on ice, remove the medium with an aspirator, and wash the cells twice with ice-cold PBS. All subsequent steps should be carried out at 4°C.
3. Scrape the cells into PBS using a plastic stirring rod (Nalgene Nunc International, Rochester, NY).
4. Pellet the cells by centrifugation in an Eppendorf tube (2 min 4000 rpm). Discard the supernatant.
5. Solubilize the cells in 50–100 µL RIPA buffer supplemented with protease inhibitors for 20 min on ice (see **Note 4**).
6. Pellet the detergent-insoluble material by centrifugation at 18,000*g* for 15 min.
7. Save the supernatant and the pellet in separate tubes (*see* **Note 5**).
8. Determine the protein concentration in the sample with the BCA protein assay, according to the manufacturer's instructions using bovine serum albumin as standard.

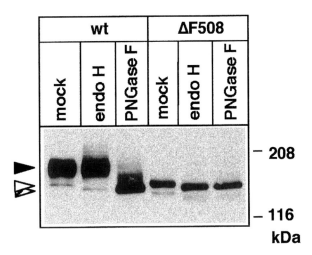

Fig. 1. Glycosidase digestion and Western blot analysis distinguish between the core- and complex-glycosylated CFTR. To monitor the core- (high-mannose) and the complex-glycosylation pattern of wt and ΔF508 CFTR, BHK cells expressing wt or mutant CFTR were solubilized with RIPA buffer. Equal amounts of lysate were digested with endoglycosidase H (endo H) and peptide N-glycosidase F (PNGase F) as described under **Subheading 3.2.2.** The mobility shift of deglycosylated CFTR was visualized with immunoblotting, using the mouse monoclonal L12B4 anti-CFTR antibody *(14)* and enhanced chemiluminescence (ECL). Filled arrowhead, complex-glycosylated form (band C); empty arrowhead, core-glycosylated form (band B); striped arrowhead, unglycosylated CFTR (band A).

9. Add 10× LSB to denature polypeptides so that a final concentration of 2× LSB will be attained and incubate the samples for 10–15 min at 37°C (*see* **Note 6**). Store the sample at –80°C until use.
10. Separate 40–100 μg of the denatured protein by SDS-PAGE according to standard protocol using a 6–7% SDS-polyacrylmide gel.
11. Transfer the polypeptides to nitrocellulose membranes at 100 V for 80 min in the cold room or by placing the transfer apparatus in ice bath.
12. Confirm the equal loading and successful transfer to the nitrocellulose membrane by staining with Ponceau S solution for 4 min.
13. To visualize the protein bands, remove the stain by washing the membrane with excess distilled water.
14. Incubate the nitrocellulose membrane in 10 mL blocking buffer for 2 h at room temperature (RT) or overnight in the cold room. This and all subsequent incubations should be performed on an orbital shaker.
15. Incubate the membrane in blocking buffer supplemented with the primary anti-CFTR antibodies (L12B4, M3A7 or 24-1) at a concentration of 0.5–1 μg/mL for 1 h at room temperature.

16. Wash the membrane with PBST six times, each for 5 min.
17. Incubate the membrane with the HRP-conjugated goat anti-mouse antibody in blocking buffer for 1 h at RT or overnight at 4°C.
18. Wash the membrane with PBST six times, each for 5 min at room temperature.
19. Visualize the secondary Ab by enhanced chemiluminescence using the ECL kit. Rinse the membrane in the 1/1 mixture of the solution A and B for 1–2 min.
20. Decant the excess solution, wrap the nitrocellulose in Saran Wrap, and expose the membrane to X-ray film in the darkroom (*see* **Note 7**).

3.2.2. Modification of the Oligosaccharide Chain of CFTR as an Indicator of Processing

The transport of CFTR from the ER through the cis/medial Golgi compartment can be followed by the maturation of the two N-linked oligosaccharides chains of CFTR *(2)*. The α-1,2-mannosidase I trims the high-mannose oligosachharides ($Man_9GlcNAc_2$) of CFTR (core-glycosylated or ER-resident form) to the $Man_5GlcNAc_2$ forms, which is then converted by the N-acetylglucosamine transferase I (GlcNac Tr I) and the α-1,2-mannosidase II to the endoglycosidase H (endo H)-resistant $GlcNAc_1Man_3GlcNAc_2$ in the cis/medial Golgi. Therefore, the ER-resident and the fully processed, complex-type N-linked oligosaccharide bearing ($GlcNAc_1Man_3GlcNAc$, which also may contain galactose, sialic acid, and additional GlcNac), can be distinguished by endo H sensitivity under denaturing conditions. Divide the lysate into three equal aliquots (each containing 50–100 µg protein), to be digested with endoglycosidase H and PNGase F. The third sample will be mock treated.

1. Prepare cell lysate from 10-cm confluent tissue culture dish by solubilyzing the cells in RIPA buffer, supplemented with protease inhibitors, as described under **Subheading 3.2.1.**
2. Denature the proteins by incubating in 1/10 dilution of the 10× denaturation buffer (5% SDS, 10% 2-mercaptoethanol), supplied with the glycosidase enzymes at 37°C for 10 min (*see* **Note 8**).
3. Adjust the pH of the samples by adding 1/10 dilution of either the 10× G5 buffer (0.5 *M* sodium citrate, pH 5.5) included with endoglycosidase H, or the 10× G7 buffer (0.5 *M* sodium phosphate, pH 7.5) supplied with PNGase F.
4. Add 1/10 dilution of 10% NP40 buffer supplied with the PNGase F sample.
5. Incubate the samples with endoglycosidase H (7 µg/mL) or PNGase F (31 µg/mL) at 37°C for 3 h. The mock treated sample is incubated in the presence of buffer only.
6. Denature the sample in 2× LSB and compare the electrophoretic mobility of the deglycosylated and mock treated CFTR by immunoblotting as described under **Subheading 3.2.1.**

The immunoblot shows the endo-H sensitivity of the core-glycosylated wt (open arrowhead, band B) and ΔF508 CFTR, indicated by the decreased apparent molecular mass upon digestion as compared to the mock-treated sample (**Fig. 1**). In contrast, the complex-glycosylated wt CFTR (filled arrowhead, band C) is resistant to endo H, but sensitive to peptide N-glycosidase F (PNGase F) digestion (**Fig. 1**). Since PNGase F cleaves between the asparagine residue and the innermost GlcNAc of both high mannose- and complex oligosaccharides, these results also show that wt CFTR is largely present as a complex-glycosylated glycoprotein in post-ER compartments, while the ΔF508 CFTR remains entrapped in the ER as a core-glycosylated intermediate.

3.3. Determination of the Processing Efficiency of CFTR by Metabolic Pulse-Chase Labeling

Since the majority of mutations impair the posttranslational conformational maturation and therefore compromise the export competence of CFTR out of the ER, determination of the maturation (or folding) efficiency is a valuable parameter to characterize the genotype phenotype relationship at the cellular level. The maturation or processing efficiency is determined by measuring the fraction of the newly synthesized, core-glycosylated CFTR that is converted into the complex-glycosylated form, using metabolic pulse-chase labeling and immunoprecipitation in conjunction with phosphorimage analysis.

1. Seed identical number of BHK-21 or CHO cells expressing CFTR into 60-mm tissue culture dishes to achieve ~80% confluence on the next day.
2. Wash the cells with αMEM lacking methionine and cysteine (αMEM-Met/Cys). Deplete the endogenous methionine and cysteine content by incubating the cells in 4 mL αMEM-Met/Cys for 40 min at 37°C.
3. Pulse label the cells in the presence of 1 mL of ^{35}S-Met and ^{35}S-Cys Pro-mix (0.1–0.2 mCi/mL) in prewarmed αMEM-Met/Cys for 15 min at 37°C (*see* **Note 9**).
4. Discard the labeling medium into a designated container for the radioactive waste.
5. Place one dish on ice and solubilize the cells to determine the total radioactivity incorporated into the newly synthesized, core-glycosylated CFTR, as described from **step 7**.
6. Chase the other monolayers in complete tissue culture medium to allow the maturation of the core-glycosylated form and the degradation of the incompletely folded form at the ER for 3 h at 37°C.
7. At the end of the chase, place the sample on ice, discard the radioactive medium, and carefully wash the cells with ice cold PBS.
8. Overlay the dish with 1 mL ice-cold RIPA buffer supplemented with protease inhibitor cocktail, and leave it on ice for 15 min. Pipet up and down the solubilization buffer to dislodge the adherent cells from the dish and transfer the lysate into an Eppendorf tube.
9. Mix the sample thoroughly and sediment the nuclei and insoluble material by centrifugation in a benchtop centrifuge (18,000g for 15 min at 4°C). Store the supernatant at –80°C.

10. Isolate CFTR by immunoprecipitation from the supernatant by incubating the lysate with the M3A7 and L12B4 (1 µg/mL from each) anti-CFTR antibodies for 2 h on a rotator at 4°C.
11. Add protein G-coated Sepharose beads (30 µL of 50% slurry/mL) to separate the immunoprecipitate and rotate the tubes for an additional hour at 4°C (*see* **Note 10**).
12. Sediment the beads (1500g for 2 min) and wash them with ice-cold RIPA buffer six times.
13. Following the final centrifugation, elute the immunoprecipitate from the beads in 50 µL of 2× LSB supplemented with 10% 2-mercaptoethanol for 20 min at 37°C.
14. After separating the samples by SDS-PAGE, incubate the gel in fixing solution (30 min) and than in Amplify for 30 min.
15. Place the gel on filter-paper support and dry it for 2–3 h at 70°C.
16. Quantify the radioactivity incorporated into the core- and complex-glycosyalted forms by phosphorimage analysis. The folding or maturation efficiency is expressed as the percentage of the core-glycosylated form converted into the complex-glycosylated CFTR, based on their radioactivity (*see* **Note 11**).
17. Visualize labeled CFTR with fluorography using Kodak X-OMAT Blue XB-1 film and intensifying screens. Expose the film for 1–3 d at –80°C.

3.4. Assessment of the Protease Susceptibility of the CFTR Cytosolic Domains by Limited Proteolysis

Limited proteolysis is a classical strategy to isolate discretely folded domains of soluble polypeptides, based on the notion that compactly folded domains, in contrast to the exposed loops and regions between folded domains, are resistant to proteolytic cleavage. This principle is applicable to the cytosolic domains of CFTR as well. Thus point mutations, which prevent the posttranslational folding or destabilize the native state, could enhance the overall protease susceptibility of CFTR by exposing proteolytic cleavage sites that are hidden in the native molecule. Limited proteolysis, in conjunction with immunoblotting, to detect the proteolytic fragments, was successfully applied to compare the folding state of the cytosolic domains of wt and mutant CFTR *(9)*. Taking into consideration the epitope specificity of the anti-CFTR antibodies, the impact of point mutations on the conformation of cytosolic domains distant from the mutation could also be assessed *(9)*. To access the cytosolic domains of CFTR, right-side-out ER, or inside-out plasma membrane vesicles are isolated (**Subheading 3.4.1.**). Following the limited proteolysis of the microsomes (**Subheading 3.4.2.**), the proteolytic digestion pattern of CFTR is probed with the NBD1-specific L12B4 and the NBD2-specific M3A7 mouse monoclonal anti-CFTR antibodies (**Subheading 3.2.1.** and **Fig. 2**). Further refinement of the method includes the limited proteolysis of metabolically labeled folding intermediates in isolated microsomes (**Subheading 3.4.3.**).

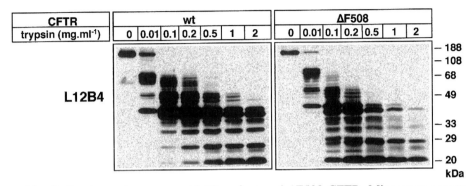

Fig. 2. *In situ* protease susceptibility of wt and ΔF508 CFTR. Microsomes were isolated with differential centrifugation from BHK cells expressing wt or ΔF508 CFTR as described under **Subheading 3.4.1.** Limited proteolysis of isolated microsomes was performed at the indicated concentrations of trypsin for 15 min at 4°C. Samples (25 μg of protein per lane for wt and 75 μg for ΔF508 CFTR) were immunoblotted with the mouse monoclonal L12B4 anti-CFTR antibody *(14)* and visualized with ECL.

3.4.1. Isolation of Microsomes

Isolation of ER, Golgi and plasma membrane-enriched microsomes from BHK-21 or CHO cells, expressing wt or mutant CFTR, is performed using nitrogen cavitation and differential centrifugation. This method had assured the generation of right-side-out ER and inside-out plasma membrane vesicles during the homogenization, exposing the cytosolic domains of CFTR to the extravesicular compartment.

1. BHK-21 or CHO transfectants are grown to confluence on twenty 150-mm tissue culture dishes. Cells are washed twice with ice-cold PBS and scraped on ice into 3 mL PBS.
2. Wash the cells with ice-cold PBS and twice in HSE-buffer in the absence of protease inhibitors in a refrigerated centrifuge (1500g for 5 min at 4°C) using 50-mL polypropylene screw top centrifuge tubes. Resuspend the pellet in 10 mL HSE-buffer.
3. Disrupt the cells by slowly releasing the pressure of the nitrogen cavitator after incubating the cell suspension at 250 psi for 3–5 min on ice. Collect the homogenate in a precooled centrifuge tube.
4. The homogenate is sedimented at 1500g for 5 min at 4°C to separate nuclei and intact cells.
5. Heavy microsomes, comprising largely of mitochondria, are separated from the postnuclear supernatant by centrifugation at 9800g for 10 min at 4°C.
6. Light microsomes, including ER, Golgi, and plasma membrane vesicles are recovered from the supernatant by ultracentrifugation at 50,000g for 50 min at 4°C.

7. The microsomal pellet is gently homogenized in 0.5 mL of ice-cold resuspension buffer, using a glass–teflon potter. Snap-freeze the microsomes in small aliquots of nitrogen and store them at –80°C. Verification of the intactness of the ER-derived vesicles has been described previously *(9)*.

3.4.2. Limited Proteolysis of Isolated Microsomes Expressing CFTR

In the following protocol, limited proteolysis of isolated microsomes is achieved by trypsinolysis. However, a wide variety of proteases, including proteinase K, chymotrypsin, thermolysine, and kallikrein, have been successfully applied to demonstrate the distinct protease susceptibility of wt and ΔF508 CFTR *(9)*. The digestion condition and the concentration range of the enzyme should be optimized individually. A detailed description of the activators and inhibitors of the most commonly used proteases have been compiled in *Proteolytic Enzymes (18)*.

1. Aliquot 0.1 mg of isolated microsomes (protein concentration of 0.8–1.5 mg/mL) in Eppendorf tubes on ice. Prepare one extra tube, which will be immediately denatured to monitor possible spontaneous proteolysis on ice.
2. Digest the microsomes in the presence of trypsin at progressively increasing concentrations (0–2 mg/mL) for 15 min at 4°C.
3. Terminate proteolysis by inhibiting the activity of trypsin with 1 m*M* PMSF.
4. Denature the sample in 2× LSB at 37°C for 20 min.
5. Proteolytic fragments are detected by immunoblotting, using the mouse monoclonal L12B4 or M3A7 anti-CFTR antibodies, as described under **Subheading 3.2.1.** To visualize low-molecular weight polypeptide fragments, the acrylamide concentration should be increased to 11–12%.

The limited proteolytic cleavage patterns of wt and ΔF508 CFTR expressing microsomes are shown on the immunoblots (**Fig. 2**), probed with the mouse monoclonal L12B4 anti-CFTR Ab, specific for the NBD1. Note the distinct protease resistance and digestion patterns of the mutant and wt CFTR. If a difference could be detected in protease susceptibility, control experiments should be performed to prove that this is not a consequence of differential localization or protein association of the wt and mutant CFTR as described previously *(9)*.

3.4.3. Limited Proteolysis of Isolated Microsomes Expressing Radioactively Labeled CFTR

To assess the conformation of transiently appearing folding intermediates in the cell (e.g., the core-glycosylated wt CFTR) by limited proteolysis, the intermediates have to be labeled radioactively before isolation of microsomes. Radioactive peptide fragments, generated by proteolytic cleavage of microsomes, are immunoprecipitated with anti-CFTR antibodies, separated by SDS-PAGE, and visualized by fluorography. This approach was successful in revealing the conformational transition between folding intermediates and the native form of wt CFTR and the similarities between the core-glycosylated wt and ΔF508 CFTR in their protease susceptibilities *(9)*.

1. Radioactively label the core-glycosylated wt CFTR in BHK-21 transfectants in the presence of 0.2 mCi/mL ^{35}S-Met and ^{35}S-Cys Pro-mix containing medium for 10 min, as described under **Subheading 3.3.**
2. Radioactively labeled cells are chilled on ice and washed with PBS. Scrape the cells carefully into ice-cold PBS and homogenize them by a ball-bearing homogenizer *(19)*.
3. Microsomes are isolated with differential centrifugation as described under **Subheading 3.4.1.**
4. Isolated microsomes are subjected to limited trypsinolysis as described for unlabeled microsomes for 15 min at 4°C (**Subheading 3.4.2.**). (Note: estimate the protein concentration and adjust the enzyme/protein ratio accordingly.)
5. The activity of trypsin is inhibited by the addition of 1 mM PMSF and microsomes are solubilized in 1 mL RIPA buffer supplemented with protease inhibitors.
6. Proteolytic fragments are immunoprecipitated with the monoclonal M3A7 and L12B4 anti-CFTR antibody and visualized by fluorography as described under **Subheading 3.3.**

4. Notes

1. Both leupeptin and pepstatin A are stored as a stock solution dissolved in dimethyl sulfoxide (DMSO) at 5-mg/mL concentration at –20°C. 100 mM PMSF is dissolved in ethanol and stored at –20°C no longer than a month.
2. Plasmid DNA for transfection can be prepared by CSCL gradient purification or by the column kit methods such as the Clontech, Qiagen Maxi/Midi, as per the manufacturer's instructions. The purity of the DNA is most critical in transient expression and should be assessed by comparing its optical density (OD) at 260 and 280 nm. The OD 260/280 nm ration should be between 1.8 and 2.0.
3. Wash the dish with PBS twice and isolate individual clones with sterile cloning rings. Detach the clones by incubating the cells with 50–100 μL 0.05% Trypsin containing PBS for 3–5 min and than pipetting a few times up and down the digestion medium. Gentle scraping can facilitate the detachment of cells, which are more adherent.
4. The solubilization volume is usually 50–200 μL for confluent 60- and 100-mm dishes, respectively. If the sample is subjected to immunoprecipitation, the solubilization volume is increaseed to 1–2 mL RIPA buffer.
5. Since mutations and pharmacological manipulations, such as inhibition of proteasomes, may induce the accumulation of CFTR aggregates, which are resistant to solubilization with RIPA buffer, higher-concentration detergent mixtures could be applied to recover CFTR from the RIPA-insoluble pellet. In our expression systems, not more than 3–4% of the total CFTR was recovered from the RIPA-insoluble fraction.
6. To avoid the formation of SDS-resistant aggregates of CFTR, denaturation should be performed below 50°C. Boiling the sample buffer induces extensive aggregation of CFTR, similarly to certain other integral membrane proteins.

7. To avoid saturation of the signal for quantitative densitometry, expose the film to various times from 15 s to 30 min, depending on the signal intensity. The linear response range of the film can be enhanced by preflashing.
8. The lysate should be denatured at 37°C but not at 50°C (as recommended in the NEB protocol), due to the thermo-aggregation tendency of CFTR.
9. To prevent the contamination of the tissue-culture incubator by radioactivity, use disposable plastic tray to hold the tissue culture-dishes. Deposit at least three carbon filters (β-Safe, Schleier & Schuell, Keene, NH), attached to the bottom of 150 × 150-mm tissue culture tray) in the incubator to adsorb radioactivity that has evaporated during the incubations. Replace the carbon filter according to the contamination level.
10. The protein G beads are supplied in a slurry containing ethanol. The beads, therefore, should be washed three times with RIPA buffer before use.
11. The assumptions that the conversion of the core-glycosyalated form is complete into the complex-glycosyalted CFTR during the 3-h chase and the complex-glycostylated form has a slow turnover, thus its degradation is negligible during the chase, have been previously verified *(3,20)*. Both assumptions have to be validated when other mutations are examined.
12. Optimization of the homogenization should be performed on nonlabeled cells by monitoring the percentage of Trypan blue-stained nuclei as a function of homogenization time. The cell nuclei with disrupted plasma membrane will stain Trypan blue-positive. Aim for 70–80% nuclear staining, since more vigorous homogenization may lead to the disruption of the chromosomal DNA. This will hamper the separation of nuclei and the isolation of microsomes with differential centrifugation.

Acknowledgments

We thank the Canadian Cystic Fibrosis Foundation, the Medical Research Council of Canada, and the National Institutes of Health, NIDDK, USA for financial support. We also thank Dr. N. Kartner for providing the L12B4 anti-CFTR antibody.

References

1. Riordan, J. R., Rommens, J. M., Kerem, B., Alon, M., Rosmahel, R., Grzelchak, Z., et al. (1989) Identification of the cystic fibrosis gene: cloning and characterization of complementary DNA. *Science* **245,** 1066–1073.
2. Cheng, S. H., Gregory, R. J., Marshall, J., Paul, S., Souza, D. W., White, G. A., et al. (1990) Defective intracellular transport and processing of CFTR is the molecular basis of most cystic fibrosis. *Cell* **63,** 827–834.
3. Lukacs, G. L., Mohamed, A., Kartner, N., Chang, X.-B., Riordan, J. R., and Grinstein, S. (1994) Conformational maturation of CFTR but not its mutant counterpart (DF508) occurs in the endoplasmic reticulum and requires ATP. *EMBO J.* **13,** 6076–6086.
4. Ward, C. L. and Kopito, R. R. (1994) Intracellular turnover of cystic fibrosis transmembrane conductance regulator. *J. Biol. Chem.* **269,** 25,710–25,718.

5. Zielenski, J. (2000) Genotype and phenotype in cystic fibrosis. *Respiration* **67,** 117–133.
6. Zielenski, J. and Tsui, L.-C. (1995) Cystic fibrosis: genotypic and phenotypic variations. *Annu. Rev. Genet.* **29,** 777–807.
7. Kerem, B., Rommens, J. M., Buchanan, J. A., Markiewicz, D., Cox, T. K., Chakravarti, A., et al. (1989) Identification of the cystic fibrosis gene: genetic analysis. *Science* **245,** 1073–1080.
8. Denning, G. M., Anderson, M. P., Amara, J. F., Marshall, J., Smith, A. E., and Welsh, M. J. (1992) Processing of mutant cystic fibrosis transmembrane conductance regulator is temperature sensitive. *Nature* **350,** 761–764.
9. Zhang, F., Kartner, N., and Lukacs, G. L. (1998) Limited proteolysis as a probe for arrested conformational maturation of ΔF508 CFTR. *Nature Struct. Biol.* **5,** 180–183.
10. Ward, C. L., Omura, S., and Kopito, R. R. (1995) Degradation of CFTR by the ubiquitin-proteasome pathway. *Cell* **83,** 121–128.
11. Jensen, T. J., Loo, M. A., Pind, S., Williams, D. B., Goldberg, A. L., and Riordan, J. R. (1995) Multiple proteolytic systems, including the proteasome, contribute to CFTR processing. *Cell* **83,** 129–135.
12. Chang, X. B., Cui, L., Hou, Y. X., Jensen, T. J., Aleksandov, A. A., Mengos, A., and Riordan, J. R. (1999) Removal of multiple arginine-framed trafficking signals overcomes misprocessing of ΔF508 CFTR present in most patients with cystic fibrosis. *Mol. Cell.* **4,** 137–142.
13. Hammond, C. and Helenius, A. (1995) Quality control in the secretory pathway. *Curr. Opin. Cell Biol.* **7,** 523–529.
14. Kartner, N., Augustinas, O., Jensen, T. J., Naismith, A. L., and Riordan, J. R. (1992) Mislocalization of DF508 CFTR in cystic fibrosis sweat gland. *Nature Genet.* **1,** 321–327.
15. Kartner, N. and Riordan, J. R. (1998) Characterization of polyclonal and monoclonal antibodies to cystic fibrosis transmembrane conductance regulator. *Meth. Enzym.* **292,** 629–653.
16. Walker, J., Watson, J., Holmes, C., Edelman, A., and Banting, G. (1995) Production and characterization of monoclonal and polyclonal antibodies to different regions of the CFTR: detection of immunologically related proteins. *J. Cell Sci.* **108,** 2433–2444.
17. Claass, A., Sommer, M., de Jonge, H., Kalin, N., and Tummler, B. (2000) Applicability of diferent antibodies for immunohistochemical localization of CFTR in sweat glands from healthy controls and from patients with cystic fibrosis. *J. Histochem. Cytochem.* **48,** 831–837.
18. Beynon, R. J. and Bond, J. S. (eds.) (1989) *Proteolytic Enzymes, A Practical Approach*, IRL Press, Oxford.
19. Balch, W. E. and Rothman, J. E. (1985) Characterization of protein transport between successive compartments of the Golgi apparatus: asymetric properties of donor and acceptor activities in a cell free system. *Arch. Biochem. Biophys.* **240,** 413–425.
20. Haardt, M., Benharouga, M., Lechardeur, D., Kartner, N., and Lukacs, G. L. (1999) C-terminal truncations destabilize the cystic fibrosis transmembrane conductance regulator without impairing its biogenesis. *J. Biol. Chem.* **274,** 21,873–21,877.

16

Isolation of CFTR

Chaperone Complexes by Co-Immunoprecipitation

Geoffrey C. Meacham and Douglas M. Cyr

1. Introduction

The cystic fibrosis transmembrane conductance regulator (CFTR) is a membrane glycoprotein that contains several large cytosolic subdomains. To progress through the secretory pathway, CFTR must fold and assemble its subdomains into stable conformations that permit exit from the endoplasmic reticulum (ER) *(1)*. ER folding of both CFTR and mutant forms of CFTR (primarily CFTR ΔF508) appears to be an inefficient step in CFTR biogenesis. Consequently, the majority of CFTR and nearly all CFTR ΔF508 is retained in the ER and degraded via the ubiquitin–proteasome pathway *(2,3)*. Molecular chaperones localized to the ER lumen (calnexin) and the cytosol (Hsp70, Hsc70, Hdj-2, Hdj-1, and Hsp90) have been shown to transiently associate with both CFTR and CFTR ΔF508 *(4–7)*. As such, these chaperones may act to survey CFTR structure as part of the ER quality control system or they may serve to facilitate the normal folding of CFTR *(8,9)*. To determine the role of chaperone proteins in CFTR biogenesis, we have developed methods to isolate complexes between CFTR and different classes of molecular chaperones. This chapter describes the methodology utilized to co-immunoprecipitate CFTR with cytosolic chaperones of the Hsp70 and Hsp40 class *(6)*.

This protocol is divided into three parts. The first section focuses on determining experimental conditions to reliably immunodeplete endogenous chaperones from cell extracts. The conditions defined in this portion of the method will be used in later protocols that describe how chaperone:CFTR complexes are isolated. Results from these immunodepletion experiments are also useful for interpreting data regarding the relative abundance of different types of chaperone:CFTR complexes.

From: *Methods in Molecular Medicine, vol. 70: Cystic Fibrosis Methods and Protocols*
Edited by: W. R. Skach © Humana Press Inc., Totowa, NJ

The second section of the method concentrates on optimizing CFTR expression in HEK293 or HeLa cells. We will describe two methods used to express CFTR in these cells: a combination transfection/viral infection system for use in HeLa cells and a straight transfection protocol for use in HEK293 cells. In both of these methods, the goal is to express CFTR to detectable levels, but to avoid high-level expression that may saturate the secretory pathway or translation machinery, or cause aggresome formation *(9,10)*. The advantage of using the transfection/viral infection system is that one can achieve high levels of CFTR expression. The strong CFTR signal from this expression system allows one rapidly to evaluate the results from co-immunoprecipitation experiments where only 5–10% of total CFTR is typically recovered in complexes with chaperones. However, a common problem observed is inefficient processing of CFTR, which appears to be due to high-level expression of membrane proteins encoded by the vaccinia virus. Thus, an alternative to expressing CFTR via the transfection/viral infection system is a one-step transfection protocol using HEK293 cells. CFTR is expressed to significant levels and processed efficiently in HEK293 cells, but total expression is much lower than in the transfection/viral infection system. The low CFTR signal from HEK293 cells is not problematic when isolating CFTR directly by immunoprecipitation, but the signal intensity becomes an issue when results are needed rapidly.

The last section outlines a method for co-immunoprecipitating CFTR in complexes that contain Hsp70 and Hsp40 proteins. This protocol utilizes a combination of the first two methods. Utilization of this protocol will enable investigators to monitor the abundance of complexes between CFTR and members of the Hsp70 and Hsp40 classes of molecular chaperones. This method can also be adapted to examine interactions between CFTR and other chaperone proteins *(4,5,7)*. Included in this protocol is discussion of controls that demonstrate the specificity of chaperone:CFTR complexes isolated. Along these same lines, we include a method to modulate ATP levels in cell extracts that enables one to demonstrate the dynamic nature of chaperone:CFTR complex formation. Finally, we outline a protocol for re-immunoprecipitation of CFTR from chaperone:CFTR complexes that were isolated by co-immunoprecipitation This is an important step in the protocol because it enables one definitively to identify CFTR as a component of chaperone complexes.

2. Materials

2.1. Immunodepletion of Chaperone Proteins from Mammalian Cell Extracts

2.1.1. Preparation of Cell Extracts

1. 70% confluent monolayer of either HeLa or HEK 293 cells (~1×10^6 cells per well of a 6-well tray).

2. Phosphate-buffered saline (PBS), pH 7.4.
3. Lysis buffer A: ice-cold PBS, pH 7.4 containing 1× protease inhibitor cocktail (Complete Tab; Roche 1697498) and 0.1 % Triton X-100.
4. Pansorbin cells (Calbiochem).
5. Detergent compatible (DC) protein assay reagent (Bio-Rad).

2.1.2. Immunoprecipitation and Detection of Chaperone Proteins

1. Chaperone antisera: Hsc 70 (Stressgen Biotechnologies; SPA-815), Hdj-1 (Stressgen Biotechnologies; SPA-840), Hdj-2 (Lab Vision; MS225-PABX). All 1 mg/mL in PBS.
2. Protein G-agarose and lysis buffer A.
3. Sodium dodecyl sulfate-polyacrylamide gel electrophoresis (SDS-PAGE) apparatus, Western blot transfer unit, and nitrocellulose membranes.
4. Reagents for Western blot analysis and detection of proteins by enhanced chemiluminescence (ECL; Amersham-Pharmacia Biotech).

2.2. Optimization of CFTR Expression in Cultured Cells

2.2.1. Transient Expression of CFTR in Mammalian Cells

1. 70% confluent monolayer of HeLa or HEK293 cells (~1 × 10^6 cells per well of a 6-well tray).
2. CFTR expression plasmid driven by a CMV promoter or a T7 and CMV promoter (pCDNA3.1; Invitrogen).
3. Effectene transfection reagent (Qiagen).
4. Growth medium: Dulbecco's modification of Eagle's medium (DMEM) + 10% fetal bovine serum + 1% penicillin/streptomycin solution) or OptiMEM (Life Technologies).
5. Vaccinia virus-expressing T7 RNA polymerase. (vTF-7.3; ATCC).

2.2.2. Metabolic Labeling of Transfected Cells and Preparation of Cell Extracts

1. Methionine-free minimal essential media (MEM; Life Technologies).
2. [^{35}S] Trans-label (1200 Ci/mmol; ICN Radiochemicals).
3. Lysis buffer: ice-cold radio-immunoprecipitation analysis (RIPA) buffer: 150 m*M* NaCl, 50 m*M* HEPES, pH 7.4, 1% NP-40, 0.5% deoxycholate, 0.2% SDS, and 1× protease inhibitor cocktail.
4. Pansorbin cells.

2.2.3. Immunoprecipitation and Detection of CFTR

1. CFTR antisera (anti-CFTR C-terminus; MAB25031; R & D Systems).
2. Protein G-agarose and RIPA buffer.
3. SDS-PAGE apparatus.

2.3. Co-Immunoprecipitation of CFTR with Chaperone Proteins

2.3.1. CFTR Expression

See **Subheading 2.2.1.**

2.3.2. Metabolic Labeling and Co-Immunoprecipitation CFTR

1. Methionine free MEM and [^{35}S] Trans-label.
2. Nondenaturing lysis buffer: ice-cold PBS, pH 7.4 containing 1× protease inhibitor cocktail, 0.1% Triton X-100 with or without 5 mM ATP (pH 7.4), 5 mM MgCl$_2$, 80 mM creatine phosphate, and 0.5 mg/mL creatine phosphokinase.
3. Chaperone antisera and CFTR antisera (*see* **Subheading 2.1.2., item 1** and **Subheading 2.2.3., item 1**).
4. Re-immunoprecipitation buffer: room-temperature PBS, pH 7.4 containing 0.1% SDS, 0.1% Triton X-100, and 0.5% bovine serum albumin.
5. Protein G-agarose.
6. SDS-PAGE apparatus.

3. Methods

3.1. Immunodepletion of Chaperone Proteins from Mammalian Cell Extracts

3.1.1. Generating and Preclearing Cell Extracts from HeLa Cells or HEK293 Cells

1. Split cell stocks, plate in 6-well trays (35 mm/well), and grow in growth medium to around 70% confluency. Choose one cell type, either HEK 293 or HeLa cells, to use throughout the entire method. See the introduction for a discussion of the advantages and disadvantages of each cell type. The amount of sera utilized for immunodepleting chaperones from each cell type may vary, but determining conditions for one cell type is a good starting point
2. Rinse each well two times with 1 mL of room-temperature PBS. All further steps are to be carried out at 4°C. Before making cell extracts, wash Pansorbin cells two times in Lysis Buffer A and resuspend to final concentration of 10% (w/v). Aspirate PBS and add 0.20 mL of ice-cold lysis buffer A to each well of a 6-well tray. Four wells will typically generate enough starting material for optimizing the immunodepletions. Scrape cells from the growth surface and transfer to a 1.5-mL tube containing 50 μL of washed Pansorbin cells. Incubate for 15 min to allow material that adheres nonspecifically to protein A or protein G to bind to the Pansorbin cells. Spin at 20,000g for 5 min.
3. Pool supernatants and set at 4°C. Remove a 25-μL aliquot for later analysis of the chaperone content in the total cell extract. Measure protein concentration of the cell extract with the DC protein assay reagent according to the manufacturer's instructions.

3.1.2. Optimization of Chaperone Immunodepletion from Cell Extracts

1. Add equal amounts of protein from the supernatant under **Subheading 3.1.1., step 3**, to four fresh 1.5-mL tubes. Under our conditions, 50 μL of a precleared cell extract typically contains around 15–20 μg of cell protein. Titrate chaperone antibodies in each tube in a total volume of 15 μL. The midpoint of the antibody titration for Hsc70, Hdj-1, and Hdj-2 should be around 12.5, 1, and 5 μg, respec-

tively. A starting range of antibody concentrations to begin with is 0, 1, 5, and 15 μg of chaperone antibody. After adding the antibody, ensure that the total volumes in each tube are identical.

2. Mix by frequent pipetting or "flicking the tube" for 30–40 min. Add 35 μL of a 70% slurry of protein G-agarose/lysis buffer A and mix for another 30–40 min. It is important to add a minimal volume of concentrated protein G-agarose to prevent further dilution of the sample. This is discussed at the end of the Methods section.

3. Spin samples for 30 s at 3000g to pellet the agarose beads. Withdraw and save supernatants and wash beads once with 600 μL of lysis buffer A. Add SDS sample buffer to a 15-μL aliquot of starting material, depleted, or mock-depleted extracts. Resuspend protein G-pellets in 65 μL SDS sample buffer, heat, and dilute as above. Separate samples on 10% SDS-PAGE gels and transfer to nitrocellulose.

4. Perform Western blot analysis of depleted extracts using the appropriate chaperone antisera. As observed in **Fig. 1**, following detection by enhanced chemiluminescence, we often observe background reactivity of the secondary antibody with the IgG that is precipitated with protein-G agarose. Quantitate the intensity of the chaperone-specific signal using densitometric analysis. Analyze the efficiency of immunodepletions by comparing the signal in total and mock-treated controls to those of experimental conditions.

3.1.3. Analysis of Depletion Efficiency

The efficiency of immunodepletion from extracts varies with the quality and quantity of the chaperone antisera. The sources of antisera suggested above are of high quality and have given reliable results in our hands. Immunodepletion efficiency may also vary from cell type to cell type due to differences in the abundance of chaperone proteins in the cells. Methods to increase the depletion efficiency include using slightly longer times for antibody incubation with more frequent mixing or adding less protein from cell extracts to the immunodepletion (*see* **Note 1**). As seen in **Fig. 1**, the conditions used for the depletion of Hdj-1, Hdj-2, or Hsc70, from HeLa cell extracts are optimized for efficiency and specificity. Once optimal experimental conditions are determined, it is essential to keep the absolute ratio of lysate protein:antibody constant in all subsequent assays.

3.2. Optimization of CFTR Expression in Cultured Cells

3.2.1. Transient Transfection of HEK 293 or HeLa Cells with CFTR Expression Plasmids

1. We will describe two transfection methods for expressing CFTR in selected mammalian cells. HeLa cells are utilized to express large quantities of CFTR and will be transfected using a combination transfection/vaccinia virus infection protocol *(6,12)*. When using this expression system, care must be taken to ensure that CFTR is expressed within the linear range. We have observed that processing of

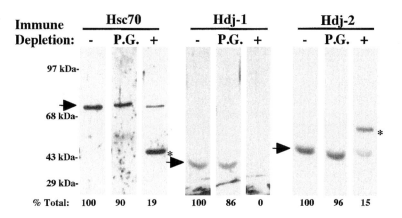

Fig. 1. Western blot analysis demonstrating the efficiency of Hsc70, Hdj-1, and Hdj-2 immunodepletion from HeLa cell extracts. P.G. indicates mock immunodepletion using protein G-agarose alone. The numbers at the bottom of the gels represent quantitation of the immunodepletion efficiency. The arrows indicate the position of the respective chaperone proteins and * indicates background reactivity of either the goat anti-rat HRP with rat anti-Hsc70 or goat anti-mouse HRP with mouse anti-Hdj-2. The migration of molecular mass markers is indicated on the left.

CFTR is relatively efficient in HEK293 cells. Thus, in experiments that monitor CFTR processing, we utilize HEK293 cells. See the introduction for further discussion of the advantages and disadvantages of each cell type.

2. Split cell stocks, plate in 6-well trays (35 mm/well), and grow in growth medium to around 70% confluency. Transfect cells with a high-quality plasmid prep of a CFTR expression vector (*see* **Note 2**). The CFTR vector used for expression in HeLa cells must contain a T7 promoter at the minimum as the recombinant vaccinia virus expresses T7 RNA polymerase. For expression in HEK293 cells, a strong promoter (e.g., CMV) must be used in order to detect CFTR expression. In general, we use the expression vector pCDNA3.1 from Invitrogen because it contains both a T7 promoter and a CMV promoter. When selecting a transfection reagent for delivery of the expression plasmid, consider both the cell toxicity and the transfection efficiency of the reagent. We use the Effectene reagent from Qiagen in this protocol because it typically gives very high transfection efficiencies. However, it can be toxic to either cells line if left on for long periods of time.

3. To optimize CFTR expression, transfect a range of CFTR cDNA from 0 to 2.5 µg. Begin with 0, 0.05, 0.1, 1, and 2.5 µg, using one well for each concentration of DNA (*see* **Note 3**). Before transfection of HeLa cells, aspirate the growth medium from each well and rinse once with 1 mL of OptiMEM. For each DNA concentration, add the transfection lipids to the CFTR cDNA in separate tubes according to the manufacturer's instructions. After incubating the lipid:DNA complexes, dilute each tube of lipid:DNA complexes with 1 mL of room-temperature

OptiMEM, mix for 5 min, and add the transfection solution to the cells. Incubate for 3 h at 37°C/5% CO_2. Transfection lipids are typically toxic to cultured cells, so ensure that each well is washed extensively (3–4 times with 1.5 mL PBS or OptiMEM) following completion of transfection. Allow for a 6–12 h postincubation in OptiMEM. When using HeLa cells in combination with vaccinia virus, proceed to **step 5**.

4. To optimize CFTR expression in HEK293 cells, transfect a range of CFTR cDNA from 0 to 2.5 μg. Begin with 0, 0.1, 0.5, 1, and 2.5 μg, using one well for each concentration of DNA. For each DNA concentration, add the transfection lipids to the CFTR cDNA in separate tubes according to the manufacturer's instructions. After incubating the lipid:DNA complexes, dilute each tube of lipid:DNA complexes with 1 mL of room temperature growth medium , mix for 5 min, and add the transfection solution to the cells. Incubate for 3 h at 37°C/5% CO_2. Wash each well extensively (3–4 times with 1.5 mL PBS or growth medium) following completion of transfection and allow for a 24-h postincubation. Proceed to **Subheading 3.1.4.**

5. Dilute stock solution of vaccinia virus expressing T7 RNA polymerase (Vtf-7-3; ATCC) in OptiMEM such that the cells are infected at a multiplicity of infection (MOI) of one in a volume of 1 mL. Incubate for 8 h at 37° C/5% CO_2. Proceed to **Subheading 3.2.4.**

3.2.2. Metabolic Labeling of Transfected Cells and Generation of Cell Extracts

1. Wash transfected cells once with 1 mL of PBS and incubate in methionine-free MEM for 45 min at 37°C/5% CO_2. Add 100 μCi of [^{35}S] Translabel per well in a total volume of 650 μL methionine-free MEM and incubate for 15 min at 37°C/5% CO_2. Withdraw labeling medium, rinse two times with 2 mL of room-temperature PBS, and put on ice. All further steps are carried out at 4°C unless indicated otherwise.

3.2.3. Immunoprecipitation of Radiolabeled CFTR

1. Before making cell extracts, wash Pansorbin cells two times in RIPA buffer and resuspend to a final concentration of 10% (w/v). Generate cell extracts by adding 0.70 mL of ice-cold RIPA buffer to each well. Scrape cells from each well and pipet cell extracts into fresh 1.5-mL tube. Add 100 μL of washed Pansorbin cells to each tube. Incubate for 15 min to allow material that adheres nonspecifically to protein A or protein G to bind to the Pansorbin cells. Spin at 20,000g for 5 min. Withdraw supernatant and remove a 10-μL aliquot from each experimental condition to monitor labeling efficiency.

2. Add CFTR antisera (2 μg of anti-CFTR C terminus) to 750 μL of lysate and incubate for one h. Add protein A-Sepharose (for rabbit antisera) or protein G-agarose (for mouse or rat antisera) in RIPA buffer and incubate for 45 min.

3. Spin samples for 30 s at 3000g to pellet the agarose beads. Wash three times with 0.75 mL of RIPA buffer and aspirate all of the supernatant from the beads. Add SDS sample buffer to beads, incubate for 10 min at 50°C, analyze on 8% SDS-PAGE gels, and visualize by autoradiography (*see* **Note 4**).

3.2.4. Analysis of Linear CFTR Expression

1. As shown in **Fig. 2A**, CFTR can be detected by immunoprecipitation using relatively small quantities of CFTR cDNA in the transfection/vaccinia virus system

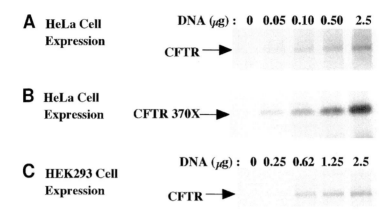

Fig. 2. Expression profile of CFTR or CFTR 370X in cultured cells. (**A**) HeLa cell expression of CFTR using the indicated amounts of CFTR expression plasmid (pCDNA3.1-CFTR) with the transfection/vaccinia virus infection protocol. Following transfection and viral infection, CFTR was immunoprecipitated from radiolabeled cell extracts as outlined under **Subheading 3.2**. (**B**) Expression profile of a CFTR fragment corresponding to amino acids 1–370. CFTR 370X was expressed in HeLa cells using the transfection/viral infection protocol as in A and CFTR 370X from these cells was immunoprecipitated from radiolabeled cell extracts using an antibody generated against the amino terminus of CFTR. (**C**) Expression profile of CFTR in HEK293 cells using the single-step transfection protocol. HEK293 cells were transfected with increasing amounts of pCDNA3.1-CFTR. The cells were metabolically labeled and CFTR was immunoprecipitated from cell extracts as outlined under **Subheading 3.2**.

with HeLa cells. Truncations of CFTR can also be expressed within a linear range using the transfection/vaccinia virus system (**Fig. 2B**). As previously mentioned, the transfection/vaccinia virus infection can potentially generate high levels of CFTR, so it is important to ensure that you are in the linear range of CFTR expression. Note the differences in the range of linear CFTR expression between HeLa and HEK293 cells. CFTR expression in HEK293 cells typically gives a much weaker signal (**Fig. 2C**), but the CFTR maturation is more efficient (data not shown). Generally, HEK293 cells present a good nonviral alternative that routinely gives subsaturating CFTR expression levels.

3.3. Co-Immunoprecipitation of CFTR with Chaperone Proteins

3.3.1. Transient Transfection of Mammalian Cells with CFTR Expression Plasmids

See **Subheading 3.2.1.**

3.3.2. Metabolic Labeling of Cells and Generating Cell Extracts

See **Subheading 3.2.2.**

3.3.3. Immunoprecipitation of CFTR: Chaperone Complexes

1. Determine the protein concentration of Pansorbin-treated cell extracts Add the predetermined amount of antisera that efficiently immunodepletes the chaperone protein from cell extracts. Carry out the co-immunoprecipitation as outlined under **Subheading 3.1.2.** Analyze co-immunoprecipitations on 8% SDS PAGE gels and visualize by autoradiography.

3.3.4. Controls and Conditions for Co-Immunoprecipitations

1. It is important to illustrate the specificity and the dynamic nature of the interactions between chaperones and CFTR. As Hsc70:substrate interactions are influenced by ATP, modifying the ATP levels in the lysis buffer demonstrates the dynamic nature of chaperone:CFTR interactions. Some suggestions include the addition of (a) 5 mM Mg-ATP, or (b) 5 mM Mg-ATP plus an ATP-regenerating system, or (c) 5 mM EDTA to lysis buffer A. The addition of 500 mM NaCl or 0.1% SDS to lysis buffer A will also influence chaperone:CFTR interactions (*see* **Note 5**).
2. To determine the relative abundance of chaperone:CFTR complexes, include a direct immunoprecipitation of CFTR under denaturing conditions in the experimental design. For this control, add SDS (0.1% final concentration) to Lysis Buffer A following the preclearing step and immunoprecipitate as indicated above. This serves as a reference for the total amount of CFTR that can be immunoprecipitated. To monitor background co-precipitation of CFTR, use nonimmune or pre-immune sera and immunoprecipitate as indicated above.

3.3.5. Identification of CFTR in Chaperone Complexes by Re-Immunoprecipitation

1. As seen in **Fig. 3**, a number of radiolabeled proteins co-precipitate with Hsc70, Hdj-1, and Hdj-2. Re-immunoprecipitation of CFTR allows one to verify the identity of CFTR isolated from these chaperone complexes. There are two methods for obtaining the starting material for the CFTR re-immunoprecipitation following the initial co-immunoprecipitation. The first is to perform the co-immunoprecipitations in duplicate: save one sample on ice (with a minimal volume of buffer) and use the other sample for the re-immunoprecipitation. The second method is to solubilize the immune complexes in SDS sample buffer and use half for the re-immunoprecipitation and save the other half on ice.
2. Add SDS sample buffer to the beads from the co-immunoprecipitation and heat for 10 min at 50°C (*see* **Notes 4** and **6**). Spin samples for 30 s at 3000g to pellet the agarose beads and withdraw the supernatant with a Hamilton syringe. Add equal amounts of the material to 0.75 mL of room-temperature re-immunoprecipitation buffer and mix (*see* **Note 7**). Add CFTR antisera and immunoprecipitate as outlined under **Subheading 3.2.3.**

3.3.6. Analysis and Quantitation of the Abundance of Chaperone: CFTR Complexes

1. For SDS PAGE analysis, load 10% of the material isolated from the direct CFTR IP (*see* **Subheading 3.2.3., step 4**). This control is important, as it is a reference

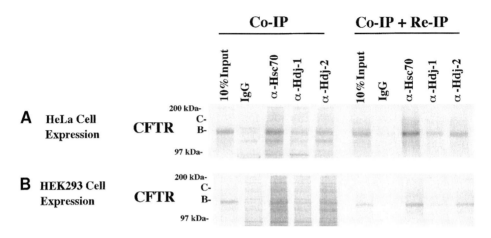

Fig. 3. Co-immunoprecipitation of immature CFTR with cytosolic Hsc70, Hdj-1, and Hdj-2. (**A**) CFTR was expressed in HeLa cells using 0.25 µg of pCDNA3.1-CFTR with the transfection/vaccinia virus protocol. Transfected cells were metabolically labeled and cell extracts were made under nondenaturing conditions as outlined under **Subheading 3.3.3.** Immune complexes between CFTR and the indicated chaperones were then harvested. A portion of the precipitated material was either saved on ice (co-IP) or subject to re-immunoprecipitation (re-IP) using CFTR specific antisera as outlined under **Subheading 3.3.5.** IgG indicates the background CFTR obtained using nonimmune mouse IgG in the co-precipitation experiments. 10% input represents 10% of the amount of CFTR that can be directly isolated by immunoprecipitation under denaturing conditions. (**B**) Co-immunoprecipitation of CFTR with Hsc70, Hdj-1, and Hdj-2. CFTR was expressed in HEK293 cells using 1 µg of pCDNA3.1-CFTR. Transfected HEK293 cells were radiolabeled and co-IPs or co-IPs plus re-IPs were carried out as detailed in A. The migration of molecular mass markers is indicated on the left. "B" denotes immature forms of CFTR and "C" denotes mature forms of CFTR.

point that indicates the abundance of chaperone:CFTR complexes. Because chaperone complexes tend to dissociate following cell lysis, a signal that corresponds to 5% or more of control is considered significant (*see* **Note 1**). As shown in **Fig. 3A**, CFTR, expressed in HeLa cells, is a substrate for Hsc70, Hdj-1, and Hdj-2. Note that there are only a small number of proteins synthesized using the vaccinia virus expression system. Our experience is that the proteins encoded by the expression plasmid and the vaccinia virus are the most prominent radiolabeled proteins. In the HEK293 expression system, however, a broad smear of proteins co-precipitate with the chaperone proteins (**Fig. 3B**). Thus, it is critical to express CFTR off a strong promoter when using this system, because the CFTR signal from the chaperone co-immunoprecipitations is masked by other radiolabeled proteins. The re-immunoprecipitation shown in the right panels is necessary to clean up the signal generated in these assays and, in this case, identifies the protein of interest as CFTR.

4. Notes

1. When initially optimizing the immunodepletions of chaperone proteins, one should consider the time required to carry out the complete method. Due to a dilution of the cellular environment, chaperone complexes from cell extracts are unstable and favor dissociation. Therefore, it is important to carry out chaperone co-immunoprecipitations as rapidly as possible to limit the dissociation of chaperone:CFTR complexes.
2. We recommend using Qiagen reagents to obtain the highest-quality CFTR expression plasmids. Because CFTR expression varies among different plasmid preps, it is helpful to purify a large quantity of DNA and use the same material for each experiment.
3. Normalize the total DNA used in each transfection with empty plasmid DNA.
4. Heat in sample buffer, before loading CFTR immunoprecipitates or co-immuno-precipitates on the gel. To prevent aggregation of CFTR, it is critical that samples containing CFTR are not heated above 60°C.
5. The method allows for the rapid isolation of preexisting CFTR:chaperone complexes formed within cells. However, CFTR:chaperone complexes could conceivably form as part of a postlysis event. One can demonstrate the specificity of chaperone complexes with CFTR by modulating ATP levels and salt concentration. Another method of demonstrating specificity is to differentiate between the forms of CFTR that are substrates for molecular chaperones. Immature (band B) and mature (band C) CFTR have different conformations inside the cell and Hsc70, Hdj-1, and Hdj-2 preferentially bind immature CFTR *(6,13)*. To examine the specificity of chaperone complexes, follow the metabolic labeling of transfected cells with a 3-h chase period to accumulate mature forms of CFTR. Then perform the co-immunoprecipitation as outlined using immature and mature CFTR as the starting material.
6. When solubilizing the immune complexes, add DTT to the SDS sample buffer to a final concentration of 20 mM. Diluting 15 μL of this material into 0.75 mL re-immunoprecipitation buffer corresponds to a final DTT concentration of 0.4 mM.
7. The hydrophobic nature of CFTR makes it is prone to aggregation following denaturation in SDS sample buffer. We have found that when verifying the identity of CFTR by re-immunoprecipitation, it is critical to include BSA in the re-immunoprecipitation buffer to maximize the recovery of CFTR.

References

1. Lukacs, G. L., Mohamed, A., Kartner, N., Chang, X. B., Riordan, J. R., and Grinstein, S. (1994) Conformational maturation of CFTR but not its mutant counterpart (DF508) occurs in the endoplasmic reticulum and requires ATP. *EMBO J.* **13,** 6076–6086.
2. Jensen, T. J., Loo, M. A., Pind, S., Williams, D. B., Goldberg, A. L., and Riordan, J. R. (1995) Multiple proteolytic systems, including the proteasome, contribute to CFTR processing. *Cell* **83,** 129–135.
3. Ward, C. L., Omura, S., and Kopito, R. R. (1995) Degradation of CFTR by the ubiquitin-proteasome pathway. *Cell* **83,** 121–127.

4. Pind, S., Riordan, J. R., and Williams, D. B. (1994) Participation of the endoplasmic reticulum chaperone calnexin (p88, IP90) in the biogenesis of the cystic fibrosis transmembrane conductance regulator. *J. Biol. Chem.* **269,** 12,784–12,788.

5. Yang, Y., Janich, S., Cohn, J. A., and Wilson, J. M. (1993) The common variant of cystic fibrosis transmembrane conductance regulator is recognized by hsp70 and degraded in a pre-Golgi nonlysosomal compartment. *Proc. Natl Acad. Sci. USA* **90,** 9480–9484.

6. Meacham, G. C., Lu, Z., King, S., Sorscher, E., Tousson, A., and Cyr, D. M. (1999) The Hdj-2/Hsc70 chaperone pair facilitates early steps in CFTR biogenesis. *EMBO J.* **18,** 1492–1505.

7. Loo, M. A., Jensen, T. J., Cui, L., Hou, Y., Chang, X.-B., and Riordan, J. R. (1998) Perturbation of Hsp90 interaction with nascent CFTR prevents its maturation and accelerates its degradation by the proteasome *EMBO J.* **17,** 6879–6887.

8. Strickland, E., Qu, B. H., Millen, L., and Thomas, P. J. (1997) The molecular chaperone Hsc70 assists the in vitro folding of the N-terminal nucleotide-binding domain of the cystic fibrosis transmembrane conductance regulator. *J. Biol. Chem.* **272,** 25,421–25,424.

9. Qu, B. H., Strickland, E., and Thomas, P. J. (1997) Cystic fibrosis: a disease of altered protein folding. *J. Bioenerg. Biomembr.* **29,** 483–490.

10. Johnston, J. A., Ward, C. L., and Kopito, R. R. (1998) Aggresomes: a cellular response to misfolded proteins. *J. Cell. Biol.* **143,** 1883–1898.

11. Garcia-Mata, R., Bebok, Z., Sorscher, E. J., and Sztul, E. S. (1999) Characterization and dynamics of aggresome formation by a cytosolic GFP-chimera. *J. Cell. Biol.* **146,** 1239–1254.

12. Fuerst, T. R., Niles, E. G., Studier, F. W., and Moss, B. (1986) Eukaryotic transient-expression system based on recombinant vaccinia virus that synthesizes bacteriophage T7 RNA polymerase. *Proc. Natl Acad. Sci. USA* **83,** 8122–8126.

13. Zhang, F., Kartner, N., and Lukacs, G. L. (1998) Limited proteolysis as a probe for arrested conformational maturation of DF508 CFTR. *Nature Struct. Biol.* **5,** 180–183.

17

CFTR Expression and ER-Associated Degradation in Yeast

Yimao Zhang, Susan Michaelis, and Jeffrey L. Brodsky

1. Introduction

The most common cause of cystic fibrosis is the deletion of a phenylalanine at position 508 (ΔF508) of the cystic fibrosis transmembrane conductance regulator (CFTR). Although the majority of wild-type CFTR is degraded in the endoplasmic reticulum (ER), suggesting that its folding efficiency is low, almost all of the ΔF508 variant is destroyed *(1–4)*. The process in which the ER quality control system ensures that misfolded or aberrant proteins, such as ΔF508 CFTR, are proteolyzed and thus prevented from entering the secretory pathway has been termed ER associated degradation, or ERAD *(5)*. It remains unclear how CFTR, or other ERAD substrates, are first selected and then targeted for destruction, but a group of factors known as molecular chaperones may play a pivotal role in this process, as they associate with CFTR in the ER and are released upon protein maturation or degradation *(6–8)*. In accordance with this hypothesis, molecular chaperones are known to aid in protein targeting to proteosome-like complexes in bacteria *(9)*.

To better define the pathway of CFTR biogenesis, Teem et al. *(10)* expressed CFTR/Ste6p fusion proteins in the budding yeast, *Saccharomyces cerevisiae*, an organism containing secretory and ERAD pathways similar to those in mammalian cells. Ste6p, the **a**-factor pheromone transporter, is homologous to CFTR and required for mating. A Ste6p-CFTR chimera was constructed in which the C-terminal portion of the first nucleotide-binding domain (NBD1) of Ste6p was replaced by the corresponding portion of CFTR. This Ste6p-CFTR chimera supported mating in yeast lacking *STE6*, but lost its ability to do so when the phenylalanine at position 508 was deleted. Using the Ste6p-ΔF508 CFTR chimera, two suppressor mutations were isolated that restored mating.

From: *Methods in Molecular Medicine, vol. 70: Cystic Fibrosis Methods and Protocols*
Edited by: W. R. Skach © Humana Press Inc., Totowa, NJ

When either of these mutations was introduced into ΔF508 CFTR and the protein was expressed in mammalian cells, the defects associated with ΔF508 CFTR were largely corrected. However, the Ste6p-ΔF508 CFTR chimera in yeast was later found to escape ER degradation *(11)*, suggesting that expression of full-length CFTR in yeast may prove better than the Ste6p-CFTR chimeras for analyzing the biogenesis of CFTR in this genetically tractable organism.

To facilitate biochemical studies of CFTR, Huang et al. *(12,13)* expressed wild-type CFTR in yeast using the promoter for the yeast plasma membrane H⁺-ATPase. Fractions enriched for CFTR were obtained which exhibited regulated chloride channel activity when reconstituted into planar lipid bilayers. By sucrose gradient centrifugation, CFTR resided in light microsomal fractions distinct from those containing plasma membrane protein. Factors required for the maturation or degradation of CFTR in this system were not examined.

To explicitly uncover the mechanism by which CFTR is targeted for degradation, we created expression plasmids in which the wild type and ΔF508 variant of CFTR can be produced in yeast. To facilitate the detection of CFTR, a triple HA (hemaglutinin) epitope was introduced at the C terminus. We have examined the degradation of CFTR in wild-type yeast strains and in those mutated for specific genes and have found that CFTR is retained in the yeast ER and, like most ERAD substrates, is degraded by the ubiquitin–proteasome pathway *(14)*. We have also determined that the cytosolic Hsc70 molecular chaperone in yeast, Ssa1p, is required to degrade CFTR *(14)*. Identical results were obtained when the fate of the ΔF508 variant of CFTR was examined. In principle, this system can be used to screen for other factors required for CFTR quality control, for small-molecule modulators of CFTR biogenesis, and given the complete sequencing of the yeast genome, for uncovering CFTR-interacting factors using large-scale immunoprecipitation and proteomics.

2. Materials
2.1. Yeast Growth and Transformation
2.1.1. Strains

The CFTR expression plasmid (see below) contains the *URA3* selectable marker. Therefore, any yeast strain that is auxotrophic for *URA3* (denoted *ura3*) can be used.

2.1.2. Media and Growth Conditions

1. YEPD: 2% Bacto-peptone, 1% yeast extract, and 2% dextrose.
2. Synthetic complete medium lacking uracil and supplemented with glucose to a final concentration of 2% (SC-ura/glucose: 0.67% Bacto-yeast nitrogen base lacking amino acids, and 0.2% of a drop-out mix that includes adenine, alanine, arginine, aspartic acid, cysteine, glutamine, glutamic acid, glycine, histidine, inositol,

isoleucine, leucine, lysine, methionine, *p*-aminobenzoic acid, phenylalanine, proline, serine, threonine, tryptophan, tyrosine, and valine).

Solid media are prepared by including Bacto-agar to a final concentration of 2%, and both solid and liquid media may be stored at 4°C for 1–2 mo after sterilization. Further details on the preparation and sterilization of yeast media can be found in **ref. 15**. For the protocol described in this chapter, cells were grown at room temperature (~26°C) in an incubator equipped with a rotating platform (set at 300 rpm). Sterile technique is required when handling yeast.

2.1.3. Yeast Transformation

1. TEL: 10 m*M* Tris-HCl, pH 7.5,1 m*M* ethylenediaminetetraacetic acid (EDTA), 0.1 *M* lithium acetate.
2. 40% polyethylene glycol MW 3350 (Sigma) in TEL.
3. High-molecular weight (salmon testes) DNA (Sigma), sheared by vigorous, repeated pipeting as described in **ref. 15**.

2.1.4. CFTR Expression Vectors

The two plasmids used in these studies, pSM1077 (*2μ URA3 PPGK-CFTR*) and pSM1152 (*2μ URA3 PPGK-CFTR-HA*), contain untagged and HA-epitope-tagged CFTR, respectively, expressed from the strong constitutive 3-phosphoglycerate kinase promoter (P_{PGK}). Their construction is described below and shown in **Fig. 1**. It is noteworthy that we and others have encountered difficulties subcloning CFTR using standard techniques requiring bacterial transformation, possibly because a low level of CFTR expression initiating from ligation products could be toxic to bacteria. We also observe that a high percentage of subclones derived from such standard ligation procedures contain substantial deletions or rearrangements in the CFTR gene; however, once a CFTR plasmid is constructed, it can be faithfully propagated in bacteria, suggesting that toxicity is a function of unligated CFTR-containing DNA.

To circumvent these difficulties, we have employed homologous recombination (HR) cloning carried out directly in yeast. The details of HR cloning are described elsewhere *(16)*, and represent an extension of the recombination-mediated healing of linearized plasmids in yeast *(17)*. HR cloning is quite powerful because of its technical simplicity and general reliability.

Plasmid pSM1077 *(2μ URA3 PPGK-CFTR)* was generated in two steps. The first step involved generating a CFTR "acceptor vector" (pSM1053) for HR. This required cloning the ends of the CFTR coding sequence into the expression plasmid pSM703 by conventional procedures. Plasmid pSM703 is composed of a standard multicopy-number yeast vector pRS426 *(18)* containing the 1.5 kb *PGK* promoter fragment *(19)* inserted into the *Hin*dIII-*Eco*RI sites of the polylinker. To construct pSM1053, 240-bp fragments containing the 5' and 3' coding ends of *CFTR*, bounded by engineered restriction sites, were generated by PCR. The 5' (N-terminal) PCR product of *CFTR* contains an

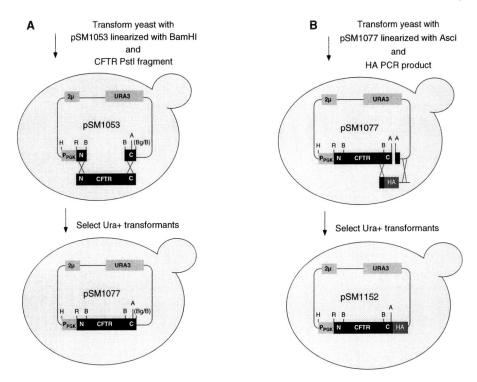

Fig. 1. Cloning by homologous recombination (HR) in yeast to generate CFTR plasmids. The approximate sites of recombination are indicated by X's. The methods used to generate pSM1077 and pSM1152 are described in the text. The restriction sites shown are A, *Asc*I; B, *Bam*HI, Bg, *Bgl*II; H, *Hin*dIII; R, *Eco*RI. Plasmids are not drawn to scale.

*Eco*RI site at the 5' end and a *Bam*HI site at the 3' end. The 3' (C-terminal) PCR product of *CFTR* contains a *Bam*HI site at the 5' end and a *Bgl*II site at the 3' end. The two PCR products were cut with *Eco*RI, *Bam*HI, and *Bgl*II, ligated together at the *Bam*HI site, and then subsequently ligated into the *Eco*RI and *Bam*HI sites of pSM703 (the resultant *Bam*HI-*Bgl*II site cannot be cleaved). The sole *Bam*H1 site in pSM1053 lies between the 5'and 3' ends of CFTR, providing a site to linearize this acceptor plasmid. The *CFTR* fragments in pSM1053 were sequenced to verify the correct orientation. The second step involved cloning the full-length *CFTR* into pSM1053 by HR (**Fig. 1A**). Specifically, the 4.7-kb *Pst*I restriction fragment containing *CFTR* from pBQ4.7 (generously supplied by J. Rommens and G. Cutting, Johns Hopkins University, Baltimore, MD) was co-transformed with *Bam*HI-linearized pSM1053 into the yeast strain SM1058 and Ura+ transformants were selected. Plasmids retrieved from yeast were amplified in bacteria, their restriction maps were verified, and one of these plasmids was designated pSM1077 (12,184 bp). The DNA sequence of the entire CFTR gene was verified by DNA sequence analysis.

To epitope tag CFTR, the triply iterated HA epitope (3x HA) was introduced into pSM1077 via HR to yield pSM1152 (**Fig. 1B**). A PCR product containing the 111 bp triple HA epitope (with a *Bam*H1 site in the middle HA repeat), followed by ~1200 bp from the 3' downstream region of the *STE6* gene was generated using pSM1052 as a template. This PCR product was cotransformed with *Asc*I-linearized pSM1077. Ura$^+$ transformants were selected, plasmids were retrieved, retransformed into *Escherichia coli*, analyzed by restriction mapping, and the region containing the HA epitope was confirmed by sequencing. The resultant plasmid, pSM1152 (13,385 bp), contains *CFTR* expressed from the *PGK* promoter with the 3x-HA epitope tag at its C terminus.

As a negative control, yeast containing the 2μ, *URA3*-marked plasmid pRS426 *(18)* lacking insert can be transformed into the desired strain when CFTR degradation is assessed.

2.2. CFTR Degradation Assay By Immunoblot Analysis

2.2.1. Solutions

1. 2 *N* NaOH/1.12 *M* β-mercaptoethanol, freshly prepared before use. Concentrated solutions of β-mercaptoethanol should be dispensed in a fume hood.
2. 50% trichloroacetic acid (TCA). TCA is extremely toxic and will cause serious burns upon contact with exposed skin. Affected areas should be rinsed thoroughly with water.
3. TCA sample buffer: 80 m*M* Tris-HCl, pH 8.0, 8 m*M* EDTA, 120 m*M* dithiothreitol (DTT), 3.5% sodium dodecyl sulfate (SDS), 0.29% glycerol, 0.08% Tris base, 0.01% Bromophenol blue.
4. Cycloheximide (Sigma) prepared in water at a final concentration of 10 mg/mL. Store at –20°C in small aliquots. Cycloheximide is poisonous if ingested.
5. SDS-polyacrylamide gels, containing 7 or 10% polyacrylamide (30/0.8 acrylamide/bis-acrylamide). Unpolymerized acrylamide is a neurotoxin.

2.2.2. Antibodies

2.2.2.1 PRIMARY ANTIBODIES

1. Monoclonal anti-HA antibody: Boehringer Mannheim, 12CA5 clone (0.4 mg/mL).
2. Monoclonal anti-C (CFTR) antibody: Genzyme (*see* **Note 1**).
3. Polyclonal anti-Sec61p antibody *(20)* (*see* **Note 2**).

2.2.2.2. SECONDARY ANTIBODIES

1. Sheep anti-mouse IgG horseradish peroxidase-conjugated antibody (Amersham) to detect the anti-HA and anti-C antibodies.
2. Donkey anti-rabbit horseradish peroxidase-conjugated antibody (Amersham) to detect the anti-Sec61p antibody.

2.2.2.3. SIGNAL DETECTION REAGENTS AND SOFTWARE

1. ^{125}I-Protein A (Amersham). [125]I is a strong gamma emitter and established radiation safety protocols for this isotope should be followed.
2. Fuji PhosphorImager and MacBas software (Koshin Graphic Systems) (*see* **Note 3**).

2.2.3. Solutions for Immunoblot analysis

1. Blotto: 50 mM Tris-HCl, pH 7.4, 150 mM NaCl, 2% nonfat dried milk, 0.1% Tween-20, 5 mM NaN$_3$. NaN$_3$ is a metabolic poison.
2. TBS-T: 50 mM Tris-HCl, pH 7.4, 150 mM NaCl, 0.2% Tween-20.

3. Methods
3.1. Yeast Growth and Transformation

The desired strain lacking the CFTR expression vector is grown on solid YEPD. From a single colony, a small (~2 mL) overnight yeast culture in YEPD is obtained which is then grown for another 2–4 h after the addition of 3 mL of fresh YEPD. The cells are harvested by centrifugation in a clinical centrifuge for 5 min at ~1800g, resuspended in an equal volume of water, recentrifuged, and then resuspended in TEL and centrifuged once again. The cells are finally resuspended in 200 μL TEL. For 100 μL of cells, 50 μg sheared salmon testes DNA, 0.2–0.5 μg plasmid DNA, and 0.7 mL 40% polyethylene glycol 3350/TEL are added. After being incubated at 30°C for 30 min, the cells are placed in a 42°C temperature-controlled heat block for 15 min. The cells are again harvested, resuspended in water, and plated on SC-ura/glucose. Single-colony transformants arise after 3–4 d and should be replated onto solid SC-ura/glucose medium (*see* **Note 4**).

3.2. CFTR Degradation Assay by Immunoblot Analysis

1. A portion of a single colony of the regrown cells is introduced into 5 mL of SC-ura/glucose medium and grown overnight. The next morning, an aliquot of the cells is inoculated into a larger culture (25–100 mL), which is then grown to logarithmic phase (*see* **Note 5**). For the degradation assay, we use CFTR expressing cells that have reached an optical density measured at 600 nm (OD$_{600}$) of ~0.50.
2. Cycloheximide is added to a final concentration of 50 mg/mL to block further protein synthesis.
3. A total of 2.5 OD$_{600}$ of cells is immediately harvested by centrifugation at ~1800g in a clinical centrifuge for 4 min. (For example, if the culture is at OD$_{600}$ = 0.5, use 5 mL of cells.) To establish a time-course of CFTR degradation, the same volume of cells is removed from the culture 0, 20, 40, 60, and 90 min after the addition of cycloheximide.
4. The pelleted cells are resuspended in 5 mL of cold water, recentrifuged, resuspended in 1 mL of cold water, and an aliquot of 150 μL of freshly prepared 2 N NaOH/1.12 M β-mercaptoethanol is added. After vigorous agitation on a Vortex mixer, the cells are left on ice for 15 min.
5. An aliquot of 150 μL of 50% TCA is added, the solution is mixed well, and the cells are left on ice for an additional 20 min.
6. Total protein is precipitated by centrifugation at 16,060g (~13,500 rpm in a microfuge) for 5 min at 4°C, and the supernatant is aspirated. The sample is briefly re-spun and the remaining supernatant is carefully removed with a gel-loading (drawn-out) pipet tip.

7. To resuspend the pellet for SDS-PAGE, 60 µL of TCA sample buffer is added and then a heat-sealed Pasteur pipet is used to grind the pellet. This takes some time and care should be exercised to ensure that the pellet is resuspended as well as possible. If the solution is yellow (acidic), ~2 µL of 1 *M* Tris (pH 8.0) may be added.

8. The cell extracts are incubated at 37°C for 30 min in a temperature-controlled heat block (*see* **Note 6**), before 2–10 µL of cell extract is resolved by 7 or 10% SDS-PAGE.

9. Total proteins are transferred to nitrocellulose membranes using a commercially available transfer apparatus and the membranes are preincubated in Blotto for 20 min with gentle shaking before the antisera are added. We use 1/200 and 1/3000 dilutions of the anti-C and anti-HA antibodies, respectively, incubated with gentle shaking overnight in TBS-T at 4°C. The next morning, the blot is washed three times for 10 min each with TBS-T at room temperature.

10. To decorate the primary antibodies, ~1 µCi of ^{125}I-Protein A in 10 mL of TBS-T is incubated with the blot with gentle shaking for 2–3 h at room temperature, after which the blots are again washed three times for 10 min in TBS-T before being wrapped in plastic and exposed to a phosphorimage screen overnight. The washes will contain a significant amount of ^{125}I, and proper handling and disposal of the isotope are essential.

11. We quantify the signal corresponding to CFTR (relative MW ~140,000) using the MacBas software supplied with our phosphorimager, but any analogous program should suffice. A region of the blot lacking signal is quantified and subtracted from the CFTR-specific signal from each time point. If the anti-Sec61p signal is constant, the results from the CFTR quantitation can be plotted. An example of a phosphorimager scan and corresponding plot demonstrating CFTR degradation in yeast is shown in **Fig. 2**. In this experiment, CFTR degradation is shown to be independent of vacuolar protease activity.

4. Notes

1. We have found that the commercially available anti-C antibody is unstable when stored for long periods at either 4°C or frozen in liquid nitrogen and stored at –70°C. Thus, we examine untagged CFTR only to confirm results obtained with the HA-tagged form of CFTR. In contrast, the anti-HA antibody is quite stable when aliquots are immediately frozen in liquid nitrogen and stored at –70°C, and then used within a few weeks after being thawed and retained at 4°C.

2. The amount of Sec61p, a component of the ER translocation pore, is measured to control for sample loading. The crude anti-serum is used at a 1/5000 dilution. However, antibodies against any ER-resident protein will suffice.

3. Although enhanced chemiluminescence (ECL) can be used to detect CFTR containing or lacking the HA epitope using the appropriate secondary antibody, the quantitation of results by ECL is irreproducible and not quantitative when compared to phosphorimage analysis of bound ^{125}I-Protein A. The linear range of signal detection by phosphorimage analysis far exceeds that when ECL and exposure of photographic films is used.

4. Once yeast transformants are regrown onto new SC-ura/glucose plates, degradation assays using these cells must be commenced within 1 wk. After this time, we

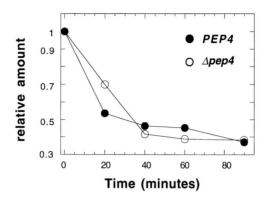

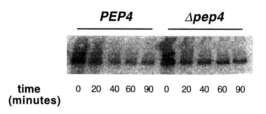

Fig. 2. The degradation of CFTR in wild-type yeast and in cells lacking the major vacuolar protease, Pep4p, is identical. Shown are the standardized results and the original immunoblot of CFTR levels in yeast measured over a 90-min cycloheximide chase assay.

have found that there may be variable expression of CFTR, especially in several mutant yeast strains we have examined.

5. To obtain cells at mid-log phase and have enough time to continue the experiments on the same day, we usually dilute the yeast overnight culture to $OD_{600} < {\sim}0.2$ with fresh medium early in the morning. This allows for at least one cell doubling to occur before the degradation of CFTR is assayed.

6. Heating CFTR-containing samples above 37°C causes a significant amount of the protein to aggregate.

References

1. Cheng, S. H., Gregory, R. J., Marshall, J., Paul, S., Souza, D. W., White, G. A., O'Riordan, C. R., and Smith, A. E. (1990) Defective intracellular transport and processing of CFTR is the molecular basis of most cystic fibrosis. *Cell* **63,** 827–834.
2. Lukacs, G. L., Mohamed, A., Kartner, N., Chang, X . B., Riordan, J. R., and Grinstein, S. (1994) Conformational maturation of CFTR but not its mutant counterpart (ΔF508) occurs in the endoplasmic reticulum and requires ATP. *EMBO J.* **13,** 6076–6086.
3. Jensen, T. J., Loo, M. A., Pind, S., Williams, D. B., Goldberg, A. L., and Riordan, J. R. (1995) Multiple proteolytic systems, including the proteasome, contribute to CFTR processing. *Cell* **83,** 129–135.

4. Ward, C. L., Omura, S., and Kopito, R. R. (1995) Degradation of CFTR by the ubiquitin-proteasome pathway. *Cell* **83,** 121–127.

5. Brodsky, J. L. and McCracken, A. A. (1999) ER protein quality control and proteasome-mediated protein degradation. *Semin. Cell Develop. Biol.* **10,** 507–513.

6. Yang, Y., Janich, S., Cohn, J. A., and Wilson, J. M. (1993) The common variant of cystic fibrosis transmembrane conductance regulator is recognized by hsp70 and degraded in a pre-Golgi nonlysosomal compartment. *Proc. Natl. Acad. Sci. USA* **90,** 9480–9484.

7. Pind, S., Riordan, J. R., and Williams, D. B. (1994) Participation of the endoplasmic reticulum chaperone calnexin (p88, IP90) in the biogenesis of the cystic fibrosis transmembrane conductance regulator. *J. Biol. Chem.* **269,** 12,784–12,788.

8. Loo, M. A., Jensen, T. J., Cui, L., Hou, Y., Chang, X., and Riordan, J. R. (1998) Perturbation of Hsp90 interaction with nascent CFTR prevents its maturation and accelerates its degradation by the proteasome. *EMBO J.* **17,** 6879–6887.

9. Wickner, S., Maurizi, M. R., and Gottesman, S. (1999) Posttranslational quality control: folding, refolding, and degradating proteins. *Science* **286,** 1888–1893.

10. Teem, J. L., Berger, H. A., Ostedgaard, L. S., Rich, D. P., Tsui, L.-C., and Welsh, M. J. (1993) Identification of revertants for the cystic fibrosis ΔF508 mutation using Ste6-CFTR chimeras in yeast. *Cell* **73,** 335–346.

11. Paddon, C., Loayza, D., Vangelista, L., Solarl, R., and Michaelis, S. (1996) Analysis of the localization of Ste6/CFTR chimeras in a *Saccharomyces cerevisiae* model for the cystic fibrosis defect CFTRΔF508. *Mol. Microbiol.* **19,** 1007–1017.

12. Huang, P., Stroffekova, K, Cuppoletti, J., Mahanty, S. K., and Scarborough G. A. (1996) Functional expression of the cystic fibrosis transmembrane conductance regulator in yeast. *Biochim. Biophys. Acta* **1281,** 80–90.

13. Huang, P., Liu, Q., and Scarborough, G. A. (1998) Lysophosphatidylglycerol: a novel effective detergent for solubilizing and purifying the cystic fibrosis transmembrane conductance regulator. *Anal. Biochem.* **259,** 89–97.

14. Zhang, Y., G. Nijbroek, M. L. Sullivan, A. A. McCracken, S. C. Watkins, S. Michaelis, and Brodsky, J. L. Distinct chaperone requirements for soluble and membrane ERAD substrates: Hsp70 facilitates the degradation of CFTR in yeast. *Mol. Biol. Cell* **12,** 1303–1314.

15. Adams, A., Gottschling, D. E., Kaiser, C., and Stearns, T. (1997) *Methods in Yeast Genetics.* Cold Spring Harbor Laboratory Press, Cold Spring Harbor, NY.

16. Oldenburg, K. R., Vo, K. T., Michaelis, S., and Paddon, C. (1997) Recombination-mediated PCR-directed plasmid construction *in vivo* in yeast. *Nucleic Acids Res.* **25,** 451,452.

17. Ma, H., Kunes, S., Schatz, P. J., Botstein, D. (1987) Plasmid construction by homologous recombination in yeast. *Gene* **58,** 201–216.

18. Christianson, T. W., Sikorski, R. S., Dante, M., Shero, J. H., and Hieter, P. (1992) Multifunctional yeast high-copy-number shuttle vectors. *Gene* **110,** 119–122.

19. Hitzeman, R. A., Chen, C. Y., Hagie, F. E., Patzer, E. J., Liu, C. C., Estell, D. A., et al. (1983) Expression of hepatitis B virus surface antigen in yeast. *Nucleic Acids Res.* **11,** 2745–2763.

20. Stirling, C. J., Rothblatt, J., Hosobuchi, M., Deshaies, R., and Schekman, R. (1992) Protein translocation mutants defective in the insertion of integral membrane proteins into the endoplasmic reticulum. *Mol. Biol. Cell* **3,** 129–142.

18

Manipulating the Folding Pathway of ΔF508 CFTR Using Chemical Chaperones

Marybeth Howard and William J. Welch

1. Introduction

Defects in protein folding constitute the basis of many genetic diseases: cystic fibrosis, alpha-1 antitrypsin deficiency, familial hypercholesterolemia, and congenital nephrogenic diabetes insipidus, to name but a few (*see* **Table 1** for a complete list). In each of these, point mutations or deletions result in a protein product that fails to achieve its properly folded state. For example, in the case of the cystic fibrosis transmembrane conductance regular protein (CFTR), the most common mutation in patients is the loss of a single phenylalanine residue (at position 508) within a polypeptide of 1480 amino acids (*1*). This seemingly minor alteration results in the newly synthesized CFTR protein being unable to fold properly and traffic to its proper destination at the plasma membrane (*2*). Instead, the vast majority of the mutant protein is retained at an early point in its maturation pathway and over time is targeted to a degradative pathway (*3–5*). As a consequence, cells expressing the mutant protein are unable to transport chloride ions across the plasma membrane in response to rises in intracellular cAMP levels.

Oftentimes the particular mutation/deletion within the affected gene is not so severe as to render the corresponding protein product entirely nonfunctional. Rather, many mutations that underlie these different genetic diseases affect the maturation pathway of the particular gene product, resulting in a reduction in the overall amount of the functional protein product. For example, Denning and colleagues were the first to realize that the ΔF508 mutation renders the folding of the CFTR protein temperature sensitive (*6*). These investigators noted that when it is expressed in either insect cells or *Xenopus* oocytes, ΔF508 CFTR protein functioned as a cAMP-regulated chloride channel (*7*). Realizing

From: *Methods in Molecular Medicine, vol. 70: Cystic Fibrosis Methods and Protocols*
Edited by: W. R. Skach © Humana Press Inc., Totowa, NJ

Table 1
Diseases Involving Protein Misfolding

Disease	Protein	Problem
α_1-Antitrypsin deficiency	α_1-Antitrypsin	Trafficking/aggregation
Cystic fibrosis	CFTR	Trafficking
Familial hypercholesterolemia	LDL receptor	Trafficking
Glanzmann's thrombasthemia	Integrin	Trafficking
Leprechaunism	Insulin receptor	Trafficking
Leukocyte adhesion deficiency	Integrin	Trafficking
Nephrogenic diabetes insipidus	Aquaporin	Trafficking
Retinitis pigmentosa	Rhodopsin	Trafficking
Tay-Sachs	β-Hexosaminidase	Trafficking
Amyotrophic lateral sclerosis	Superoxide dismutase	Misfolding
Cancer	p53 (other oncogenes?)	Misfolding
Marfan syndrome	Fibrillin	Misfolding
Osteogenesis imperfecta	Procollagen	Misfolding
Alzheimer's	β-amyloid	Aggregation
Cataracts	Crystallins	Aggregation
Familial amyloidosis	Transthyretin	Aggregation
Scrapie	Prion	Aggregation
Creutzfeldt-Jakob		
Familial insomnia		

that oocytes and insects cells are incubated at lower temperatures, Denning et al. (*6*) examined the effect of incubating mammalian cells expressing ΔF508 CFTR at 26°C instead of 37°C. Now correct folding of the ΔF508 CFTR mutant was observed. Moreover, and like the situation with the insects cells and oocytes, cAMP-regulated chloride transport was observed in those cells expressing the mutant protein. Thus, we now know that the loss of a single phenylalanine residue at position 508 within the CFTR protein results in a newly synthesized protein whose maturation is temperature-dependent.

Prompted by the observations of Denning and colleagues, our laboratory set out to identify other ways to manipulate the folding pathway of the ΔF508 CFTR protein. Here we were aided by a number of previous studies, dating back to the 1960s and 1970s, showing that a number of different low-molecular-weight compounds were effective in correcting the folding pathway of mutant proteins. For example, in both bacteria and yeast, addition of various polyols (sucrose, glycerol) was found to be an effective way to correct the folding of different proteins containing missense mutations (*8–10*). Interestingly, a large percentage of these missense mutants also exhibited temperature sensitivity in their folding pathway. Consequently, we wondered whether a similar approach might be effective for the temperature-sensitive ΔF508 CFTR folding mutant. Cells expressing the ΔF508 CFTR mutant were incubated in media supplemented with varying concentrations of glycerol for 24–72 h. Via Western blotting, along with functional studies examining chloride transport, we demonstrated that glycerol treatment indeed was effective in correcting the folding of at least some of the mutant CFTR protein *(11)*. At around the same time, work from Ron Kopito's laboratory confirmed our observations; glycerol treatment of cells could in fact rescue the folding of the mutant CFTR protein *(12)*.

Subsequent work has shown that a similar strategy is effective for many proteins that display temperature sensitivity in their folding pathway. Inclusion of different low-molecular-weight compounds into the growth medium is an effective method for correcting the folding of many different proteins that display temperature sensitivity in their folding pathway *(13–17)*. It is worth noting that many of these compounds represent a larger class of compounds referred to as cellular osmolytes (*see* **Table 2**). Osmolytes accumulate within cells, primarily those of epithelia origin, in response to osmotic stress. They help stabilize cell volume and, in a mechanism still under study by physical chemists, somehow protect proteins (and perhaps other macromolecules) against thermal and/or chemical denaturation. We refer the reader to some excellent reviews of this fascinating area of cell biology and biochemistry *(18–21)*.

1.1. Parameters Affecting Efficient Rescue of ΔF508 CFTR Misfolding and Detection of the Mature Protein

We have found in the course of our studies that the choice of two important reagents will influence the final results and thus merits mentioning.

1.1.1. Cell Type

Epithelial cells are more amenable to the study of correcting protein misfolding using osmolytes than fibroblast cells. As such, it is the epithelial cell that is the first line of defense to the extracellular environment. These cells have evolved to adapt readily to osmotic changes in the environment via accumulation of osmolytes from the extracellular environment, via specific transporters, as well the synthesis and intracellular accumulation of their own osmolytes. Since endogenous CFTR is expressed only in epithelial cells, the use of this cell type is compatible with the study of CFTR synthesis and protein folding after osmolyte treatment.

1.1.2. Antibody and CFTR Expression Levels

The detection of the CFTR protein using an antibody against the native protein is not a trivial undertaking. While many antibodies against the CFTR protein have been developed, the quality of the data, the ability to detect endogenous CFTR, and the availability of the antibodies as a general reagent make the study of CFTR difficult. We have tested various antibodies for the

Table 2
Common Cellular Osmolytes

Amino acids and derivatives	Carbohydrates	Methylamines
Alanine	Arabitol	Betaine
Glutamic acid	Glycerol	Glycerophosphorylcholine
Proline	Mannitol	Sarcosine
γ-Aminobutyric acid	Mannose	Trimethylamine N-oxide
Taurine	Sorbitol	
Sucrose		
Trehaolse		
Myo-inositol		

detection of CFTR using a heterologous expression system and Western blot. Our data indicate that an antibody raised against a recombinant protein representing amino acids 590–830 (within the R domain) has proven to be the most effective. Having said that, the sensitivity of this antibody to detect the endogenous CFTR protein in cells and tissues is still poor. Hence, for most of our work we exploit the use of transient and/or stable transfection to increase the relative levels of the wild-type and mutant CFTR proteins. In addition, we are also looking at various epitope-tagged CFTR constructs. Epitope-tagging proteins has become quite common. The advantage is the commercial availability of the antibody to the tag and the sensitivity and specificity found using various detection methods—for example, immunoprecipation, Western blot, immunofluorescence. For CFTR, however, placement of the epitope tag has shown to be critical in two ways: (1) it can interfere with the maturation of the protein and (2) because CFTR cannot be completely denatured by boiling, detection of the epitope can be problematic. However, success of this approach with other proteins still lends credence to further investigation of epitope tagging for the CFTR protein.

Here we summarize some of the methods thatwe and others have developed to manipulate protein folding pathways in mammalian cells using osmolytes. While much of the emphasis here concerns the ΔF508 CFTR mutant, we remind the reader that this approach appears to be effective for many different protein folding mutants (especially those that display temperature sensitivity in their folding pathway). Because of the fairly high concentrations required to correct the folding pathway, one has to question whether the use of osmolytes will ever be clinically useful. Instead we suggest that osmolytes can help reveal whether a particular protein folding mutant is amenable for correction. Once that is established, then the search for small molecules that at clinically relevant concentrations bind to the mutant protein and promote folding of that protein can begin.

2. Materials

2.1. Transfection of MammalianCells

1. HEK 293 cells (*see* **Note 1**).
2. Cell culture medium: minimum essential medium (MEM) (Gibco-BRL) with 10% fetal bovine serum (FBS) (Hyclone) and 1% penicillin-streptomycin (Gibco-BRL).
3. Plasmid DNA containing the full-length CFTR wild-type and ΔF508 cDNA subcloned downstream of the CMV promoter (*see* **Note 2**).
4. Lipofectamine and plus reagent (Gibco-BRL).

2.2. Osmolyte Treatment and Induction of CFTR Expression

1. Betaine (Sigma, 99% purity) (*see* **Note 3**).
2. Glycerol (Fisher, enzyme grade).
3. Myo-inositol (Sigma, 99% purity).
4. Sorbitol (Sigma, 99% purity).
5. Taurine (Sigma, 99% purity) (*see* **Note 4**).
6. Sodium salt of butyric acid (Sigma) dissolved in media, stored at –20°C.

2.3. Preparation of Cell Lysates

1. PBS (Cellgro).
2. RIPA buffer (1% sodium deoxycholate, 1% Triton X-100, 0.1% sodium dodecyl sulfate [SDS] in phosphate-buffered saline [PBS]).
3. Protein determination kit (Bio-Rad).
4. Protease inhibitors (Calbiochem) (100× = 500 μ*M* AE135F, 150 n*M* aprotinin, 1 μ*M* E-64, 0.5 m*M* ethylenediaminetetraactic acid (EDTA), 1 μ*M* leupeptin, 0.1 mg/mL pepstatin).
5. 5× Laemmli sample buffer: 0.2*M* Tris-HCl, pH 6.8, 5% SDS, 0.25 *M* dithiothreitin (DTT), 37.5% glycerol, 0.15% bromophenol blue.

2.4. Western Blot Analysis of CFTR Protein Expression

1. 1× Ponceau Red stain (0.2% Ponceau, 1% acetic acid).
2. 10% normal goat serum (*see* **Note 5**).
3. Wash buffer: 0.1% Tween/PBS.
4. 2% BSA in 0.1% Tween/PBS.
5. CFTR R-domain antibody: polyclonal antibody made against a recombinant protein consisting of amino acids 590–830 fused to glutathione S-transferase *(11)*. Dilute antibody in 2% BSA.
6. Horseradish peroxidase (HRP)-goat anti-rabbit (ICN). Diluted in 2% BSA.
7. Chemiluminescent reagent: Super Signal (Pierce).
8. Fluorescent crayon.

3. Methods

3.1. Transfection of Mammalian Cells

1. Eighteen to twenty-four hours before transfection, plate 1.5×10^6 HEK 293 cells in 60-mmol dishes.

2. Prepare transfection reactions using serum-free MEM. Dilute 32 μL of lipofectamine in 1 mL of MEM using a sterile tube (*see* **Note 6**). Incubate for 15 min at room temperature.
3. In a second tube, mix 3.2 μg of plasmid DNA with 32 mL of plus regent in 1 mL of MEM. Incubate for 15 min at room temperature.
4. Combine the two solutions. Incubate for 15 min at room temperature.
5. Wash the cells twice with serum-free MEM and add the transfection reaction to the cells.
6. Incubate the cells at 37°C and 5% CO_2 for 3 h.
7. Remove the transfection media, wash the cells twice with MEM containing 5% FBS, and incubate the cells in media for 1 h.

3.2. Osmolyte Treatment and Induction of CFTR Expression

1. Add myo-inositol, sorbitol, and taurine to the tissue culture media to a final concentration of 100 *M*.
2. For the addition of betaine and glycerol, the cells need to be slowly acclimated to these compounds—otherwise cell death can occur. For betaine, 25 mmol is added every 2 h to a final concentration of 100 m*M*. For glycerol, 250 mmol is added every 2 h to a final concentration of 750 m*M*.
3. At 48 h posttransfection, 10 mmol sodium butyrate is added to the cells to increase transcription of the CFTR gene from the CMV promoter.

3.3. Preparation of Cell Lysates

1. At 18 h postinduction, place cells on ice and wash twice with PBS.
2. For 60mm plates, add 200 μL of RIPA buffer containing 1× protease inhibitors.
3. Scrape cells from the plate, transfer to a 1.5-mL Eppendorf tube, and incubate on ice for 20 min.
4. Pellet cell debris by centrifugation at 14,000*g* for 5 min.
5. Transfer the supernatant to a clean Eppendorf tube on ice and sample 8 μL from each tube for protein lysate determination.
6. Add equal volume of 5× Laemmli sample buffer to the remaining supernatants.

3.4. Western Blot Analysis of CFTR Protein Expression

1. Samples are heated at 50°C for 10 min (*see* **Note 7**) and an equal concentration of total protein from each sample is electrophoresed through a 7.5% polyacrylamide gel.
2. The dye front is electrophoresed off the gel and electrophoresis continued for another 20 min (*see* **Note 8**).
3. Transfer the proteins from the acrylamide gel to a nitrocellulose membrane using a standard protein transfer apparatus at either 0.2 mV overnight or 0.6 mV for 3 h.
4. The membrane is washed twice in distilled water to get rid of residual SDS and stained with 1× Ponceau Red for determination of protein transfer for all lanes as well as marking lanes and molecular-weight markers.
5. Destain the membrane in 1× PBS
6. Block in 10% normal goat serum/0.1% Tween/PBS for 1 h at room temperature on a shaker.

7. Wash 3× for 5 min in PBS.
8. Incubate with GST-R antibody diluted at 1/1000 in 2% BSA/0.1% Tween/PBS for 1 h. Another CFTR antibody, M3A7, became commercially available in 2001 (Upstate Biotechnology). We found this antibody to be better for detecting CFTR in western blots, use according to manufacturer's protocol.
9. Wash 6× for 5 min in 0.1% Tween/PBS.
10. Incubate with HRP-goat anti-rabbit antibody diluted at 1/10,000 in 2% BSA/ 0.1% Tween/PBS for 1 h at room temperature.
11. Wash 6× for 5 min in 0.1% Tween/PBS.
12. A final wash of 3× for 5 min in PBS eliminates detergent prior to incubation with chemiluminescence solution.
13. The membrane is incubated in Super Signal (Pierce) for 5 min, placed between plastic sheet protectors, and molecular-weight markers identified using fluorescent crayon markings on tape. The membrane is exposed to UV light in the darkroom for 1 s and various exposure times to film are acquired starting with a 30-s exposure.

4. Notes

1. The use of osmolytes to rescue protein misfolding as described in this chapter is not specific for HEK 293 cells. The optimal transfection protocol for 293 cells was determined using pCMVβ-gal as a reporter gene and various commercially available lipid reagents. Our transfection effeciency for 293 cells using the protocol described in this chapter is 40%.
2. For transfections, high-purity plasmid DNA is required. Various kits are available to isolate and purify plasmid DNA. We use the Qiagen Maxi Prep kit.
3. All osmolyte stock solutions are 1 *M*, dissolving the solute in serum-free medium. Stocks are stored at –20°C. Betaine is acidic and potassium hydroxide is used to adjust the pH of the solution.
4. Heat (45°C) is required to dissolve 1 *M* stock solutions of taurine. Storage at –20°C results in taurine precipitating out of solution and thus requires reheating the solution.
5. Various reagents have been used to block the membrane; we have found that using normal goat serum and the GST-R antibody gives us little or no background.
6. For lipofectamine, there is no specification for the type of tube required, for example, polypropylene or polystyrene.
7. Heating CFTR protein to high temperature to achieve complete denaturation results in aggregation and precipitation of the protein. As a consequence, the protein will not show up on the gel and/or will not be properly resolved.
8. Under these gel electrophoresis conditions, CFTR migrates within the top third of the gel.

References

1. Kerem, B., Rommens, J. M., Buchanan, J. A., Markiewicz, D., Cox, T. K., Chakravarti, A., Buchwald, M., and Tsui, L. (1989) Identification of the cystic fibrosis gene: genetic analysis. *Science* **245,** 1073–1080.

2. Cheng, S. H., Gregory, R. J., Marshall, J., Paul, S., Souza, D. W., White, G. A., O'Riordan, C. R., and Smith, A. E. (1990) Defective intracellular transport and processing of CFTR is the molecular basis of most cystic fibrosis. *Cell* **63,** 827–834.
3. Ward, C. L. and Kopito, R. R. (1994) Intracellular turnover of cystic fibrosis trnasmembrane conductance regulator. *J. Biol. Chem.* **269,** 25,710–25,718.
4. Jensen, T. J., Loo, M. A., Pind, S., Williams, D. B., Goldberg, A. L., and Riordan, J. R. (1995) Multiple proteolytic systems, including the proteasome, contribute to CFTR processing. *Cell* **83,** 129–135.
5. Ward, C. L., Omura, S., and Kopito, R. R. (1995) Intracellular turnover of cystic fibrosis transmembrane conductance regulator: inefficient processing and rapid degradation of wild-type and mutant proteins. *Cell* **83,** 121–127.
6. Denning, G. M., Anderson, M. P., Amara, J. F., Marshallo, J., Smith, A. E., and Welsh, M. J. (1992) Processing of mutant cystic fibrosis transmembrane conductance regulator is temperature sensitive. *Nature* **358,** 761–764.
7. Drumm, M. L., Wilkinson, D. J., Smit, L. S., Worrell, R. T., Strong, T. V., Frizzell, R. A., Dawson, D. C., and Collins, F. S. (1991) Chloride conductance expressed by ΔF508 and other mutant CFTRs in *Xenopus* oocytes. *Science* **254,** 1797–1799.
8. Hawthorne, D. C. and Friis, J. (1964) Osmotic-remedial mutants. A new classification for nutritional mutants in yeast. *Genetics* **50,** 829–839.
9. Russell, R. R. B. (1972) Temperature-sensitive osmotic remedial mutants of *Escherichia coli. J. Bact.* **112,** 661–665.
10. Singer, M. A. and Lindquist, S. (1998) Multiple effects of trehalose on protein folding in vitro and in vivo. *Mol. Cell* **1,** 639–648.
11. Brown, C. R., Hong-Brown, L. Q., Biwersi, J., Verkman, A. S., and Welch, W. J. (1996) Chemical chaperones correct the mutant phenotype of the DF508 cystic fibrosis transmembrane conductance regulator protein. *Cell Stress Chaperones* **1,** 117–125.
12. Sato, S., Ward, C. L., Krouse, M. E., Wine, J. J., and Kopito, R. R. (1996) Glycerol reverses the misfolding phenotype of the most common cystic fibrosis mutation. *J. Biol. Chem.* **271,** 635–638.
13. Tatzelt, J., Prusiner, S. B., and Welch, W. J. (1996) Chemical chaperones interfere with the formation of scrapie prion protein. *EMBO J.* **15,** 6363–6373.
14. Brown, C. R., Hong-Brown, L. Q., and Welch, W. J. (1997) Correcting temperature-sensitive protein folding defects. *J. Clin. Invest.* **99,** 1432–1444.
15. Tamarappoo, B. K. and Verkman, A. S. (1998) Defective aquaporin-2 trafficking in nephrogenic diabetes insipidus and correction by chemical chaperones. *J. Clin. Invest.* **101,** 2257–2267.
16. Yang, D., Yip, C. M., Huang, T. H. J., Chakrabartty, A., and Fraser, P. E. (1999) Manipulating the amyloid-β aggregation pathway with chemical chaperones. *J. Biol. Chem.* **274,** 32,970–32,974.
17. Burrows, J. A. J., Willis, L. K., and Perlmutter, D. H. (2000) Chemical chaperones mediate increased secretion of mutant alpha-1-antitrypsin Z: a potential pharmacological strategy for prevention of liver injury and emphysema in alpha-1-antitrypsin deficiency. *Proc. Natl. Acad. Sci. USA* **97,** 1796–1801.

18. Gekko, K. and Timasheff, S. N. (1981) Mechanism of protein stabilization by glycerol: preferential hydration in glycerol-water mixtures. *Biochemistry* **20,** 4667–4676.
19. Somero, G. N. (1986) Protons, osmolytes, and fitness of internal milieu for protein function. *Am. J. Physiol.* **251,** R197–R213.
20. Schein, C. H. (1990) Solubility as a function of protein structure and solvent components. *Bio/Technology* **8,** 308–316.
21. Burg, M. B. (1995) Molecular basis of omotic regulation. *Am. J. Physiol.* **268,** F983–F996.

19

CFTR Degradation and Aggregation

Michael J. Corboy, Philip J. Thomas, and W. Christian Wigley

1. Introduction

Defective protein folding is becoming increasingly recognized as a significant cause of human disease, and cystic fibrosis (CF) is a prime example. A number of CF-causing mutations in the cystic fibrosis transmembrane conductance regulator (CFTR) result in a CFTR protein that does not reach the plasma membrane but is instead retained by the cellular quality control system and degraded by the ubiquitin–proteasome system. Misfolded CFTR that cannot be degraded accumulates in the cell as centrosome-associated inclusions of aggregated protein that are replete with proteasome components. In fact, the centrosomal region is a significant site of proteasome concentration in resting cells, suggesting a novel role for this subcellular location in the quality control of protein expression. This chapter gives an overview of CFTR misfolding, degradation, and aggregation, and provides details of methods used in our laboratory to study these processes.

1.1. CFTR Folding and Misfolding

CFTR folding and maturation, and the role of molecular chaperones in these processes, are described in detail in Chapters 15 and 16, and will only be covered briefly here. CFTR, a member of the ABC (<u>A</u>TP <u>B</u>inding <u>C</u>assette) transporter supergene family, is a polytopic membrane protein composed of two nucleotide-binding domains (NBDs), two transmembrane domains (TMDs), and a PKA-sensitive regulatory domain *(1)*. In addition to its role in chloride conductance *(2–4)*, CFTR regulates the activity of several other critical transport systems in the apical membrane of epithelial cells *(5,6)*. Disease-causing mutations in CFTR lead to loss of one or more of these activities due to a variety of molecular mechanisms, the most common of which is defective fold-

From: *Methods in Molecular Medicine, vol. 70: Cystic Fibrosis Methods and Protocols*
Edited by: W. R. Skach © Humana Press Inc., Totowa, NJ

ing *(7)*. Several mutations, including the common ΔF508 mutation, result in misfolded CFTR proteins that never reach their proper location in the apical membrane.

Both wild-type and ΔF508 CFTR are initially synthesized in the endoplasmic reticulum (ER) membrane as essentially indistinguishable ~140-kDa coreglycosylated immature species *(8–10)* that associate with the molecular chaperones Hsp70 *(11–13)*, Hsp90 *(14)*, and calnexin *(15)*. Some fraction of the wild-type precursor traffics to the Golgi apparatus, after its increase in stability and release from chaperones, where it is processed to a mature ~160-kDa species carrying complex oligosaccharides. The processing and maturation of even wild-type CFTR is inefficient, with <30% of the wild-type molecules ever reaching mature form in cultured cells *(8–10)*. In contrast, most of the immature wild-type (~70%) and nearly all of the immature ΔF508 CFTR never reach the Golgi but are instead detained by the ER quality control system and degraded.

1.2. Quality Control and CFTR Degradation

The ER is the site of synthesis and initial maturation of integral membrane proteins such as CFTR as well as secreted proteins. A critical role of the ER is to ensure that these nascent proteins achieve their native conformation before being allowed to traffic through the secretory pathway to their ultimate subcellular destination. In general, correctly folded, processed, and assembled proteins are transported, whereas misfolded proteins and persistently unassembled subunits are retained and subsequently degraded *(16)*, although the actual site of degradation within the cell is unclear—that is, at the ER membrane, in the cytosol, or at another subcellular location. For CFTR, this is apparent in the ER-like distribution seen in cells expressing folding mutants such as ΔF508 and P205S *(8,17)*. In contrast, cells expressing wild-type CFTR show, in addition to the ER pattern, a peripheral distribution indicative of trafficking of the mature protein to the plasma membrane *(8)*. Strictly speaking, ER retention may be somewhat of a misnomer, though, as ΔF508 has been reported to visit, at least transiently, the ER–Golgi intermediate compartment *(18)*. However, whether this represents "leaky" retention or a bona-fide part of the ER degradation pathway is not currently known.

Misfolded CFTR is degraded in a ubiquitin-dependent manner by the 26S proteasome *(19,20)*. The 26S proteasome is composed of two major subcomplexes, the 20S proteasome and PA700. The 20S proteasome, a 700-kDa cylinder, constitutes the catalytic core of the protease *(21,22)*. The catalytic sites are located within a hollow cavity of the cylinder, and narrow openings at the ends of the cylinder limit substrates to short peptides and unfolded proteins *(23–25)*. The PA700 regulatory complex (also called the 19S cap) associates with the ends of the 20S proteasome cylinder to form the 26S complex *(21,26,27)*. Misfolded proteins are targeted for degradation by the covalent attachment of poly-ubiquitin chains by cytosolic and/or membrane-bound ubiquitin conjugating enzymes *(28,29)*. The poly-ubiquitinated substrates are then recognized by the 26S proteasome, followed by de-ubiquitination and the degradation of the substrate by the multiple proteolytic activities of the catalytic core. PA700 imparts specificity for ubiquitinated substrates at least in part through its established poly-ubiquitin binding and cleavage activities *(30)*. PA700 also has multiple ATPase activities *(21)*, and likely enhances degradation of ubiquitinated proteins by unfolding substrates and facilitating their translocation into the central cavity of the protease *(27,31)*. A second regulatory complex, PA28 (11S cap), also associates with the 20S proteasome in vivo *(32–34)*. PA28 does not require ubiquitinated substrates for activity and apparently functions to increase proteasome processing of short peptides—for example, in antigen presentation *(35,36)*.

Cytosolic proteasomes degrade ER-associated misfolded CFTR, and indeed numerous medically relevant secretory and membrane proteins, via a process termed ER-associated degradation, or ERAD. ERAD is a multistep process beginning with recognition and retention of misfolded proteins in the ER, ubiquitination, dislocation from the membrane, deglycosylation, and finally de-ubiquitination and degradation by the 26S proteasome. CFTR has been used as a model system for the investigation of the ERAD pathway (*see also* Chapter 15), although the molecular mechanisms of several individual steps are still not well understood. For example, although it is clear that CFTR is poly-ubiquitinated *(19,37,38)* and poly-ubiquitination is involved in CFTR degradation by the proteasome *(19)*, the initial recognition events leading to the retention of misfolded CFTR in the ER are undefined. ΔF508 CFTR exhibits prolonged interaction with both Hsp70 and calnexin in vivo *(11,13,15)*, but it is not known whether extended chaperone binding actually participates in recognition and/or mediates retention, or is merely a consequence of persistence of the immature form of CFTR. In addition, nearly a third of the CFTR sequence is embedded in the membrane, and it is not known if the recognition of transmembrane folding mutations (such as P205S, in TMD1) is distinct from the recognition of folding mutations in soluble domains (such as ΔF508, in NBD1).

Similarly, the mechanism of extraction of misfolded CFTR from the membrane is unclear. The current model for dislocation of misfolded proteins from the ER involves retrograde transport of ubiquitinated substrates through the Sec61 translocon channel *(39–41)*, and there is evidence for such a mechanism in CFTR degradation *(37,42,43)*. However, it is unclear if polytopic membrane proteins such as CFTR are degraded as they are extracted from the ER membrane, or if they proceed through cytosolic intermediates. While many lumenal ERAD substrates (such as carboxypeptidase Y) appear to be completely extracted from the ER prior to proteolysis *(44)*, for polytopic ERAD substrates (such as CFTR), studies in yeast suggest that the dislocation and proteolytic activities are more tightly coordinated *(45)*. Such synchronized extraction and degradation would likely serve to prevent cytosolic accumulation of aggregation-prone, potentially toxic hydrophobic transmembrane regions.

1.3. Misfolding and Aggregation at Centrosome

The initial defect of protein misfolding is typically the undesired surface exposure of normally buried hydrophobic regions *(46,47)*. Left unattended, these exposed hydrophobic patches can associate and drive aggregation of the nonnative proteins into insoluble inclusions. Since such surfaces are potentially toxic *(48)*, it is not surprising that cells have evolved quality control mechanisms to recognize misfolded proteins and either repair or eliminate them. Both chaperones and regulatory components of the proteasome rely mostly on binding to the same or similar determinants on the misfolded protein, namely, the surface-exposed hydrophobic regions. Thus, the decision between repair and elimination has been proposed to be a kinetic competition between binding by molecular chaperones, leading to refolding, and binding by regulatory components of the proteasome, leading to degradation *(46,49)*. The distinction between the two systems is not quite so clear, however. For example, in addition to its role in preventing aggregation and promoting folding, the chaperone Hsp70 is also required for the ubiquitination and degradation of several proteins *(50)*. Conversely, PA700 exhibits a chaperone-like binding mode in vitro, perhaps related to its role in degradation *(51)*. In any case, when neither the salvage nor degradation system is capable of dealing with the misfolded protein, the usual result is aggregation.

A number of biochemical studies have shown that misfolded CFTR is prone to aggregation. Inhibition of the proteasome in cells expressing ΔF508 CFTR leads to the formation of high-molecular-weight, detergent-insoluble complexes of poly-ubiquitinated CFTR *(19,52)*. In the absence of degradation, CFTR forms similar complexes when expressed in a cell-free system designed to reconstitute ERAD *(37)* (*see also* Chapter 20). CFTR aggregation in vivo can be visualized by immunocytochemistry. When the degradation capacity of the proteasome is overwhelmed in vivo by either proteasome inhibition or overexpression of mutant CFTR, the misfolded CFTR that cannot be degraded accumulates as a large perinuclear inclusion (**Fig. 1**) that colocalizes with γ-tubulin at and proximal to the centrosome *(17,52)* (**Fig. 2**). These inclusions also occasionally arise from high-level expression of even wild-type CFTR *(17)*, and are likely a reflection of CFTR's intrinsic folding inefficiency under these conditions. The centrosome-associated CFTR inclusions are also enriched in proteasome components, such as the 20S proteasome, PA700, PA28, and ubiquitin, and relevant chaperones, such as Hsp70 and Hsp90 *(17,53–55)*. The formation of these inclusions is consistent with an ER dislocation process in

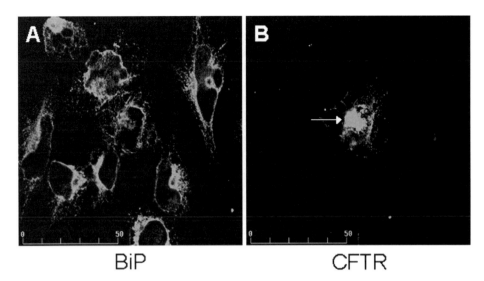

Fig. 1. Intracellular localization of misfolded CFTR. HEK 293 cells expressing ΔF508 CFTR were treated for 12 h with 10 μ*M* lactacystin, beginning 48 h posttransfection. Following fixation and permeabilization with methanol as described in **Methods**, cells were immunostained with mouse monoclonal anti-BiP and rabbit polyclonal anti-CFTR and visualized by confocal microscopy. The arrow indicates the perinuclear inclusion of misfolded CFTR. Scale bar indicates size in μm.

which extraction from the membrane and degradation, while likely coordinated, are not explicitly coupled *(37,45)*. Inhibition of proteasome activity with inhibitors such as lactacystin would not necessarily inhibit extraction of the ubiquitinated protein. If extraction of CFTR from the membrane is not quickly followed by or linked to proteolysis, then exposure of the large hydrophobic transmembrane domains could drive the protein into a nonnative conformation that could be recognized by packaging machinery and/or rapidly form an insoluble aggregate. This process is consistent with the models presented by Bebok et al., *(42)* and by Johnston et al., *(52)*, in which dislocation and inclusion formation, respectively, proceed via a deglycosylated cytosolic intermediate. In contrast, recent studies by Chen et al., *(56)* indicate that in COS cells treated with the proteasome inhibitor MG132, immature CFTR remains in the membrane and is not deglycosylated, consistent with results from ERAD of polytopic substrates in yeast *(45)*. Clearly, more work is needed to clarify these discrepancies.

This centrosomal association of proteasomes is not strictly a function of CFTR overexpression, but also a general feature of resting cells *(17)*. 20S proteasomes, PA700, PA28, ubiquitin, Hsp70, and Hsp90 have all been shown by immunocytochemistry to co-localize with centrosomes in several different

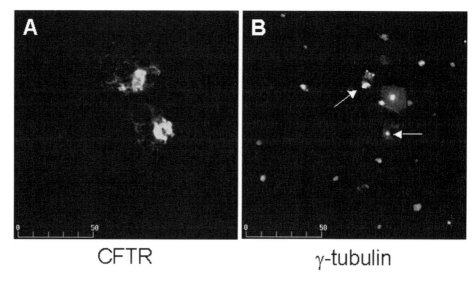

CFTR   γ-tubulin

Fig. 2. Intracellular inclusions of misfolded proteins arise from the centrosome. HEK 293 cells expressing ΔF508 CFTR were treated with 10 μ*M* lactacystin for 12 h and immunostained with rabbit polyclonal anti-CFTR and mouse monoclonal anti-γ-tubulin. Arrows indicate γ-tubulin-visualized centrosomes from which mutant CFTR aggregates appear to form. The scale bar indicates size in μm. (Reproduced from Wigley et al. [1999] *J. Cell Biol.* **145,** 481–490, by permission of The Rockefeller University Press.)

cultured cell lines under basal conditions (**Fig. 3**). The association is stable, as these proteasome components and chaperones also cosediment with centrosomes in sucrose density gradients *(17)*. In addition, the purified centrosome-associated proteasomes are active in degrading ubiquitinated proteins and proteasome-specific peptide substrates, and demonstrate the same ATP dependence and inhibitor profile as soluble proteasomes *(57)*. When combined with mutant CFTR overexpression, pharmacological inhibition of the proteasome results in striking recruitment of cytosolic proteasome components to the centrosomal inclusions. This recruitment is accompanied by appreciable expansion of the centrosome *(17)* and redistribution of proteasomes, γ-tubulin, and chaperones to an insoluble fraction (**Fig. 4**). Thus, the centrosomal proteasomes may not be a distinct population, but more likely represent dynamic partitioning of proteasomes from the cytosolic pool to the centrosome and/or ER membrane, analogous to the mobilization of cytosolic ribosomes to the rough ER membrane during the translation of secreted proteins.

The centrosome has been primarily regarded in terms of its role in microtubule assembly and organization of the mitotic spindle during cell division *(58–60)*.

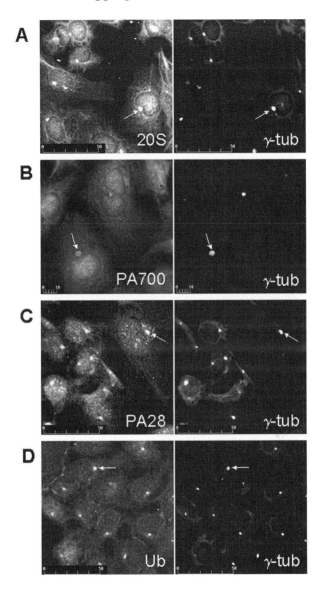

Fig. 3. Localization of proteasome components at the centrosome. HEK 293 cells were immunostained with mouse monoclonal anti-γ-tubulin and either rabbit polyclonal anti-20S proteasome, chicken polyclonal anti-PA700, rabbit polyclonal anti-PA28, or mouse monoclonal anti-ubiquitin antibodies, as indicated in each panel. Arrows indicated locations of perinuclear proteasome-enriched centrosomes. Scale bars indicate size in μm. (Reproduced from Wigley et al. [1999] *J. Cell Biol.* **145,** 481–490, by permission of The Rockefeller University Press.)

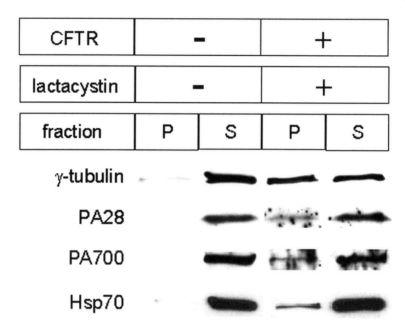

CFTR		−		+	

lactacystin		−		+	

fraction	P	S	P	S

γ-tubulin

PA28

PA700

Hsp70

Fig. 4. Co-redistribution of the centrosome Hsp70 and the proteasome in response to inclusion formation. HeLa cells expressing P205S CFTR and treated with 10 μ*M* lactacystin for 12 h and untreated mock-transfected control cells were lysed and separated into supernatant (S) and pellet (P) fractions as described in **Methods**. Fractions were separated by SDS-Page and analyzed by Western blotting using the indicated antibodies. (Repoduced from Wigley et al. [1999] *J. Cell Biol.* **145,** 481–490, by permission of The Rockefeller University Press.)

In addition to its function as the microtubule-organizing center, however, a growing list of proteins that localize to the centrosome suggests additional important roles for this dynamic organelle *(59,60)*. The observations regarding centrosomal inclusions of misfolded CFTR and the centrosomal association of proteasome components highlight a novel function of the centrosome as a site of proteolysis, where significant protein turnover occurs as part of the cellular quality control of protein expression *(17,52)* (**Fig. 5**). A significant benefit of such a system could be to accumulate proteolytic substrates at a site of proteasome concentration, thereby offering an additional means of regulating protein turnover. A diverse group of proteasome substrates that undergo regulated proteolysis has been localized to the centrosome, including cyclins *(61,62)*, p53 *(63)*, and IκB *(64)*, suggesting additional roles for the centrosome-associated proteasome in cell cycle regulation, tumor suppression, and antiviral defense and inflammation. This chapter focuses on techniques used to study these phenomena using a combination of immunocytochemical and biochemi-

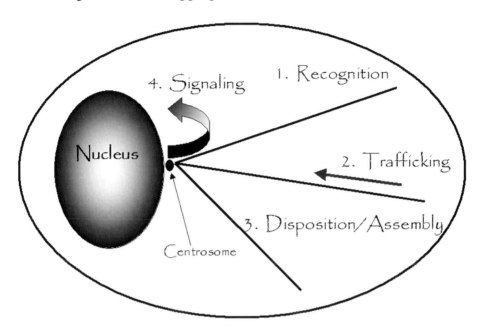

Fig. 5. Schematic of a eukaryotic cell. The nucleus (gray) and centrosome (black) are as indicated. Black lines represent microtubules radiating from the centrosome to the cell periphery. The schematic is drawn to highlight several important questions that remain regarding the centrosomal inclusions described herein and elsewhere: **1**. How is the substrate recognized and what proteins are involved? **2**. Does trafficking to the centrosome serve to simply deposit aggregated substrates, or also to concentrate them, thereby increasing their exposure/susceptibility to the centrosome-associated proteasomes? **3**. Is assembly into vimentin-surrounded perinuclear centrosomal inclusions an active, protein-mediated process, or simply a result of aggregation? **4**. What signals arise from the processes, occurring at this location and what are their targets?

cal methods to visualize and characterize the centrosome-associated inclusions of misfolded CFTR and the centrosomal proteasome.

2. Materials
2.1. Centrosome-Associated CFTR Inclusions
2.1.1. Formation: Cell Lines, Plasmids, and Transfection

1. Human embryonic kidney (HEK) 293 cells, HeLa cells (American Type Culture Collection).
2. Dulbecco's modified Eagle's medium (DMEM) (Gibco).
3. Fetal calf serum (Gibco).
4. Tissue culture antibiotics (streptomycin, penicillin) (Gibco).
5. Standard tissue-culture plastic ware, glass cover slips.

Corboy, Thomas, and Wigley

6. pCMVNot6.2 containing full-length human CFTR cDNA (generous gift of Dr. Johanna Rommens, The Hospital For Sick Children, Toronto).
7. Quick Change Mutagenesis System (Stratagene).
8. Fugene 6 Mammalian Transfection Reagent (Boehringer Mannheim).
9. Lactacystin (10 m*M*) and MG132 (50 m*M*) (Calbiochem) as stocks in dimethyl sulfoxide (DMSO), stored at –20°C.

2.1.2. Immunocytochemistry

1. Phosphate-buffered saline (PBS), methanol (100%, stored at –20°C).
2. 50 m*M* glycine in PBS.
3. Blocking medium: 5% goat serum, 1% bovine serum albumin (BSA), 0.1% gelatin in PBS.
4. Primary antibodies: anti-CFTR mouse mAb 24-1 (R&D Systems); anti-CFTR rabbit pAb R3194 *(65)*; anti-GRP78 (BiP) pAb SPA-826 (StressGen); anti γ-tubulin mouse mAb (Sigma).
5. Appropriate fluorescently labeled secondary antibodies (Jackson Immunoresearch).
6. Fluorescent microscope (we routinely use a Bio-Rad MRC 1024 confocal microscope).

2.1.3. Characterization of Soluble and Insoluble Fractions

1. Trypsin in Hank's balanced salt solution (HBSS) (Gibco).
2. PBS.
3. PBS supplemented with Complete™ Protease Inhibitor Cocktail (Roche).
4. Syringes fitted with 27-gauge needles.
5. Standard protein gel electrophoresis setup, transfer apparatus, and nitrocellulose.
6. Transfer buffer: 25 m*M* Tris, 192 m*M* glycine, pH 8.3, and 20% methanol.
7. TTBS: 20 m*M* Tris-HCl, pH 7.6, 137 m*M* NaCl, 0.05% Tween 20.
8. Blocking buffer: 10% nonfat milk in TTBS.
9. Primary antibodies: anti-γ-tubulin mouse mAb (Sigma); anti-Hsp70 mouse mAb MA3-006 (Affinity Bioreagents); anti-PA700 chicken pAb *(17)*, and anti-PA28 rabbit pAb *(66)*, prepared as described.
10. Appropriate horseradish peroxidase (HRP)-labeled secondary antibodies (Jackson Immunoresearch), ECL detection reagents, and Hyperfilm (Amersham).

2.2. Centrosome-Associated Proteins

2.2.1. Immunocytochemistry

1. Solutions as in **Subheading 2.2.2.**
2. Primary antibodies: anti-γ-tubulin mouse mAb and anti-ubiquitin mouse mAb (Sigma); anti-GRP78 (BiP) pAb SPA-826 (StressGen); anti-Hsp70 mouse mAb MA3-006 (Affinity Bioreagents); anti-20S proteasome rabbit pAb *(31)*, anti-PA700 chicken pAb *(17)*, and anti-PA28 rabbit pAb *(66)*, prepared as described.
3. Labeled secondary antibodies and fluorescent microscope as under **Subheading 2.1.2.**

2.2.2. Immunoblot Analysis of Purified Centrosomes

1. Cytochalasin D (10 mg/mL), Nocodazole (1 m*M*) (Sigma) as stocks in DMSO, stored at –20°C

2. Trypsin in HBSS (Gibco).
3. TBS.
4. 8% sucrose in 0.1× TBS.
5. Lysis buffer: 1 mM HEPES, pH 7.2, 0.5% NP-40, 0.5 mM MgCl$_2$, 0.1% β-mercaptoethanol, 1 μg/mL leupeptin, 1 μg/mL pepstatin, 1 μg/mL aprotinin, 1 mM PMS.F Add NP-40 and protease inhibitors fresh just before use. (alternatively, use Complete™ Inhibitor Cocktail tablets, Roche).
6. 1 M HEPES, pH 7.4.
7. 10 mg/mL DNAse I (Roche) in TBS (store aliquots at –20°C).
8. 40, 50, 60, and 70% sucrose solutions (wt/wt) in 10 mM PIPES, pH 7.2; 0.1% Triton X-100; 0.1% β-mercaptoethanol (add β-mercaptoethanol fresh).
9. Electrophoresis and immunoblotting reagents and supplies as under **Subheading 2.1.2., item 2.**
10. Primary antibodies: anti-γ-tubulin mouse mAb (Sigma); anti-Hsp70 mouse mAb MA3-006 and anti-Hsp90 mouse mAb MA3-011 (Affinity Bioreagents); anti-GRP78 (BiP) pAb SPA-826 (StressGen); anti-20S proteasome rabbit pAb *(31)*, anti-p31 *(17)*, and anti-PA28 rabbit pAb *(66)*, prepared as described. (To establish purity of the centrosome preparations, we also immunoblot for cytosolic [aldolase], nuclear [lamin B1], and Golgi markers [β-cop].)

3. Methods

3.1. Centrosome-Associated CFTR Inclusions

3.1.1. Formation: Cell Lines, Plasmids, and Transfection

HEK 293 and HeLa cells are maintained in DMEM supplemented with 10% FCS, 50 μg/mL streptomycin, and 50 U/mL penicillin at 37°C in humidified 95% air/5% CO (*see* **Note 1**). Plasmids pCMVNot6.2 and pCMVNot6.2-ΔF containing expressible human CFTR cDNAs are purified using standard plasmid purification kits supplied by either Qiagen or Clontech, following protocols supplied by the manufacturer. Additional CFTR mutations (e.g., P205S) are introduced using a suitable mutagenesis method (we prefer the Quick Change Site-Directed Mutagenesis System from Stratagene). The following protocol is for transfecting cells in 35-mm dishes or 6-well plates. Reagent volumes and DNA amounts are per well. Scale up or down accordingly for different sized dishes.

1. Plate cells: Plate cells 1 d before transfection to achieve ~50% confluence. For example, split a confluent 60-mm dish 1/12 into 6-well cluster plates, using 2 mL complete DMEM per well.
2. Form DNA-Fugene complexes: For each well, add 12 μL Fugene directly to 88 μL serum-free DMEM in an Eppendorf tube and mix by tapping. Do not allow undiluted Fugene to touch the walls of the tube. In a separate tube, place 1 μg CFTR vector. Add Fugene–DMEM mixture to DNA and mix by tapping. Incubate at room temperature for 15 min. After incubation, add 900 μL complete DMEM per tube. We frequently perform a transfection control using, for example, 1 μg GFP vector.

3. Aspirate medium from cells and replace with 1 mL of complete DMEM. Add DNA–Fugene–DMEM complex mixture (now 1 mL volume, giving 2 mL total per well) directly to wells and swirl gently to mix. Return to incubator for appropriate time.
4. Check transfection efficiency, for example, by examining cells for GFP fluorescence.
5. For proteasome inhibition, add lactacystin to final concentration of 10 μM and continue incubation for 2–12 h.

3.1.2. Immunocytochemistry and Inclusion Morphometry

Approximately 24 h posttransfection:

1. Release cells from dishes by trypsinization and re-plate onto glass coverslips. (alternatively, transfection and analysis can all be performed on cover slips).

Approximately 72 h posttransfection:

2. Rinse cells 3× with PBS.
3. Fix and permeabilize cells with 1 mL of ice-cold methanol for 10 min at –20°C (see **Note 2**).
4. Rinse 3× with PBS.
5. Incubate in 1 mL of 50 mM glycine in PBS for 10 min (this and all subsequent steps at room temperature).
6. Block nonspecific sites with 0.1 mL blocking medium (*see* **Materials**) for 1 h.
7. Remove blocking medium and add primary antibody for either CFTR, centrosomes (γ-tubulin), proteasomes (20S, PA700, PA28), or ER (BiP) as 1/100 dilution in 0.1 mL blocking medium; incubate 1 h.
8. Remove primary antibody and wash cells 3× with blocking medium.
9. Add fluorescently labeled secondary antibody as 1/100 dilution in 0.1 mL blocking medium; incubate 1 h.
10. Remove secondary antibody and wash cells 3× with blocking medium.
11. Repeat **steps 7–10** with appropriate antibodies for counterstaining.
12. Visualize cells and obtain images using Bio-Rad MRC1024 confocal microscope.

3.1.3. Characterization of Soluble and Insoluble Fractions

Approximately 48 h posttransfection:

1. Add lactacystin to one plate of each set to final concentration of 10 μM; return to incubator and continue growth for 12 h.
2. Wash cells 2× with PBS, harvest by trypsinization, and pellet by centrifugation at 4°C.
3. Wash cell pellet 2× with PBS and resuspend in 100 μL PBS with Complete Protease Inhibitor Cocktail (supplemented PBS).
4. Lyse by multiple (10–20×) passage through a 27-gauge needle.
5. Centrifuge lysate (14,000g, 4°C, 1 h); remove and save supernatant (can be stored at –70°C until analysis).
6. Wash pellets 1× with supplemented PBS.

7. Recentrifuge (14,000g, 4°C, 30 min); remove and discard supernatant.
8. Resuspend pellets in 100 µL supplemented PBS (store at –70°C until analysis).
9. Separate pellet and supernatant fractions by electrophoresis on 4–20% SDS-PAGE gels.
10. Transfer proteins to nitrocellulose using transfer buffer (*see* **Materials**) with 20% methanol, and block with blocking buffer (*see* **Materials**).
11. Perform immunoblotting using γ-tubulin, PA28, PA700, and Hsp70 antibodies.

3.2. Centrosome-Associated Proteins

3.2.1. Immunocytochemistry

1. Plate cells onto glass cover slips.

Approximately 48 h after plating:

2. Fix, permeabilize, and block cells as under **Subheading 3.1.2., step 2.**
3. Remove blocking medium and add primary antibody centrosomes (γ-tubulin), proteasomes (20S, PA700, PA28), chaperones (Hsp70, Hsp90), ubiquitin, and control subcellular markers (BiP) as 1/100 dilution in 0.1 mL blocking medium; incubate 1 h.
4. Remove primary antibody and wash cells 3× with blocking medium.
5. Add fluorescently labeled secondary antibody as 1/100 dilution in 0.1 mL blocking medium; incubate 1 h.
6. Remove secondary antibody and wash cells 3× with blocking medium.
7. Repeat **steps 7–10** with appropriate antibodies for counterstaining.
8. Visualize cells and obtain images using Bio-Rad MRC1024 confocal microscope.

3.2.2. Immunoblot Analysis of Purified Centrosomes

1. Treat exponentially growing 293 or HeLa cells for 1 h with 1 µg/mL cytochalasin D and 0.2 µM nocodazole to disrupt cytoskeleton.
2. Release cells by trypsinization and collect by centrifugation.
3. Wash cell pellet 1× in TBS, and 1× in 0.1× TBS/8% sucrose, collecting cells by centrifugation between washes. Resuspend cells in 2 mL 0.1× TBS/8% sucrose.
4. Add 8 mL lysis buffer (*see* **Materials**). Gently shake suspension and pass 5× through a narrow-mouth 10-mL serological pipet to lyse cells.
5. Centrifuge lysate (2,500g, 10 min, room temperature) to remove swollen nuclei, chromatin aggregates, and unlysed cells.
6. Add HEPES to 10 mM and DNAse I to 1 µg/mL from concentrated stocks, and incubate 30 min on ice.
7. Gently underlay solution with 1 mL 60% sucrose solution (*see* **Materials**) and centrifuge (10,000g, 30 min, room temperature) to sediment centrosomes onto the cushion.
8. Remove the upper 8 mL of the supernatant and discard. Load the remainder, including the cushion (~3 ml, ~30% sucrose, containing the concentrated centrosomes), onto a discontinuous sucrose gradient consisting of 70%, 50%, and 40% sucrose solutions (1 mL ea) from the bottom, respectively. Centrifuge gra-

dient (120,000*g*, 1 h, 4°C). Poke a small hole in the bottom of the tube and collect 300-µL fractions; proceed to **step 9** or store at –70°C.

9. Dilute gradient fractions into 1 mL of 10 m*M* PIPES, pH 7.2 and pellet centrosomes in microfuge (14,000 rpm, 15 min, 4°C). Resuspend centrosome pellets in SDS-PAGE sample buffer, boil 5 min, and separate samples by electrophoresis on 10% SDS-PAGE gels.

10. Transfer to nitrocellulose as under **Subheading 3.1.2., step 3** and perform immunoblot using antibodies against centrosome (γ-tubulin) and proteins of interest, for example, proteasome (20S, PA700, PA28), chaperones (Hsp70, Hsp90), and control subcellular markers (e.g., BiP, aldolase, Lamin-B1, β-cop).

4. Notes

1. Cell lines selected for transfection analysis of CFTR expression and localization should be at a passage number of between approximately 35 and 55 for best results. The reasons for this are twofold. First, at higher passage numbers, transformed cell lines tend to grow much more rapidly than at lower passages, and this can cause cells to form highly confluent cell layers in the time frame of the experiment that may detach, en masse, from the cover slips during the methanol permeablization and fixation procedure. This is especially problematic when analyzing HEK 293 cells. Second, cell crowding (not to be confused with cell–cell contacts important for the growth of some lines) can distort cell morphologies and impair interpretation of subcellular staining patterns. This is particularly important for colocalization experiments. For example, the cis-Golgi is in close proximity to the centrosome and may appear to colocalize with perinuclear inclusions such as those described here and elsewhere.

2. Methanol fixation, a technique long used by researchers investigating the cytoskeleton, is useful for the analysis of some cytoskeletal staining patterns such as the centrosome and microtubular and actin filament networks. This fixation procedure extracts a significant fraction of the cytoplasm, revealing subtle staining patterns, which would otherwise be masked by large signals originating in the cytoplasmic compartment. For example, staining for 20S proteasomes in detergent-permeabilized and paraformaldehyde-fixed cells is inadequate to visualize the fraction of this complex that associates with the ER membrane, cytoskeleton, or centrosome.

Acknowledgments

This work was supported by research grants from the American Heart Association and the NIH-NIDDK to PJT, the Cystic Fibrosis Foundation to MJC and PJT, and the Haberecht Foundation to WCW.

References

1. Riordan, J. R., Rommens, J. M., Kerem, B.-S., Alon, N., Rozmahel, R., Grzelczak, Z., Zielenski, J., Lok, S., Plavsic, N., Chou, J.-L., Drumm, M. L., Iannuzzi, M. C., Collins, F. S., and Tsui, L.-C. (1989) Identification of the cystic fibrosis gene: cloning and characterization of complementary DNA. *Science* **245**, 1066–1073.

2. Anderson, M. P., Gregory, R. J., Thompson, S., Souza, D. W., Paul, S., Mulligan, R. C., Smith, A. E., and Welsh, M. J. (1991) Demonstration that CFTR is a chloride channel by alteration of its anion selectivity. *Science* **253,** 202–205.

3. Bear, C. E., Duguay, F., Naismith, A. L., Kartner, N., Hanrahan, J. W., and Riordan, J. R. (1991) Cl- channel activity in Xenopus oocytes expressing the cystic fibrosis gene. *J. Biol. Chem.* **266,** 19,142–19,145.

4. Sheppard, D. N. and Welsh, M. J. (1999) Structure and function of the CFTR chloride channel. *Physiol. Rev.* **79,** S23–S45.

5. Lee, M. G., Wigley, W. C., Zeng, W., Noel, L. E., Marino, C. R., Thomas, P. J., and Muallem, S. (1999) Regulation of Cl^-/HCO_3^- exchange by cystic fibrosis transmembrane conductance regulator expressed in NIH 3T3 and HEK 293 cells. *J. Biol. Chem.* **274,** 3414–3421.

6. Schwiebert, E. M., Benos, D. J., Egan, M. E., Stutts, M. J., and Guggino, W. B. (1999) CFTR is a conductance regulator as well as a chloride channel. *Physiol. Rev.* **79[1],** S145–S166.

7. Thomas, P. J., Ko, Y. H., and Pedersen, P. L. (1992) Altered protein folding may be the molecular basis of most cases of cystic fibrosis. *FEBS Lett.* **312,** 7–9.

8. Cheng, S. H., Gregory, R. J., Marshall, J., Paul, S. , Souza, D. W., White, G. A., O'Riordan, C. R., and Smith, A. E. (1990) Defective intracellular transport and processing of CFTR is the molecular basis of most cystic fibrosis. *Cell* **63,** 827–834.

9. Lukacs, G. L., Mohamed, A., Kartner, N., Chang, X.-B., Riordan, J. R., and Grinstein, S. (1994) Conformational maturation of CFTR but not its mutant counterpart (F508) occurs in the endoplasmic reticulum and requires ATP. *EMBO J.* **13,** 6076–6086.

10. Ward, C. L. and Kopito, R. R. (1994) Intracellular turnover of cystic fibrosis transmembrane conductance regulator. Inefficient processing and rapid degradation of wild-type and mutant proteins. *J. Biol. Chem.* **269,** 25,710–25,718.

11. Yang, Y., Janich, S., Cohn, J. A., and Wilson, J. M. (1993) The common variant of cystic fibrosis transmembrane conductance regulator is recognized by hsp70 and degraded in a pre-Golgi nonlysosomal compartment. *Proc. Natl. Acad. Sci. USA* **90,** 9480–9484.

12. Strickland, E., Qu, B.-H., Millen, L., and Thomas, P. (1997) The molecular chaperone Hsc70 assists the *in vitro* folding of the N-terminal nucleotide-binding domain of the cystic fibrosis transmembrane conductance regulator. *J. Biol. Chem.* **272,** 25,421–25,424.

13. Meacham, G. C., Lu, Z., King, S., Sorscher, E., Tousson, A., and Cyr, D. M. (1999) The Hdj-2Hsc70 chaperone pair facilitates early steps in CFTR biogenesis. *EMBO J.* **18,** 1492–1505.

14. Loo, M. A., Jensen, T. J., Cui, L., Hou, Y.-X., Chang, X.-B., and Riordan, J. R. (1998) Perturbation of Hsp90 interaction with nascent CFTR prevents its maturation and accelerates its degradation by the proteasome. *EMBO J.* **17,** 6879–6887.

15. Pind, S., Riordan, J. R., and Williams, D. B. (1994) Participation of the endoplasmic reticulum chaperone calnexin (p88, IP90) in the biogenesis of the cystic fibrosis transmembrane conductance regulator. *J. Biol. Chem.* **269,** 12,784–12,788.

16. Ellgaard, L., Molinari, M., and Helenius, A. (1999) Setting the standards: quality control in the secretory pathway. *Science* **286,** 1882–1888.

17. Wigley, W. C., Fabunmi, R. P., Lee, M. G., Marino, C. R., Muallem, S., DeMartino, G. N., and Thomas, P. J. (1999) Dynamic association of proteasomal machinery with the centrosome. *J. Cell Biol.* **145,** 481–490.

18. Gilbert, A., Jadot, M., Leontieva, E., Wattiaux-De Coninck, S., and Wattiaux, R. (1998) F508 CFTR localizes in the endoplasmic reticulum-golgi intermediate compartment in cystic fibrosis cells. *Exp. Cell. Res.* **242,** 144–152.

19. Ward, C. L., Omura, S., and Kopito, R. R. (1995) Degragation of CFTR by the ubiquitin-proteasome pathway. *Cell* **83,** 121–127.

20. Jensen, T. J., Loo, M. A., Pind, S., Williams, D. B., Goldberg, A. L., and Riordan, J. R. (1995) Multiple proteolytic systems, including the proteasome, contribute to CFTR processing. *Cell* **83,** 129–135.

21. Coux, O., Tanaka, K., and Goldberg, A. L. (1996) Structure and functions of the 20S and 26S proteasomes. *Annu. Rev. Biochem.* **65,** 801–847.

22. Baumeister, W., Walz, J., Zuhl, F., and Seemuller, E. (1998) The proteasome: paradigm of a self-compartmentalizing protease. *Cell* **92,** 367–380.

23. Wenzel, T. and Baumeister, W. (1995) Conformational constraints in protein degradation by the 20S proteasome. *Nat. Struct. Biol.* **2,** 199–204.

24. Lowe, J., Stock, D., Jap, B., Zwickl, P., Baumeister, W., and Huber, R. (1995) Crystal structure of the 20S proteasome from the archaeon T. acidophilum at 3. 4 A resolution. *Science* **268,** 533–539.

25. Groll, M., Ditzel, L., Lowe, J., Stock, D., Bochtler, M., Bartunik, H. D., and Huber, R. (1997) Structure of 20S proteasome from yeast at 2. 4 A resolution. *Nature* **386,** 463-471.

26. Yoshimura, T., Kameyama, K., Takagi, T., Ikai, A. , Tokunaga, F., Koide, T., Tanahashi, N., Tamura, T., Cejka, Z., Baumeister, W., Tanaka, K., and Ichihara, A. (1993) Molecular characterization of the "26S" proteasome complex from rat liver. *J. Struct. Biol.* **111,** 200–211.

27. Adams, G. M., Falke, S., Goldberg, A. L., Slaughter, C. A., DeMartino, G. N., and Gogol, E. P. (1997) Structural and functional effects of PA700 and modulator protein on proteasomes. *J. Mol. Biol.* **273,** 646–657.

28. Hochstrasser, M. (1996) Ubiquitin-dependent protein degradation. *Annu. Rev. Genet.* **30,** 405–439.

29. Ciechanover, A. (1994) The ubiquitin-proteasome proteolytic pathway *Cell* **79,** 13–21.

30. Lam, Y. A., Xu, W., DeMartino, G. N., and Cohen, R. E. (1997) Editing of ubiquitin conjugates by an isopeptidase in the 26S proteasome. *Nature* **385,** 737–740.

31. Ma, C.-P., Vu, J. H., Proske, R. J., Slaughter, C. A., and DeMartino, G. N. (1994) Identification, purification, and characterization of a high molecular weight ATP-dependent activator (PA700) of the 20S proteasome. *J. Biol. Chem.* **269,** 3539–3547.

32. Gray, C. W., Slaughter, C. A., and DeMartino, G. N. (1994) PA28 activator protein forms regulatory caps on proteasome stacked rings. *J. Mol. Biol.* **236,** 7–15.

33. Dubiel, W., Pratt, G., Ferrell, K., and Rechsteiner, M. (1992) Purification of an 11S regulator of the multicatalytic protease. *J. Biol. Chem.* **267,** 22,369–22,377.

34. Ma, C.-P., Slaughter, C. A., and DeMartino, G. N. (1992) Identification, purification, and characterization of a protein activator (PA28) of the 20 S proteasome (macropain) *J. Biol. Chem.* **267,** 10,515–10,523.
35. Groettrup, M., Soza, A., Eggers. M., Kuehn, L., Dick, T. P., Schild, H., Rammensee, H.-G., Koszinowski, U. H., and Kloetzel, P.-M. (1996) A role for the proteasome regulator PA28a in antigen presentation. *Nature* **381,** 166–168.
36. Kloetzel, P. M., Soza, A., and Stohwasser, R. (1999) The role of the proteasome system and the proteasome activator PA28 complex in the cellular immune response. *Biol. Chem.* **380,** 293–297.
37. Xiong, X., Chong, E., and Skach, W. R. (1999) Evidence that endoplasmic reticulum (ER)-associated degradation of cystic fibrosis transmembrane conductance regulator is linked to retrograde translocation from the ER membrane. *J. Biol. Chem.* **274,** 2616–2624.
38. Sato, S., Ward, C. L., and Kopito, R. R. (1998) Cotranslational ubiquitination of cystic fibrosis transmembrane conductance regulator in vitro. *J. Biol. Chem.* **273,** 7189–7192.
39. Plemper, R. K. and Wolf, D. H. (1999) Retrograde protein translocation: ERADication of secretory proteins in health and disease. *Trends Biochem. Sci.* **24,** 266–270.
40. Plemper, R. K. and Wolf, D. H. (1999) Endoplasmic reticulum degradation. Reverse protein transport and its end in the proteasome. *Mol. Biol. Rep.* **26,** 125–130.
41. Sommer, T. and Wolf, D. H. (1997) Endoplasmic reticulum degradation: reverse protein flow of no return. *FASEB J.* **11,** 1227–1233.
42. Bebok, Z., Mazzochi, C., King, S. A., Hong, J. S., and Sorscher, E. J. (1998) The mechanism underlying cystic fibrosis transmembrane conductance regulator transport from the endoplasmic reticulum to the proteasome includes Sec61beta and a cytosolic deglycosylated intermediary. *J. Biol. Chem.* **273,** 29,873–29,878.
43. Xiong, X., Bragin, A., Widdicombe, J. H., Cohn, J., and Skach, W. R. (1997) Structural cues involved in endoplasmic reticulum degradation of G85E and G91R mutant cystic fibrosis transmembrane conductance regulator. *J. Clin. Invest* **100,** 1079–1088.
44. Plemper, R. K., Deak, P. M., Otto, R. T., and Wolf, D. H. (1999) Re-entering the translocon from the lumenal side of the endoplasmic reticulum. Studies on mutated carboxypeptidase yscY species. *FEBS Lett.* **443,** 241–245.
45. Plemper, R. K., Egner, R., Kuchler, K., and Wolf, D. H. (1998) Endoplasmic reticulum degradation of a mutated ATP-binding cassette transporter Pdr5 proceeds in a concerted action of Sec61 and the proteasome. *J. Biol. Chem.* **273,** 32,848–32,856.
46. Wickner, S., Maurizi, M. R., and Gottesman, S. (1999) Posttranslational quality control: folding, refolding, and degrading proteins. *Science* **286,** 1888–1893.
47. Agashe, V. R. and Hartl, F. U. (2000) Roles of molecular chaperones in cytoplasmic protein folding. *Semin. Cell Dev. Biol.* **11,** 15–25.
48. Thomas, P. J., Qu, B.-H., and Pedersen, P. L. (1995) Defective protein folding as a basis of human disease. *TIBS* **20,** 456–459.
49. Gottesman, S., Wickner, S., and Maurizi, M. R. (1997) Protein quality control: triage by chaperones and proteases. *Genes Dev.* **11,** 815–823.
50. Bercovich, B., Stancovski, I., Mayer, A., Blumenfeld, N., Laszlo, A., Schwartz, A., and Ciechanover, A. (1997) Ubiquitin-dependent degradation of certain protein substrates *in vitro* requires the molecular chaperone Hsc70. *JBC* **272,** 9002–9010.

51. Strickland, E., Hakala, K., Thomas, P. J., and DeMartino, G. N. (2000) Recognition of misfolding proteins by PA700, the regulatory subcomplex of the 26 S proteasome. *J. Biol. Chem.* **275**, 5565–5572.
52. Johnston, J. A., Ward, C. L., and Kopito, R. R. (1998) Aggresomes: A Cellular Response to Misfolded Proteins. *J. Cell Biol.* **143**, 1883–1898.
53. Lange, B. M., Bachi, A., Wilm, M., and Gonzalez, C. (2000) Hsp90 is a core centrosomal component and is required at different stages of the centrosome cycle in Drosophila and vertebrates. *EMBO J.* **19**, 1252–1262.
54. Brown, C. R., Doxsey, S. J., Hong-Brown, L. Q., Martin, R. L., and Welch, W. J. (1996) Molecular chaperones and the centrosome. A role for TCP-1 in microtubule nucleation. *J. Biol. Chem.* **271**, 824–832.
55. Brown, C. R., Hong-Brown, L. Q., Doxsey, S. J., and Welch, W. J. (1996) Molecular chaperones and the centrosome. A role for HSP 73 in centrosomal repair following heat shock treatment. *J. Biol. Chem.* **271**, 833–840.
56. Chen, E. Y., Bartlett, M. C., and Clarke, D. M. (2000) Cystic fibrosis transmembrane conductance regulator has an altered structure when its maturation is inhibited. *Biochemistry* **39**, 3797–3803.
57. Fabunmi, R. P., Wigley, W. C., Thomas, P. J., and DeMartino, G. N. (2000) Activity and regulation of the centrosome-associated proteasome. *J. Biol. Chem.* **275**, 409–413.
58. Doxsey, S. J. (1998) The centrosome—a tiny organelle with big potential. *Nature Genetics* **20**, 104–106.
59. Zimmerman, W., Sparks, C. A., and Doxsey, S. J. (1999) Amourphous no longer: the centrosome comes into focus. *Curr. Opin. Cell Biol.* **11**, 122–128.
60. Urbani, L. and Stearns, T. (1999) The centrosome. *Curr. Biol.* **9**, R315–R317.
61. Koepp, D. M., Harper, J. W., and Eledge, S. J. (1999) How the Cyclin Became a Cyclin: Tegulated Proteolysis in the Cell Cycle. *Cell* **97**, 431–434.
62. Bailly, E., Pines, J., Hunter, T., and Bornens, M. (1992) Cytoplasmic accumulation of cyclin B1 in human cells: association with a detergent-resistant compartment and with the centrosome. *J. Cell. Sci.* **101**, 529–545.
63. Brown, C. R., Doxsey, S. J., White, E., and Welch, W. J. (1994) Both viral (adenovirus E1B) and cellular (hsp70, p53) components interact with centrosomes. *J. Cell. Physiol.* **160**, 47–60.
64. Crepieux, P., Kwon, H., Leclerc, N., Spencer, W., Richard, S., Lin, R., and Hiscott, J. (1997) IKBa physically interacts with a cytoskeleton-associated protein through its signal response domain. *Mol. Cell. Biol.* **17**, 7375–7385.
65. Zeng, W., Lee, M. G., Yan, M., Diaz, J., Benjamin, I., Marino, C. R., Kopito, R., Freedman, S., Cotton, C., Muallem, S., and Thomas, P. (1997) Immuno and functional characterization of CFTR in submandibular and pancreatic acinar and duct cells. *Am. J. Physiol.* **273**, C442–C455.
66. Ma, C.-P., Willy, P. J., Slaughter, C. A., and DeMartino, G. N. (1993) PA28, an activator of the 20s proteasome, is inactivated by proteolytic modification of its carboxyl terminus. *J. Biol. Chem.* **268**, 22,514–22,519.

20

In Vitro Reconstitution of CFTR Biogenesis and Degradation

Jon Oberdorf and William R. Skach

1. Introduction

1.1. Proteasome-Mediated Protein Degradation

The regulated degradation of cellular proteins occurs primarily through the ATP-dependent ubiquitin/proteasome pathway (*1*). One function of this pathway is to control the quality of nascent proteins (*2*). In this process ubiquitin-conjugating enzymes and ubiquitin-protein ligases create isopeptide bonds linking the 8-kDa ubiquitin polypeptide to lysine residues on the target protein. Additional ubiquitin molecules are added via ubiquitin–ubiquitin isopeptide bonds until the resulting chain is recognized by a large multicatalytic protease, the 26S proteasome. This proteolytic machine is formed through the ATP-dependent association of two multimeric components, the 20S proteasome and the 19S regulatory subunit. The 19S subunit recognizes the polyubiquitinated protein, removes the ubiquitin chains, and feeds the protein into the 20S proteasome, a toroidal cylinder composed of four stacked heptameric rings (*3*). The two outer rings are comprised of α subunits that bind the 19S particles. The inner rings consist of ß subunits, three of which exhibit distinct protease activities. These Pup1/Z/beta$_2$, Pre2/X/beta$_5$, and Pre3/Y/beta$_1$ subunits preferentially cleave substrates after basic, hydrophobic, or acidic residues, respectively (*4,5*). These cleavage specificities are responsible for the trypsin-like (T-L), chymotrypsin-like (ChT-L), and caspase-like (CP-L) activities characteristic of eukaryotic proteasomes. The hallmark of proteasome-mediated degradation is ATP-dependent conversion of substrate into small peptide fragments 6–20 amino acids in length (*6*).

From: *Methods in Molecular Medicine, vol. 70: Cystic Fibrosis Methods and Protocols*
Edited by: W. R. Skach © Humana Press Inc., Totowa, NJ

1.2. Endoplasmic Reticulum-Associated Degradation (ERAD)

In the endoplasmic reticulum (ER), misfolded transmembrane and secreted proteins are degraded by the ubiquitin–proteasome pathway via a process referred to as ER-associated degradation (ERAD) *(7)*. In most individuals with cystic fibrosis, inherited mutations in the cystic fibrosis transmembrane conductance regulator (CFTR) gene result in enhanced degradation of newly synthesized CFTR protein by the ERAD pathway *(8,8a)*. Current evidence suggests that these mutations disrupt CFTR folding and lead to an alternate or intermediate protein structure that is recognized by ER quality control machinery *(9,10)*. Precisely how cells recognize and degrade mutant CFTR remains unknown. However, cellular chaperones that participate in nascent protein folding appear to either promote CFTR maturation *(11)* or direct CFTR toward ERAD degradation *(12,12a)*. The net result of these, and possibly additional, interactions, therefore determines the balance of CFTR that is successfully packaged in the ER and delivered to the plasma membrane.

To understand better how the fate of CFTR is determined, we have reconstituted the ERAD pathway in vitro using CFTR synthesized in native ER membranes *(13)*. This chapter describes techniques for the in vitro expression of full-length, glycosylated and membrane-integrated CFTR using a rabbit reticulocyte lysate expression system. Although the procedures described here use canine pancreas rough microsomes (CRM) as a source of ER, functional ER membranes from other sources (e.g., *Xenopus laevis* oocytes *[14,15]* or semipermeabilized cells *[16]*) could potentially be used as well. Once translation is complete, microsomes containing newly synthesized CFTR are used to follow proteasome-mediated degradation. Because only the protein of interest contains incorporated radioisotope, it is possible to monitor the direct conversion of CFTR into trichloroacetic acid (TCA)-soluble peptide fragments. This technique therefore provides a significant advantage over cell-based degradation assays that detect the loss of specific epitopes. The in vitro system is also more flexible because microsomes and lysate can be modified pharmacologically and/or biochemically either before or during the degradation reaction. Finally, because ER membranes are the only cellular organelle present, CFTR processing is limited to early events localized to the ER compartment. While this latter point has proven to be a distinct advantage in studying many ER-related processes, it should be noted that in reconstituted systems, certain events may occur more slowly or less efficiently than in intact cells. It is therefore important to correlate in-vitro and in-vivo results when possible.

We will also describe the use of fluorogenic peptide substrates to assay the individual protease activities of the 26S proteasome. This technique has enabled us to determine the relative contribution of specific beta subunits toward CFTR degradation. The fluorogenic assays can also be used to track proteasome activity during fractionation protocols. Used together, peptidase and degradation assays can more accurately determine now the proteasome facilitates protein degradation in the ERAD pathway.

2. Materials

2.1. Preparation of RRL

2.1.1. Rabbit Injection to Induce Reticulocyte Formation

1. New Zealand White rabbits (~6 mo old, ≥ 3 kg).
2. 3-mL syringes (no. of rabbits $\times$ 3).
3. 26-gage needles.
4. Clinical centrifuge with rotor suitable for hematocrit determination (e.g., IEC rotor 927).
5. Hematocrit reader, hematocrit tubes, and clay to plug tubes.
6. Acetyl phenyl hydrazine (APH) solution: Add 2.5 g of APH to 20 mL of ethanol, then add 50 mL of water. pH to 7.0 with ~1 mL of 1 M KOH, and bring to 100 mL with water. Filter solution (0.22 μm), aliquot, and store at –20°C.

2.1.2. Collection and Processing of Reticulocyte Lysate

1. Rabbit restrainer.
2. Pentobarbital/nembutal (50 mg/mL, 4–5 mL per rabbit).
3. Heparin (1000 U/mL, 2 mL per rabbit).
4. 70% isopropanol.
5. Syringes, 10 mL, 30 mL, 60 mL.
6. Three-way stop valve.
7. Butterfly needles (23-gage).
8. Hypodermic needles (16-gage).
9. IV tubing (e.g., extension set no. ET-20L (472010) from B/Braun: 21-in.-long tubing.
10. Small surgical instruments: forceps, scalpel, and blades.
11. Gauze wipes.
12. Diethyl pyrocarbamate (DEPC, Sigma, St. Louis MO).
13. 250-mL centrifuge bottles (1 per rabbit).
14. 50-mL polypropylene centrifuge tubes (DEPC-treated).
15. Filtered RNAse-free, double-distilled, ice-cold water.
16. Reticulocyte wash buffer: 5 mM glucose, 0.14 M NaCl, 0.05 M KCl, 5 mM MgCl$_2$ (~500 mL per rabbit).
17. Micrococcal nuclease (US Biochemicals), 15 U/μL in 10 mM Tris-HCl (pH 8.0) or RNAse-free water. Store in aliquots at –80°C.
18. 0.1 M CaCl$_2$.
19. 0.1 M EGTA.
20. 1 mM hemin stock solution. Combine reagents in the following order: 6.44 mg hemin (Sigma, bovine crystalline type I), 0.25 mL of 1 M KOH, 0.5 mL of 0.2 M Tris-HCl, pH 7.0–8.0, 8.9 mL of ethylene glycol, 0.19 mL of 1 N HCl, 0.05 mL of H$_2$O. Filter (0.22-μm) and store at –20°C.

2.2. Fluorogenic Proteasome Assay

2.2.1. AMC Assay Substrates

AMC assay substrates are prepared at 10 mM in DMSO and stored at –80°C.

1. N-succinyl-leu-leu-val-tyr amido-methylcoumarin (LLVY-AMC) (Sigma, St. Louis, MO).
2. N-t-boc-leu-arg-arg amido-methylcoumarin (LRR-AMC) (Sigma).
3. 7-Amido-4-methylcoumarin (AMC) (Sigma).
4. Z-leu-leu-glu amido-methylcoumarin (LLE-AMC), (CalBiochem, San Diego, CA, listed as "proteasome substrate II").

2.2.2. Solutions

1. Buffer A: 100 mM Tris-HCl, pH 8.0, 1 mM ATP, 1 mM dithiothreitol (DTT).
2. Buffer B: mix 10 μL of 10× degradation buffer (**Subheading 2.5., item 1**), 20 μL of sucrose buffer (**Subheading 2.5., item 2**), 2 μL of creatine kinase (**Subheading 2.4.2., item 6**).
3. Dilution buffer: 100 mM Tris-HCl, pH 9.0.
4. Sedimentation buffer: 20 mM Tris-HCl, pH 7.5, 1 mM ATP, 1 mM MgCl$_2$, 1 mM DTT.
5. 10% sodium dodecyl sulfate (SDS) in water.
6. Untreated RRL or a 290K pellet from RRL (**Subheading 3.1., step 6**).
7. 96-well opaque plates (Costar, cat. no. 3915).
8. Bio-Rad FluoroMark plate reader (355Ex/460Em).

2.3. Preparation of ER Microsomal Membranes

1. Pancreas tissue source (*see* **Subheading 3.3., step 1**).
2. 50-mL Potter-Elvehem tissue homogenizer with Teflon pestles (one loose-fitting and one snug).
3. 25-mL Potter-Elvehem tissue homogenizer (Teflon pestle).
4. Electric drive for homogenizer.
5. Surgical instruments: scalpel, forceps, large scissors, small scissors, 3 hemostats.
6. Hand-held food processor or parsley grinder.
7. Baked or DEPC-treated glassware and centrifuge tubes.
8. 10× stock buffer (100 mL): 0.5 M K acetate, 60 mM Mg acetate, 10 mM EDTA, and 0.5 M triethanolamine acetate, pH 7.5.
9. Buffer C: 1/10 dilution of 10× stock buffer containing 0.25 M sucrose, 1 mM DTT and 0.5 mM phenylmethylsulfonyl fluoride (PMSF). Add DTT and PMSF immediately before use.
10. Buffer D: 1/10 dilution of 10× stock buffer containing 1.3 M sucrose
11. Buffer E (100 mL): 50 mM triethanolamine, 0.25 M sucrose. Add 1 mM DTT immediately before using.

2.4. In Vitro Transcription and Translation

All reagents, solutions, and containers used for transcription and translation must be kept RNAse-free.

2.4.1. Transcription Buffers

1. 5× transcription buffer: 30 mM MgCl$_2$, 10 mM spermidine, 200 mM Tris-HCl (pH 7.5).
2. 10× NTPs: 5 mM ATP, 5 mM CTP, 5 mM UTP, 1 mM GTP, 20 mM Tris-HCl, pH 8.0. Nucleotides were purchased from Roche Molecular Biochemicals (Indianapolis, IN).
3. Diguanosine triphosphate (GpppG, Promega): Dissolve 25 U in 300 μL water (~ 5 mM) and store at –80°C.
4. 0.1 M DTT (Roche Molecular Biochemicals).
5. tRNA (10 mg/mL, bovine liver type XI, Sigma).
6. RNAse inhibitor (20 U/mL, Promega).
7. SP6 polymerase (20 U/mL, Epicenter).

2.4.2. Translation Reagents

1. 20× translation buffer: 2 M K acetate, 16 mM Mg acetate, and 40 mM Tris-acetate, pH 7.5.
2. Emix: 5 mM ATP, 5 mM GTP, 60 mM creatine phosphate, 0.2 mM of all 19 amino acids except methionine, and 5 μCi/μL Trans^{35}S-label (ICN, Costa Mesa, CA). Aliquots are typically made in volumes of 100–200 μL, adjusted to pH 7.4 with Tris base, and stored at –80°C.
3. Rabbit reticulocyte lysate (hemin and nuclease treated—*see* **Subheading 3.1., step 7**).
4. 10 mg/mL tRNA (from bovine liver type XI, Sigma).
5. 20 U/mL RNAse inhibitor (Promega).
6. Creatine kinase (CK): Dissolve creatine kinase (Sigma) 4 mg/mL in 50% glycerol, 10 mM Tris-acetate, pH 7.5. Store at –20°C.
7. Microsomal membranes (nuclease treated—see **Subheading 3.3.**).
8. SDS loading buffer (SDS-LB): 4% SDS, 2 mM EDTA, 10% sucrose, 0.05% bromophenol blue, 1 M DTT, and 100 mM Tris-HCl, pH 8.9.
9. Aurin tricarboxylic acid (ATA): 1–2 mM aurin tricarboxylic acid (adjusted to pH ~7.0 with Tris base).

2.5. In Vitro Degradation Assay

1. 10× degradation buffer: 10 mM ATP, 120 mM creatine phosphate, 30 mM DTT, 50 mM MgCl$_2$, 100 mM Tris-HCl, pH 7.5.
2. 0.1 M sucrose buffer: 0.1 M sucrose, 100 mM KCl, 5 mM MgCl$_2$ 1 mM DTT, and 50 mM HEPES-KOH, pH 7.5.
3. 0.5 M sucrose buffer: 0.5 M sucrose, 100 mM KCl, 5 mM MgCl$_2$, 1 mM DTT, and 50 mM HEPES-KOH, pH 7.5.
4. Creatine kinase (CK) (*see* **Subheading 2.4.2., item 6**).
5. Hexokinase stock: dissolve in water at 2000 U/mL (Sigma).
6. 2 M deoxyglucose.
7. 20% trichloroacetic acid.
8. Ready-Safe scintillation fluid (Beckman, Fullerton, CA).
9. 1 mM hemin stock solution (*see* **Subheading 2.1.2., item 21**).

10. MG132 (10 mM in DMSO—from Sigma, listed as "*n*-cbz-leu-leu-leu-al").
11. Scintillation counter (e.g., LS 6500, Beckman, Fullerton, CA).
12. Tabletop ultracentrifuge (e.g., Optima TLX, Beckmann).

3. Methods

3.1. Preparation of RRL

A significant advantage of *de novo* RRL preparation is that the composition and quality of reaction conditions can be controlled and optimized when assembled from its component parts. Several commercial preparations of RRL are available for in-vitro translation (e.g., Promega). However, if large numbers of experiments are to be performed it is often more economical to prepare this reagent. The following procedure is used routinely in our laboratory. It is based on protocol previously described by Jackson et al. *(17)* and takes roughly 1 wk from start to finish. Typically 5–10 rabbits are processed simultaneously, which generates enough reagent to last for several months to a year or more (*see* **Note 1**).

1. All steps involving the handling and care of animals should be approved by the institutional animal review board.
2. Inject rabbits subcutaneously in scruff of neck on three consecutive days (d 1, 2, and 3) with 2 mL of APH solution.
3. On d 4–7, monitor animals for health, activity, and food intake. Hematocrits may be measured in selected animals by collecting blood samples in a capillary tube (via ear vein puncture). Centrifuge blood at ~8000g for 5 min and read hematocrit directly. The hematocrit should normally not fall below 20%.
4. On d 8, place rabbits in a restrainer, cannulate an ear vein with a 23-gage butterfly needle connected to a three-way stopcock, and inject 2 mL of heparin (2000 U), followed by a lethal dose of pentobarbital (200–250 mg) 1 min later. When rabbit has lost eyelid reflex and respiration has ceased, remove the animal from restrainer, transect left ribs with a scalpel, open chest cavity and puncture left ventricle directly with 16-gage needle attached to IV extension tubing. Collect blood in 250-mL centrifuge bottle on ice and collect any remaining pooled venous blood in chest cavity. Perform all subsequent steps on ice.
5. Centrifuge blood at 2500g at 4°C for 10 min and discard supernatant (and buffy coat layer of white blood cells). Wash cells three times with 150 mL of ice-cold reticulocyte wash buffer, collecting cells each time by centrifugation at 2500g for 10 min. After the third wash resuspend cells in small volume of wash buffer, transfer to 50-mL conical tube, centrifuge at 3000g for 10 min, and remove supernatant. Add equal volume of ice-cold H_2O and shake very vigorously for 30 s to lyse cells. Repeat shaking every 5 min, three times. Centrifuge lysate at 15,000g for 10 min and carefully decant supernatant. Lysate can be frozen in liquid nitrogen at this stage (15- to 50-mL conical tubes) and stored at –80°C for several years with minimal loss of activity. We typically aliquot several additional small samples (~0.5 mL) to determine relative activity in translation and/or degradation assays (*see* **Note 1**).

6. For degradation reactions, the lysate is used without further modification (*see* **Note 2**).

7. For translation reactions, hemin is added to a final concentration of 40 µM and endogenous RRL RNA is digested by nuclease treatment. To perform the latter, a 1-mL aliquot of RRL is quickly thawed in a 25°C water bath. Then, 10 µL of 0.1 M $CaCl_2$ and 10 µL of micrococcal nuclease are added and the sample is incubated for 8–10 min at 25°C. Then 20 µL of 0.1 M EGTA is added and the sample is aliquoted, frozen in liquid nitrogen, and stored at –80°C for 2–3 mo.

3.2. Analysis of RRL Proteasome Activity Using Fluorogenic Peptide Assay

A major advantage of using an in vitro system to reconstitute ERAD is that the reaction conditions are directly amenable to manipulation by proteasome inhibitors and other agents *(13)*. Moreover, the effect of inhibitors on ChT-L, T-L, and PGPH activities of the 20S and 26S proteasome can be measured directly using a relatively simple fluorogenic assay *(18)*. Here amido-methylcoumarin (AMC) becomes highly fluorescent when it is cleaved from the carboxy terminus of short peptide sequences that are specific for each beta-subunit activity. Specificity depends primarily on the carboxy-terminal amino acid of the peptide (*see* **Note 3**).

1. Assay of diluted RRL according to Kanayama et al. *(19)*: Initial operations are performed at 4°C. For ChT-L assay dilute untreated RRL 1/100 with assay buffer A containing 100 µM LLVY-AMC. For T-L and CP-L activities, dilute untreated RRL 1/30 with buffer A containing 100 µM LRR-AMC and 100 µM LLE-AMC, respectively. While samples are still on ice, take 10-µL aliquots and add to 10 µL of 10% SDS (pre-aliquot the SDS into a 96-well opaque plate at room temperature). Wait ~1 min and dilute the SDS-inactivated samples with either 200 µL of dilution buffer alone (to determine background fluorescence), or 200 µL of dilution buffer containing AMC at a concentration that generates a desired reference value (e.g., 2.5 µM AMC in 200 µL of dilution buffer will be the equivalent of 500 pmol or 50 µM AMC in a 10-µL sample volume). Transfer remaining sample mixtures to a 37°C water bath, and take timed samples (10 µL of sample into 10 µL of 10% SDS followed by 200 µL of dilution buffer) at 10, 20, and 30 min for ChT-L activity and at 30, 60, and 90 min for T-L and CP-L activities. (The adjustments in RRL concentration and length of incubation are made because LLVY-AMC is hydrolyzed more readily than the other substrates. For all conditions, however, hydrolysis should be linear with time.)

2. Assay RRL proteasome activity under conditions used to measure CFTR degradation (*see* **Subheading 3.5.2.**). To compensate for the high level of proteasome activity in undiluted RRL, the procedure in **step 1** must be modified. Add 1 µL of 10 mM AMC-coupled substrate (LLVY, LLE, or LRR) to 32 µL of assay buffer B. Background and reference samples are acquired by sequentially adding 3.2 µL of this solution (buffer B + AMC) and 6.8 µL of untreated RRL to 10 µL of 10% SDS before diluting with 200 µL of dilution buffer. Warm remaining buffer B + AMC and untreated RRL in separate tubes to 37°C and combine at a 33/67 ratio to

start assay. Add 10-μL to aliquots of this RRL mixture to 10 μL of 10% SDS at 20, 40, and 60 s for LLVY-AMC assay, or at 1, 2, and 3 min for LLE-AMC and LRR-AMC, before diluting with 200 μL of dilution buffer.

3. Quantitation: When all samples are processed, read the fluorescence of free AMC in a fluorescent plate reader (e.g., Bio-Rad FluoroMark) at 355Ex/460Em. Dilute reactions (**step 1**) can be referenced to a predetermined AMC standard curve, but parallel background and standard determinations are recommended when the fluorescence of added agents or the quenching by the RRL may be significant (The high concentration of RRL used in **step 2** quenches 80% of AMC fluorescence, but background fluorescence of the standard curve is similarly quenched, so accuracy is not significantly compromised).
   Results are calculated according to the formula:

(Sample value – background value) × (ref. amount of AMC [500 pmoles]/ref. value)

4. Separation of proteasomes from low-molecular-weight proteases: Proteasome fluorogenic substrates may also be hydrolyzed by other cellular proteases. Most other proteases, however, will have a molecular weight of <200 kDa and can be separated from the proteasome by either glycerol gradient or differential centrifugation (*see* **Note 3**). To perform the latter, dilute untreated RRL 1/5 with sedimentation buffer and centrifuge at 290,000*g* for 2 h. Resuspend the resulting pellet in a small volume of the same buffer, split into aliquots, flash-freeze in liquid nitrogen, and store at –80°C. This material can subsequently be used to measure proteasome activities according to the procedure described in **step 1**. Although this 290K pellet may more accurately measure proteasome activity in the RRL, the extent to which it measures 26S vs 20S proteasome activity will depend on the substrate used (*see* **Note 4**).

3.3. Preparation of ER Microsomes

Our canine pancreas microsome preparation is based on the procedure described by Walter and Blobel *(20)*. Because microsomal preparations are used for cell-free translation, all solutions and supplies must be RNAse-free.

1. Remove pancreas from euthanized animal and immediately place into 100 mL of ice-cold buffer C (*see* **Note 5**). Trim away fat, connective tissue, and blood vessels, and record dry weight. Grind pancreas by hand using an ice-cold food mill or parsley grinder (or equivalent), until a coarse pulpy consistency is achieved. Collect fragments in a 500-mL beaker together with 4 vol (4 mL/g of original tissue) of ice cold buffer C.

2. Homogenize this mixture in a 50-mL Potter-Elvehem tissue homogenizer attached to a high-speed motor with 3–4 passes of a loose-fitting Teflon pestle. Homogenize solution a second time with three passes of a tight-fitting Teflon pestle. Sample must be kept ice-cold during the entire procedure.

3. Divide homogenate into 50-mL polyallomer tubes and centrifuge at 600*g* for 10 min. Decant supernatant into fresh 50-mL polyallomer tubes and centrifuge at 10,000*g* for 10 min. Decant the resulting supernatant into a 150-mL beaker, taking care not to dislodge the loose pellet.

4. Carefully layer ~15–20 mL of supernatant fraction over a 5-mL cushion of buffer D and centrifuge at 150,000g for 3 h. Carefully aspirate supernatant. Transfer pellets to a baked 25-mL homogenizer and gently resuspend microsomes (by hand) in buffer E (0.5 mL/g of starting material. When the solution is uniform, aliquot and freeze 1-mL aliquots in liquid nitrogen. Microsomes are stable for several years in this state when stored at –80°C.
5. Determine the OD$_{280}$ by dissolving 10 μL of membrane suspension in 990 μL of 20 mM Tris-HCl (pH 8.0), 1% SDS. This provides a useful reference to determine the relative translocation efficiency of different microsomal preps.
6. Before use, endogenous mRNA is digested with micrococcal nuclease via the same procedure described for RRL (*see* **Subheading 3.1., step 7**). Typically, 1 mL of microsomes are treated, frozen in liquid nitrogen as 50- to 100-μL aliquots, and stored at –80°C for up to 3 mo.
7. Test microsomes for their efficiency at translocation and glycosylation by titrating membranes into translation reactions expressing appropriate control secretory and/or membrane proteins. Optimal preparations yield ≥90% membrane integration and ~80% core glycosylation of in vitro-synthesized CFTR (*see* **Note 6**).

3.4. Cell-Free Transcription and Translation

Transcription reactions are usually made up fresh in 10–50 μL volumes or stored as aliquots at –80°C. The following conditions can be used for either SP6 or T7 RNA polymerase.

1. To assemble a 20-μL transcription reaction, the following reagents are combined on ice: 4 μL of 5× transcription buffer, 2 μL of 10× NTPs, 2 μL of 0.1 M DTT, 2 μL of GpppG, 0.4 μL tRNA, 0.8 μL of RNase inhibitor, 0.8 μL of SP6 polymerase, and 8 μL of plasmid DNA (1 mg/mL). Incubate for 1 h at 40°C (37°C for T7 polymerase) and transfer immediately to ice.
2. Translation reactions are linked to transcription so that no purification or extraction of RNA is necessary. The composition of translation buffers takes into account the ionic contributions of the transcript which under normal conditions constitutes 20% of the translation volume. To assemble a 100-μL translation reaction, combine 5 μL of 20× translation buffer, 20 μL Emix, 40 μL RRL (nuclease treated with hemin), 1 μL RNAse inhibitor, 1 μL CK, 20 μL transcription mixture, 10 μL microsomes (actual volume is determined empirically), and 3 μL H$_2$O. Incubate at 24°C for 15 min. Add 5 μL of ATA (0.05–0.1 mM final concentration), and incubate for an additional 1 h and 45 min. Transfer reaction to ice (*see* **Note 7**).
3. Certain components may need to be titrated for optimal translation of individual transcripts. Typical concentrations for potassium and magnesium vary between 50–150 mM and 0.5–2.5 mM, respectively. High concentrations of microsomes inhibit translation, whereas low concentrations yield low translocation and glycosylation efficiencies. For large proteins such as CFTR (140 kDa), ATA (an inhibitor of translation initiation) is added (~50–100 μM) to synchronize transla-

tion and increase the ratio of full-length protein to partially synthesized fragments. Optimal concentration of Mg, K, and the timing of ATA addition should be determined empirically to maximize translation efficiency (*see* **Note 8**). For small proteins, ATA is usually not needed.

3.5. In Vitro Reconstitution of ERAD

The RRL translation system provides a ready source of core glycosylated CFTR integrated in native ER membranes. Following translation, ER microsomes are first isolated from the translation reaction by pelleting through a sucrose cushion and then reconstituted in degradation reactions of defined composition.

3.5.1. Collection and Resuspension of Microsomal Membranes

1. Dilute translation mixture with two volumes of 0.1 *M* sucrose buffer and layer mixture onto a cushion (0.3–0.7 mL) containing 0.5 *M* sucrose buffer. Centrifuge at 180,000g for 10 min, and wash membrane pellet by carefully overlaying and immediately aspirating 1 mL of 0.1 *M* sucrose buffer. This should remove nearly all of the free ^{35}S-methionine present in the translation reaction.
2. Physically dislodge the membrane pellet in 40 µL (~1/2 of original translation volume) of 0.1 *M* sucrose buffer with a 200-µL pipet tip. Vigorously titurate the solution with the end of the pipet tip placed tightly against the bottom of the tube so that the buffer (and pellet) slowly squeezes through the opening. It is critical to continue tituration until the entire pellet is completely resuspended. Recool the tube on ice if necessary (*see* **Note 9**).

3.5.2. Monitoring Substrate Degradation

For CFTR degradation, individual reactions as small as 25 µL can be used, although 50-µL reactions seem to give more reproducible results. Our usual protocol is to divide a single large reaction mixture into equal aliquots to test several conditions simultaneously—ATP depletion, proteasome inhibition, and so on. For a 200-µL total volume:

1. Combine on ice, 20 µL of 10× degradation buffer, 136 µL of untreated RRL (*see* **Subheading 3.1., step 6**), 40 µL of resuspended microsomes containing radiolabeled CFTR (from **Subheading 3.4.**). For ATP depletion, remove 49 µL and to this aliquot add 0.5 µL hexokinase and 0.5 µL deoxyglucose. To the remaining 147 µL sample, add 3 µL of creatine kinase and split into three additional 50-µL samples. Use one sample for control degradation (no additional changes), and use the remaining samples for desired experimental conditions (e.g., proteasome inhibition).
2. At time $T = 0$, remove 3 µL aliquots from each 50-µL reaction mixture and place one in 2.5 mL of scintillation fluid containing 250 µL of 20% TCA, another in 300 µL of 20% TCA (on ice), and a third in 30 µLof SDS-LB.

3. Transfer remaining reaction mixtures to a 37°C incubator (*see* **Note 7**). At desired time points, remove two 3-μL aliquots and place one in SDS-LB and the other into 300 μL of 20% TCA (*see* **Note 10**).

4. At the completion of the time course, centrifuge all TCA samples at 15,000*g* for 15 min (4°C), and transfer 250 μL of supernatant to 2.5 mL of scintillation fluid. Count samples in scintillation counter (e.g., Beckman LS6500 or equivalent).

5. Substrate degradation can be monitored by either of two techniques: (a) direct visualization by sodium dodecyl sulfate-polyacrylamide gel electrophoresis (SDS-PAGE) or (b) scintillation counting. For SDS-PAGE, samples collected into SDS-LB are incubated for 30 min at 37°C, centrifuged at 15,000*g* for 2 min, separated on a 7% acrylamide gel, and processed for autoradiography using EN³HANCE fluorography according to the manufacturer's instructions (NEN Life Science Products, Boston, MA).

6. To determine the extent of CFTR conversion into TCA-soluble fragments, TCA soluble counts are first multiplied by 1.2 to correct for the fraction of TCA sample recovered (e.g., 250 μL of 300 μL). The percent of CFTR degradation is then calculated using the following formula:

$$\text{CFTR degraded} = [\text{counts}(T_n) - \text{count/hex}(T_n)] \div \{[\text{total counts} \cdot \text{correction factor}] - [\text{counts}(T_0)]\} \cdot 100$$

where counts(T_n)	= corrected TCA soluble counts measured for samples taken at each time point (T_n)
count/hex(T_n)	= corrected TCA soluble counts measured in presence of hexokinase at each time point (T_n)
total counts	= total radioactivity in the sample (e.g., measured at time 0)
correction factor	= (CFTR − mock)/(CFTR), where CFTR = radioactivity of microsomes containing radiolabeled CFTR and mock = radioactivity of microsomes from mock translations (see next section)

3.5.3. Data Analysis

A small component of TCA-soluble radioactivity is released from membranes in the absence of ATP. This results from nonspecific association of Trans³⁵S-Label with microsome components. The relative contribution of ATP-independent release is assessed by comparing CFTR and "mock" translations (i.e., transcription/translation reactions that omit DNA template). Microsomes from mock translations typically contain ~22% of the radiolabel incorporated during a normal CFTR translation. Membrane-associated radioactivity actually incorporated into CFTR is therefore ~78% of the total (in our hands) *(28)*. When analyzed under reducing conditions by SDS-PAGE, microsomes from mock translations appear devoid of radiolabeled protein. Moreover, release of these nonspecific counts into the TCA-soluble fraction is independent of ATP and RRL and thus is likely due to reversible association of Trans³⁵S-Label with components with microsomal membranes. Importantly, release of TCA-soluble radioactivity from mock reactions is equivalent to the

ATP-independent release of radioactivity from CFTR translations. In other words, radioactivity released nonspecifically under conditions of ATP depletion (e.g., hexokinase/deoxyglucose) is not related to CFTR degradation, and is subtracted from each corresponding sample (*see* **Note 11**).

4. Notes

1. Repeated freeze-thaw cycles will decrease RRL activity. Three or four cycles are generally well tolerated as long as samples are thawed quickly, and refrozen by submersion in liquid nitrogen. For unclear reasons the quality of RRL may vary substantially between rabbits. Therefore we store lysate from each rabbit separately and analyze each for translation and degradation efficiency. Only the most active preparations are used. A single rabbit will normally yield between 20 and 40 mL of lysate. Lower yields can result from failure to completely exanguinate the animal or failure to lyse all of the reticulocytes. The latter problem is usually due to inadequate shaking of the lysate and will be manifest by a very large pellet in the second 15,000g spin of the RRL protocol.
2. Most commercial RRL preparations are designed for performing translations and therefore contain added hemin. These preparations are incompatible with proteasome degradation assays because hemin inhibits ATPase activity of the 19S proteasome subunit *(21)*. Some "untreated" RRL preparations may still contain hemin, so contact the manufacturer before using. In the presence of hemin, degradation is inhibited but ubiquitination is not, so degradation substrates accumulate as ubiquitinated intermediates. RRL without added hemin contains some endogenous free hemin. This is usually not enough to inhibit degradation but may account for differences in degradation efficiency observed for different rabbits.
3. RRL components may be separated by glycerol gradient centrifugation and fractions assayed for substrate hydrolysis in the absence and presence of known proteasome inhibitors, (e.g., 100 μM MG132). We have found that LLE-AMC and LLVY-AMC hydrolyzing activity is specific for the proteasome because this activity sediments at the predicted size of the proteasome on glycerol gradients and is abolished by specific proteasome inhibitors. However, RRL contains additional low-molecular-weight protease(s) (<200 kDa) capable of cleaving LRR-AMC that are resistant to proteasome inhibitors *(28)*.
4. Being the immediate precursors of erythrocytes, reticulocytes are unlikely to contain immunoproteasomes *(22)* so all fluorogenic peptidase activities of the RRL should derive from the ß subunits of standard proteasomes. RRL contains approximately equal amounts of 20S and 26S proteasomes (not shown), but the latter hydrolyzes LLVY-AMC 10-fold faster *(23,24)*. Therefore, ChT-L activity primarily reports the form of the proteasome that is directly involved in ubiquitin-mediated degradation. However, the degree to which the 26S proteasome preferentially hydrolyzes other fluorogenic substrates may vary *(24)*.
5. Traditionally canine pancreatic microsomes have been used to study in vitro translation of secreted and transmembrane proteins. However, preparations can also be made from pig or sheep pancreas by following essentially the same procedure *(25)*. Proteolysis or autolysis of the pancreas can be a significant problem,

so the pancreas should be removed as quickly as possible following euthanasia. All steps are performed on ice and/or in a cold room.

6. Like RRL, canine pancreas membrane preparations vary widely in their efficiency, and it may take several attempts to achieve a preparation with satisfactory function. A suitable preparation, however, generates 10–30 mL of microsomes and is sufficient for thousands of typical translation and/or degradation reactions.

7. Ubiquitination of CFTR should not occur at 24°C (temperature used for translation) if CFTR is properly inserted into the ER membrane. Cotranslational ubiquitination of CFTR has been reported to occur at 30°C but was observed for only a small fraction of total protein (26).

8. A common problem in translating large proteins such as CFTR is the generation of incomplete translation products. This can occur if (a) insufficient ATA is added, (b) ATA is added too late, or (c) transcript concentration is too high. One way to increase the relative yield of full-length CFTR products is to reduce the amount of transcript to 2% and increase the RRL concentration to 60% (27). For these conditions, transcription is carried out as described but the 20× translation buffer is modified as follows: 1 *M* KCl, 38 m*M* MgCl$_2$, 36 m*M* DTT, and 184 m*M* Tris-HCl, pH 7.5. For maximal translation efficiency, samples should be incubated for 1 minute at 37°C before being shifted to 24°C. Then, 50 μ*M* ATA is added at 20 min and translation is continued for a total of 2 h. We have found that this alternative procedure gives similar yields of full-length CFTR with fewer incomplete translation products. Additional articles by Jackson and Hunt (17) and Promega's technical manual part TM232 (downloadable through their Web site) contain further information concerning the optimization of RRL translation.

9. Uniform resuspension of microsomes is necessary to avoid scatter in experimental results. This is the most difficult step in the degradation procedure and may require significant practice to master. When resuspension is complete, the solution should appear faintly opalescent, and no particulate membrane clumps should be visible. If foaming of the solution occurs, transfer the liquid portion to a fresh tube when resuspension is complete. If the resuspended microsomes have significantly less radiolabeled protein than the original translation (as determined by SDS-PAGE autoradiography), the following should be considered: (a) The microsomal pellet may have been lost during resuspension; (b) CFTR was synthesized but did not insert into the membranes. The latter can occur if microsomes are suboptimal or if the translation reaction was not mixed sufficiently.

10. Because RRL is so concentrated, the protein will rapidly precipitate in 20% TCA. Therefore tubes should be vortexed immediately after addition of sample to TCA to assure adequate dispersion of TCA-soluble peptide fragments.

11. Under our conditions, 50–70% of total CFTR should be converted to TCA soluble fragments. Lower values may result if: (a) ATP regenerating system is not working (remake 10× buffer with fresh creatine phosphate); (b) RRL contains an inhibitory factor(s) (e.g., most commercial RRL preparations contain hemin); (c) translation efficiency is very low. Release of TCA soluble radioactivity in the absence of ATP should be ≤10% of the total counts incorporated into membranes. When translation efficiency is very low this percentage becomes much higher

(~30%) and only about 10–20% of total counts become degraded. To improve translation, *see* **Subheading 3.4.** RRL degradation activity can be easily assessed using commercially available radiolabeled substrates such as ^{14}C-lysozyme *(13)*.

References

1. Hershko, A. and Ciechanover, A. (1998) The ubiquitin system. *Annu. Rev. Biochem.* **67,** 425–479.
2. Kopito, R. (1997) ER quality control: the cytoplasmic connection. *Cell* **88,** 427–430.
3. Ferrell, K., Wilkinson, C., Dubiel, W., and Gordon, C. (2000) Regulatory subunit interactions of the 26S proteasome, a complex problem. *TIBS* **25,** 83–88.
4. Dick, T., Nussbaum, A., deeg, M., Heinemeyer, W., Groll, M., Schirle, M., et al. (1998) Contributions of proteasomal beta-subunits to the cleavage of peptide substrates analyzed with yeast mutants. *J. Biol. Chem.* **273,** 25,637–25,646.
5. Arendt, C. and Hochstrasser, M. (1997) Identification of the yeast 20S proteasome catalytic centers and subunit interactions required for active-site formation. *Proc. Nat. Acad. Sci. USA* **94,** 7156–7161.
6. Wang, R., Chait, B., Wolf, I., Kohanski, R., and Cardozo, C. (1999) Lysozyme degradation by the bovine multicatalytic complex (proteasome): evidence for a nonprocessive mode of degradation. *Biochemistry* **38,** 14,573–14,581.
7. Brodsky, J. and McCracken, A. (1997) ER-asociated and proteasome-mediated protein degradation: how two topologically restricted events came together. *Trends Cell Biol.* **7,** 151–155.
8. Jensen, T., Loo, M., Pind, S., Williams, D., Goldberg, A., and Riordan, J. (1995) Multiple proteolytic systems, including the proteosome, contribute to CFTR processing. *Cell* **83,** 129–136.
8a. Ward, C., Omura, C., and Kopito, R. (1995) Degradation of CFTR by the ubiquitin-proteasome pathway. *Cell* **83,** 121–128.
9. Qu, B., Strickland, E., and Thomas, P. (1997) Localization and suppression of a kinetic defect in cystic fibrosis transmembrane conductance regulator folding. *J. Biol. Chem.* **272,** 15739–15744.
10. Qu, B. and Thomas, P. (1996) Alteration of the cystic fibrosis transmembrane conductance regulator folding pathway. *J. Biol. Chem.* **271,** 7261–7264.
11. Loo, M., Jensen, T., Cui, L., Hou, Y., Chang, X., and Riordan, J. (1998) Perturbation of Hsp90 interaction with nascent CFTR prevents its maturation and accelerates its degradation by the proteasome. *EMBO J.* **17,** 6879–6887.
12. Jiang, C., Fang, S., Xiao, Y., O'Connor, S., Nadler, S., Lee, D., et al. (1996) Partial restoration of cAMP-stimulated CFTR chloride channel activity in DeltaF508 cells by deoxyspergulin. *Am. J. Physiol.* **275,** C171–178.
12a. Meacham, G., Va Herson, C., Zhang, W., Younger, J., and Cyr, D. (2001) The Hsc70 co-chaperone CHIV targets immature CFTR for proteasomal degradation. *Nature Cell Biol.* **3,** 100–105.
13. Xiong, X., Chong, E., and Skach, W. (1999) Evidence that endoplasmic reticulum (ER)-associated degradation of cystic fibrosis transmembrane conductance regulator is linked to retrograde translocation from the ER membrane. *J. Biol. Chem.* **274,** 2616–2624.

14. Lu, Y., Turnbull, I., Bragin, A., Carveth, K., Verkman, A., and Skach, W. (2000) Reorientation of Aquaporin-1 topology during maturation in the endoplasmic reticulum. *Mol. Biol. Cell* **11**, 2973–2985.

15. Kobilka, B. (1990) The role of cytosolic and membrane factors in processing of the human beta-2 adrenergic receptor following translocation and glycosylation in a cell free system. *J. Biol. Chem.* **265**, 7610–7618.

16. McLaughlin, S., Conn, S., and Bulleid, N. (1999) Folding and assembly of type X collagen mutants that cause metphyseal chondrodysplasia-type Schmid. *J. Biol. Chem.* **274**, 7570–7575.

17. Jackson, R. and Hunt, T. (1983) Preparation and use of nuclease-treated rabbit reticulocyte lysates for the translation of eukaryotic messenger RNA. *Meth. Enzymol.* **96**, 50–74.

18. Bogyo, M., McMaster, J., Gaczynska, M., Tortorella, D., Goldberg, A., and Ploegh, H. (1997) Covalent modification of the active site threonine of proteasomal beta subunits and the *Escherichia coli* homolog HsIV by a new class of inhibitors. *Proc. Natl. Acad. Sci. USA* **94**, 6629–6634.

19. Kanayama, H., Tamura, T., Ugai, S. Kagawa, S., Tanahashi, N., Yoshimura, S., et al. (1992) Demonstration that a human 26S proteolytic complex consists of a proteasome and multiple associated protein components and hydrolyzes ATP and ubiquitin-ligated proteins by closely linked mechanisms. *Eur. J. Biochem.* **206**, 567–578.

20. Walter, P. and Blobel, G. (1983) Preparation of microsomal membranes for cotranslational protein translocation, in *Methods in Enzymology*, vol. 96 (Fleischer, S. and Fleischer, B., eds.), Academic Press, New York, pp. 84–93.

21. Hoffman, L. and Rechsteiner, M. (1996) Nucleotidase activities of the 26 S proteasome and its regulatory complex. *J. Biol. Chem.* **271**, 32,538–32,545.

22. Ustrell, V., Realini, C., Pratt, G., and Rechsteiner, M. (1995) Human lymphoblast and erythrocyte multicatalytic proteases: differential peptidase activities and responses to the 11S regulator. *FEBS Lett.* **376**, 155–158.

23. Ugai, S., T. Tamura, N. Tanahashi, S. Takai, N. Komi, C. chung, K. tanaka, and A. Ichihara, 1993. Purification and characerization of the 26S proteasome complex catalyzing ATP-dependent breakdown of ubiquitin-ligated proteins from rat liver. J. Biochem., 113:754-768.

24. Reidlinger, J., A. Pike, P. Savory, R. Murray, and Rivett, A. J. (1997) Catalytic properties of 26S and 20S proteasomes and radiolaveling of MB1, LMP7, and C7 subunits associated with trypsin-like and chymotrypsin-like activities. *J. Biol. Chem.* **272**, 24,899–24,905.

25. Kaderbhai, M., Harding, V., Karim, A., Austen, B., and Kaderbhai, N. (1995) Sheep pancreatic microsomes as an alternative to the dog source for studying protein translocation. *Biochem. J.* **15**, 57–61.

26. Sato, S., Ward, C., and Kopito, R. (1998) Cotranslational ubiquitination of cystic fibrosis transmembrane conductance regulator *in vitro*. *J. Biol. Chem.* **273**, 7189–7192.

27. Dasso, M. and Jackson, R. (1989) On the fidelity of mRNA translation in the nuclease-treated rabbit reticulocyte lysate system. *Nucleic Acids Res.* **17,** 3129–3244.

28. Oberdorf, J., Carlson, E., and Skach, W. (2001) Redundancy of mammalian proteasome β-subunit function during endoplasmic reticulum associated degradation. *Biochemistry, in press.*

21

In Vitro CFTR Folding Assays

Rhesa D. Stidham, W. Christian Wigley, and Philip J. Thomas

1. Introduction

Cystic fibrosis (CF), a severe autosomal recessive disorder, is marked by reduced regulated chloride conductance across the apical membrane of affected epithelia. This reduction is attributable to mutations in the cystic fibrosis transmembrane conductance regulator (CFTR), which acts as an ATP-dependent cAMP-regulated chloride channel. As shown in **Fig. 1**, CFTR is a multidomain membrane protein composed of five functional domains: two nucleotide-binding domains (NBD), two transmembrane domains (TMD), and a regulatory domain (R). The most prevalent cystic fibrosis-causing mutation is the deletion of the F508 residue in NBD1 of CFTR *(1,2)*. This deletion affects the ability of the domain, and thus the CFTR protein, to fold into its native state *(3)*, leading to its retention in the endoplasmic reticulum (ER) and subsequent degradation *(4)*.

Notably, when this mutant protein is induced to fold, by either altering conditions of temperature *(5,6)*, introducing second site supressor mutations *(7,8)*, or adding osmolytes to the medium *(7,9,10)*, the protein regains significant function. These results suggest that correcting the folding defect may be of therapeutic benefit. To date, only manipulations that have a general effect on protein folding have been utilized to increase the folding yield of CFTR. Such manipulations lack specificity, and therefore may not be viable therapeutic options for cystic fibrosis patients. However, these results do lead to the intriguing suggestion that a pharmacological agent could effect a similar correction of the CFTR folding defect *(3,11)*. The basic premise is to couple the energetically favorable binding reaction to the disfavored folding reaction; such an approach offers an important advantage in that it targets the primary defect (misfolding) rather than the secondary loss of function. Several recent precedents in the literature support the utility of this approach.

From: *Methods in Molecular Medicine, vol. 70: Cystic Fibrosis Methods and Protocols*
Edited by: W. R. Skach © Humana Press Inc., Totowa, NJ

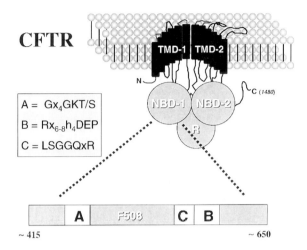

Fig. 1. Schematic of the cystic fibrosis transmembrane conductance regulator. CFTR is comprised of two transmembrane domains (TMD1 and TMD2), two nucleotide-binding domains (NBD-1 and NBD-2), and a cytosolic regulatory domain (R). The nucleotide-binding domains contain the Walker A and B consensus sequences common to nucleotide-binding proteins as well as the C consensus sequence. The most prevalent CF-causing mutation, the deletion of F508, is located in NBD-1 between the A and C consensus sites.

Small molecules have been found that bind to and increase the stability of the native state of p53 folding mutants (*12,13*). Significantly, the steady-state levels of the folded protein are increased in direct correlation with the amelioration of the disease phenotype in an animal model (*13*). In addition, ligand binding energy can be used to rescue the folding defects of two mutant membrane proteins, the V2 vasopressin receptor (*14*) and human P-glycoprotein (*15*). The G-protein-coupled V2 vasopressin receptor is composed of several transmembrane spans and, like CFTR, a number of mutations lead to its defective folding and disease. Preincubation of cells expressing maturation/folding mutants of the V2 vasopressin receptor in the presence of a known, permeant, high-affinity ligand has been shown to increase the cell-surface expression of the receptor and to restore partial function (*14*). Similarly, the defective folding of several mutants of the human P-glycoprotein, a homolog of CFTR, can be overcome by binding of the solutes that it normally pumps across the membrane (*15*). Unfortunately, high-affinity CFTR-specific ligands that could be used to increase the folding yield of the protein are currently lacking. Thus, robust assays would be required to identify possible starting structures and for the development of improved compounds that serve as folding assistants.

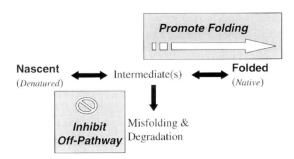

Fig. 2. General schematic of the folding pathway of a protein. The nascent protein passes through a series of transient intermediate states en route to the native, folded structure. Reactions such as aggregation and proteolysis compete for these intermediates, funneling them off the productive folding pathway. The ΔF508 mutation increases the rate of off-pathway associations and thus decreases the productive folding yield of the protein, perhaps through its destabilizing effect on one of the on-pathway intermediates. Strategies aimed at correcting the defective folding caused by ΔF508 could act either by shifting the equilibrium toward productive folding or away from unproductive off-pathway reactions.

1.1. Biochemical-Based Folding Assays

The folding of a protein can be viewed as a trajectory along which the denatured protein (many conformations) moves through a series of intermediate states (a limited set of conformations) to reach the final native structure (single conformation). During this process, "off-pathway" reactions such as aggregation or interaction with the proteolytic machinery compete with the folding reaction for the "on-pathway" folding intermediates (**Fig. 2**). Such a view of protein folding yields two general mechanisms for altering the folding pathway, one thermodynamic in nature and the other kinetic.

A protein's sequence encodes both the stability of the native state relative to the unfolded state (the thermodynamic) and the relative rates of the multitude of steps both on and off the folding pathway (the kinetic). Not surprisingly, alterations in sequence (mutations) or environment (ligands, pH, etc.) can lead to changes in stability and/or pathway. In this regard, disease-associated mutations that decrease native state stability have been identified *(16,17)*. In contrast, the cystic fibrosis-causing ΔF508 mutation confers a temperature sensitive phenotype on the folding of CFTR without dramatic effect on the native state stability. At reduced temperature, there is a partial correction of the folding defect and a subsequent increase in the folding yield of the mutant protein both in vivo and in vitro *(5,6)*. Such a temperature sensitive for folding (tsf) phenotype indicates that F508 is critical for defining an efficient folding pathway (the kinetics).

This result has important implications for small-molecule binding to the CFTR native state as a possible therapy; any such ligand must interact with a species that is kinetically accessible to the critical, effected step in the folding pathway in order to be successful. Since the pathway from the critical intermediate to the native state is currently unknown for maturation-defective CFTR mutants, the ideal search for molecules that correct the folding defect should involve a screen for compounds that affect the kinetics of the folding reaction as well as those that affect the thermodynamic stability of the native state.

Binding studies to CFTR, or a domain of CFTR, would yield candidates for testing the ability to stabilize the native state. However, monitoring the folding kinetics of a large membrane protein such as CFTR in vitro is currently beyond our experimental capabilities. Additional difficulties arise with the domain-based approach, namely, in the choice of the fragment used for binding studies, the compatibility of the binding assay with the conditions required for folding, and the considerable manual manipulation that would complicate the screening process. In spite of these issues, a model of the first nucleotide-binding domain (NBD1) of CFTR should prove more tenable than the full-length protein for such a study. For example, it has been shown that the rate of formation of higher-molecular-weight aggregates, an "off-pathway" reaction, has a shorter lag phase and is faster for an NBD1 model containing the prevalent ΔF508 mutation *(6)*, indicating that the mutation destabilizes a critical intermediate on the folding pathway of the NBD1, making it more prone to off-pathway reactions. Compounds that decrease the concentration of the species that are prone to proteolysis or aggregation would thus shift the kinetic balance toward productive folding. Such an effect of test compounds on the kinetics of folding could be conveniently monitored by their ability either to increase the folding yield or to decrease the rate of the "off-pathway" aggregation reaction.

1.1.1. Native State Stability

The native state stability of a protein domain is typically determined by chemical denaturation. A folded domain is only marginally stable even under optimal conditions; as denaturant concentration is increased, the domain undergoes a cooperative unfolding transition over a narrow range of denaturant (**Fig. 3**). The concentration dependence of chemical denaturant required to induce the transition is related directly to the stability of the folded protein. When unfolding is reversible and two-state, the fraction folded over the transition region can be used to calculate the free energy for denaturation of the protein (ΔG_D). The fraction unfolded/fraction folded is used to determine an equilibrium constant at each denaturant concentration and the corresponding $\Delta G_{D\,[\text{denaturant}]}$ (**Eqs. 1** and **2**).

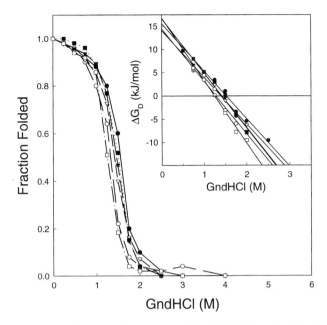

Fig. 3. Representative denaturation curve of the NBD1 domain. The folded domain was denatured by addition of guanidine HCl and the unfolding of the protein monitored by the decrease in fluorescence of the single tryptophan (Trp[496]) as it is exposed to solvent. NBD1 domain at a concentration of 1.8 μM in 30 mM Tris-HCl, pH 8.0, 40 mM arginine, 0.2 mM EDTA, and 0.1 mM dithiothreitol was incubated with denaturant at the indicated concentrations for 2 h. Fluorescence was excited at 282 nm and the emission recorded. The wavelength maximum was used to calculate the fraction folded at each denaturant concentration. NBD1 wild-type (residues 404–589) (●), NBD1ΔF (○), NBD1-R553M (▼), NBD1ΔF-R553M (▽), NBD1-G551D (■), NBD1D-S549R (□). For this reversible, two-state process, the fraction folded over the transition region can be used to calculate a free energy of denaturation (ΔGD) at each concentration of GdnHCl and this information used to extrapolate to obtain a free energy of denaturation in the absence of denaturant (ΔG_0) (*inset*). Reproduced from *J. Biol. Chem.* (1997) **272**, 15,739–15,744.

$$K_{eq} = [\text{unfolded}]/[\text{folded}] \tag{1}$$

$$\Delta G_D = -RT \ln K_{eq} \tag{2}$$

These values are then used to determine a free energy for denaturation (ΔG_D) for unfolding in the absence of denaturant by extrapolation. The difference in the ΔG_D for the mutant NBD1 vs. the wild-type NBD1 or vs the mutant NBD1 in the presence of a pharmaceutical agent ($\Delta\Delta G_D$) allows a comparison of the effect of the mutation or drug on the native state stability of the domain. Often the amount of denaturant required to reach the inflection of the transition, C_m, is used to compare the wild-type and mutant protein as well *(17,18)*. The denaturation curves for a variety of constructs predicted to contain the entire NBD1 of CFTR have been monitored by fluorescence of a single tryptophan at position 496 *(6)*. In the folded domain, the relatively apolar environment of this side chain is reflected in the 324-nm emission maximum.

1.1.2. Folding Yield

A variety of evidence suggests that the *tsf* mutation, ΔF508, affects an intermediate on the folding pathway of CFTR rather than the native state stability of the protein *(6)*. The mutation results in an increase in the concentration of an intermediate that is prone to aggregation. Aggregation, a concentration-dependent, associative process, effectively competes this intermediate away from productive folding, decreasing the final folding yield of the protein. A comparison of the relative efficiency of folding to the native state for the wild type and the ΔF508 NBD1 at various temperatures has been used to demonstrate this kinetic defect (**Fig. 4A**). The protein is solubilized and unfolded in denaturant and then induced to fold by dilution into a refolding buffer that contains L-arginine and low denaturant concentration. When the reaction is complete, the insoluble, misfolded protein is pelleted by centrifugation, the supernatant containing the folded protein removed, and the relative fraction of the two forms determined. The partitioning between the two forms reflects the concentration of the critical kinetic-branchpoint intermediate. This approach does not require the critical step to be monitored directly, which is difficult or impossible if it is very fast, sparsely populated, and/or spectrally silent.

1.1.3. "Off-Pathway" Aggregation

Since kinetic competition between productive folding and off-pathway reactions determines the final folding yield of the protein, monitoring the rate of the slow off-pathway reactions is also a useful means of assessing these folding defects. It has been shown that the rate of formation of higher-molecular-weight aggregates by the ΔF508 NBD1, an off-pathway reaction, has a shorter lag phase and is accelerated relative to the wild-type *(6)* (**Fig. 4B**). The rate of aggregate formation can be easily monitored by measuring the turbidity (or light scattering) of the protein over time once refolding has been initiated. Typically the NBD1 protein is solubilized and unfolded in denaturant and the protein then rapidly diluted into a buffer containing L-arginine under conditions at which the final folding yield is less than one and the rate of off-pathway aggregation is monitored. Such an aggregation assay has been used to monitor the effect of mutations *(6,7)*, chaperones *(19,20)*, and osmolytes *(7)* on NBD1 folding and is readily amenable to a high-throughput 96-well plate format.

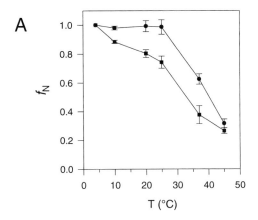

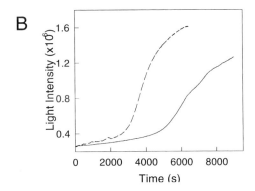

Fig. 4. Kinetic competition between off-pathway associations and productive folding. **(A)** NBD1 domain (residues 404–589) was solubilized in 6 M guanidine HCl and then diluted into refolding buffer preequilibrated at the indicated temperatures to a final concentration of 2 μM. Samples were incubated at the appropriate temperature overnight and the fraction of soluble protein determined by the intrinsic tryptophan fluorescence of the single Trp at position 496. Wild-type NBD1 domain (●), NBD1ΔF (■). **(B)** NBD1 domain solubilized in 6 M guanidine HCl was diluted into refolding buffer to a concentration of 18 μM at room temperature and the kinetics of off-pathway aggregation monitored by light scattering due to the aggregates at 400 nm at an angle of 90° to the incident beam. NBD1 is depicted with a solid line; NBD1ΔF is depicted with a dashed line. Reproduced from *J. Biol. Chem.* (1996) **271**, 7261–7264.

2. Materials

2.1. Native State Stability

2.1.1. Protein Preparation

1. Bacterial growth medium (Luria broth, etc.).
2. 1 M isopropylthio-β-ᴅ-galactoside (IPTG).

3. Overnight cultures of BL21 *Escherichia coli* bacteria transformed with the pET28a plasmid containing CFTR sequence with an N-terminal polyhistidine tag under control of a T7 promoter (*see* **Note 1**).
4. 10 mg/mL kanamycin sulfate.
5. Binding buffer: 5 mM imidazole, 20 mM Tris-HCl, pH 7.9, 0.5 M NaCl, (+) and (–) 6 M guanidine HCl (*see* **Note 2**).
6. Strip buffer: 20 mM Tris-HCl, pH 7.9, 100 mM ethylenediaminetetraacetic acid (EDTA), 0.5 M NaCl.
7. Distilled water.
8. Charge buffer: 50 mM NiSO$_4$.
9. Wash buffer: 30 mM imidazole, 20 mM Tris-HCl, pH 7.9, 0.5 M NaCl, 6 M guanidine HCl.
10. Elution buffer: 0.4 M imidazole, 20 mM Tris-HCl, pH 7.9, 6 M guanidine HCl.
11. Dialysis buffer: 100 mM Tris-HCl, pH 7.4, 2 mM EDTA.
12. Novagen "His·Bind" resin.
13. 12–14,000 mW cutoff dialysis tubing.

2.1.2. Native State Stability

1. Protein pellet (*see* **Subheading 3.1.1.**).
2. 6 M Guanidine HCl or other appropriate denaturant (8 M urea) (*see* **Note 2**).
3. Refolding buffer: 0.4 M L-arginine HCl. 0.1 M Tris-HCl, pH 8.0, 2 mM EDTA.
4. 10 mM dithiothreitol (DTT) (*see* **Note 3**).
5. Fluorometer.

2.2. Folding Yield

1. Protein pellet (*see* **Subheading 3.1.1.**).
2. 6 M Guanidine HCl (*see* **Note 2**).
3. Refolding buffer (*see* **Note 3**).
4. Heat blocks preequilibrated to various temperatures.
5. Fluorometer.

2.3. "Off-Pathway" Aggregation

1. Protein pellet (*see* **Subheading 3.1.1.**).
2. 6 M Guanidine HCl (*see* **Note 2**).
3. Refolding buffer: (*see* **Note 3**).
4. Spectrophotometer/Fluorometer.

3. Methods
3.1. Native State Stability
3.1.1. Protein Preparation

1. Innoculate 1 L of sterile Luria broth containing 10 µg/mL kanamycin sulfate with BL21 *E. coli* overnight culture. Allow the bacteria to grow to O.D. ≈0.4 at 37°C on a shaker.
2. Protein expression is induced by the addition of IPTG to a final concentration of 0.1 M.

3. Allow the culture to grow at 37°C on a shaker for at least another 4 h.
4. Pellet bacteria at 3200g for 20 min. Pour off the supernatant.
5. Resuspend the bacterial pellet in ~300 mL binding buffer without denaturant.
6. Sonicate the resuspended pellet with a Branson sonicator at high power output 5× for 45 s. Cool the sample on ice during sonication.
7. Pellet the insoluble material (inclusion bodies enriched in the NBD1) at 15,000g for 30 min. Discard supernatant.
8. Resuspend the pellet in ~30 mL of binding buffer that has 6 M guanidine HCl (*see* **Note 4**). Pellet the insoluble material at 39,000g for 30 min. At this point the NBD1 protein should remain soluble in the denaturant, giving a nonturbid, yellowish supernatant.
9. Prepare Novagen "His·Bind" (Ni^{2+}) column as per Novagen directions using the strip buffer, water, charge buffer, and binding buffer.
10. Equilibrate the column with binding buffer, which contains the 6 M guanidine HCl.
11. Load crude, unfolded NBD1 sample from **step 8** onto the column.
12. Once the sample is loaded, wash the column extensively with binding buffer containing 6 M guanidine HCl (*see* **Note 5**).
13. Wash the column with wash buffer containing imidazole and guanidine HCl to remove nonspecific binding.
14. Elute the protein with elution buffer containing guanidine HCl.
15. Pool the protein fractions into 12–14,000 mW dialysis tubing. Dialyze at 4°C against several changes (1 L) of dialysis buffer to remove the guanidine. The NBD1 protein forms a white precipitate as denaturant is removed in the dialysis.
16. Aliquot the protein into microfuge tubes. Centrifuge at 14,000g for 15 min at 4°C. Speed-vac to concentrate and dry the sample. Freeze pellet at –20°C for later use.

3.1.2. Native State Stability

1. Resuspend the precipitated protein pellet (from **Subheading 3.1.1., step 16**) in 6 M guanidine HCl. Incubate the tube on ice for 10 min to ensure that most of the protein is unfolded and resolubilized.
2. Pellet any remaining insoluble protein for 15 min by spinning at 14,000g in a microfuge at 4°C. Remove the supernatant from the pellet to a fresh tube.
3. Determine protein concentration using the absorbance at 280 nm of the protein in 6 M guanidine HCl. The extinction coefficient used to calculate the protein concentration will depend on the particular NBD1 construct used (*see* **Note 6**).
4. Dilute the unfolded protein sample in 4°C refolding buffer to give a final protein concentration of 2 μM and a final guanidine HCl concentration of 200 mM.
5. Incubate at 4°C overnight.
6. Pellet any insoluble/misfolded material at 14,000g for 15 min at 4°C. Carefully remove the supernatant to a fresh microfuge tube.
7. To determine a denaturation curve, the protein is incubated for 2 h in the appropriate denaturant concentration to allow the unfolding to come to equilibrium. The denaturant concentrations chosen bracket the C_m (*see* **Subheading 1.1.1.**) and define the top and bottom of the sigmoid.

8. Using an excitation wavelength of 282 nm, the emission spectrum of the refolding buffer alone is taken, followed by the emission spectra of the protein samples at each denaturant concentration. The buffer-alone emission is then subtracted from the sample spectra.

3.2. Folding Yield

1. Equilibrate heat blocks at the desired temperatures (for example, 4, 30, 37, and 42°C).
2. Resuspend the protein pellet (from **Subheading 3.1.1., step 16**) in 6 *M* guanidine HCl. Incubate the tube on ice for 10 min to ensure that the protein is resolubilized. Pellet any insoluble protein for 15 min at 14,000*g* in a microfuge at 4°C. Remove the supernatant from the pellet to a fresh tube.
3. Determine the protein concentration using the absorbance at 280 nm of the protein in 6 *M* guanidine HCl. The extinction coefficient used to calculate the protein concentration will depend on which NBD1 construct is used (*see* **Note 6**).
4. Calculate the amount of protein required to give a final protein concentration of 2 µ*M* and a final guanidine HCl concentration of 200 m*M* in refolding buffer.
5. Add refolding buffer into each of several microfuge tubes and allow tubes to equilibrate at the appropriate temperatures for the yield experiment.
6. Add the amount of protein calculated in **step 4** to each of the preequilibrated tubes and mix by vortex. Incubate at the designated temperatures overnight.
7. Pellet the insoluble/unfolded material at 14,000*g* for 15 min at 4°C. Carefully (so the pellet is not disturbed) remove the supernatant and measure the fraction of folded protein (relative to wild-type using the intrinsic tryptophan 496 fluorescence). This is the concentration of protein that productively folds at the given temperature. Alternatively, the soluble and insoluble fractions can be analyzed by sodium dodecyl sulfate-polyacrylamide gel electrophoresis (SDS-PAGE) after solubilization in sample buffer *(19)*.

3.3. "Off-Pathway" Aggregation

1. Preincubate the UV spectrophotometer sample holder at 37°C. Also preheat a heat block at 37°C.
2. Repeat **steps 2–4** under **Subheading 3.2.** calculating for 18 µ*M* final protein concentration.
3. Incubate refolding buffer at 37°C in the heat block.
4. Quickly add the calculated amount of protein to the preheated buffer while vortexing continuously. Transfer the sample to the cuvet and monitor the aggregation (at 400 nm by turbidity in a spectrophotometer or light-scattering in a fluorometer).

4. Notes

1. The pET28a expression plasmid is purchased from Novagen; subsequent cloning allows for the expression of an N- or C-terminal polyhistidine fusion with the protein of interest for ease of purification. Subsequent purification steps use this polyhistidine tag. Various constructs predicted to contain the entire NBD1 of CFTR have been cloned into the expression system and purified by this method.

2. The final concentration of guanidine HCl (or urea) stock should by assessed by its refractive index and adjusted accordingly *(21)* using **Eq. 3**, where ΔN is the reflective index increment at 589 nm and 20°C.

$$[GdnHCl] = 57.147(\Delta N) + 38.68(\Delta N^2) - 91.60(\Delta N^3) \qquad (3)$$

3. Arginine is not stable for long-term storage. Although it is unnecessary to make the refolding buffer fresh before use, care should be taken with refolding buffer that has been stored for a long time. Dithiothreitol should be made fresh every time and added to premade buffer stock minus the reductant.
4. The guanidine HCl is included in the binding buffer in order to solubilize the inclusion bodies formed from the overexpressed NBD1.
5. The column should be washed until the absorbance at 280 nm has reached a stable baseline.
6. The extinction coefficient as calculated for the NBD1 construct is different for the folded and the unfolded protein. Thus, protein concentration determinations are performed under denaturing conditions *(22)*.

Acknowledgments

This work was supported by grants from the NIH-NIDDK, the Welch Foundation and the Cystic Fibrosis Foundation, as well as the UTSW Molecular Biophysics Training Grant. The authors wish to thank Elizabeth Strickland and Patrick Thibodeau for helpful comments.

References

1. Tsui, L.-C. (1992) The spectrum of cystic fibrosis mutations. *TIG* **8**, 392–398.
2. Cutting, G. R. (1994) Mutations that cause cystic fibrosis. NIDDK Workshop #9.
3. Thomas, P. J., Shenbagamurthi, P., Sondek, J., Hullihen, J. M., and Pedersen, P. L. (1992) The cystic fibrosis transmembrane conductance regulator. *J. Biol. Chem.* **267**, 5727–5730.
4. Cheng, S. H., Gregory, R. J., Marshall, J., Paul, S., Souza, D. W., White, G. A., O'Riordan, C. R., and Smith, A. E. (1990) Defective intracellular transport and processing of CFTR is the molecular basis of most cystic fibrosis. *Cell* **63**, 827–834.
5. Denning, G. M., Anderson, M. P., Amara, J. F., Marshall, J., Smith, A. E., and Welsh, M. J. (1992) Processing of mutant cystic fibrosis transmembrane conductance regulator is temperature-sensitive. *Nature* **358**, 761–764.
6. Qu, B.-H. and Thomas, P. J. (1996) Alteration of the cystic fibrosis transmembrane conductance regulator folding pathway: effects of the ΔF508 mutation on the thermodynamic stability and folding yield of NBD1. *J. Biol. Chem.* **271**, 7261–7264.
7. Qu, B.-H., Strickland, E., and Thomas, P. J. (1997) Localization and suppression of a kinetic defect in cystic fibrosis transmembrane conductance regulator folding. *J. Biol. Chem.* **272**, 15,739–15,744.
8. Teem, J. L., Berger, H. A., Ostedgaard, L. S., Rich, D. P., Tsui, L.-C., and Welsh, M. J. (1993) Identification of revertants for the cystic fibrosis ΔF508 mutation using STE6-CFTR chimeras in yeast. *Cell* **73**, 335–346.

9. Sato, S., Ward, C. L., Krouse, M. E., Wine, J. J., and Kopito, R. R. (1996) Glycerol reverses the misfolding phenotype of the most common cystic fibrosis mutation. *J. Biol. Chem.* **271,** 635–638.

10. Brown, C. R., Hong-Brown, L. Q., Biwersi, J., Verkman, A. S., and Welch, W. J. (1996) Chemical chaperones correct the mutant phenotype of the deta-F508 cystic fibrosis transmembrane conductance regulator protein. *Cell Stress Chaperones* **1,** 117–125.

11. Thomas, P. J., Ko, Y. H., and Pedersen, P. L. (1992) Altered protein folding may be the molecular basis of most cases of cystic fibrosis. *FEBS Lett.* **312,** 7–9.

12. Bullock, A. N., Henckel, J., DeDecker, B. S., Johnson, C. M., Nikolova, P. V., Proctor, M. R., Lane, D. P., and Fersht, A. R. (1997) Thermodynamic stability of wild-type and mutant p53 core domain. *Proc. Natl. Acad. Sci. USA* **94,** 14,338–14,342.

13. Foster, B. A., Coffey, H. A., Morin, M. J., and Rastinejad, F. (1999) Pharmacological rescue of mutant p53 conformation and function. *Science* **286,** 2507–2510.

14. Morello, J. P., Salahpour, A., Laperriere, A., Bernier, V., Arthus, M. F., Lonergan, M., Petaja-Repo, U., Angers, S., Morin, D., Bichet, D. G., and Bouvier, M. (2000) Pharmacological chaperones rescue cell-surface expression and function of misfolded V2 vasopressin receptor mutants. *J. Clin. Invest* **105,** 887–895.

15. Loo, T. W. and Clarke, D. M. (1997) Correction of defective protein kinesis of human P-glycoprotein mutants by substrates and modulators. *J. Biol. Chem.* **272,** 709–712.

16. Thomas, P. J., Qu, B.-H., and Pedersen, P. L. (1995) Defective protein folding as a basis of human disease. *TIBS* **20,** 456–459.

17. Strickland, E., Thomas, P. J., and Li, M. (2000) Folding polypeptides for drug production and discovery, in *Peptide and Protein Drug Analysis* (Reid, R. E., ed.), Marcel Dekker, New York, pp. 235–255.

18. Shirley, B. A. (1995) Urea and guanidinium hydrochloride denaturation curves, in *Protein Stability and Folding: Theory and Practice* (Shirley, B. A., ed.,) Humana, Totowa, NJ, pp. 177–190.

19. Strickland, E., Qu, B.-H., Millen, L., and Thomas, P. (1997) The molecular chaperone Hsc70 assists the *in vitro* folding of the N-terminal nucleotide-binding domain of the cystic fibrosis transmembrane conductance regulator. *J. Biol. Chem.* **272,** 25,421–25,424.

20. Strickland, E., Hakala, K., Thomas, P. J., and DeMartino, G. N. (2000) Recognition of misfolding proteins by PA700, the regulatory subcomplex of the 26 S proteasome. *J. Biol. Chem.* **275,** 5565–5572.

21. Pace, C. N. (1986) Determination and analysis of urea and guanidine hydrochloride denaturation curves. In: *Methods in Enzymology, vol. 131* (Hirs, C. H. W. and Timashef, S. N., eds.) Academic Press, New York pp. 266–280.

22. Gill, S. C. and von Hippel, P. H. (1989) Calculation of protein extinction coefficients from amino acid sequence data. *Anal. Biochem.* **182,** 319–326.

22

Analysis of CFTR Endocytosis by Cell Surface Biotinylation

Kelly Weixel and Neil A. Bradbury

1. Introduction

Correct localization of cystic fibrosis transmembrane conductance regulator (CFTR) is critical to its function. Although an intracellular role for CFTR is still somewhat controversial (*1*), there is clear agreement on an important role for CFTR in the plasma membrane. However, it is not only important that CFTR be inserted into the plasma membrane, it has to stay there the requisite amount of time. Although many CFTR mutations result in CFTR molecules that reach the plasma membrane (with altered conductance or regulation), the most clinically important mutation, ΔF508 CFTR, fails to reach the plasma membrane in physiologically relevant quantities. The precise amount of ΔF508 CFTR that reaches the plasma membrane remains controversial (*2,3*). Even so, until the "holy grail" of gene therapy is realized, therapeutic strategies to augment plasma membrane expression of mutant CFTR remain important. Indeed, many laboratories, both academic and commercial, are currently engaged in screening endeavors to identify pharmacological agents capable of improving the folding and traffic of mutant CFTR molecules (especially ΔF508 CFTR) leading to their insertion into the plasma membrane.

Strategies aimed at getting ΔF508 CFTR to the plasma membrane (either by chemical chaperones or by manipulation of endogenous chaperones) address only one aspect of CFTR trafficking, namely, the biosynthetic/exocytic trafficking of CFTR to the cell surface. As with many cell surface proteins, its residence time in the plasma membrane is as important as whether the protein is inserted into the plasma membrane in the first place. This is particularly important for CFTR, since recent studies by Marino (*4*) have suggested that ΔF508 CFTR is very rapidly removed from the plasma membrane by endocy-

From: *Methods in Molecular Medicine, vol. 70: Cystic Fibrosis Methods and Protocols*
Edited by: W. R. Skach © Humana Press Inc., Totowa, NJ

tosis (at a rate faster than that observed for wild-type CFTR). Clearly, a better understanding of the mechanisms by which CFTR is removed from the plasma membrane and the molecular interactions that CFTR undergoes during its internalization is needed. The aim of this chapter is to provide a description of the methods employed to study CFTR endocytosis. In addition, methods to inhibit endocytosis are described, along with background information necessary to interpret the experimental results. To introduce the subject, we provide a brief description of the mechanisms of signal-mediated endocytosis as they are currently understood, and provide a contextual framework within which the study of CFTR endocytosis is performed.

1.1. Endocytosis

Endocytosis is a process whereby cells internalize a large assortment of macromolecules from the extracellular environment (including nutrients, growth hormones, toxins, and viruses) *(5–7)*. Endocytosis also plays an important role in the constitutive and regulated targeting of proteins among various cellular membrane compartments such as the plasma membrane, endosomes and the *trans* Golgi network (TGN). The term endocytic trafficking describes the process of sequestration and internalization from the cell surface into intracellular endocytic vesicles (endosomes), trafficking of endosomes among intracellular organelles, and recycling back to the cell surface. Despite the observation that many plasma membrane proteins undergo endocytic internalization, most exhibit long half-lives (typically >24 h) and escape degradation by recycling back to the cell surface. Indeed, many receptors have been estimated to be internalized and recycled back to the plasma membrane as many as 10 times an hour. For example, individual low-density lipoprotein (LDL) receptors are internalized from the plasma membrane with a half-life of ~5 min, yet the half-life of the total LDLR protein pool is ~25 h *(8)*.

1.2. Endocytic Signals

In most cases, rapid internalization of membrane proteins occurs at select areas of the plasma membrane that are associated with the protein clathrin (i.e., clathrin-coated pits). Concentration of many receptors, as well as other membrane proteins, within clathrin-coated pits at the cell surface is dependent on localization signals encoded in short amino acid sequence motifs. Currently, the two best-defined internalization signals include critical aromatic residues (usually tyrosine) in the context of one or more bulky hydrophobic amino acids *(9–11)* and dileucine/leucine–isoleucine signals (**Table 1**). The endocytic sorting signal in the tail of the LDL receptor was the first endocytic signal identified *(12)* and has the motif NPXY (where X can be any amino acid). Although it was the first sequence identified, it is perhaps the least well characterized and is rarely used as a sorting signal. An alternate tyrosine-based sorting signal

Table 1
Tyrosine- and Dileucine-Based Endocytosis Signals Found in Rapidly Endocytosed Integral Membrane Proteins

Endocytosed molecule	Endocytic signal
YXXΦ signals	
TGN38	YQRL
LAMP-1	YQTI
CFTR	YDSI
Transferrin receptor	YTRF
LDL receptor	NPVY[a]
Dileucine signals	
CD3-γ	SDKQTLLPN
GLUT4	RRTPSLLEQ

[a]Although it is a tyrosine-based signal, the LDL receptor conforms to the sequence NPXY rather than YXXΦ.

is the YXXΦ motif *(13)*, where Φ is an amino acid with a bulky hydrophobic side chain (**Table 1**). It was originally proposed that tyrosine-based endocytosis motifs adopted a tight- or β-turn structure, exposing the tyrosine residue on the apex of the turn *(13)*. Support for such a model was provided by two-dimensional nuclear magnetic resonance (NMR) *(14,15)*. However, recent crystallographic data showed that the tyrosine-based motif of TGN38 (DYQRLN) adopts an extended conformation rather than a β-turn *(16)*. The dileucine motif conforms to the canonical sequence $X^{-1}XLL$ or $X^{-1}XIL$, where X is usually a polar residue, and X^{-1} is a negatively charged residue. First identified in the cytoplasmic tail of CD3-γ, the dileucine motif has now been shown to direct traffic of a number of proteins including the insulin-responsive glucose transporter Glut4 and CD4, the co-receptor for HIV *(17,18)*.

1.3. Clathrin Adaptors

Targeting of proteins bearing endocytic motifs to clathrin-coated pits is mediated by the actions of protein complexes referred to as adaptors *(19)*. Although localized to different regions of the cell, the adaptors have a similar composition and apparent structure (**Fig. 1**). There are two well-characterized clathrin adaptor complexes, AP-1 and AP-2, each of which consists of two heavy chains, a medium chain, and a small chain. AP-1 facilitates clathrin-mediated budding and sorting in the TGN and comprises two heavy chains (γ and β1) of ~100 kDa, a medium chain (μ1), ~47 kDa, and a small chain (σ1) ~20 kDa. AP-2 is similarly comprised of four subunits, (α1, β2, μ2, and σ2) and functions to select cargo for endocytic clathrin coated vesicles formed at

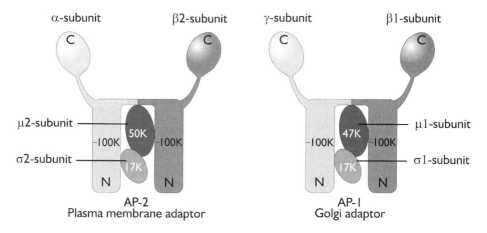

α-subunit   β2-subunit   γ-subunit   β1-subunit

μ2-subunit
σ2-subunit

μ1-subunit
σ1-subunit

AP-2
Plasma membrane adaptor

AP-1
Golgi adaptor

Fig. 1. Schematic representation of the subunit organization of the clathrin-associated adaptors. The β1, μ1, and σ1 subunits of the TGN-associated AP-1 complex share homology with the β2, μ2, and σ2 subunits of the endocytic adaptor complex AP-2. The α subunit of AP-2 and the γ subunit of AP-1 are distantly related.

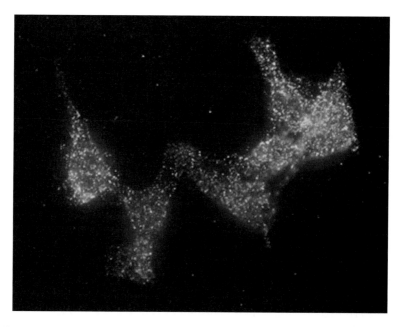

Fig. 2. Immunofluorescent localization of AP-2 in HEK-CFTR cells. The endocytic coated pits and vesicles, stained for α-adaptin, are distributed all over the plasma membrane.

```
HUMAN     (1410) CQQFLVIEENKVRQYDSIQKLLNERSLFRQAISPSDRVKLFPHR--NSSKCKSKP---QIAALKEETEE
Killifish (1428) CQSFLMIEKSSVKSYDSIQKLMNEMSHLKQAISPADRLHLFPTPHRLNSIKRPQPQTTKISSLPEEAED
Rat       (1408) CQRFLVIEQGNVWQYESLQALLSEKSVFQRALSSSEKMKLFHGR--HSSKQKPRT---QITAVKEETEE
Cow       (1411) CQRFFVIEENKVRQYDSIQRMLSEKSLFRQAISPADRLKLLPHR--NSSRQRSRS---NIAALKEETEE
Frog      (1413) CQRFLVIEDNTVRQYDSIQKLVNEKSFFKQAISHSDRLKLFPLHRRNSSKRKSRP---QISALQEETEE
Monkey    (1411) CQQFLVIEENKVRQYDSIQKLLNERSLFRQAISPSDRVKLFPHR--NSSKCKTQP---QIAALKEETEE
Mouse     (1406) CQRFLVIEESNVWQYDSLQALLSEKSIFQQAISSSEKMRFFQGR--HSSKHKPRT---QITALKEETEE
Rabbit    (1380) CQRFLVIEENTVRQYESIQKLLSEKSLFRQAISSSDRAKLFPHR--NSSKHKSRP---QITALKEEAEE
Sheep     (1411) CQRFLVIEENKVRQYDSIQRMLSEKSLFRQAISPADRLKLLPHR--NSSRQRSRA---NIAALKEETEE
Dogfish   (1420) CQQFLVIEGCSVKQFDALQKLLTEASLFKQVFGHLDRAKLFTAHRRNSSKRKTRP---KISALQEEAEE
```

Fig. 3. Comparison of the amino acid sequences of CFTR carboxyl-terminal tails from various species. Sequence alignment was generated using the AlignX™ algorithm of the Vector NTI suite (Bethesda, MD). Amino acid sequence alignment of CFTR from human (P13569), monkey (AAC14012), sheep (Q0055), rabbit (AAC48608), frog (AAC60023), mouse (M60493), dogfish (P26362), killifish (AF000271), and cow (P35071) are shown. The tyrosine residue is conserved among all of the species except the dogfish, which has a phenylalanine residue. Phenylalanine residues have been shown to substitute for tyrosine residues and still maintain wild-type internalization activity for the transferrin receptor *(36)*. Sequences conform to the YXXΦ motif (underlined) common to internalization signals, where X can be any amino acid and Φ is a bulky hydrophobic residue.

the plasma membrane (**Fig. 2**). While AP-2 complexes bind to both tyrosine-based and dileucine-based signals, they do so through different subunits. Tyrosine-based signals interact with the μ2 chain, whereas dileucine-based signals interact selectively with the β-2 subunit. Consistent with this observation, tyrosine-based signals do not compete with dileucine signals for AP binding, nor does saturation of the tyrosine-based trafficking pathway affect the sorting of dileucine-containing proteins *(20)*.

1.4. CFTR

CFTR functions to regulate chloride ion permeability at the apical membrane of polarized epithelial cells *(21)*. CFTR can also be found in endosomal and recycling compartments *(1)*. Several studies have shown that CFTR undergoes endocytosis *(22,23)* via clathrin coated vesicles *(23–25)*. Indeed, it appears that CFTR contains clathrin-mediated endocytosis signals in both the amino and carboxyl termini *(26)*. Examination of the carboxyl terminal tail of CFTR across several species reveals the presence of a conserved YXXΦ motif (**Fig. 3**), a motif that is specifically recognized by the AP-2 clathrin adaptor complex *(27)*. Mutation of the Y^{1424}DSI motif to A^{1424}DSI, as expected, inhibits AP-2 binding *(27)* and CFTR endocytosis *(26)*. A model for clathrin-mediated endocytosis of CFTR is presented in **Fig. 4**.

1.5. Techniques to Study Endocytosis

Much information regarding the endocytosis of integral membrane proteins has been garnered from the use of radiolabeled ligands, such as transferrin and

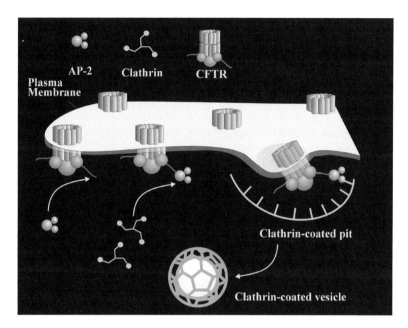

Fig. 4. Model for clathrin-mediated endocytosis of CFTR. Endocytic signals in the carboxyl-terminal domain of CFTR are recognized by the AP-2 endocytic adaptor complex. Binding of AP-2 to CFTR causes localization of CFTR into clathrin-coated pits which invaginate and eventually pinch off to form clathrin-coated vesicles. These vesicles rapidly uncoat to yield soluble adaptors and clathrin to initiate new rounds of endocytosis, and an uncoated vesicle, or endosome, containing CFTR.

LDL. Exposure of cells to labeled ligands at 4°C is followed by the endocytic uptake of the ligand upon rewarming. Cell surface ligand is easily removed by mild acid washes, and the amount of cell associated radioactivity is thus a measure of endocytosis. Such an approach permits both specificity and, provided the ligand can be labeled to a high specific activity, a large signal-to-noise ratio. These techniques are described in detail by McGraw and Subtil *(28)*. Radiolabeled antibodies to extracellular domains of CFTR offer a potential analogous approach to studying CFTR endocytosis, but the lack of high-affinity/high-specificity antibodies to extracellular domains of CFTR makes this approach untenable at the present time.

An alternative approach, outlined in detail in the present chapter, is to biotinylate cell surface proteins with a cleavable biotinylating reagent (**Fig. 5**). Following endocytosis, the cells are cooled to 4°C and remaining cell surface biotin is cleaved using membrane-impermeant reagents. In this way, proteins remaining on the cell surface are no longer labeled, whereas endocytosed proteins sequestered within intracellular endosomes remain biotinylated. Following cell lysis and solubilization, streptavidin-agarose is used to isolate endocytosed

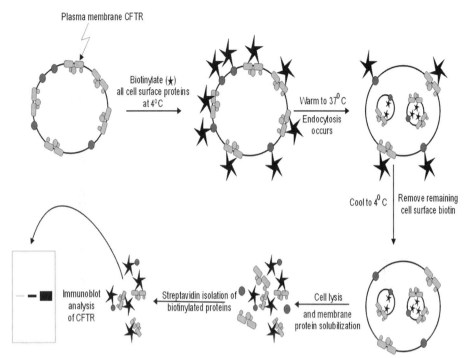

Fig. 5. Model for monitoring CFTR endocytosis using a cleavable biotinylating reagent. Cell surface proteins are biotinylated using a cleavable biotin moiety. Cell surface proteins are allowed to undergo endocytosis. Exposure of the cell surface to a membrane-impermeant thiol reducing agent removes biotin from cell surface proteins but is unable to do so from internalized proteins.

material, and the recovered material is subject to immunoblot analysis using antibodies against the protein of interest, in this case CFTR. As endocytosis proceeds, the amount of biotinylated CFTR that is resistant to cleavage will increase. At early time points, the amount of CFTR detected in intracellular compartments will increase linearly. At later time points deviations are expected due to recycling back to the plasma membrane and protein degradation.

2. Materials

2.1. Tissue Culture

1. Flp-In™ HEK cells stably expressing CFTR (*see* **Note 1**).
2. Dulbecco's mModified Eagle medium (DMEM) (high glucose) (Invitrogen, cat. no. 11965-092) prepared as described by the manufacturer.
3. Fetal bovine serum (FBS) (Hyclone, cat. no. SH30070.03).
4. Glutamine (Life Technologies, cat. no. 25030081).
5. Hygromycin (Life Technologies, cat. no. 10687010).
6. HEK-CFTR medium (DMEM—high glucose): 10% FBS, 2.0 mM L-glutamine, 150 µg/mL hygromycin.

7. Phosphate-buffered saline (PBS) (Sigma, cat. no. P4417).
8. Trypsin-EDTA (Life Technologies, cat. no. 25200-056).
9. T75-cm^2 flasks (Fisher, cat. no. 10-126-10).

2.2. Cell Surface Biotinylation

1. PBS-CM: 137 mM NaCl, 2.7 mM KCl, 0.1 mM CaCl$_2$, 1.0 mM MgCl$_2$, 4.3 mM Na$_2$HPO$_4$, 1.4 mM KH$_2$PO$_4$. Adjust pH to 7.4, if needed, with NaOH.
2. PBS-8: 137 mM NaCl, 2.7 mM KCl , 4.3 mM Na$_2$HPO$_4$, 1.4 mM KH$_2$PO$_4$. Adjust pH to 8.0 with 0.5 M NaOH.
3. Biotinylating solution: 1 mg/mL EZ-Link™ NHS-SS biotin in PBS-8 (*see* **Note 2**) (Pierce, cat. no. 21331).
4. PBS + 1% (w/v) bovine serum albumin (BSA).
5. Stripping solution: 100 mM MESNA (mercaptoethanesulphonic acid; Sigma, cat. no. M1511), 50 mM Tris, 100 mM NaCl, 1 mM EDTA, 0.2% (w/v) BSA. Adjust pH to 8.6 with HCl.
6. Lysis buffer: 50 mM Tris, 150 mM NaCl, 10 mM NH$_4$MoO$_4$, 0.1% (v/v) NP-40. Adjust pH to 7.4 with HCl.
7. Protease inhibitors (Complete™ EDTA-free protease inhibitor cocktail, Calbiochem, cat. no. 1873580).
8. Streptavidin agarose (ImmunoPure™ streptavidin gel, Pierce, cat. no. 20349).
9. 2X Laemmli sample buffer: 125 mM Tris-HCl, pH 6.7, 5% v/v β-mercaptoethanol, 2.5% (w/v) sodium dodecyl sulfate (SDS), 25% (v/v) glycerol, 0.01% (w/v) bromophenol blue.
10. CFTR antibody (Chemicon, Anti NBF-2, cat. no. MAb 3480; or R & D, Anti-C terminus, cat. no. MAb 25031).
11. ECL reagent (SuperSignal chemiluminescent substrates, Pierce, cat. no. 34080).
12. X-ray film (Kodak X-OMAT AR film).
13. Transfer buffer: 25 mM Tris, 190 mM glycine, 20% (v/v) methanol.
14. TBS-BLOTTO: 10 mM Tris-HCl, pH 7.4, 137 mM NaCl, 0.1% (v/v) Tween-20, 5% (w/v) nonfat dry milk.

3. Methods
3.1. HEK-CFTR Cell Culture

As with all cell culture, all solutions and equipment that come in contact with the cells must be sterile. Proper sterile technique should be observed, and all procedures carried out in a laminar-flow hood. HEK-CFTR cells were generated using Invitrogen's FlpIn system (*see* **Note 1**), with CFTR being driven off a cytomegalovirus (CMV) promoter. HEK293 cells containing a Flp recombinant target (FRT) site in a transcriptionally active genome locus were co-transfected with plasmids containing CFTR (along with a hygromycin resistance gene) and a yeast recombinase. Expression of the recombinase results in homologous recombination events between the FRT site and Flp sites in the CFTR plasmid. Thus each cell incorporates the CFTR gene in the same locus with the same transcriptional activity. For maintenance, HEK-CFTR cells (*see* **Note 1**) should be passaged when they are 80–90% confluent (3–4 d if split at a 1:5 to 1:10 dilution). Trypan blue is used to determine cell viability. Log-phase cultures should be >90% viable.

1. HEK-CFTR cells are maintained in DMEM plus 10% FBS and hygromycin (150 μg/mL). We typically add 200 mL of FBS and 6 mL of hygromycin to 1800 mL DMEM. The DMEM is prepared as described by the manufacturer.
2. Cells are kept in an incubator at 37°C in 5% CO_2 and passaged once to twice a week. It is important not to let the cells become overly confluent before passage and therefore avoid the need for excessive exposure to the trypsin-EDTA solution. Cells are passaged when 80–90% confluent.
3. The cells are washed once in PBS to remove excess media and serum (serum contains inhibitors of trypsin). Trypsin-EDTA solution (5 mL) is added to the monolayer, followed by incubation at room temperature for 1–5 min until the cells start to detach.
4. Once the cells are detached, they are briefly passed up and down in a sterile pipet to break up clumps of cells. Complete medium (5 mL) is added to prevent further trypsin activity. For maintenance of cells in 75-cm² tissue culture flasks, 1 mL of the 10-mL cell suspension is added to a new 75-cm² flask and 15 mL of fresh medium containing 150 μg/mL hygromycin added. Flasks are incubated in a 37°C humidified chamber containing 5% CO_2.

3.2. Cell Surface Biotinylation

Note: All procedures are performed at 4°C unless otherwise noted.

1. HEK-CFTR cells are grown in tissue culture-treated 100-mm dishes (*see* **Note 2**) until they reach 80–90% confluence.
2. The culture medium is removed by aspiration and the cells rinsed three times with PBS-CM to remove contaminating proteins. Since the biotinylation reagent cross-links primarily through lysine residues, residual serum protein will effectively inhibit cell surface biotinylation (*see also* **Note 3**).
3. Cells are rinsed once in PBS-8, and cell surface proteins are biotinylated by incubating the cells with EZ-Link NHS-SS Biotin (1 mg/mL) (see **Note 4**). For 100-mm culture dishes, 3 mL of biotinylating reagent in PBS-8 is adequate to cover the surface of the cells. Different volumes can be applied depending upon the size of culture dish used; we find that 100-mm dishes yield good reproducible signals.
4. Cells are then incubated on ice for 30 min to facilitate cell surface biotinylation (*see* **Note 5**). Following biotinylation, cells are then rinsed with PBS-BSA (4°C) and incubated with 5 mL of PBS-BSA on ice for 10 min to quench any residual NHS-SS biotin. The cells are now ready for experimental manipulation.

3.3. Endocytosis

Endocytosis is monitored by allowing cell surface proteins to enter endocytic compartments that are inaccessible to extracellular reducing agents. Since the NHS-SS biotin contains a reducible disulfide bond, membrane impermeant reducing agents are able to remove remaining cell surface biotin while leaving internalized biotin intact.

1. To monitor the internalization of cell surface CFTR, cells are warmed back to 37°C for varying periods of time. A 100-mm dish is sufficient for each time point using HEK-CFTR cells. The amount of material needed for other cell types will depend upon the expression level of CFTR, and will have to be determined empirically by the investigator.
2. Cells are rinsed once with culture medium (prewarmed to 37°C) and incubated in 37°C culture media following return to the incubator. Time points of 1, 2.5, 7.5, and 15 min are convenient time points to evaluate CFTR endocytosis.
3. At each time point, cells are cooled rapidly to 4°C by washing once in ice-cold PBS-CM. Biotinylated proteins remaining on the cell surface are cleaved by membrane-impermeant thiol reducing agents (*see* **Note 6**).
4. Cells are incubated with 5 mL of stripping buffer at 4°C for 15 min without shaking.
5. The stripping buffer is then aspirated and replaced with fresh stripping buffer for a further 15-min incubation at 4°C without shaking. A final third wash of stripping buffer for 15 min results in removal of >90% of all cell surface biotin (**Fig. 6**).
6. The efficiency of biotin stripping is evaluated by measuring the relative amount of biotinylated CFTR both before and after the reduction of the disulfide bonds on cells kept at 4°C.
7. Unreacted mercaptoethanesulfonic acid (MESNA) is quenched prior to cell lysis by rinsing cells with 5 mL of PBS-BSA followed by incubation in 5 mL of PBS-BSA for a further 10 min at 4°C.

3.4. Cell Lysis and Biotin Recovery

1. Washed cells are lysed and solubilized by the addition of 500 μL of ice-cold lysis buffer (containing protease inhibitors) to each 100-mm dish of cells.
2. The dishes are placed on ice for 2 min, and then the cells are scraped off with a rubber policeman and transferred to a 1.5-mL centrifuge tube.
3. The samples are vortexed rapidly and placed on ice for a further 15 min.
4. Insoluble material is removed by centrifugation at 4°C for 1 min at 12,000g. The supernatant is carefully removed without disturbing the pellet and transferred to a fresh 1.5-mL centrifuge tube. The pellet is discarded.
5. Protein concentration in all samples is normalized by standard protein assay protocols. Equivalent amounts of protein for each data point (~3 mg protein) are incubated with 60 μL of packed ImmunoPure streptavidin gel and samples rotated at 4°C overnight.
6. Biotin conjugates are precipitated by centrifugation at 12,000g for 30 s at 4°C. The supernatant is aspirated and discarded, and the pellet is resuspended in 1 mL of lysis buffer. The wash is repeated twice more.
7. Following the final wash, the supernatant is carefully aspirated and the pellet resuspended in 30 μL of 5× Laemmli sample buffer. Samples are heated to 30°C for 5 min then subject to centrifugation for 2 min at 12,000g.

3.5. SDS-PAGE and Immunoblot

1. Denaturing electrophoresis in sodium dodecyl sulfate (SDS) slab gels (7.5% acrylamide) (SDS-PAGE) is performed according to the method of Laemmli *(29)*.
2. CFTR is transferred to nitrocellulose using a transfer buffer without SDS (25 m*M* Tris, 190 m*M* glycine, and 20% (v/v) methanol). Using the Bio-Rad MiniBlot™ transfer system, we find transfer of CFTR to be essentially complete at power settings of 100 V and 250 mA for a 100-min transfer.
3. Following transfer, the blot is blocked in TBS-BLOTTO for 1 h at room temperature.
4. CFTR primary detecting antibodies, diluted 1:1000 in TBS-BLOTTO, are added to the blot with gentle shaking overnight at 4°C.
5. The nitrocellulose blots are rinsed 6× for a total of 30 min in TBS-BLOTTO. Secondary goat-anti mouse antibodies conjugated to horseradish peroxidase (HRP) are diluted 1:2000 in TBS-BLOTTO and added to the blot for 60 min at room temperature with gentle shaking (*see* **Note 7**). The blots are then rinsed 6× in TBS without milk for a total of 30 min.
6. Nitrocellulose blots are immersed in fresh ECL reagent for 4 min. Excess fluid is drained off (but do not dry the blot) and the nitrocellulose sandwiched between two sheets of overhead transparency film.
7. Blots are exposed to X-ray film for an appropriate time.

3.6. Data Analysis

1. Developed X-ray film is scanned using a flat-bed scanner. There are a large variety of scanner types and models currently available. Virtually all scanners include their own scanning and image editing software.
2. Gel images are scanned and saved in *8-bit gray-scale* mode. Scanning in *line art* mode results in loss of information, and scanning in *colour* mode uses additional computer memory without increasing the amount of useful information.
3. Quantitation of scanned images is performed using software designed for densitometric analysis. Quantitation of "band" parameters, including pixel intensity and number of pixels, is achieved using the various algorithms supplied in the software packages. We have found *Un-Scan-It* (Silk Scientific, Orem UT) to be straightforward to use, providing a simple yet flexible set of options for densitometric analysis of films and gels.

3.7. Critical Parameters

The protocol described in the current chapter has been optimized for monitoring CFTR endocytosis in HEK-CFTR cells. While it is equally applicable to monitoring CFTR endocytosis in other cell types, conditions for each cell type will have to be optimized. The efficiency of cell surface biotinylation needs to be determined by examining the effects of increasing biotinylation time to find the minimal period required to achieve steady-state CFTR labeling. Similarly, the efficiency of thiol reduction/stripping should be determined by comparing cell surface CFTR signal before and after stripping. Loss of CFTR-biotin signal following stripping should be at least 90%.

3.8. Anticipated Results

It is critical that residual biotin remaining on the cell surface following endocytosis be efficiently cleaved. Such thiol cleavage should be at least 90% efficient (**Fig. 6**). On average, we obtain a cleavage efficiency of 93.5% ± 3.2 ($n = 3$) compared to total cell surface biotin from unstripped cells. The values obtained from the stripped samples are subtracted from all time points as a background value. With increasing time, there should be an increase in biotinylated CFTR signal (**Fig. 7**). Each time point is expressed as a fraction of the total cell surface CFTR pool present at time zero (**Fig. 8**). It should be realized that the extent and rate of CFTR endocytosis will, to some extent, depend upon the CFTR expression level (since AP-2 binding is saturable; *see* **Note 8**) and upon the cell type expressing CFTR. Mutation of motifs in CFTR which interact with the clathrin mediated machinery should also inhibit CFTR endocytosis. For example, a Y1424A mutation in CFTR which occurs in the carboxyl terminal YXXΦ motif (Y^{1424}DSI) results in a marked reduction (~60–80%) in CFTR/AP-2 interactions *(27)* and CFTR endocytosis (**Fig. 9**) *(26)*.

3.9. Alternative Strategies

While the strategy described above has proven to be robust and reproducible in our hands, variations of this protocol have been utilized by other investigators with similar results. Lukacs et al. *(23)* have metabolically labeled CFTR with ^{35}S methionine prior to biotinylating cell surface proteins with sulpho-NHS-SS biotin (EZ-Link NHS-SS biotin). Endocytosed material is resistant to membrane-impermeant thiol reducing agents. Following cell lysis, total CFTR (both biotinylayted and nonbiotinylated) is first immunoprecipitated using CFTR antibodies. The precipitates are solubilized in SDS buffer and biotinylated-CFTR is reprecipitated using streptavidin agarose. SDS-PAGE followed by autoradiography provides a monitor of endocytosed CFTR. Biotinylation of oligosaccharide moieties of cell surface proteins can also be employed to study endocytosis *(4,22)*. Such a strategy uses a two-step procedure to label glycoconjugates, which requires an initial periodate oxidation step followed by exposure to biotin-LC-hydrazide. Endocytosis of CFTR is monitored by including a 37°C incubation step following periodate oxidation but before biotinylation. After the 37°C incubation step remaining cell surface oxidized glycoconjugates are biotinylated. Following cell lysis biotinylated and nonbiotinylated proteins are separated by streptavidin agarose and CFTR detected by immunoprecipitation of streptavidin bound and unbound fractions followed by in vitro phosphorylation of CFTR by protein kinase A and (^{32}P)-γ-ATP. Phosphorylated CFTR is resolved by SDS-PAGE and subject to autoradiographic analysis. Using this approach, endocytosis of CFTR is monitored as a loss of signal.

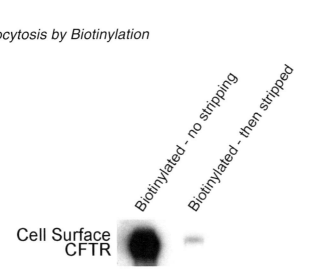

Fig. 6. Thiol reduction of remaining cell surface biotin. Following uptake of cell surface proteins by endocytosis, residual cell surface biotin must be efficiently removed. One should expect >90% efficiency of stripping. This important control should be present in each experiment.

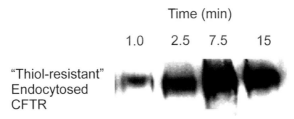

Fig. 7. Scanned image of lumigram from an endocytosis experiment.

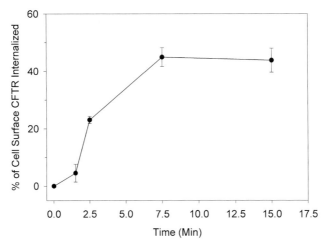

Fig. 8. Time course of CFTR endocytosis.

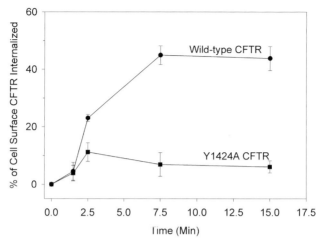

Fig. 9. Endocytosis of wild-type and Y1424A CFTR.

3.10. Inhibition of Clathrin-Mediated Endocytosis

All endocytic mechanisms are temperature and energy dependent, and are blocked at 4°C. At present, there are no pharmacological agents that block clathrin-mediated endocytosis, but such processes can be inhibited by intracellular potassium depletion *(30)*, hypertonic sucrose media *(31)*, and cytosol acidification *(32)*. While such approaches have proven useful in determining the internalization pathways of proteins, including CFTR *(23,25)*, conclusions must be drawn cautiously as the extent and specificity of endocytic inhibition varies greatly among cell types *(33)*.

4. Notes

1. HEK-CFTR cells generated using Invitrogen's Flp-In system are available from the authors upon request. The Flp-In system from Invitrogen is designed for rapid generation of isogenic stable expression cell lines. Invitrogen's Flp-In system utilizes a *Saccharomyces cervisiae*-derived DNA recombination system that uses a recombinase (Flp) and site-specific recombination to make possible integration of genes of interest (i.e., wild-type or mutant CFTR) into a specific site into mammalian cell genomes. Flp-In HEK-293 cells (Invitrogen, cat. no. R750-07) contain a single Flp recombinase target (FRT) site and stably express the *lacZ-Zeocin*™ gene under the control of the SV40 promoter. CFTR was cloned into the pcDNA5/FRT expression vector, which contains the human CMV promoter and the hygromycin resistance gene. When Flp-In HEK293 cells are co-transfected with pcDNA5/FRT/CFTR and a plasmid that constitutively expresses Flp recombinase (pOG44), the Flp recombinase mediates a homologous recombination event between FRT sites in the pcDNA5/FRT/CFTR plasmid and the FRT sites already integrated into the genome. This system affords the advantage of

having expression vectors integrating at the same unique locus in every trans-fected cell. Moreover, since all Flp-In cell lines are isogenic, all transfected clones produce equivalent levels of protein. For more information on this system, the reader is directed to www.Invitrogen.com.

2. We have noted that occasionally, despite careful washing, cells detach from the cell culture dish. This is usually most apparent for cultures that have become overconfluent. Corning "Tissue Culture Treated" dishes (Corning, cat. no. 430167) are coated and provide a reasonably good adherence matrix for the cells. Neverthe-less, it is advisable not to use cultures that have exceeded 90% confluency.

3. Biotinylation of many membrane proteins is enhanced at alkaline pH *(34)*. This is consistent with the chemistry of reactive NHS esters of biotin, which react with the ε amino groups of lysines or amino acyl α-amino groups when they are in the unprotonated or neutral NH_2 form. Since the pK_a of the ε-amino group of lysine is ~10.5, it follows that lysine residues will have a greater likelihood of being available for cross-linking at elevated rather than neutral pH.

4. EZ-Link NHS-SS biotin should be made fresh each day. Although the cross-linker is water soluble, it is prone to hydrolysis; such hydrolysis increases at elevated pH, so long-term storage is not recommended.

5. There is a great deal of flexibility in the actual conditions that promote protein biotinylation. We have varied incubation temperatures from 4 to 18°C, pH of the biotinylation buffer from pH 7.0 to pH 9.0, and incubation time from 5 minutes to overnight. For the HEK-CFTR cells described in this chapter, we have found that pH 8.0 for 30 min at 4°C yields good reproducible signals. Investigators will have to determine empirically the most suitable conditions for CFTR biotinylation with their particular cell line, since such conditions are cell type dependent.

6. We have tried several membrane-impermeant thiol reducing agents including MESNA and glutathione. We have found MESNA to yield the most reproducible results. It is also important to perform 15-min washes three times rather than one 45-min wash. The efficiency of stripping is much greater with repetitive washes rather than a single wash of similar total time. We have not found that performing more than three washes significantly reduces the cell surface signal any further.

7. There are many methods available for the detection of immunoreactive proteins on immunoblots. We routinely use enhanced chemiluminescence (ECL), which offers a high degree of sensitivity without the need to use radiolabeled reagents. The actual combination of horseradish peroxidase-linked secondary antibodies and ECL reagents are matters of personal preference and experience. We have found consistent results using goat-anti mouse peroxidase-linked secondary anti-bodies from Becton-Dickinson (cat. no. M15345) and ECL reagents from Pierce (SuperSignal Chemiluminescent substrates, cat. no. 34080).

8. Care should be exercised when comparing CFTR endocytosis rates among dif-ferent constructs, cell lines, and stable vs transient expression systems. Transient overexpression of proteins can result in reduced rates of endocytosis, as has been shown for the transferrin receptor *(35)* and CFTR *(26)*, consistent with the notion that the cellular machinery for endocytosis is limiting and saturable.

Acknowledgments

The authors wish to thank Mr. Mark Silvis for his excellent technical assistance and for generating the HEK-CFTR cell lines. The financial support of the Cystic Fibrosis Foundation and the National Institute of Health are also gratefully acknowledged.

References

1. Bradbury, N. A. (1999) Intracellular CFTR: localization and function. *Physiol. Rev.* **79,** S175–S191.
2. Cheng, S. H., Claass, A., Sommer, M. et al. (1990) Defective intracellular transport and processing of CFTR is the molecular basis of most cystic fibrosis. *Cell* **63,** 827–834.
3. Kalin, N., Claass, A., Sommer, M. et al. (1999) DeltaF508 CFTR protein expression in tissues from patients with cystic fibrosis. *J. Clin. Invest.* **103,** 1379–1389.
4. Heda, G. H., Tanwani, M., and Marino, C. R. (2001) The ΔF508 mutation shortens the biochemical half-life of plasma membrane CFTR in polarized epithelial cells. *Am. J. Physiol.* **280,** C166–C174.
5. Metchnikoff, E. (1893) *Lectures on the Comparative Pathology of Inflammation.* Paul, Kegan, Trench, Trabner, and Co, London.
6. Mellman, I. (1996) Endocytosis and molecular sorting. *Annu. Rev. Cell Dev. Biol.* **12,** 575–625.
7. Mukherjee, S., Ghosh, R. N., and Maxfield, F. R. (1997) Endocytosis. *Physiol. Rev.* **77,** 759–803.
8. Steinman, R. M., Mellman, I. S., Muller, W. A. et al. (1983) Endocytosis and the recycling of plasma membrane. *J. Cell Biol.* **96,** 1–27.
9. Trowbridge, I. S. and Collawn, J. F. (1993) Signal-dependent membrane protein trafficking in the endocytic pathway. *Annu. Rev. Cell Biol.* **9,** 129–161.
10. Heilker, R., Spiess, M., and Crottet, P. (1999) Recognition of sorting signals by clathrin adaptors. *Bioessays* **21,** 558–567.
11. Bonifacino, J. S. and Dell'Angelica, E. C. (1999) Molecular bases for the recognition of tyrosine-based sorting signals. *J. Cell Biol.* **145,** 923–926.
12. Anderson, R. G. W., Goldstein, J. L., and Brown, M. S. (1977) A mutation that impairs the ability of lipoprotein receptors to localize in coated pits on the cell surface of human fibroblasts. *Nature* **270,** 695–699.
13. Collawn, J. F., Stangel, M., Kuhn, L. A. et al. (1990) Transferrin receptor internalization sequence YXRF implicates a tight turn as the structural recognition motif for endocytosis. *Cell* **63(5),** 1061–1072.
14. Bansal, A. and Gierasch, L. M. (1991) The NPXY internalization signal of the LDL receptor adopts a reverse-turn conformation. *Cell* **67,** 1195–1201.
15. Eberle, W., Sander, C., Klaus, W. et al. (1991) The essential tyrosine of the internalization signal in lysosomal acid phosphatase is part of a β turn. *Cell* **67,** 1203–1209.
16. Owen, D. J. and Evans, P. R. (1998) A structural explanation for the recognition of tyrosine-based endocytic signals. *Science* **282,** 1327–1332.
17. Letourner, F. and Klausner, R. D. (1992) A novel di-leucine motif and a tyrosine-based motif independently mediate lysosomal targeting and endocytosis of CD3 chains. *Cell* **69(7),** 1143–1157.

18. Haft, C. R., De La Luz Sierra, M., Hamer, I., et al. (1998) Analysis of the juxtamembrane dileucine motif in the insulin receptor. *Endocrinology* **139,** 1618–1629.
19. Kirchhausen, T. (1999) Adaptors for clathrin-mediated traffic. *Annu. Rev. Cell Dev. Biol.* **15,** 705–732.
20. Marks, M. S., Woodruff, L., Ohno, H., et al.(1996) Protein targeting by tyrosine- and di-leucine-based signals: evidence for distinct saturable components. *J. Cell Biol.* **135,** 341–354.
21. Sheppard, D. N. and Welsh, M. J. (1999) Structure and function of the CFTR chloride channel. *Physiol. Rev.* **79,** S23–S46.
22. Prince, L. S., Workman, R. B. J., and Marchase, R. B. (1994) Rapid endocytosis of the cystic fibrosis transmembrane conductance regulator chloride channel. *Proc. Natl. Acad. Sci. USA* **91,** 5192–5196.
23. Lukacs, G. L., Segal, G., Kartner, N., et al. (1997) Constitutive internalization of cystic fibrosis transmembrane conductance regulator occurs via clathrin-dependent endocytosis and is regulated by protein phosphorylation. *Biochem. J.* **328,** 353–361.
24. Bradbury, N. A., Cohn, J. A., Venglarik, C. J., et al. (1994) Biochemical and biophysical identification of cystic fibrosis transmembrane conductance chloride channels as components of endocytic clathrin coated vesicles. *J. Biol. Chem.* **269,** 8296–8302.
25. Bradbury, N. A., Clark, J. A., Watkins, S. C., et al. (1999) Characterization of the internalization pathways for the cystic fibrosis transmembrane conductance regulator (CFTR). *Am. J. Physiol.* **276,** L659–688.
26. Prince, L. S., Peter, K., Hatton, S. R., et al. (1999) Efficient endocytosis of the cystic fibrosis transmembrane conductance regulator requires a tyrosine-based signal. *J. Biol. Chem.* **274,** 3602–3609.
27. Weixel, K. and Bradbury, N. A. (1999) The carboxy terminus of CFTR binds the AP-2 endocytic adaptor complex. *J. Biol. Chem.* **275,** 3655–3660.
28. McGraw, T. E. and Subtil, A. (1999) Endocytosis: biochemical analyses, in *Current Protocols in Cell Biology* (Bonifacino, J. S., et al., eds.), John Wiley & Sons, New York. p. 15.3.1.
29. Laemmli, U. K. (1970) Cleavage of structural proteins during the assembly of bacteriophage T4. *Nature* **277,** 680–685.
30. Larkin, J. M., Brown, M. S., Goldstein, J. L., et al. (1983) Depletion of intracellular potassium arrests coated pit formation and receptor-mediated endocytosis in fibroblasts. *Cell* **33,** 273–285.
31. Sandvig, K., Olsnos, S., Petersen, O. W., et al. (1989) Control of coated pit function by cytoplasmic pH. *Methods Cell Biol.* **32,** 365–382.
32. Sandvig, K., et al. (1987) Acidification of the cytosol inhibits endocytosis from coated pits. *J. Cell Biol.* **105,** 679–689.
33. Moya, M., Dautry-Varsat, A., Goud, B., et al. (1985) Inhibition of coated pit formation in Hep2 cells blocks the cytotoxicity of diptheria toxin but not that of ricin toxin. *J. Cell Biol.* **101,** 548–559.
34. Gottardi, C. J. and Caplan, M. J. (1992) Cell surface biotinylation in the determination of epithelial membrane polarity. *J. Tissue Cult. Methods* **14,** 173–180.

35. Warren, R. A., Green, F. A., and Enns, C. A. (1996) Saturation of the endocytic pathway for the transferrin receptor does not affect the endocytosis of the epidermal growth factor receptor. *J. Biol. Chem.* **272,** 2116–2121.
36. McGraw, T. E. and Maxfield, F. R. (1990) Human transferrin receptor internalization is partially dependent upon an aromatic amino acid on the cytoplasmic domain. *Cell Regul.* **1(4),** 369–377.

II

CFTR Structure and Function:
Regulatory Complexes

23

CFTR Regulation of ENaC

Scott H. Donaldson, Elaine G. Poligone, and M. Jackson Stutts

1. Introduction
1.1. ENaC Dysregulation in Cystic Fibrosis

The idea that cystic fibrosis (CF) results from dysregulation of ion channels, including the epithelial Na^+ channel (ENaC), evolved from observations made before the cloning of the CF gene in 1989. Multiple laboratories had reported that protein kinase A (PKA) stimulated a Cl^- channel called the ORCC (outward rectifying Cl^- channel) in cells from normal, but not CF, epithelial tissues *(1–3)*. We had also reported that amiloride-sensitive Na^+ absorption was elevated in the airway epithelia of CF patients *(4–6)*. Once cloned, sequences within the CF gene identified it as a member of the ATP-binding cassette (ABC) transporter superfamily *(7)*. Surprisingly, the CF gene product was found to form a Cl^- channel with distinctly different properties from the ORCC *(8,9)*. Because ABC proteins were known to function as both transporters and regulators of other processes *(10)*, and because the regulation of ORCC and amiloride-sensitive Na^+ absorption were affected in CF, the CF gene product was named the cystic fibrosis transmembrane conductance regulator (CFTR) *(11)*. Subsequently, CFTR has been reported to affect the activity of a large number of other ion channels and solute transporters *(12)*.

The chief interest in CFTR's ability to affect the function of other ion channels and transporters is the possibility that such secondary functions contribute in an organ-specific fashion to the pathogenesis of CF. The organ-specific ion transport abnormalities observed in CF are highly variable, ranging from decreased salt and water secretion in pancreatic *(13)* and bile ducts *(14)* to decreased salt absorption by sweat ductal epithelium *(15)*. In order to understand how a CFTR function other than Cl^- conductance contributes to pathophysiology at an affected site, it is helpful to identify the molecular basis of the

From: *Methods in Molecular Medicine, vol. 70: Cystic Fibrosis Methods and Protocols*
Edited by: W. R. Skach © Humana Press Inc., Totowa, NJ

putative secondary function and define its role in normal physiology. Despite serious efforts, this level of understanding has not yet been achieved for CFTR's apparent functional interactions with other ion channels and transporters, including ENaC.

Lung disease is the primary cause of disability and death in CF patients, yet the nature of the relationship between CFTR function(s) and the maintenance of lung health remains controversial. In normal individuals, the removal of inhaled pathogens from the airway surface by mucociliary clearance (MCC) forms a major line of lung defense *(16,17)*. In addition, the antimicrobial properties of airway surface liquid (ASL) contribute to the maintenance of a sterile airway environment *(18,19)*. In CF patients, innate lung defense mechanisms become overwhelmed, and chronic infection and inflammation lead to the destruction of conducting airways. The precise defect in innate defense that results from CFTR mutations is a matter of intense investigation and debate. One school of thought holds that CFTR Cl⁻ channel activity determines the salt composition of airway surface liquid *(20)*. This theory proposes that normal airway epithelia utilize CFTR as the exclusive path for Cl⁻ absorption to extract salt from the ASL, leaving a hypotonic luminal solution, much like a sweat duct. As a consequence, this model projects that CF airway surface liquid is relatively hypertonic. It was further hypothesized that a higher salt concentration in CF ASL interferes with the antimicrobial action of natural defensin molecules, leading to a breech in airway defense. Although this is an attractive model for the pathogenesis of CF lung disease, recent reports on the ionic composition of ASL in normal and CF using noninvasive ion-selective electrodes and fluorescent dyes have concluded that both normal and CF ASL are nearly isotonic and not different *(21,22)*. This conclusion is compatible with independent assessments of the high water permeability of normal and CF airway epithelia, which suggest that neither epithelium can maintain a hypotonic ASL fluid *(23–25)*.

An alternative hypothesis relating CFTR mutations to the development of lung disease proposes that regulation of ENaC by CFTR is required to maintain an ASL height that is adequate for MCC to proceed. MCC is a complex process, involving coordinated functions of ciliary beating, salt and water transport, and mucus secretion. Central to the MCC process is the maintenance of a low-viscosity periciliary liquid layer on the airway surface that enables cilia to beat effectively and propel mucus out of the lung *(26,27)*. The depth of this periciliary liquid layer is determined by net salt and water movements across airways epithelia, and thus is strongly influenced by ion channel activity *(21,25)*. The ion channels in the apical membrane of airway epithelia that are rate limiting for net salt movement are CFTR and ENaC *(28,29)*. The abnormal CFTR and ENaC activities observed in CF may, therefore, account for a reduced MCC rate and the subsequent onset of airway infection. Support for this theory includes the repeated observation that Na^+ absorption in CF airways is two- to threefold greater than in normal airways in vivo *(30,31)*, in freshly excised tissues *(5)*, and in various cultured airway epithelial preparations *(32–34)*. Recent studies utilizing highly differentiated airway epithelial cultures that develop rotational mucus transport further demonstrated that the hyperabsorption of Na^+ by CF airway epithelia diminished the periciliary liquid layer and caused mucostasis *(25)*. Therefore, the drastic consequences of CF lung disease appear to originate from the abnormal pattern of ion transport that results from mutations in the CF gene. Moreover, available data strongly suggest that negative modulation of ENaC by CFTR in human airways is a normal function of CFTR and relevant to CF lung disease pathogenesis. It is important to establish the molecular basis of this relationship between CFTR and ENaC, and methods that may help in this effort are the subject of this chapter.

1.2. Test Systems for Studying CFTR and ENaC

Numerous test systems have been used for study of CFTR–ENaC interactions. Normal and CF airway epithelia, studied in vivo or in vitro soon after excision, comprise the "gold standard" for demonstrating a negative influence of CFTR on ENaC *(4,5,30,31,35)*. However, maneuvers to explore the molecular basis of the phenomenon in fresh tissues are limited. To circumvent this limitation, several heterologous expression systems are available.

1.2.1. Xenopus *Oocytes*

The *Xenopus* laevis oocyte system has been used to study the expression of foreign mRNA and cDNA for more than two decades *(36)*. This single-cell, eukaryotic system has been popularized for the study of plasma membrane proteins for several reasons. Being exceptionally large (~1 mm diameter), injection of RNA and placement of intracellular recording electrodes is technically easy. To a great extent, heterologously expressed proteins are properly processed such that cytoplasmic, membrane, and even secreted proteins reach their usual cellular destination and are functionally active. In the case of heteromeric proteins, proper subunit assembly into a functionally active molecule is usually observed. Expression of foreign proteins is also remarkably robust, both in terms of the quantity of protein produced and the proportion of injected oocytes that ultimately express the desired construct. Finally, oocytes lend themselves to a wide variety of assays ranging from basic biochemical techniques to electrophysiological studies.

Drawbacks to using the *Xenopus* oocyte expression system should also be considered. These include the presence of seasonal variability of oocyte quality, the transient duration of heterologous protein expression (days), and the relatively small number of cells that can be studied in a single experiment. In addition, even when a channel is expressed reliably, the dominant means of regulation in the oocyte may be via mechanisms that are different from the native tissue of interest. Therefore, the decision to utilize this system for the study of plasma membrane ion channels, such as ENaC and CFTR, depends largely on the experimental questions being asked.

A vast amount of data in the areas of CFTR and ENaC biology has already been accrued using the *Xenopus* oocyte system. After the molecular cloning of the CFTR gene in 1989 *(11)*, this system was used to demonstrate that the resulting protein product functioned directly as a chloride channel *(37)*, while later studies examined CFTR activation, regulation *(38,39)*, and the behavior of mutant CFTR channels *(38,40–42)*. Further, the cloning of all three ENaC subunits was accomplished with a functional complementation assay in oocytes by Canessa et al. in 1994 *(43,44)*. Since then, the *Xenopus* oocyte system has been a mainstay for the study of ENaC, and has contributed to our understanding of channel regulation and structure–function relationships. In addition, the nature of interactions between CFTR and ENaC has been widely studied in this system *(45–52)*. These groups uniformly reproduced negative regulation of ENaC by CFTR, and have additionally addressed specific questions, such as the domains of ENaC and CFTR *(46,47)* or the ionic conditions *(50)* that are required for interaction.

1.2.2. Mammalian Cells

Although *Xenopus* oocytes have proven to be a remarkably useful system for the study of CFTR and ENaC, the ability to perform functional studies in mammalian cells is desirable. Epithelial cells that natively express both CFTR and ENaC, such as airway or sweat duct epithelia, are useful for determining the role of each ion channel in tissue-specific patterns of ion transport. However, to probe the ability of CFTR to affect ENaC function, one approach has been to express CFTR and ENaC stably, separately or together in cells that do not express either channel natively *(53–56)*. The creation of stable cell lines and the ability to study function in a polarized mammalian cell system are significant advantages over oocytes. Weighing against these benefits are considerable problems. Whereas there has been widespread success in heterologous expression of CFTR, three gene products must be expressed to observe amiloride sensitive Na^+ conductance. Generation of stable cell lines can be time consuming and costly. Once cell lines expressing ENaC are successfully derived, additional genetic manipulations become increasingly difficult. However, the advantages offered by stable cell lines for patch clamp and biochemical approaches make the effort worthwhile. We have used an NIH 3T3 fibroblast cell model system because it is relatively easy to co-express stably multiple foreign genes, though is limited by being a nonpolarized system *(53,54)*. Epithelial cells are a more relevant model for studying CFTR–ENaC interactions, but it is more difficult to express multiple proteins in this system.

2. Materials

2.1. Xenopus *Oocytes*

2.1.1. Oocyte Harvesting

1. 3-Aminobenzoic acid ethyl ester (methanesulfonate salt).
2. Collagenase type IA.
3. Calcium-free/replete modified Barth's solution: 88 mM NaCl, 1.0 mM KCl, 2.4 mM NaHCO$_3$, 0.82 mM MgSO$_4$, 20 mM HEPES, ± 0.41 mM CaCl$_2$, 0.33 mM Ca(NO$_3$), pH 7.5; supplemented with 10 mg/mL penicillin, 5 mg/mL streptomycin, ± 2.5 mM sodium pyruvate, and 0.5 mM theophylline.
4. #11 scalpel.
5. 4-O silk suture on curved needle.
6. Dissecting instruments (scissors, sharp #5 forceps, needle driver).
7. Dissecting microscope.
8. Low-temperature incubator.

2.1.2. RNA Preparation and Injection

1. cDNA encoding gene of interest (with upstream RNA polymerase-binding site and downstream polyA tail).
2. In vitro transcription kit and m^{7}G(5')pppG cap nucleotide analog (Roche Molecular Biochemicals).
3. Chloroform/phenol/isoamyl alchohol, 25/24/1, v/v/v.
4. 70 and 100% ethanol.
5. Agarose gel electrophoresis unit.
6. Microinjector (Dagan Instruments; Drummond Scientific).
7. Coarse micromanipulator.
8. Pipet puller.
9. Small-internal-diameter pipet glass (Microcaps, Drummond Scientific).
10. Injecting platform (polypropylene mesh attached to 75-mm culture dish).
11. Dissecting microscope.

2.1.3. Electrophysiological Studies in Oocytes

1. Pipet puller (DMZ-Universal Puller).
2. Thin-walled borosilicate glass pipets (Warner Instrument).
3. Micromanipulators (Newport; Narashige).
4. Patch clamp amplifier (Geneclamp 500, Axon Instruments).
5. Computer.
6. Data digitizer (Digidata 1200, Axon Instruments).
7. Electrophysiology acquisition and analysis software (pClamp 8.0, Axon Instruments).
8. Amiloride.

2.1.4. Biochemical Analyses in Oocytes

1. Homogenization buffer: 150 mM NaCl, 10 mM Mg-acetate, 20 mM Tris-HCl, pH 7.6.
2. Protease inhibitors: 20 µg/mL phenylmethylsulfonyl fluoride, 5 µg/mL leupeptin, 5 µg/mL pepstatin.

3. Triton X-100.
4. Sucrose.
5. Glass-teflon homogenizer or hypodermic needles (22 and 27 gage).
6. Sodium dodecyl sulfate-polyacrylamide gel electrophoresis (SDS-PAGE) and electrophoretic transfer units.
7. Nitrocellulose or PVDF membranes.
8. Appropriate primary and secondary antisera.
9. ECL reagent (Amersham Pharmacia).
10. Sulfo-NHS-LC-Biotin (Pierce).
11. Magnabind Streptavidin beads (Pierce).
12. Stepped sucrose gradient: 50–20% sucrose dissolved in 50 mM NaCl, 10 mM Mg-acetate, 20 mM Tris-HCl, pH 7.6, + protease imhibitors.

2.2. Mammalian Cells

2.2.1. Transfection and Selection

1. Retroviral vectors containing genes encoding CFTR or αβγ ENaC subunits, as well as genes for resistance to G418 or puromycin.
2. Selection medium containing G418 and/or puromycin (or appropriate antibiotic for vector chosen).
3. Cloning rings.
4. Tissue culture plates.
5. Dexamethasone, sodium butyrate for inducing media.

2.2.2. Biochemical Expression

1. Specific antibodies directed against CFTR or αβγ ENaC subunits for Western blot analysis.
2. SDS-PAGE gel box.
3. Lysis buffer: 62.5 mM Tris-HCl, pH 6.5, 2% SDS, 6 M urea, 160 mM dithiothreitol (DTT), and 0.01% bromophenol blue.
4. Electrophoretic transfer unit.
5. Precast 4–15% gradient acrylamide gels (Bio-Rad).
6. Power supply.
7. Nitrocellulose or PVDF (Immobilon) membrane.
8. Enhanced chemiluminesence reagent for detection of horseradish peroxidase-conjugated secondary antibodies.
9. Radiolabeled probe complementary to specific sequences in CFTR or ENaC subunits for Northern blot analysis.
10. Agarose gel box for RNA gel.
11. Autoradiography film (Kodak).
12. Film developer.

2.2.3. Functional Expression/Characterization

1. Pipet puller (DMZ-Universal Puller).
2. Air table.

3. Faraday cage.
4. Micromanipulator (Newport).
5. Computer.
6. Electrophysiology acquisition and analysis software (pClamp 8.0 software suite, Axon Instruments).
7. Thin-wall borosilicate glass capillary tubes with filament for patch pipets, 1.5-mm outside diameter (Warner Instrument).
8. Patch clamp solutions for bath and pipet (Li^+-containing gluconate salts for study of ENaC; ATP-containing solutions for whole-cell pipet solutions).
9. Amiloride.
10. Patch clamp amplifier (Axopatch-1C or equivalent, Axon Instruments).
11. Data digitizer (Digidata 1200 or equivalent, Axon Instruments).
12. Ussing chambers (Easy Mount Diffusion Chambers, Physiologic Instruments).
13. Multichannel voltage/current clamp (Physiologic Instruments).
14. Software for analysis of Ussing chamber studies (Acquire and Analyze, Physiologic Instruments).

3. Methods

3.1. Xenopus *Oocytes*

3.1.1. Oocyte Harvesting

1. *Xenopus laevis* are indigenous to South Africa, air breathing, but entirely aquatic. Care and maintenance has been extensively reviewed elsewhere *(57)*. Prior to surgery for oocyte removal, the frog is anesthetized by placing it in a 0.1–0.2% solution of the methane sulfonate salt of 3-aminobenzoic acid ethyl ester ("tricaine") for 15–30 min.
2. One should test for the adequacy of anesthesia by dripping a small amount of water into the mouth of the frog (held on its back), and observing for the absence of the swallow reflex. During anesthesia and recovery, care should be taken to prevent drowning by maintaining the animal's nose above the level of water using an inclined holding container.
3. Once the frog is fully anesthetized, it is placed in the supine position on a clean surface. A small (~1-cm) diagonal incision is made through the skin layer in either lower abdominal quadrant with a scalpel. The underlying fascia is grasped with forceps and cut with scissors parallel to the skin incision. Oocytes should be readily visible and are harvested by simply pulling them through the incision with forceps and excising as much of the ovarian tissue as is required. The remaining ovarian tissue can then be placed back into the abdomen, and the fascia and skin are closed separately with ~2 stitches per layer. Although sterile surgical instruments should be used in this procedure, the animal's skin does not need to be disinfected and the incidence of wound infection is very low due to the presence of natural antimicrobial peptides present in the frog's skin.
4. Surgically harvested oocytes must have the outer follicular layer removed in order to facilitate penetration of the egg with injecting/measuring pipets. Defolliculation of a relatively small number of oocytes may be done manually

with fine forceps after shrinking the cells in a hypertonic solution (200 m*M* K⁺-aspartate, 10 m*M* HEPES, pH 7.4). Alternatively, enzymatic digestion with collagenase allows the defolliculation of a large number of oocytes but can reduce their viability if overdigestion occurs (*see* **Note 1**).

5. The oocytes are then extensively washed with calcium-free MBS, transferred to MBS containing calcium and antibiotics and maintained at 16–19°C. Some investigators also advocate the addition of theophylline and sodium pyruvate in order to improve the duration of oocyte viability. Individual, healthy, Stage V–VI oocytes are selected and moved into a separate container from the larger pool of oocytes to maintain their viability. Waiting overnight before injecting these oocytes improves the likelihood of survival, and allows the elimination of oocytes destined to die as a result of the defolliculation process. Removal of deteriorating oocytes and replacement of the bathing solution with fresh MBS should be performed daily.

3.1.2. RNA Preparation and Injection

1. Although cDNA can be injected into the oocyte nucleus, with successful RNA transcription and protein translation *in ovo*, most investigators favor intracytoplasmic injection of RNA. Total or poly-A RNA isolated from tissues or synthesized cRNA can be used successfully, although the subsequent level of protein expression will depend on the abundance of the RNA species of interest.

2. In-vitro transcribed cRNA encoding genes of interest are synthesized using a vector that contains a prokaryotic RNA polymerase site (e.g., SP6 or T7) upstream of the coding sequence, which has been linearized downstream of the 3' terminus (*see* **Note 2**).

3. After degrading the cDNA template with RNase-free DNase I and purifying the in vitro transcribed cRNA with phenol/chloroform extraction and ethanol precipitation, the integrity of the transcript and its quantity must be determined with denaturing agarose gel electrophoresis and spectrophotometry. Then 50–100 nL of the desired RNA solution is injected into the oocyte's vegetal pole. In general, 1–20 ng/oocyte of a purified RNA transcript is used for expression studies (*see* **Note 3**).

4. The technical aspects of cytoplasmic injection are generally straightforward. Necessary equipment includes a coarse micromanipulator to position the injection pipet, a microinjector, a dissecting stereomicroscope, and a pipet puller. Narrow-internal-diameter injection pipets (to contain ~ 1 µL/cm) are pulled in a single step with the pipet puller, and the tips broken off to diameters of ~10–20 µm. The outer surface of the pipet is marked in 1-mm increments to aid in visually confirming the volume of injection (~100 nL/mm with Drummond Microcaps).

5. A small aliquot of RNA (2 µL) is then placed onto an RNase-free surface (parafilm) and drawn into the pipet with vacuum pressure.

6. Oocytes are placed in a small amount of MBS on a 75-mm culture dish, to which a piece of polypropylene mesh has been glued in order to keep the oocytes stationary during injection.

7. The injection pipet is positioned over the oocyte's vegetal pole and lowered until it pierces the oocyte. Injection of 50–100 nL of RNA is performed while visually

confirming the movement of the RNA solution through the pipet, as clogging of the pipet tip is not an uncommon event. When using a pressure microinjector, 10 psi of pressure will usually deliver the desired volume of solution within 2–5 s if the pipet tip has been broken off to the appropriate diameter and is not clogged (*see* **Note 4**).

3.1.3. Two-Electrode Voltage Clamping

The large size of *Xenopus* oocytes and their reliable expression of heterologous proteins have made them useful systems for the study of ion channels and electrogenic transporters, including CFTR and ENaC. Two-electrode voltage clamping (TEVC) is the most basic experimental configuration, which provides a measurement of total cellular current while maintaining the membrane potential at a fixed voltage. This is accomplished through the use of an intracellular electrode that records the actual membrane potential, and a second electrode that is used to pass current, so that the membrane potential remains at the level set by the operator.

1. Intracellular electrodes are pulled using a standard electrode puller with capillary glass containing a thin filament. The electrode pipets are backfilled with 3 *M* KCl, and electrical contact to the headstage is made with a chlorinated silver wire. Electrode resistances below 2 MΩ are ideal. The pipette electrodes may be reused for the study of several oocytes as along as the pipet resistance remains low (< 3 MΩ).
2. Positioning of the electrode pipets is easily accomplished with coarse mechanical manipulators under low magnification (5–10×). Neither a vibration-isolated table nor a Faraday cage is usually necessary for TEVC, although a heavy table may be needed to dampen floor vibrations in some buildings, and standard grounding techniques must be used.
3. Before impaling the oocyte, with both pipets in the bath solution, the electrode offset is negated to ± 1 mV. Electrode entry into the oocyte can then be monitored both visually and by the measurement of a negative resting potential (–20 to –80 mV) as the pipets enter the oocyte. In the absence of exogenously expressed ion channels, the amount of current required to voltage clamp the oocyte membrane potential at –100 mV ranges from ~80 to 200 nanoamperes (*see* **Note 5**).
4. Once clamped at the desired membrane potential, the oocyte preparation is generally very stable (>1 h) and tolerates continuous perfusion/solution changes (*see* **Note 6**). When recording very large ionic currents (e.g., >5 µA), special consideration of the series resistance through the bath-grounding electrode should be given *(58)*. Under these circumstances, a significant voltage drop across the grounding electrode may result in a significant error in the measurement of the transmembrane potential. To avoid this problem, either the resistance of the bath grounding electrode should be minimized (to ≤ 1 kΩ, by utilizing a short/large-diameter agar bridge containing 3 *M* KCl, or directly grounding the bath with a Ag/AgCl pellet if appropriate) or by actively controlling the bath potential through the use of a separate virtual ground circuit.

3.1.4. Patch Clamp Recording from Oocytes

1. Patch clamp recordings from oocytes require removal of the vitelline membrane. This membrane is beneath the overlying follicular layer and is in direct contact with the plasma membrane. To facilitate its removal, the exposure to hypertonic solution is used to widen the space between the plasma and vitelline membranes, thus allowing careful mechanical stripping. This approach is hindered by adhesions between these layers, and subsequent damage to the plasma membrane when attempting to remove the vitelline membrane.

2. Recently, we adopted an improved approach for the preparation of oocytes for patch clamp studies *(59)*. This method utilizes strong enzymatic digestion after oocyte harvesting (4 mg/mL type II collagenase and 4 mg/mL type II hyaluronidase in MBS for 1 h at room temperature), mechanical defolliculation using fine forceps, and prescreening for oocytes with good plasma membrane–vitelline membrane separation with a 15-min exposure to MBS/sucrose (sucrose added to increase osmolarity to 460 mosmol/L).

3. Oocytes that demonstrate a clear separation between the vitelline and plasma membranes are selected and returned to isosmotic MBS overnight before injection with RNA.

4. After RNA injection and an appropriate incubation period, the oocyte is again exposed to hyperosmolar MBS/sucrose solution for 10–15 min, and the vitelline membrane carefully removed with fine forceps.

5. The denuded oocyte is then briefly washed in isosmotic MBS, and placed into a small plastic culture dish containing the desired "bath solution" for patch clamp recording. Within several minutes, the oocyte will stick to the bottom of the plastic dish, and is ready for patch clamp recording. Movement of the recording chamber should be avoided at this point, as the denuded oocyte is extremely fragile (*see* **Note 7**).

6. Details regarding the preparation of patch pipets and seal formation are no different than with techniques for patch clamping small cells. Seal formation for macropatches, using pipettes with 0.6–2 $M\Omega$ resistances, can be slow and uses very little suction. Endogenous stretch-activated channels, with a conductance of approx 40 pS, can confound recordings of the desired population of channels and are often activated at positive membrane potentials. Gadolinium (100 μM) in the pipet solution largely blocks these channels, though their presence appears to be sporadic within a given batch of oocytes (*see* **Note 8**).

3.1.5. Biochemical Analyses in Oocytes

Biochemical assays are often used to confirm protein expression when an electrophysiological signal is not present (e.g., a putative channel regulator, or a mutated channel without measurable current). Alternatively, an observed change in the magnitude of current through a channel, under a given set of experimental conditions, may result from a change in the translational efficiency of the RNA species, from an effect on the number of channels that reach the plasma membrane, or from altered gating behavior of the channel itself.

These possibilities may be addressed with the addition of biochemical analyses to functional electrophysiological studies. The principles underlying biochemical analyses in oocytes, including protein preparation, isolation, and detection are largely similar to those used in other cellular systems, though a few caveats that are worth noting.

1. Oocytes are homogenized with a glass-Teflon homogenizer, or by repeated aspiration through hypodermic needles (22 gage × 5, 27 gage × 1).
2. Homogenization buffer (~ 20 µL/oocyte) should contain antiproteases and detergents (e.g., 1% Triton X-100 for nondenaturing solubilization) appropriate to the application. It is often desirable to remove yolk and pigment-containing granules, which are the major proteins in the crude cell homogenate. This is accomplished by centrifuging the homogenized sample at 10,000g for 10 min in a 4°C microcentrifuge.
3. The desired supernatant, lying between pelleted yolk and pigment granules and a floating lipid layer, is then aspirated carefully and used for gel electrophoresis.
4. Enrichment of membrane proteins *(60,61)* is accomplished by homogenizing oocytes in homogenization buffer containing 10% w/v sucrose, layering the lysate onto a 50–20% stepped sucrose gradient and centrifuging the sample at 15,000g for 30 min in a swinging bucket rotor at 4°C. A membrane-enriched fraction will then be found at the interface between the 20 and 50% sucrose layers.
5. Because oocytes will take up exogenous amino acids, newly synthesized proteins may be labeled by the addition of [³H]leucine or [³⁵S]methionine to the incubating medium after RNA injection. Proteins may then be detected by denaturing polyacrylamide gel electrophoresis (SDS-PAGE) and autoradiography, with/without a prior purification step via immunoprecipitation.
6. Direct injection of labeled amino acids may also be done at the time of RNA injection, and will provide higher specific activity labeling of *de novo*-synthesized proteins. Alternatively, when appropriate antiserum is available, proteins separated with SDS-PAGE may be transferred to a nitrocellulose filter and subjected to immunodetection (Western blotting).
7. Immunocytochemical staining of oocytes provides another approach to the detection of heterologously expressed proteins. This method allows not only confirmation of expression, but also gives information regarding the ultimate cellular localization of the foreign protein. Immunostaining is carried out on oocytes that have been fixed in 3% PFA for 4 h, frozen and sectioned (6–10 µm thick). Further technical details will depend primarily on the target protein and the performance characteristics of the available antibodies.
8. Quantitation of channels at the plasma membrane surface enables the relationship between current magnitude (by two-electrode voltage clamping) and relative channel number to be established. This is typically the case when studying the mechanism of action of a channel regulator or environmental condition that alters the magnitude of the observed macroscopic current. This has been carried out, in the case of CFTR and ENaC, with various techniques that complement the biochemical approaches outlined above. One such approach involves specific

binding between a radiolabeled antibody (e.g., via [125I]-iodination) and the target protein, and has been used to quantitate surface expression of ENaC subunits *(62)*. Another approach employed confocal microscopy to detect CFTR channels at the cell surface of nonpermeablized oocytes *(63)*. A third useful technique entails biotinylation of cell surface proteins with a cell-impermeant biotinylation reagent (Sulfo-NHS-LC-Biotin; Pierce), purification of these surface proteins with streptavidin-coated beads (Pierce), and subsequent immunodetection with SDS-PAGE and appropriate antisera *(64)*. Regardless of the approach chosen, careful controls (oocytes injected with water or cRNA encoding an unrelated protein) need to be included in each experiment, and thorough blocking/washing steps are needed to avoid the problem of nonspecific signal. Finally, complete defolliculation of oocytes should be ensured, as this complex cellular layer can frequently be the source of nonspecific signal.

3.2. Mammalian Cells

3.2.1. Transfection and Selection

1. NIH 3T3 fibroblasts are a convenient mammalian model system that are null for CFTR and ENaC expression, easily infected with retrovirus, and amenable to study with conventional patch clamp methods.
2. Murine amphotropic retroviral vectors encoding normal human CFTR (LCFSN) or ENaC subunits (LISN) were used in our studies to infect the parental cells *(65)* (*see* **Note 9**).
3. The three rat ENaC subunits were expressed from infection with LISN, which contains α, β, and γ rENaC cDNA in the viral LTR. ENaC subunits are expressed as a tricistronic mRNA containing α, β, and γ from 5' to 3'. At the 5' end of the α– and β-subunit sequences, internal ribosome entry-site sequences from encephalomyocarditis and polio virus, respectively, were included to increase translation. Additionally, an SV40 promoter was added 3' to the α subunit to increase transcription of a puromycin-selectable marker.
4. Cells are infected with LCFSN and or empty vector and passaged into medium containing G418 to select for cells expressing neomycin resistance. After confirmation of CFTR expression by Northern blot analysis, clonal cell lines were infected with LISN. Cells expressing α,β,γ-rENaC were selected by growth in puromycin-containing medium. Puromycin- and neomycin-resistant cells were expanded and clonal cell lines were obtained . Expression of genes under the transcriptional control of the viral LTR are increased by the addition of 1 μM dexamethasone *(66)* and 2 mM sodium butyrate *(67)* to the culture medium 1 d before studying the cells biochemically or functionally.

3.2.2. Biochemical Expression of CFTR

Expression of CFTR and α,β,γ-rENaC subunit mRNAs are confirmed by standard Northern blot analysis. Protein expression of CFTR is assessed by Western blot using affinity-purified rabbit polyclonal antibodies generated against peptides in the regulatory (R) domain or COOH terminus of CFTR *(68)*.

1. Cells expressing CFTR are grown to confluence, washed with phosphate-buffered saline, and solubilized directly from culture wells with lysis buffer. Electrophoresis of solubilized protein is performed on precast 4–15% gradient acrylamide gels. Transfer of proteins to PVD membranes (Bio-Rad) and subsequent immunoblotting has been described previously *(68)*.

2. Stable protein expression of ENaC subunits is assessed by Western blot and immunoprecipitation using polyclonal antibodies generated against the cytosolic amino or carboxyl terminus of α, β, or γENaC. In some cases, detection of ENaC protein expression by Western blot can be difficult due to low expression level and/or due to low-affinity antibodies. In these cases, immunoprecipitation using specific ENaC antisera in metabolically labeled cells followed by autoradiography can significantly increase the sensitivity for protein detection over that for Western blotting.

3.2.3. Whole-Cell Patch Clamp Technique

1. In whole-cell recording, a gigaohm seal is first formed between a patch pipet and a cell *(69)*. The cell-attached membrane patch is then disrupted by pulses of voltage and/or negative pressure applied to the pipet. Subsequently, the cytosol of the patched cell becomes continuous with the solution inside the pipet. Pipet and bath solution composition are designed to achieve specific goals, e.g., solutions composed of gluconate salts of Na^+ or Li^+ decrease the relative contribution of non-ENaC mediated currents, although nonselective cation channels exist in most cells that support some non-ENaC-mediated whole-cell currents *(70)*. However,

2. ENaC-mediated conductance is readily identified as the difference between current voltage (IV) plots taken before and during exposure to 10 μ*M* amiloride *(71–73)* (*see* Note 10). Proteins, peptides, or pharmacological reagents included in the pipet solution diffuse into the cell and can manipulate the activity of transmembrane proteins, as well as cytoskeletal or lipid-bound proteins. Thus, the involvement of specific signaling pathways implicated in channel regulation can be tested through whole-cell patch clamp.

3. Whole-cell patch clamp experiments are caried out on fibroblasts expressing CFTR and α,β,γ rENaC or α,β,γ rENaC alone *(71)*. Patch pipets are pulled from glass capillary tubes to achieve electrodes with resistances of 3–8 MΩ. Gigaohm seal formation is monitored by measuring changes in pipet resistance with the pClamp 8.0 software system. Use of negative pipet potentials after initial contact with the cell membrane often increases the frequency of seal formation.

4. Once access to the cytosol is achieved, a depolarized whole-cell potential difference is the first indication of ENaC expression. A typical whole-cell voltage clamp protocol used for measuring whole-cell currents is as follows. Cells are voltage clamped at 0 mV and pulsed to –40 mV for 0.40-s intervals. This sequence is repeated for 90 s to ensure that the pipet–membrane seal under whole-cell conditions is stable.

5. At defined intervals, the cell is voltage clamped at 0 mV and pulsed from –80 mV to +80 mV, in 20-mV increments, with 0.45 s at each voltage *(71)*.

6. Average currents recorded at each clamp voltage are used to generate current–voltage (IV) plots. Whole-cell conductance is measured from the slope of the IV

plot. Because whole-cell experiments provide information for total cellular currents, it is important to determine what portion of those currents is attributed to ENaC activity. Therefore, current–voltage tracings are obtained in the absence and presence of 10 μ*M* amiloride *(73)* (*see* **Note 10**). The difference in IV curves generated in the presence and absence of amiloride reflects the amiloride-sensitive current. As the only amiloride-sensitive channel in these cells, we can equate amiloride-sensitive current with ENaC activity.

7. Differences in amiloride-sensitive currents in cells expressing CFTR and ENaC vs those expressing ENaC alone can be used to determine if CFTR expression affects ENaC function in these 3T3 fibroblasts. Cells that express ENaC alone exhibit basal inward currents that are inhibited by amiloride. Treatment of these cells with cpt-cAMP, a nonhydrolyzable cAMP analog, produces increased amiloride-sensitive currents *(71)*. In cells coexpressing CFTR and ENaC, treatment with cpt-cAMP inhibits amiloride-sensitive currents. Because these cells are bathed in solutions containing impermeant anions, the apparent inhibition of ENaC by coexpressed CFTR cannot be attributed to changes in membrane potential or ion driving forces. Similar results were reported using M1 cells *(74)*. Although the precise pathways that account for CFTR inhibition of ENaC have not been fully described, these model systems provide a useful means for testing potential candidates.

3.2.4. Single-Channel Analyses

The magnitude of amiloride sensitive whole currents are determined by both the number (N) of ENaC and the open probability (P_o) of individual ENaC present in the membrane. Each component of ENaC currents is targeted by intracellular regulatory pathways, although the best-identified mechanisms affect the number of ENaC present on the plasma membrane *(75,76)*. Therefore, the study of single-channel characteristics of ENaC in cells expressing ENaC alone or ENaC in combination with CFTR is a fundamental approach to identifying the molecular basis for CFTR's modulation of ENaC.

1. Because ENaC has been studied extensively in both natively and heterologously expressing cells, the single-channel characteristics of ENaC are well known. ENaC exhibits a low single-channel conductance (typically 3–6 pS), slow gating characteristics (transitions of the order of seconds), and modest voltage-dependent gating. Single-channel analyses of NIH 3T3 cells expressing ENaC alone reveal high probability of single-channel openings in the cell attached configuration *(71)*.

2. After excision to achieve an inside-out patch, these channels exhibit rundown in which the channel open probability (P_o) gradually decreases. Exposure of the cytosolic side of the membrane to the catalytic subunit of PKA and ATP effectively activates ENaC and returns P_o to prerundown levels. Similar experiments performed in cells coexpressing ENaC and CFTR reveal substantial decreases in ENaC P_o upon exposure to PKA and ATP.

3. Careful observation of ENaC single channel gating kinetics in the presence of maximal PKA activity reveal a marked reduction in mean open time (MOT) in

cells coexpressing CFTR as compared to cells expressing ENaC alone *(71)*. Thus, CFTR-mediated inhibition of ENaC can be observed at both the whole-cell and single-channel levels, and likely involves changes in ENaC gating as one component.

3.2.5. Mammalian Cell Functional Expression by Ussing Chamber Assays

Polarized epithelial tissues expressing ENaC and CFTR in a highly differentiated state may constitute a more relevant model for discovering a molecular basis for the CFTR-ENaC interaction.

1. Madin-Darby canine kidney (MDCK) cells stably expressing ENaC or ENaC and CFTR are generated using the retroviral vectors described above *(65,72)*.
2. Cells are grown to confluence on permeable supports capable of being mounted into Ussing chambers.
3. Studies are performed in the presence of bilateral chloride-free solutions to further isolate and enhance detection of sodium currents. Use of cell-permeable reagents (forskolin) to increase levels of cAMP show dramatic increases in amiloride-sensitive short-circuit currents (Isc) in cells expressing ENaC alone *(54)*.
4. In sharp contrast, cells coexpressing CFTR and ENaC display decreases in amiloride-sensitive Isc upon treatment with forskolin. This observation is similar to what was observed in freshly excised human airway epithelia *(5)*. The key finding from those studies was that forskolin markedly stimulated the already enhanced amiloride-sensitive Isc in CF tissues (lacking CFTR function), an observation that has since ignited a search for regulatory mechanisms linking CFTR and ENaC function.

3.3. Conclusions

Several model systems allow the profitable study of CFTR and ENaC channels, each with relative advantages and drawbacks. The negative modulation of ENaC function by CFTR that is observed in vivo has been recapitulated in several of these systems, thus providing the platform from which we may explore the molecular mechanisms that support this important functional interaction. Although critical questions remain unresolved, it is through this research that we may come to understand the pathophysiology underlying cystic fibrosis and thus better target the development of novel therapeutics.

4. Notes

1. When collagenase treatment is used for defolliculation, ovarian lobes should first be teased apart into small clusters of oocytes with forceps and scissors. Incubation in a 1–2 mg/mL solution of collagenase (containing minimal trypsin activity) in nominally calcium-free modified Barth's solution (MBS) at room temperature for 60–90 min on a gently rotating platform is generally adequate to provide enough oocytes to work with, without excessive cell death.
2. When the 5' and 3' flanking regions of the original cDNA (including a polyA sequence) are not contained in the cDNA of interest, the coding sequence may be

inserted into an "oocyte expression vector" that provides 5' and 3' untranslated regions from a well-translated *Xenopus* gene (e.g., β-globin) and a 3' polyA tail. The use of m^{7}G(5')ppp(5')G capped nucleotide *(77)* in the transcription reaction also improves cRNA stability and protein expression.

3. Any number of individual transcripts may be mixed together before injection for coexpression studies, but the total amount of injected RNA should not exceed 50 ng/oocyte, as higher amounts may have adverse effects on oocyte health and individual transcript expression. Our experience with ENaC suggests that robust expression occurs within 24 h after injecting ≥1 ng of RNA/oocyte (0.3 ng of each subunit). Expression of CFTR may require somewhat larger amounts of cRNA (~10 ng/oocyte), and is usually observed 24–48 h after injection.

4. Careful, nontraumatic removal of the pipet from the oocyte is a key step in obtaining reproducible injections, and is facilitated by using the surface tension at the air-liquid interface to gently pull the oocyte off the pipet. Placing the freshly injected oocytes on ice for 10–30 min before returning them to the 16–19°C incubator may aid closure of the punctured plasma membrane, and thus limit cytoplasmic leakage and cell death

5. Current values greater than 200 nA usually indicate a "leaky" plasma membrane, poor seal around the pipet entry site, or constitutive activity of an exogenously expressed ion channel. Clamping the oocyte to values greater than +20 mV often results in a large outward current due to voltage activation of endogenous calcium-activated chloride channels, which may complicate measurement of the desired channel activities.

6. We have observed changes in current in relationship to the rate of perfusion, so a constant perfusion rate and solution depth should be maintained. A gravity-driven perfusion system with a suction pipet to control the level of the solution is simple and works well on both accounts. Creation of a small-volume perfusion chamber ($3 \times 3 \times 20$ mm, with a port for the placement of a grounding electrode) facilitates rapid solution changes, while the shallow chamber depth limits the risk of capacitance coupling between electrodes.

7. Once prepared, the oocyte is amenable to cell-attached recording, the formation of excised patches, and macropatch recording. These approaches complement two-electrode voltage clamping, as they allow single-channel analyses when using small pipet tip diameters, and analysis of small channel groupings when employing large macropatch pipets. While similar information is obtained in the two-electrode voltage clamp and macropatch modes, the macropatch configuration allows greater temporal resolution of channel kinetics (owing to the small membrane area being studied) and the ability to control both intracellular and extracellular bath composition when in the excised configuration. The formation of macropatches, however, is technically much more difficult than the two-electrode configuration.

8. Investigators have commonly noted the topographical clustering of channels, though the likelihood of this phenomenon may vary, depending on the channel being studied. Fortunately, a single oocyte will survive the formation of several seals, allowing one to probe several different regions if the desired channel activ-

ity is not observed initially. Seasonal variation in the quality of ion channel recordings has also been noted, with improved results during winter months being reported *(78)*.

9. LCFSN contains CFTR cDNA under the transcriptional control of the retroviral long terminal repeat (LTR) and a gene encoding neomycin resistance under control of an internal SV40 promoter.

10. The relatively specific inhibition of ENaC by micromolar concentrations of amiloride provides a reliable means to identify ENaC expression functionally. As a consequence, ENaC activity is typically expressed as the amiloride-sensitive Na$^+$ current and/or the single-channel activity of amiloride-sensitive Na$^+$ channels. Because native epithelial cells that express ENaC are typically difficult to patch, heterologous expression of ENaC subunits in easily patched mammalian cells, such as 3T3 fibroblasts, has been a useful approach. CFTR expression is detected by functional assays of chloride currents activated in response to agents that increase cellular levels of cAMP. These agents include forskolin *(7)*, which increases the activity of adenylate cyclase and isobutyl-methylxanthine (IBMX) *(40)*, which inhibits phosphodiesterase activity.

References

1. Hwang, T. C., Lu, L., Zeitlin, P. L., Gruenert, D. C., Huganir, R., and Guggino, W. B. (1989) Cl- channels in CF: lack of activation by protein kinase C and cAMP-dependent protein kinase. *Science* **244,** 1351–1353.
2. Jetten, A. M., Yankaskas, J. R., Stutts, M. J., Willumsen, N. J., and Boucher, R. C. (1989) Persistence of abnormal chloride conductance regulation in transformed cystic fibrosis epithelia. *Science* **244,** 1472–1475.
3. Welsh, M. J., Li, M., and McCann, J. D. (1989) Activation of normal and cystic fibrosis Cl- channels by voltage, temperature, and trypsin. *J. Clin. Invest.* **84,** 2002–2007.
4. Knowles, M., Gatzy, J., and Boucher, R. (1983) Relative ion permeability of normal and cystic fibrosis nasal epithelium. *J. Clin. Invest.* **71,** 1410–1417.
5. Boucher, R. C., Stutts, M. J., Knowles, M. R., Cantley, L., and Gatzy, J. T. (1986) Na+ transport in cystic fibrosis respiratory epithelia. Abnormal basal rate and response to adenylate cyclase activation. *J. Clin. Invest.* **78,** 1245–1252.
6. Cotton, C. U., Stutts, M. J., Knowles, M. R., Gatzy, J. T., and Boucher, R. C. (1987) Abnormal apical cell membrane in cystic fibrosis respiratory epithelium. An in vitro electrophysiologic analysis. *J. Clin. Invest.* **79,** 80–85.
7. Rommens, J. M., Dho, S., Bear, C. E., Kartner, N., Kennedy, D., Riordan, J. R., Tsui, L. C., and Foskett, J. K. (1991) cAMP-inducible chloride conductance in mouse fibroblast lines stably expressing the human cystic fibrosis transmembrane conductance regulator. *Proc. Natl. Acad. Sci. USA* **88,** 7500–7504.
8. Gabriel, S. E., Clarke, L. L., Boucher, R. C., and Stutts, M. J. (1993) CFTR and outward rectifying chloride channels are distinct proteins with a regulatory relationship. *Nature* **363,** 263–268.
9. Egan, M., Flotte, T., Afione, S., Solow, R., Zeitlin, P. L., Carter, B. J., and Guggino, W. B. (1992) Defective regulation of outwardly rectifying Cl- channels by protein kinase A corrected by insertion of CFTR. *Nature* **358,** 581–584.

10. Mimmack, M. L., Gallagher, M. P., Pearce, S. R., Hyde, S. C., Booth, I. R., and Higgins, C. F. (1989) Energy coupling to periplasmic binding protein-dependent transport systems: stoichiometry of ATP hydrolysis during transport in vivo. *Proc. Natl. Acad. Sci. USA* **86,** 8257–8261.

11. Rommens, J. M., Iannuzzi, M. C., Kerem, B., Drumm, M. L., Melmer, G., Dean, M., Rozmahel, R., Cole, J. L., Kennedy, D., Hidaka, N., and et al. (1989) Identification of the cystic fibrosis gene: chromosome walking and jumping. *Science* **245,** 1059–1065.

12. Greger, R., Mall, M., Bleich, M., Ecke, D., Warth, R., Riedemann, N., and Kunzelmann, K. (1996) Regulation of epithelial ion channels by the cystic fibrosis transmembrane conductance regulator. *J. Mol. Med.* **74,** 527–534.

13. Nousia-Arvanitakis, S. (1999) Cystic fibrosis and the pancreas: recent scientific advances. *J. Clin. Gastroenterol.* **29,** 138–142.

14. Colombo, C., Battezzati, P. M., Strazzabosco, M., and Podda, M. (1998) Liver and biliary problems in cystic fibrosis. *Semin. Liver Dis.* **18,** 227–235.

15. Quinton, P. M. and Reddy, M. M. (1991) Regulation of absorption in the human sweat duct. *Adv. Exp. Med. Biol.* **290,** 159–170.

16. Rennard, S. I. and Romberger, D. J. (2000) Host defenses and pathogenesis. *Semin. Respir. Infect.* **15,** 7–13.

17. Wanner, A., Salathe, M., and O'Riordan, T. G. (1996) Mucociliary clearance in the airways. *Am. J. Respir. Crit. Care Med.* **154,** 1868–1902.

18. Wilmott, R. W., Khurana-Hershey, G., and Stark, J. M. (2000) Current concepts on pulmonary host defense mechanisms in children. *Curr. Opin. Pediatr.* **12,** 187–193.

19. DeLong, P. A. and Kotloff, R. M. (2000) An overview of pulmonary host defense. *Semin. Roentgenol.* **35,** 118–123.

20. Singh, P. K., Tack, B. F., McCray, P. B., Jr., and Welsh, M. J. (2000) Synergistic and additive killing by antimicrobial factors found in human airway surface liquid. *Am. J. Physiol. Lung Cell Mol. Physiol.* **279,** L799–805.

21. Matsui, H., Grubb, B. R., Tarran, R., Randell, S. H., Gatzy, J. T., Davis, C. W., and Boucher, R. C. (1998) Evidence for periciliary liquid layer depletion, not abnormal ion composition, in the pathogenesis of cystic fibrosis airways disease. *Cell* **95,** 1005–1015.

22. Jayaraman, S., Song, Y., Vetrivel, L., Shankar, L., and Verkman, A. S. (2001) Noninvasive in vivo fluorescence measurement of airway-surface liquid depth, salt concentration, and pH. *J. Clin. Invest.* **107,** 317–324.

23. Verkman, A. S., Matthay, M. A., and Song, Y. (2000) Aquaporin water channels and lung physiology. *Am. J. Physiol. Lung Cell Mol. Physiol.* **278,** L867–879.

24. Pedersen, P. S., Holstein-Rathlou, N. H., Larsen, P. L., Qvortrup, K., and Frederiksen, O. (1999) Fluid absorption related to ion transport in human airway epithelial spheroids. *Am. J. Physiol.* **277,** L1096–1103.

25. Matsui, H., Davis, C. W., Tarran, R., and Boucher, R. C. (2000) Osmotic water permeabilities of cultured, well-differentiated normal and cystic fibrosis airway epithelia. *J. Clin. Invest.* **105,** 1419–1427.

26. Houtmeyers, E., Gosselink, R., Gayan-Ramirez, G., and Decramer, M. (1999) Regulation of mucociliary clearance in health and disease. *Eur. Respir. J.* **13,** 1177–1188.

27. Gueron, S. and Levit-Gurevich, K. (1998) Computation of the internal forces in cilia: application to ciliary motion, the effects of viscosity, and cilia interactions. *Biophys. J.* **74,** 1658–1676.

28. Boucher, R. C. (1994) Human airway ion transport. Part one. *Am. J. Respir. Crit. Care Med.* **150,** 271–281.

29. Boucher, R. C. (1994) Human airway ion transport. Part two. *Am. J. Respir. Crit. Care Med.* **150,** 581–593.

30. Knowles, M., Gatzy, J., and Boucher, R. (1981) Increased bioelectric potential difference across respiratory epithelia in cystic fibrosis. *N. Engl. J. Med.* **305,** 1489–1495.

31. Knowles, M. R., Stutts, M. J., Spock, A., Fischer, N., Gatzy, J. T., and Boucher, R. C. (1983) Abnormal ion permeation through cystic fibrosis respiratory epithelium. *Science* **221,** 1067–1070.

32. Willumsen, N. J. and Boucher, R. C. (1989) Shunt resistance and ion permeabilities in normal and cystic fibrosis airway epithelia. *Am. J. Physiol.* **256,** C1054–1063.

33. Willumsen, N. J., Davis, C. W., and Boucher, R. C. (1989) Cellular Cl- transport in cultured cystic fibrosis airway epithelium. *Am. J. Physiol.* **256,** C1045–1053.

34. Clarke, L. L. and Boucher, R. C. (1992) Chloride secretory response to extracellular ATP in human normal and cystic fibrosis nasal epithelia. *Am. J. Physiol.* **263,** C348–356.

35. Alton, E. W., Rogers, D. F., Logan-Sinclair, R., Yacoub, M., Barnes, P. J., and Geddes, D. M. (1992) Bioelectric properties of cystic fibrosis airways obtained at heart- lung transplantation. *Thorax* **47,** 1010–1014.

36. Mertz, J. E. and Gurdon, J. B. (1977) Purified DNAs are transcribed after microinjection into Xenopus oocytes. *Proc. Natl. Acad. Sci. USA* **74,** 1502–1506.

37. Bear, C. E., Duguay, F., Naismith, A. L., Kartner, N., Hanrahan, J. W., and Riordan, J. R. (1991) Cl- channel activity in Xenopus oocytes expressing the cystic fibrosis gene. *J. Biol. Chem.* **266,** 19,142–19,145.

38. Fulmer, S. B., Schwiebert, E. M., Morales, M. M., Guggino, W. B., and Cutting, G. R. (1995) Two cystic fibrosis transmembrane conductance regulator mutations have different effects on both pulmonary phenotype and regulation of outwardly rectified chloride currents. *Proc. Natl. Acad. Sci. USA* **92,** 6832–6836.

39. Smit, L. S., Wilkinson, D. J., Mansoura, M. K., Collins, F. S., and Dawson, D. C. (1993) Functional roles of the nucleotide-binding folds in the activation of the cystic fibrosis transmembrane conductance regulator. *Proc. Natl. Acad. Sci. USA* **90,** 9963–9967.

40. Drumm, M. L., Wilkinson, D. J., Smit, L. S., Worrell, R. T., Strong, T. V., Frizzell, R. A., et al. (1991) Chloride conductance expressed by delta F508 and other mutant CFTRs in Xenopus oocytes. *Science* **254,** 1797–1799.

41. Smit, L. S., Strong, T. V., Wilkinson, D. J., Macek, M., Jr., Mansoura, M. K., Wood, D. L., et al. (1995) Missense mutation (G480C) in the CFTR gene associated with protein mislocalization but normal chloride channel activity. *Hum. Mol. Genet.* **4,** 269–273.

42. Hipper, A., Mall, M., Greger, R., and Kunzelmann, K. (1995) Mutations in the putative pore-forming domain of CFTR do not change anion selectivity of the cAMP activated Cl- conductance. *FEBS Lett.* **374,** 312–316.

43. Canessa, C. M., Horisberger, J. D., and Rossier, B. C. (1993) Epithelial sodium channel related to proteins involved in neurodegeneration. *Nature* **361,** 467–470.
44. Canessa, C. M., Schild, L., Buell, G., Thorens, B., Gautschi, I., Horisberger, J. D., and Rossier, B. C. (1994) Amiloride-sensitive epithelial Na+ channel is made of three homologous subunits. *Nature* **367,** 463–467.
45. Mall, M., Hipper, A., Greger, R., and Kunzelmann, K. (1996) Wild type but not deltaF508 CFTR inhibits Na+ conductance when coexpressed in Xenopus oocytes. *FEBS Lett.* **381,** 47–52.
46. Briel, M., Greger, R., and Kunzelmann, K. (1998) Cl- transport by cystic fibrosis transmembrane conductance regulator (CFTR) contributes to the inhibition of epithelial Na+ channels (ENaCs) in Xenopus oocytes co-expressing CFTR and ENaC. *J. Physiol.* **508,** 825–836.
47. Schreiber, R., Hopf, A., Mall, M., Greger, R., and Kunzelmann, K. (1999) The first-nucleotide binding domain of the cystic-fibrosis transmembrane conductance regulator is important for inhibition of the epithelial Na+ channel. *Proc. Natl. Acad. Sci. USA* **96,** 5310–5315.
48. Hopf, A., Schreiber, R., Mall, M., Greger, R., and Kunzelmann, K. (1999) Cystic fibrosis transmembrane conductance regulator inhibits epithelial Na+ channels carrying Liddle's syndrome mutations. *J. Biol. Chem.* **274,** 13,894–13,899.
49. Chabot, H., Vives, M. F., Dagenais, A., Grygorczyk, C., Berthiaume, Y., and Grygorczyk, R. (1999) Downregulation of epithelial sodium channel (ENaC) by CFTR co-expressed in Xenopus oocytes is independent of Cl- conductance. *J. Mem. Biol.* **169,** 175–188.
50. Jiang, Q., Li, J., Dubroff, R., Ahn, Y. J., Foskett, J. K., Engelhardt, J., and Kleyman, T. R. (2000) Epithelial sodium channels regulate cystic fibrosis trans-membrane conductance regulator chloride channels in Xenopus oocytes. *J. Biol. Chem.* **275,** 13,266–13,274.
51. Kunzelmann, K., Kiser, G. L., Schreiber, R., and Riordan, J. R. (1997) Inhibition of epithelial Na+ currents by intracellular domains of the cystic fibrosis trans-membrane conductance regulator. *FEBS Lett.* **400,** 341–344.
52. Ji, H. L., Chalfant, M. L., Jovov, B., Lockhart, J. P., Parker, S. B., Fuller, C. M., Stanton, B. A., and Benos, D. J. (2000) The cytosolic termini of the beta- and gamma-ENaC subunits are involved in the functional interactions between cystic fibrosis transmembrane conductance regulator and epithelial sodium channel. *J. Biol. Chem.* **275,** 27,947–27,956.
53. Stutts, M. J., Gabriel, S. E., Olsen, J. C., Gatzy, J. T., O'Connell, T. L., Price, E. M., and Boucher, R. C. (1993) Functional consequences of heterologous expression of the cystic fibrosis transmembrane conductance regulator in fibroblasts. *J. Biol. Chem.* **268,** 20,653–20,658.
54. Stutts, M. J., Canessa, C. M., Olsen, J. C., Hamrick, M., Cohn, J. A., Rossier, B. C., and Boucher, R. C. (1995) CFTR as a cAMP-dependent regulator of sodium chan-nels. *Science* **269,** 847–850.
55. Lukacs, G. L., Chang, X. B., Kartner, N., Rotstein, O. D., Riordan, J. R., and Grinstein, S. (1992) The cystic fibrosis transmembrane regulator is present and functional in endosomes. Role as a determinant of endosomal pH. *J. Biol. Chem.* **267,** 14,568–14,572.

56. Kartner, N., Hanrahan, J. W., Jensen, T. J., Naismith, A. L., Sun, S. Z., Ackerley, C. A., Reyes, E. F., Tsui, L. C., Rommens, J. M., Bear, C. E., and et al. (1991) Expression of the cystic fibrosis gene in non-epithelial invertebrate cells produces a regulated anion conductance. *Cell* **64,** 681–691.

57. Goldin, A. L. (1992) Maintenance of Xenopus laevis and oocyte injection. *Methods Enzymol* **207,** 266–279.

58. Nagel, G., Szellas, T., Riordan, J. R., Friedrich, T., and Hartung, K. (2001) Non-specific activation of the epithelial sodium channel by the CFTR chloride channel. *EMBO Rep.* **2,** 249–254.

59. Choe, H. and Sackin, H. (1997) Improved preparation of Xenopus oocytes for patch-clamp recording. *Pflugers Arch.* **433,** 648–652.

60. Gurdon, J. B. and Melton, D. A. (1981) Gene transfer in amphibian eggs and oocytes. *Annu. Rev. Genet.* **15,** 189–218.

61. Lane, C., Shannon, S., and Craig, R. (1979) Sequestration and turnover of guinea-pig milk proteins and chicken ovalbumin in Xenopus oocytes. *Eur. J. Biochem.* **101,** 485–495.

62. Firsov, D., Schild, L., Gautschi, I., Merillat, A. M., Schneeberger, E., and Rossier, B. C. (1996) Cell surface expression of the epithelial Na channel and a mutant causing Liddle syndrome: a quantitative approach. *Proc. Natl. Acad. Sci. USA* **93,** 15,370–15,375.

63. Peters, K. W., Qi, J., Watkins, S. C., and Frizzell, R. A. (1999) Syntaxin 1A inhibits regulated CFTR trafficking in xenopus oocytes. *Am. J. Physiol.* **277,** C174–180.

64. Pajor, A. M., Sun, N., and Valmonte, H. G. (1998) Mutational analysis of histidine residues in the rabbit Na+/dicarboxylate co-transporter NaDC-1. *Biochem. J.* **331,** 257–264.

65. Olsen, J. C., Johnson, L. G., Stutts, M. J., Sarkadi, B., Yankaskas, J. R., Swanstrom, R., and Boucher, R. C. (1992) Correction of the apical membrane chloride permeability defect in polarized cystic fibrosis airway epithelia following retroviral-mediated gene transfer. *Hum. Gene. Ther.* **3,** 253–266.

66. Groner, B., Hynes, N. E., Rahmsdorf, U., and Ponta, H. (1983) Transcription initiation of transfected mouse mammary tumor virus LTR DNA is regulated by glucocorticoid hormones. *Nucleic Acids Res.* **11,** 4713–4725.

67. Barka, T. (1998) Effect of sodium butyrate on the expression of genes transduced by retroviral vectors. *J. Cell Biochem.* **69,** 201–210.

68. Sarkadi, B., Bauzon, D., Huckle, W. R., Earp, H. S., Berry, A., Suchindran, H., Price, E. M., Olson, J. C., Boucher, R. C., and Scarborough, G. A. (1992) Biochemical characterization of the cystic fibrosis transmembrane conductance regulator in normal and cystic fibrosis epithelial cells. *J. Biol. Chem.* **267,** 2087–2095.

69. Neher, E. and Sakmann, B. (1976) Single-channel currents recorded from membrane of denervated frog muscle fibres. *Nature* **260,** 799–802.

70. Koch, J. P. and Korbmacher, C. (2000) Mechanism of shrinkage activation of nonselective cation channels in M-1 mouse cortical collecting duct cells. *J. Membr. Biol.* **177,** 231–242.

71. Stutts, M. J., Rossier, B. C., and Boucher, R. C. (1997) Cystic fibrosis transmembrane conductance regulator inverts protein kinase A-mediated regulation of epithelial sodium channel single channel kinetics. *J. Biol. Chem.* **272,** 14,037–14,040.

72. Ishikawa, T., Marunaka, Y., and Rotin, D. (1998) Electrophysiological character-ization of the rat epithelial Na+ channel (rENaC) expressed in MDCK cells. Effects of Na+ and Ca2+. *J. Gen. Physiol.* **111,** 825–846.

73. Chalfant, M. L., O'Brien, T. G., and Civan, M. M. (1996) Whole cell and unitary amiloride-sensitive sodium currents in M-1 mouse cortical collecting duct cells. *Am. J. Physiol.* **270,** C998–1010.

74. Letz, B. and Korbmacher, C. (1997) cAMP stimulates CFTR-like Cl- channels and inhibits amiloride-sensitive Na+ channels in mouse CCD cells. *Am. J. Physiol.* **272,** C657–666.

75. Staub, O., Abriel, H., Plant, P., Ishikawa, T., Kanelis, V., Saleki, R., Horisberger, J. D., Schild, L., and Rotin, D. (2000) Regulation of the epithelial Na+ channel by Nedd4 and ubiquitination. *Kidney Int.* **57,** 809–815.

76. Alvarez de la Rosa, D., Zhang, P., Naray-Fejes-Toth, A., Fejes-Toth, G., and Canessa, C. M. (1999) The serum and glucocorticoid kinase sgk increases the abundance of epithelial sodium channels in the plasma membrane of Xenopus oocytes. *J. Biol. Chem.* **274,** 37,834–37,839.

77. McCaman, R. E., Carbini, L., Maines, V., and Salvaterra, P. M. (1988) Single RNA species injected in Xenopus oocyte directs the synthesis of active choline acetyltransferase. *Brain Res.* **427,** 107–113.

78. Stuhmer, W. (1992) Electrophysiological recording from Xenopus oocytes. *Methods Enzymol.* **207,** 319–339.

24

Yeast Two-Hybrid Identification and Analysis of Protein Interactions with CFTR

Viswanathan Raghuram, Kenneth R. Hallows, and J. Kevin Foskett

1. Introduction

The discovery of the cystic fibrosis transmembrane conductance regulator (CFTR) as the gene product mutated in cystic fibrosis and its identification as a cAMP-dependent protein kinase-regulated Cl^- channel have provided important insights into its role in transepithelial fluid and salt transport and into the bases for channel dysfunction in the disease. Nevertheless, many pathophysiological and cell-biological features associated with expression of normal and mutant CFTR remain unexplained. The identification of novel protein–protein interactions involving CFTR has become important in the process of discovery and characterization of mechanisms involved in the regulation of CFTR as well as in its regulation of other membrane transport proteins and cellular processes.

Since its introduction over a decade ago (*1,2*), yeast two-hybrid analysis has emerged as a powerful and sensitive method to screen for novel proteins that interact with a protein of interest, to then grade the strength of the interaction, and to identify important regions and residues involved in the interaction. The yeast two-hybrid assay takes advantage of the fact that yeast transcription factors are composed of separable independent domains. Specifically, many regulators contain a DNA-binding domain (DNA-BD), which binds to a specific promoter sequence, and a transcriptional activation domain (AD), which directs the RNA polymerase complex to transcribe the gene downstream of the DNA-binding site (*3,4*). Both domains are required to activate gene transcription, and both domains must be present together in close physical proximity for this activation to occur. Normally, this proximity requirement is accomplished by the presence of both domains within the same protein. If the DNA-BD and AD

From: *Methods in Molecular Medicine, vol. 70: Cystic Fibrosis Methods and Protocols*
Edited by: W. R. Skach © Humana Press Inc., Totowa, NJ

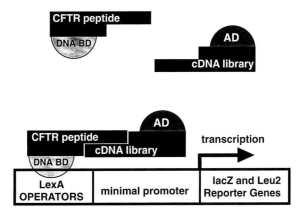

Fig. 1. Schematic of the LexA two-hybrid system. The example shown has a peptide sequence from CFTR fused in frame to the LexA DNA-binding domain (DNA BD), and a tissue-specific cDNA library fused in frame with the B42 transcriptional activation domain (AD). Interaction of the CFTR peptide with a protein sequence in the library enables transcriptional activation of reporter genes.

are separated onto different proteins and then expressed in the same cell, they fail to interact with each other and thus cannot activate target genes *(5,6)*. However, transcriptional activity can be restored if the DNA-BD and -AD are brought into close physical proximity (*see* **Fig. 1**). The yeast two-hybrid system employs two different cloning vectors (termed "bait" and "prey" vectors) to generate fusions of these domains to genes encoding proteins to be tested for interaction with each other. Generally, for the initial yeast two-hybrid screen, the gene encoding the protein of interest (for which one is seeking interacting partners) is cloned downstream of the gene encoding the DNA-BD in the bait vector. A cDNA library is cloned into the prey vector downstream of the AD. The library proteins are then co-expressed with the bait in yeast in an "interactor hunt." If the bait and prey proteins interact in vivo, a novel transcriptional activator is created, which allows transcription of reporter genes so that the protein–protein interactions are phenotypically detectable.

1.1. Overview of Available Two-Hybrid Systems

Our laboratory has successfully employed the Matchmaker LexA two-hybrid system (cat. no. K1609-1, Clontech Laboratories, Palo Alto, CA), based on the methodology originally used by Gyuris et al. *(7)* to screen for novel proteins that interact with either the CFTR R domain or C-terminal tail *(8,9)*. This system utilizes a yeast strain called EGY48, an auxotroph that cannot grow in the absence of histidine, tryptophan, and uracil. However, the presence of the bait (pLexA) and prey (pB42AD) cloning plasmids and the p8op-lacZ reporter plasmid allows the growth of EGY48 in the absence of these nutrients due to complementation by specific genes encoded on these plasmids (see below).

The DNA-BD in the bait vector is provided by the prokaryotic LexA protein *(10)*. This 10.2-kb pLexA bait vector is used to generate fusions of the 202-residue LexA protein with a bait protein, whose cDNA is cloned in frame downstream of it. The strong yeast *ADH1* promoter drives the constitutive expression of fusion protein. The *HIS3* gene allows for EGY48 growth on His-deficient media, serving as a transformation marker for selection in yeast.

The AD in the prey vector (pB42AD) is an *Escherichia coli* peptide (B42) that activates transcription in yeast *(11)*. The 6.45-kb prey vector expresses as fusion proteins cDNAs cloned in frame downstream of a cassette consisting of the SV40 nuclear localization sequence, the 88-residue B42AD, and the hemagglutinin (HA) epitope tag. The vector contains *TRP1* as a selection marker. The inducible yeast *GAL1* promoter is used to drive expression of the fusion proteins. Therefore, the prey fusion protein will be expressed only in glucose-free growth media containing galactose as the carbon source.

The LexA two-hybrid system contains two reporter genes. p8op-lacZ is a 10.3-kb reporter plasmid that carries the β-galactosidase-producing *lacZ* reporter gene under the control of eight *LexA* operators. It also contains the *URA3* gene as a selection marker. The *LEU2* reporter gene is integrated into the EGY48 genome, but is under the control of six *LexA* operators. Thus, the reporter genes will be expressed only if the bait and prey proteins interact, thereby reconstituting a functional LexA transcription factor. Reporter gene (*LEU2* and *lacZ*) transcriptional activation is assayed by the ability of transformed yeast to grow on leucine-deficient plates or demonstrate β-galactosidase activity (blue color) on X-gal plates (*see* **Fig. 1**).

This LexA-based two-hybrid system is only one of several that are currently available commercially. Other two-hybrid systems employ either the DNA-binding and activation domains of *GAL4* to confer activation of *HIS3* and *lacZ* reporter genes *(2,12)*, the DNA-binding domain of *LexA* and activation domain of VP16 to confer activation of *HIS3* and *lacZ* reporter genes *(13)*, or the DNA-binding domain of *GAL4* and the activation domain of VP16 to confer activation of the chloramphenicol transferase gene (*CAT*) and the hygromycin resistance gene (*hyg*^{r}) *(14)*. Specific examples of interaction trap components within the LexA two-hybrid system (LexA fusion plasmids, activation domain fusion plasmids, and *LacZ* reporter plasmids) and an overview of their attributes are listed in **Table 1**.

1.2. Applications of Yeast Two-Hybrid Assays

Yeast two-hybrid methodology is useful to both screen for novel proteins that interact with a protein region of interest, as well as for then identifying the important interacting regions and residues in both proteins. In addition, the two-hybrid assays can be used to explore whether any two peptides or peptide regions interact with each other (e.g., whether two different regions of CFTR interact).

Table 1
Selected Interaction Trap Components

Plasmid name	Selection in yeast	Comments/description
Lex A fusion plasmids (baits)		
pEG202 (pLexA)	*HIS3*	Contains *ADH* promoter that expresses LexA followed by polylinker
pJK202	*HIS3*	Like pEG202, but has nuclear localization sequences between LexA and polylinker to enhance translocation of bait to nucleus
pNLexA	*HIS3*	Contains *ADH* promoter that expresses polylinker followed by LexA; for baits whose NH$_2$-terminal residues must remain unblocked
pGilda	*HIS3*	Contains *GAL1* promoter that expresses LexA followed by polylinker; for use with baits that are toxic to yeast when expressed continuously
pRFHM1	*HIS3*	Contains *ADH* promoter that expresses LexA fused to homeodomain of bicoid to produce nonactivating fusion; negative control for activation and interaction assays
pSH17-4 (pLexA-Pos)	*HIS3*	Contains *ADH* promoter that expresses LexA fused to GAL4 activation domain; used as positive control for activation
Activation domain fusion plasmids (preys)		
pJG4-5 (pB42AD)	*TRP1*	Contains *GAL1* promoter that expresses nuclear localization domain, transcriptional activation domain, HA epitope tag, and polylinker; used to express cDNA libraries (Clontech)
pYESTrp	*TRP1*	Contains *GAL1* promoter that expresses nuclear localization domain, transcriptional activation domain, V5 epitope tag, f1 ori and T7 promoter/flanking site, and polylinker; used to express cDNA libraries (Invitrogen)

(continued)

Table 1 *(continued)*

Plasmid name	Selection in yeast	Comments/description
LacZ reporter plasmids		
pSH18-34 (p8op-LacZ)	*URA3*	Contains eight *LexA* operators controlling *lacZ* gene transcription; highly sensitive indicator plasmid for transcriptional activation
pJK103	*URA3*	Contains two *LexA* operators controlling *lacZ* gene transcription; moderately sensitive indicator plasmid for transcriptional activation
pRB1840	*URA3*	Contains one *LexA* operator controlling *lacZ* gene transcription; least sensitive (most stringent) indicator plasmid for transcriptional activation
pJK101	*URA3*	Contains *GAL1* upstream activating sequence and two *LexA* operators followed by *lacZ* gene; control used in repression assay to assess bait binding to operator sequences

Note: All plasmids are suitable for expression in both yeast and *E. coli*. Ampicillin resistance is the *E. coli* selection marker for all plasmids listed. Plasmid names given in parentheses are those used in our protocol. Condensed from **ref. *15***.

1.2.1. Overview

In this chapter we describe how to perform an initial yeast two-hybrid screen using a specific domain or region of CFTR as bait and a specific cDNA library cloned into the prey vector. The first step is to construct a bait plasmid that expresses LexA fused to the peptide of interest. Ideally, the bait peptide should be a soluble, cytoplasmic region of CFTR. In our experience, shorter fragments that contain a minimally sufficient region for interaction will be more sensitive than longer fragments, with bait peptides preferably shorter than ~300 residues. The bait construct is then transformed into yeast containing *Leu2* and *lacZ* reporter genes. A series of control experiments is performed to ensure that the bait protein is stably expressed in yeast, and more important, that it by itself does not appreciably activate transcription. After the suitability of the bait construct has been confirmed, the yeast strain containing the bait plasmid is transformed with high efficiency using a cDNA library made in the prey vector. Yeast cells expressing library proteins that interact

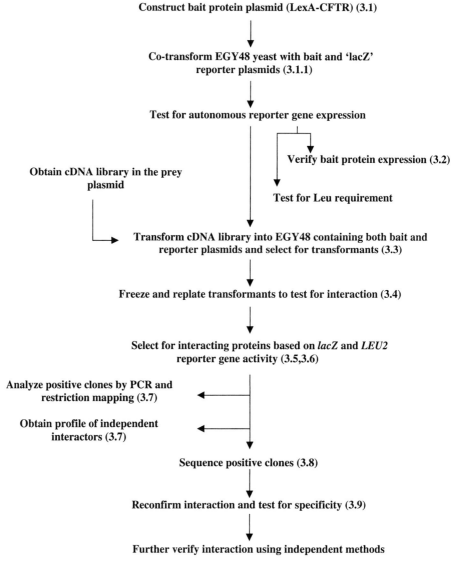

Fig. 2. Steps involved in a two-hybrid screen.

with the bait protein are selected on leucine-deficient medium. The leucine-positive colonies are further tested for their ability to turn blue on medium containing X-gal. Once specific interacting prey plasmids are identified, they are isolated and characterized by a series of tests to confirm specificity of the interaction with the bait protein. Those found to be specific are then analyzed by sequencing (*see* **Fig. 2**).

An alternative method of performing an interactor hunt is through interaction mating, whereby a strain that expresses the bait protein is mated with a strain that has been pretransformed with the library DNA, and then the resulting diploid cells are screened for interaction. This technique is particularly useful when more than one bait will be used to screen a single library. The details of this technique are available elsewhere *(15)*.

1.2.2. Interpretation of Two-Hybrid Screening Data

Although the two-hybrid system is a powerful and sensitive method to detect protein–protein interactions, false positive or artifactual interactions may occur. Therefore, after an interaction has been discovered and characterized using the yeast two-hybrid system, it is important to confirm it using independent methods. Even for true positives, the problem of determining which interactions are biologically relevant or interesting may not be trivial. Prioritization of discovered interactions for further analysis is often subjective and difficult, and it may depend on the perceived relevance of the interaction to the research interests and goals of the investigator. Nevertheless, certain guidelines may be helpful. For example, interacting peptides that contain specific protein–protein interaction domains are more likely to be true positives that are biologically relevant and interesting. In contrast, identification of proteins known to be "sticky" or involved in routine cellular housekeeping functions (e.g., ribosomal proteins, chaperone proteins, or ubiquitination proteins) may be less interesting unless one is specifically involved in studying these cellular functions with respect to CFTR.

In attempts to prioritize, it is important not to place undue emphasis on the apparent strengths of interaction as assayed by the initial two-hybrid screen. Although it is possible to derive some insights into the quantitative strength of interaction (e.g., by measuring the β-galactosidase activity—*see* **Subheading 3.10.**), many variables such as the stability of fusion proteins, their transport to the nucleus, and their ability to bind to DNA can affect the interaction's phenotype. Hence, it is not advisable to use two-hybrid data to compare affinities of unrelated proteins with a bait protein. However, it is possible to make meaningful comparisons of the affinities of a single bait protein with several related prey proteins (and vice versa).

1.2.3. Characterization of Important Interaction Determinants and Domains

After an interacting prey protein has been identified by a yeast two-hybrid screen and confirmed with appropriate controls, further two-hybrid analyses can then be used to characterize positive interactions. Specifically, the important interaction determinants and domains on both CFTR and the interacting protein can be identified by generating site-specific deletion, truncation, or substitution mutants of both proteins and repeating the two-hybrid analysis.

1.3. Confirmation and Further Characterization of Interactions Identified by Two-Hybrid Analysis Using Independent Methods

Several independent techniques can be used to confirm and further characterize proteins found to interact with CFTR by yeast two-hybrid analysis. Co-immunoprecipitation and in vitro protein "pull-down" methodologies are relatively straightforward biochemical techniques that are well described elsewhere (*see* **ref. 15** for detailed protocols). Surface plasmon resonance (SPR) is a powerful tool to determine the quantitative affinities and kinetic parameters of association and dissociation of interacting proteins *(9,16)*. Demonstration of co-localization by immunofluorescence or immunohistochemistry in native tissue sections or CFTR-expressing cell lines can provide supporting evidence for interaction of the two proteins in vivo. Finally, the physiological relevance and functional significance of a novel CFTR-interacting protein can be ascertained by identifying functional effects of the interaction between CFTR and the interacting protein. For example, the interacting protein may modulate the localization, trafficking, or channel properties of CFTR, or conversely, association with CFTR may modulate the function of the interacting protein.

2. Materials

2.1. Transformation of Yeast

2.1.1. Carbon Source Stock Solutions

1. 40% Dextrose (20×). Dissolve 400 g/L dextrose in deionized water. It may be necessary to warm the solution to promote solubility. Autoclave at 121°C for 15 min. Store at room temperature.
2. 20% Gal/Raff (10×). Dissolve 200 g/L galactose and 100 g/L raffinose in deionized water. Autoclave to sterilize and store at room temperature.

2.1.2. Yeast Growth Media

1. YPD medium: 10 g/L yeast extract, 20 g/L peptone, 15 g/L bacto-agar (for plates only). Sterilize by autoclaving. Add 50 mL of sterile 40% dextrose (20×) solution per liter to give a final concentration of 2%.
2. Synthetic dropout (SD) medium. This medium is used to test for genes involved in specific biosynthetic pathways and to select for gene function in transformation experiments. Dropout powder lacks one or more nutrients but contains all other nutrients. For example, –Ura, –His dropout powder contains all other nutrients except uracil and histidine. Different types of dropout powder are available from Clontech. To prepare, add 6.7 g/L yeast nitrogen base without amino acids, 15.0 g/L bacto-agar (for plates), Dropout powder (*see* Clontech package for instructions) and 90 mL of H_2O. Adjust pH to 5.6–5.8 for highest efficiency transformation, and autoclave. Add 100 mL of the appropriate sterile carbon source. Pour plates and allow medium to harden at room temperature. Store plates inverted, in a plastic sleeve at 4°C.

3. SD/X-gal plates:
   a. 10× buffered (BU) salt solution: 70 g/L $Na_2HPO_4 \cdot 7H_2O$, 30 g/L NaH_2PO_4. Adjust pH to 7.0, then autoclave and store at room temperature.
   b. X-gal stock solution: dissolve in N,N-dimethylformamide (DMF) at a concentration of 20 mg/mL. Store in the dark at –20°C.
   Prepare SD medium as described above except use 800 mL of H_2O and do not adjust pH. Autoclave, cool to 55°C, and add 100 mL of 10× carbon source (final concentration 2%), 100 mL of 10× BU salts (final concentration 1×),and 4 mL of X-gal (final concentration 80 mg/L). Store X-gal-containing plates at 4°C, wrapped in aluminum foil.

2.1.3. Transformation Mix

1. Stock solutions
   a. 50% PEG 4000 (polyethylene glycol, avg mol wt = 3350): prepare with deionized water. Warm the solution to help dissolve PEG. Filter sterilization is recommended. It can also be autoclaved.
   b. 1 *M* lithium acetate (LiAc), pH 7.5 adjusted with dilute acetic acid and autoclaved.
   c. SS-DNA: Sonicated herring testis carrier DNA (Clontech; cat. no. K1606-A), diluted to 2 mg/mL in Tris-EDTA (TE). Denature the carrier DNA by placing it in a boiling water bath for 10 min and immediately cooling it on ice. Store the carrier DNA at –20°C. As long as it is thawed on ice, the carrier DNA only needs to be denatured every fourth or fifth time.
2. Transformation mix (prepared fresh before use): 240 μL PEG (50% w/v), 36 μL of 1 *M* LiAc, 25 μL SS-DNA (2.0 mg/mL), 40 μL sterile H_2O. We usually transform 50 μL of yeast in a 1.5-mL tube using 340 μL of transformation mix. Each transformation requires 340 μL of transformation mix.
3. 42°C heat block.
4. 30°C incubator.
5. Positive and negative (nonspecific bait) control plasmids (*see* **Table 1**).

2.2. Western Analysis

1. SDS-PAGE gel apparatus.
2. 2× Laemmli sample buffer.
3. LexA antibody (Clontech 5397-1, Invitrogen R990-25).

2.3. Library Transformation

1. YPAD medium: prepare YPD medium as described (*see* **Subheading 2.1.2.**), and add 15 mL of sterile 0.2% adenine hemisulfate solution per liter of medium.
2. Dropout selection plates (24 × 24 cm and 100 mm).
3. Prey library (different libraries available from Clontech).
4. Transformation mix.
5. 42°C heat block.
6. 30°C incubator.
7. 50-mL conical sterile tubes.
8. Spectrophotometer.

2.4. Recovery of Transformants

1. Glycerol solution (sterile): 65% (v/v) glycerol, 0.1 M MgSO$_4$, 25 mM Tris-HCl, pH 8.0. It can be stored at room temperature.

2.5. Screen for Interaction Positive Colonies

1. YPAG medium: YPAD solution containing 2% galactose instead of glucose.

2.6. Galactose-Dependent Interaction

1. 30°C incubator.

2.7. Characterization of Interacting Clones

1. Lysis solution: 50 mM Tris-HCl, pH 7.5, 10 mM EDTA pH 7.5, 0.3% (v/v) β-mercaptoethanol added immediately before use, 2% (v/v) β-glucoronidase (type HP-2; Sigma) prepared fresh before use.
2. Acid-washed glass beads (212–300 μm; Sigma).
3. PCR thermal cycler and reagents.
4. 10 μM forward primer (FP): 5'-CGT AGT GGA GAT GCC TCC.
5. 10 μM reverse primer (RP): 5'-CTG GCA AGG TAG ACA AGC CG.
6. Standard agarose DNA gel electrophoresis system.

2.8. Isolation of Interacting Clones

1. *E. coli* strains:
   a. KC8 (carries the *trpC, leuB,* and *hisB* mutations for complementation to yeast *TRP1, LEU2,* and *HIS3* genes, respectively. Constructed by K. Struhl and available from Clontech, cat. no. C2023-1.)
   b. DH5α or other strain suitable for high quality plasmid DNA preparation.
2. M9–Trp Plates. To 750 mL of deionized H$_2$O, add 15 g of bacto-agar and autoclave to sterilize. To this solution (cooled to 55°C) add 200 mL 5 × M9 salt solution (sterile; 5 × M9 salt solution is made by dissolving the following in deionized water to final volume of 1 L and sterilized by autoclaving 64 g Na$_2$HPO$_4$·7H$_2$O, 15 g KH$_2$PO$_4$, 2.5 g NaCl, 5.0 g NH$_4$Cl, 2 mL of 1 M MgSO$_4$, 10 mL of 40% glucose, 0.1 mL of 1 M CaCl$_2$, 1 mL of 1 M thiamine-HCl, and supplemented with 40 mg/mL each uracil, histidine, and leucine.
3. LB/ampicillin plates.
4. 30°C and 37°C incubators.
5. Electroporator.

2.9. Confirmation of Interaction Positive Clones

1. EGY48 containing the lacZ reporter plasmid.
2. 30°C incubator.

2.10. β-Galactosidase Liquid Assay

1. Z buffer: 60 mM Na$_2$HPO$_4$, 40 mM NaH$_2$PO$_4$, 10 mM KCl, 1 mM MgSO$_4$, 50 mM β-mercaptoethanol. Prepare 1 L, adjust to pH 7.0. Do not autoclave.

2. Sodium dodecyl sulfate (SDS), 0.1%.
3. *o*-Nitrophenyl-β-D-galactoside (ONPG). 4 mg/mL in Z buffer. Prepare fresh.
4. Na$_2$CO$_3$: 1 *M* stock solution.
5. 30°C water bath.
6. Spectrophotometer.

3. Methods

3.1. Transformation of Yeast with the Bait Plasmid

1. Using routine cloning techniques, insert DNA encoding the protein region of interest into the polylinker of pLexA, or other LexA fusion plasmids to make an in-frame fusion protein (bait plasmid).
2. Using the Quick and Easy transformation method outlined below, co-transform EGY48 with:
   a. "Bait" plasmid + p8op-lacZ;
   b. Positive control (pLexA-Pos) + p8op-lacZ;
   c. Negative control (pRFHM1) + p8op-lacZ;
   d. pLexA + p8op-lacZ (*see* **Note 1**).
3. Plate each transformation mixture on Glu/SD –Ura, –His dropout plates. Incubate for 2–3 d at 30°C.
4. Restreak at least 10 different single-colonies on
   a. Glu/SD –Ura, –His
   b. Glu/SD –Ura, –His, –Leu
   c. Glu/SD –Ura, –His, X-gal
5. Incubate at 30°C and monitor growth and color for 2–3 d. Ideal baits will be white on X-gal plates and will not grow on –Leu media (*see* **Note 2**).

3.1.1. Quick and Easy Transformation (17)

1. Inoculate EGY48 in 10 mL of YPD. Incubate overnight (o/n) at 30°C.
2. Each transformation requires about 1 mL of overnight culture. Pellet the cells at 6000 rpm for 2 min in a microfuge.
3. Resuspend cells in 1 mL of 100 m*M* LiAc and incubate for 5 min at 30°C.
4. Spin at top speed for 10 s and remove supernatant with a micropipet.
5. Add 340 µL of transformation mix and 10 mL of plasmid DNA (100 ng to 2 µg).
6. Resuspend cell pellets by vortexing, and incubate at 42°C for 20 min.
7. Pellet cells at top speed for 10 s and remove supernatant.
8. Gently resuspend pellet in 100–200 µL of sterile H$_2$O by slowly pipeting up and down.
9. Plate the cell suspension on to appropriate dropout SD plates. Incubate at 30°C for 2–4 d.

3.2. Confirmation of Bait Protein Expression by Western Analysis

1. Inoculate 5 mL of Glu/SD/ –His, –Ura liquid medium with yeast colonies for each bait plasmid and pLexA as positive control. Incubate at 30°C o/n with shaking.
2. Dilute o/n culture 1/10 in to 2 mL of Glu/SD –Ura, –His dropout medium and incubate for 2–3 h at 30°C.

3. Centrifuge 1.5 mL of the culture in a microfuge at maximum speed for 1 min. Discard supernatant.
4. Add 50 μL of 2× Laemmli sample buffer and resuspend the pellet by vortexing.
5. Lyse cells by transferring the tube to a boiling water bath for 5 min.
6. Centrifuge at maximum speed for 30 s to pellet the cellular debris.
7. Resolve 20–30 μL of lysate by SDS-PAGE analysis.
8. Perform a standard Western analysis to detect the expression using antibodies to either LexA or the bait protein (CFTR).

3.3. Large-Scale Yeast Library Transformation (Sufficient for 20 Transformations; Modified from ref. 18)

1. Inoculate 50 mL of Glu/SD –Ura, –His dropout medium with EGY48 containing the bait and reporter plasmids, and incubate o/n at 30°C with shaking at 200 rpm.
2. Dilute o/n culture into 100 mL of YPAD (prewarmed) to a density of $OD_{600} = 0.2$ (~4 × 10^6 cells/mL). Incubate at 30°C for 3–5 h with shaking until an $OD_{600} = 0.8$–1.0 is reached.
3. Harvest cells in sterile 50-mL centrifuge tubes at 3000g for 5 min.
4. Discard supernatant, and resuspend and pool cells in 50 mL of sterile H_2O, and centrifuge again.
5. Resuspend cell pellet in 1.0 mL of 100 mM LiAc and transfer to a microfuge tube. Pellet cells at 8000 rpm for 1 min and remove supernatant.
6. Resuspend cells in 1.0 mL of LiAc (100 mM). Aliquot 50 μL into 20 microfuge tubes. Pellet cells at top speed for 20 s, and remove supernatant with a micropipet.
7. Boil a sample of SS-DNA for 5 min and quickly chill on ice.
8. Prepare transformation mix (TM) (*see* **Note 3**).
9. Add 340 μL of transformation mix (TM) to cell pellet, and then add 10 μL of plasmid DNA (0.5–5 μg).
10. Resuspend pellet first by pipetting up and down, followed by vigorous vortexing. Incubate at 30(C for 30 min.
11. Heat-shock at 42°C for 20–30 min (see **Note 4**).
12. Microfuge at 6000 rpm for 30 s and remove the supernatant with a pipette.
13. Resuspend the cells gently by pipetting it up and down in 1.0 mL of sterile water.
14. (a) Serial dilutions are used to estimate accurately the number of transformants obtained and to assess the efficiency of transformation. Aliquot 20 μL each from five tubes and transfer them to another tube containing 900 μL of sterile water. Make a series of 1/10 dilutions in 1 mL sterile water (up to 10^{-6}). Plate 100 μL of dilutions (10^{-6}–10^{-2}) on Glu/SD –His, –Ura, –Trp dropout plates (100 mm). Count the number of colonies to determine the total number of transformants obtained. The total number of transformants = number of colonies × 100 × dilution factor × total number of transformation tubes.
14. (b) Plate the entire remaining contents of each tube onto Glu/SD –Ura, –His, –Trp dropout plates (one tube per 24 × 24-cm plate).
15. Incubate the plates for 2–4 d at 30°C to recover transformants.

3.4. Recovery of Transformants

1. Cool all the plates for 2 h at 4°C.
2. Add 5 mL of sterile water to each plate and, using a sterile glass slide, gently scrape yeast cells off the plate. Pool the cells from all the plates into three or four sterile 50-mL conical tubes.
3. Centrifuge at 3000g for 5 min, remove and discard supernatant. Resuspend cells in 50 mL of water and recentrifuge.
4. Resupend cell pellet in an equal volume of sterile glycerol solution, mix well. Store in aliquots of 1 mL at –70°C up to 1 yr.

3.5. Screen for Interaction Positive Colonies

1. Dilute an aliquot of frozen yeast cells to 1/50 with YPAG medium. Incubate at 30°C for 2 h with shaking to induce the expression of cDNA under the control of *GAL1* promoter on the library plasmid.
2. Make serial dilutions of yeast cells and plate on 100-mm Gal/Raff –His, –Ura, –Trp dropout plates. Incubate at 30°C for 2–3 d. Count the number of colonies and determine the number of colony-forming units (cfu) per aliquot of frozen yeast.
3. Thaw an appropriate aliquot of yeast cells, which is equal to 10 times the total number of transformants obtained (as determined in **Subheading 3.3., step 14a**).
4. Dilute thawed cells to 1/50 in prewarmed YPAG medium and incubate at 30°C for 2–3 h.
5. Centrifuge cells at 3000g for 5 min and resuspend cells in 1.0 mL of sterile water.
6. Plate 100-µL aliquots on 10 100-mm Gal/Raff –His, –Ura, –Trp, –Leu plates. Incubate at 30°C for 2–5 d until colonies appear.
7. Pick individual colonies and streak on 100-mm Glu/SD –His, –Ura, –Trp master plates (plates that that are divided into grids of 100). It is advantageous to make master plates on each day (i.e., d 2, d 3, and so on) (*see* **Note 5**).

3.6. Verification of Galactose-Dependent Interaction

1. Restreak from Glu/SD –His, –Ura, –Trp master dropout plates to the following plates:
   a. Gal/Raff/SD –His, –Ura, –Trp, –Leu
   b. Gal/Raff/SD –His, –Ura, –Trp, X-Gal
   c. Glu/SD –His, –Ura, –Trp, –Leu
   d. Glu/SD –His, –Ura, –Trp, X-Gal
2. Incubate at 30°C for 2–5 d.
3. Monitor and document the relative growth and color of the colonies on –Leu and X-Gal plates, respectively, on each day. The colonies are considered positive if they are blue on Gal/Raf/X-Gal/ plates but not on Glu/X-Gal plates, and if they grow on Gal/Raf/SD –Leu plates but not on Glu/SD –Leu plates (*see* **Note 6**).

3.7. Characterization of Interacting Clones

1. Restreak positive yeast colonies onto Glu/SD –Ura, –His, –Trp dropout plates. Incubate at 30°C overnight.
2. Use an inoculating loop or toothpick to transfer the yeast colonies to a microfuge tube or 96-well microtiter plate containing 25 µL of lysis solution. Incubate at 37°C for 2–3 h with shaking.

3. Add 0.1 g of acid-washed glass beads to each tube and vortex for 5 min.
4. Add 100 µL of sterile water to each tube and mix gently. Centrifuge at 6000 rpm for 1 min and transfer the supernatant to labeled microfuge tube. Freeze the tubes at –20°C.
5. Using standard PCR protocols, amplify 5 µL of the sample in a 50-µL volume using the forward primer FP and the reverse primer RP.
6. Resolve 10 µL of PCR reaction products on a 1% agarose gel.
7. Digest 10 µL of PCR reaction product with a "4 base cutter" such as *Hae*III in a total volume of 20 µL. Analyze the digested products on a 2.0–2.5% agarose gel. Based on insert size and the restriction pattern, group the obtained interactors into families (*see* **Note 7**).

3.8. Isolation of Interaction Positive Plasmids

1. Use 2–5 µL of lysed yeast (**Subheading 3.7., step 4**) to electroporate into KC8 *E. coli* , or use any standard *E. coli* transformation protocol to transform KC8. Incubate overnight on LB/ampicillin plates at 37°C.
2. Restreak the colonies from LB/ampicillin plates onto bacterial minimal (M9) medium lacking Trp. Incubate overnight at 37°C. The yeast *TRP1* gene can be used to complement the bacterial *trpC-9830* mutation in KC8. This procedure allows easy the isolation of library prey plasmid from other plasmids.
3. Isolate plasmid DNA from two or three individual colonies from each bacterial transformation and analyze the plasmids by digesting them with restriction enzymes that will release the inserted cDNA from the vector.
4. Transform DH5α with the isolated plasmid DNA. Plasmid DNA isolated from DH5α can be used for sequencing using the forward primer (FP1).

3.9. Confirmation of Interaction Positive Clones

1. Using the protocol outlined under **Subheading 3.1., step 1,** co-transform EGY48 containing the lacZ reporter plasmid (p8op-lacZ) with:
   a. Bait plasmids + prey plasmid (interaction trap positives).
   b. Negative control + prey plasmid.
   c. Prey plasmid alone (*see* **Note 8**).
2. Plate each transformation mixture on appropriate dropout plates and incubate for 2–3 d at 30°C.
3. Restreak at least 10 different colonies for each transformation on:
   a. Glu/SD –Ura, –His, –Trp.
   b. Gal/Raff/SD –Ura, –His, –Trp, –Leu.
   c. Gal/Raff/SD –Ura, –His, –Trp, X-gal.
   d. Glu/SD –Ura, –His, –Trp, –Leu.
   e. Glu/SD –Ura, –His, –Trp, X-gal.
4. The following procedure is necessary to eliminate false-positive preys that have the ability to bind to LexA operator. Test the transformants containing the prey plasmid alone on:
   a. Glu/SD –Ura, –Trp.
   b. Gal/Raff/SD –Ura, –Trp, –Leu.
   c. Gal/Raff/SD –Ura, –Trp, X-gal.

5. Monitor and document the growth and color of the colonies to reconfirm the interaction-trap positive clones.

3.10. Quantitative Analysis of Interactions: β-Galactosidase Liquid Assay

1. Inoculate two or three independent single-colonies for each interaction-positive clone in 2 mL of liquid SD medium to maintain selection on the plasmids. Grow o/n at 30°C.
2. Vortex o/n culture tube and spin at 6000g for 5 min. Resuspend pellet in 1 mL of sterile H_2O.
3. Repeat above step to remove any residual glucose and transfer 100 μL of cell suspension to 2 mL of SD/Gal/Raf medium.
4. Incubate cultures at 30°C for 4–6 h with shaking. Harvest cells by centrifugation and resuspend them in 1 mL Z Buffer by vortexing.
5. Centrifuge cells again and resuspend in 1 mL of Z buffer. 100 μL of cell suspension can be used to measure OD_{600}.
6. Transfer 100 mL of cell suspension to a fresh tube containing 0.9 mL Z buffer. Add 1–2 drops of chloroform and 0.1% SDS to each tube. Incubate at 30°C with shaking for 15 min.
7. Add 200 μL of freshly prepared ONPG in Z buffer to each tube and blank tubes. Start the timer. Vortex and incubate the samples at 30°C.
8. After yellow color develops, add 0.5 mL of 1 M Na_2CO_3 to the tubes and vortex. Record elapsed time in minutes (*see* **Note 9**).
9. Centrifuge at 14, 000 rpm to remove cellular debris, and transfer 1 mL of supernatant to a cuvet.
10. Measure OD_{420} of samples relative to blank.
11. Calculate ×-galactosidase units: ×-gal (units) = $1000 \times OD_{420} / (t \times V \times OD_{600})$, where t = elapsed time in minutes, V = volume of cells and OD_{600} = absorbance of 1 mL of culture.

4. Notes

1. pLexA has weak transcriptional activity. Thus, it is not a good negative control, although it can used for comparisons with weak interactors.
2. The *LEU2* reporter on EGY48 is more sensitive than the *lacZ* reporter for some baits. Therefore, the test for Leu requirement is the most important test to determine the background.
3. The transformation mix will be very viscous, hence pipet it carefully. Prepare at least 10% more transformation mix than the required amount.
4. The duration of heat shock will vary and needs to be optimized.
5. It is necessary to pick a sufficient number of Leu+ colonies to ensure that the entire library has been screened. In our experience, a bait to be useful in an interaction screen should not produce more than 1 Leu+ colony per 10^4 library transformants. Therefore, the minimum number of Leu+ colonies that should be picked is given by 10^{-4} x (# library transformants screened).
6. Always restreak colonies previously grown on glucose plates on Gal/Raff plates. A strong two-hybrid interaction will give a blue color the next day. Weaker two-

hybrid interactions will usually require 2–3 d. Colonies that turn blue after 2 d are not very reliable. Growth on –Leu plates can be monitored up to 5 d, with strong interactors usually growing by the second day.

7. Restriction endonuclease digestion and PCR analysis are highly predictive for estimating cDNA identity, but are not absolute methods.

8. Some of the interaction-trap positive clones can code for proteins that have the ability to bind to the LexA operator and hence activate transcription. The LexA fusion protein expressed by the nonspecific bait plasmid can some times mask such false-positive interactions by outcompeting the library-encoded cDNAs that bind weakly to the LexA operator. To rule out such false positives, the failure of the prey plasmid to activate transcription needs to be verified in the absence of any bait plasmid.

9. Length of the reaction will be between 30 min and 4 h. Adjust the reaction time by adjusting the volume of resuspended cells in Z buffer.

References

1. Fields, S. and Song, O. (1989) A novel genetic system to detect protein-protein interaction. *Nature* **340,** 245,246.

2. Chien, C.-T., Bartel, P. L., Sternglanz, R., and Fields, S. (1991) The two-hybrid system: a method to identify and clone genes for proteins that interact with a protein of interest. *Proc. Natl. Acad. Sci. USA* **88,** 9578–9582.

3. Keegan, L., Gill, G., and Ptashne, M. (1986) Separation of DNA binding from the transcription-activating functionof a eucaryotic regulary protein. *Science* **231,** 699–704.

4. Hope, I. A. and Struhl, K. (1986) Functional dissection of a eukaryotic transcriptional protein, GCN4 of yeast. *Cell* **46,** 885–894.

5. Brent, R. and Ptashne, M. (1985) A eukaryotic transcriptional activator bearing the DNA specificity of a procaryotic repressor. *Cell* **43,** 729–736.

6. Ma, J. and Ptashne, M. (1988) Converting an eukaryotic transcriptional inhibitor into an activator. *Cell* **55,** 443–446.

7. Gyuris, J., Golemis, E., Chertkov, H., and Brent, R. (1993) Cdi1, a human G1 and S phase protein phosphatase that associates with Cdk2. *Cell* **75,** 791–803.

8. Hallows, K. R., Raghuram, V., Kemp, B. E., Witters, L. A., and Foskett, J. K. (2000) Inhibition of cystic fibrosis transmembrane conductance regulator by novel interaction with the metabolic sensor AMP-activated protein kinase. *J. Clin. Invest.* **105,** 1711–1721.

9. Raghuram, V., Mak, D.-O. D., and Foskett, J. K. (2001) Regulation of cystic fibrosis transmembrane conductance regulator single-channel gating by bivalent PDZ-domain-mediated interaction. *Proc. Natl. Acad. Sci. USA* **98,** 1300–1305.

10. Ebina, Y., Takahara, Y., Kishi, F., and Nakazawa, A. (1983) LexA protein is a repressor of the colicin E1 gene. *J. Biol. Chem.* **258,** 13,258–13,261.

11. Ma, J. and Ptashne, M. (1987) A new class of yeast transcriptional activators. *Cell* **51,** 113–119.

12. Durfee, T., Becherer, K., Chen, P. L., Yeh, S. H., Yang, Y., Kilburn, A. E., Lee, W. H., and Elledge, S. J. (1993) The retinoblastoma protein associates with the protein phosphatase type 1 catalytic subunit. *Genes Dev.* **7,** 555–569.
13. Vojtek, A. B., Hollenberg, S. M., and Cooper, J. A. (1993) Mammalian Ras interacts directly with the serine/threonine kinase Raf. *Cell* **74,** 205–214.
14. Fearon, E. R., Finkel, T., Gillison, M. L., Kennedy, S. P., Casella, J. F., Tomaselli, G. F., Morrow, J. S., and Dang, C. V. (192) Karyoplasmic interaction selection strategy: a general strategy to detect protein-protein interactions in mammalian cells. *Proc. Natl. Acad. Sci. USA* **89,** 7958–7962.
15. Golemis, E. A., Serebriiskii, I., Finley Jr., R. L., Kolonin, M. G., Gyuris, J., and Brent, R. (1999) Interaction trap/two-hybrid system to identify interacting proteins, in *Current Protocols in Molecular Biology* (Ausubel, F. M., Brent, R., Kingston, R. E., Moore, D. D., Seidman, J. G., Smith, J. A., and Struhl, K., eds.), John Wiley and Sons, pp. 20.1.1–20.1.40.
16. Schuck, P. (1997) Use of surface plasmon resonance to probe the equilibrium and dynamic aspects of interactions between biological macromolecules. *Annu. Rev. Biophys. Biomol. Struct.* **26,** 541–566.
17. Gietz, R. D. and Woods, R. A. (1994) High efficiency transformationof yeast, in *Molecular Genetics of Yeast: Practical Approaches* (Johnson, J. A., ed.), Oxford University Press, London, pp. 121–134.
18. Gietz, R. D., Schiesdtl, R. H., Willems, A., and Woods, R. A. (1995) Studies on the transformation of intact yeast cells by the LiAc/SS-DNA/PEG procedure. *Yeast* **11,** 355–360.

25

Biochemical Assays for Studying Indirect Interactions Between CFTR and the Cytoskeleton

Peter J. Mohler, Patricia L. Kultgen, M. Jackson Stutts, and Sharon L. Milgram

1. Introduction

One approach for understanding the regulation of CFTR and determining how CFTR regulates the activity of other ion channels is to identify CFTR-associated proteins at the apical membrane of airway epithelia. The development of improved methods for studying protein interactions has led to the identification of cytoskeletal-associated scaffolding proteins involved in organizing plasma membrane microdomains and forming multiprotein complexes important for efficient regulation of ion channels and transporters. Many plasma membrane-associated scaffolding proteins contain one or more PDZ domains, conserved 90–100-amino acid protein interaction modules first described in the postsynaptic density protein P̲SD95, the *Drosophila* tumor suppressor d̲lg-A, and the tight junction protein Z̲O-1 (reviewed in **refs.** *1* and *2*). PDZ domains typically mediate interactions with the COOH termini of proteins terminating in consensus PDZ-binding sequences (E–S/T–X–V/I), although other types of interaction also occur. While some data suggest that CFTR may bind directly to the actin cytoskeleton *(3)*, recent experiments indicate that CFTR interacts indirectly with the cytoskeleton via subapical scaffolding proteins that contain PDZ domains *(4–7)*. In this chapter we review in vitro binding assays for studying interactions between CFTR and epithelial scaffolding proteins.

ERM-binding phosphoprotein 50 (EBP50) was the first PDZ protein demonstrated to be accumulated at the apical membrane of epithelial tissues *(4,8)*. EBP50 contains two tandem PDZ domains and a COOH-terminal domain that associates with the NH_2 terminus of ezrin, radixin, and moesin (ERM proteins;

From: *Methods in Molecular Medicine, vol. 70: Cystic Fibrosis Methods and Protocols*
Edited by: W. R. Skach © Humana Press Inc., Totowa, NJ

A

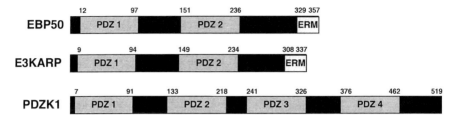

B

EBP50 PDZ1	EBP50 PDZ2	E3KARP PDZ1	E3KARP PDZ2	PDZK1 PDZ1	PDZK1 PDZ2	PDZK1 PDZ3	PDZK1 PDZ4	
	60.5	73.3	64.0	45.9	46.5	48.3	44.8	EBP50 PDZ1
		60.5	69.8	34.1	36.5	51.2	38.4	EBP50 PDZ2
			65.1	41.2	40.7	45.3	45.3	E3KARP PDZ1
				32.9	43.0	45.3	39.5	E3KARP PDZ2
					30.6	34.1	36.5	PDZK1 PDZ1
						39.5	38.4	PDZK1 PDZ2
							36.8	PDZK1 PDZ3

Fig. 1. Domain organization and comparison of PDZ domains of EBP50, E3KARP, and PDZK1. (**A**) Domain organization of EBP50, E3KARP, and PDZK1. EBP50 and E3KARP each contain two PDZ domains and a COOH terminal ERM-family binding domain. PDZK1 contains four PDZ domains. Amino acid residues defining each domain are indicated. (**B**) Comparison of percent identity between the isolated PDZ domains of EBP50, E3KARP, and PDZK1. Amino acids defining the aligned PDZ domains are noted in part A. Sequences were aligned by the Clustal method using Lasergene software.

Fig. 1A) *(8)*. EBP50 associates with ezrin, and ezrin associates with actin *(9)*; therefore EBP50 is a cytoskeletal-associated scaffolding protein that may link CFTR (and other membrane proteins) to the apical cytoskeleton. To better understand the function of EBP50, Wang et al. used peptide phage display to identify COOH-terminal sequences that associate with each of the EBP50 PDZ domains *(7)*. The consensus binding sequence of the first PDZ domain of EBP50 was shown to be X–[T>S]–R–L, identical to D–T–R–L at the COOH terminus of human CFTR. EBP50 is the human ortholog of Na⁺/H⁺ exchanger regulatory factor (NHERF), which was identified based on its ability to interact with, and to regulate, the Na^+/H^+ exchanger 3 *(10)*, a protein at the brush border of intestinal and kidney epithelium *(11)*. A second family member, E3KARP (NHERF2), also contains two PDZ domains, binds ezrin with a similar affinity, and can inhibit NHE3 activity *(12)*. While EBP50 and E3KARP share a similar domain structure and significant sequence identity (**Fig. 1**), subtle differences may explain the unique function of each protein. For example, unlike EBP50, E3KARP is not phosphorylated by PKA in vivo and mRNAs encoding the two proteins are differentially expressed in some tissues (reviewed in **refs.** *13* and *14*). Furthermore, phospholipase C-beta 3 associates with E3KARP but not EBP50, suggesting that the two proteins do not have identical binding partners in cells *(15)*. Finally the PDZ domains of PDZK1, a human protein expressed at high levels in kidney epithelial cells *(16)*, shares significant sequence identity with EBP50 and E3KARP (**Fig. 1B**). PDZK1 is highly homologous with rat diphor, a protein whose expression is regulated by changes in dietary phosphate *(17,18)*. PDZK1 and diphor each contain four PDZ domains (**Fig. 1**). It is not yet known whether PDZK1 and diphor associate with ERM family members.

To date, the functional relationships among EBP50, E3KARP, and PDZK1/diphor are unknown. One approach to comparing the functions of these three related proteins is to use in vitro binding assays to study their ability to associate with proteins via their PDZ domains. For example, using radiolabeled PDZ proteins and biotinylated CFTR peptides, we asked whether multiple EBP50-related proteins could associate with the COOH-terminus of CFTR. A biotinylated peptide corresponding to the COOH-terminal 10 amino acids of CFTR was immobilized on streptavidin-agarose. Next, radiolabeled PDZ proteins (EBP50, E3KARP, and diphor), generated by coupled in vitro transcription/translation, were incubated with the biotinylated peptide for several hours at 4°C. After extensive washing, the associated proteins (bound fraction) were analyzed by sodium dodecyl sulfate-polyacrylamide gel electrophoresis (SDS-PAGE) and phosphorimaging. We found that EBP50, E3KARP, and diphor bound to the CFTR COOH-terminal peptide (**Fig. 2**). In this particular experiment we used mutant CFTR peptide, where the final four amino acids implicated in the PDZ-specific interaction were substituted by glycine, as a negative control (**Fig. 2**). EBP50, E3KARP, and diphor did not associate with the CFTR mutant peptide, providing an important demonstration of specificity in the assay. Based on the peptide mapping data of Wang et al., we further asked whether EBP50, E3KARP, and diphor could associate with the COOH-termini of other proteins that terminated in the consensus sequence for association with PDZ1 or PDZ2 of EBP50. The peptides we tested include YAP65, an adaptor protein cloned based on its ability to associate with the Src family kinase c-Yes

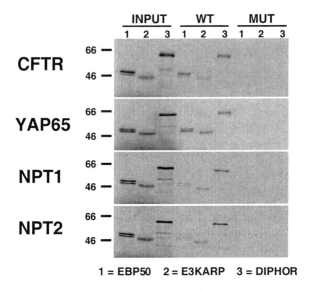

1 = EBP50   2 = E3KARP   3 = DIPHOR

PEPTIDES USED FOR BINDING:

CFTR WT: BIOTIN-SGSGREEEVQDTRL
CFTR MUT: BIOTIN-SGSGREEEVQGGGG
YAP65 WT: BIOTIN-SGSGLDKESFLTWL
YAP65 MUT: BIOTIN-SGSGLDKESFGGGG
NPT1 WT: BIOTIN-SGSGWAKEKQHTRL
NPT1 MUT: BIOTIN-SGSGWAKEKQGGGG
NPT2 WT: BIOTIN-SGSGLPAHHNATRL
NPT2 MUT: BIOTIN-SGSGLPAHHNGGGG

Fig. 2. EBP50, E3KARP, and diphor all specifically bind the COOH terminus of CFTR, YAP65, NPT1, and NPT2. Biotinylated peptides were immobilized on streptavidin-agarose beads and incubated with radiolabeled, in vitro translated EBP50, E3KARP, or diphor for 2 h at 4°C. After washing the beads to remove nonspecifically bound proteins, the bound fraction was eluted in Laemmeli buffer, separated by 10% SDS-PAGE, and analyzed by phosphorimage analysis. The sequences of all wild-type and mutant peptides used are shown.

(19), and the Na^+/P_I co-transporters NPT1 and NPT2. Using in vitro binding assays we found that each of the scaffolding proteins was capable of interaction with COOH-terminal peptides encompassing the last 10 amino acids of YAP65, NPT1, and NPT2 (**Fig. 2**). Although these data indicate that many different protein interactions can occur in vitro, it will be critical to use cell-based assays to determine which interactions occur in vivo.

In vitro binding assays can also be developed in which the PDZ protein is immobilized on beads, and interactions can be studied using specific recombinant proteins or whole-cell lysates from an appropriate tissue. For example, we

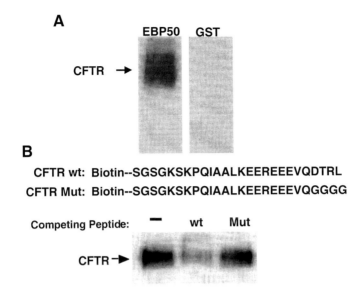

Fig. 3. Affinity precipitation of EBP50 and CFTR from CalU3 cell lysates. (**A**) GST or GST-EBP50 were immobilized on glutathione agarose beads and incubated with ~500 μg of CalU3 cell lysate for 2 h at 4°C. The bound fraction was separated on 7% SDS-PAGE, and immuoblotted with rabbit anti-CFTR R domain (1:200). (**B**) Binding of CFTR to GST-EBP50 was assayed as described in (A) in the presence of 400 n*M* wild-type CFTR or CFTRmut peptide. Binding of CFTR to GST-EBP50 in the presence of CFTR or CFTRmut peptides was determined by immunoblot analysis as described above. The sequences of wild-type CFTR and CFTR mutant (CFTRmut) peptides are shown.

used a GST-EBP50 fusion protein and CalU3 cell lysates to ask whether full-length native CFTR could associate with EBP50 (*4*). To do this we incubated detergent-soluble proteins extracted from CalU3 cells with GST or GST-EBP50 fusion protein immobilized on glutathione-sepharose beads, and analyzed the bound fraction by western blot with CFTR antibodies. As seen in **Fig. 3A**, CFTR associates with GST-EBP50 but not with GST, indicating that the full-length proteins are capable of interaction. The interaction between EBP50 and CFTR can be blocked by the addition of a peptide encompassing the last 14 amino acids of CFTR, but not by a CFTR COOH-terminal peptide in which the last four amino acids were substituted with glycine (**Fig. 3B**). This simple additional step further demonstrates that the association between EBP50 and CFTR is mediated by the COOH-terminus of CFTR. Similar types of in vitro binding assays were used to show that CFTR associates with E3KARP (*5*), and that YAP65 associates with EBP50 (*20*).

In vitro binding assays can also be used to study binding specificities within multidomain proteins such as EBP50 and E3KARP. This can be easily accom-

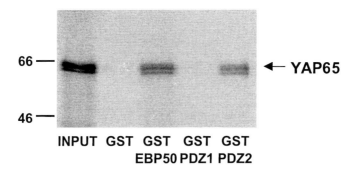

Fig. 4. Identification of the YAP65-binding site in EBP50. Ten micrograms of GST, GST-EBP50, GST-PDZ1, or GST-PDZ2 were immobilized on glutathione agarose beads and incubated with 5 μL of radiolabeled YAP65 generated by coupled in vitro transcription/translation. After washing in buffers containing 1 *M* NaCl, bound proteins were eluted from the beads and analyzed by SDS-PAGE and phosphorimage analysis.

plished by generating GST fusion proteins of individual PDZ domains for in vitro binding assays. For example, we showed that CFTR preferentially associated with PDZ1 of EBP50, while YAP65 preferentially associated with PDZ2 *(4,20)*. Experiments mapping the binding specificity of the EBP50–YAP65 interaction are briefly described. GST fusion proteins corresponding to PDZ1 and PDZ2 domains of EBP50 were immobilized on glutathione agarose; full-length GST-EBP50 and GST were included as positive and negative controls, respectively. Radiolabeled in vitro translated YAP65 was incubated with each immobilized GST affinity resin, the columns were washed, and the bound proteins analyzed by SDS-PAGE and phosphorimage analysis (**Fig. 4**); this approach clearly showed that YAP65 preferentially associates with PDZ2 of EBP50.

Apical membrane scaffolding proteins may serve multiple regulatory functions in epithelial cells, from stabilizing proteins at the appropriate cell surface to forming regulatory networks important for efficient regulation of ion transport *(10–14,20)*. To elucidate these functions it will be critically important to compare the cellular expression, subcellular distribution, and cellular binding partners of EBP50, E3KARP, and PDZK1. Although in vitro binding assays cannot be used as a measure of in vivo protein association, they are often the first step in the characterization of protein–protein interactions. Further in vivo assays including co-immunoprecipitations and co-localization experiments are necessary to further demonstrate in vivo protein associations.

2. Materials

2.1. Generation and Expression of GST Fusion Protein

1. cDNA-encoding protein sequence of interest subcloned in-frame into the appropriate pGEX vector (Pharmacia).

2. Luria broth (LB): 10 g/L peptone, 5.0 g/L yeast extract, 10 g/L NaCl.
3. 50 mg/mL ampicillin (1000× stock) in water.
4. Competent BL21 (DE3) pLys S *Escherichia coli* (Life Technologies).
5. Protease inhibitor cocktail: standard inhibitor cocktail (Sigma) is supplemented with phenylmethylsulfonyl fluoride (PMSF). The latter is made up as a 30 mg/mL (1000×) stock solution in ethanol (*see* **Note 1**).
6. Isopropyl-1-thio-ß-D-galactopyranoside (IPTG; Sigma).

2.2. Binding of Recombinant Protein or Peptide to Agarose Beads

1. Recombinant GST-fusion protein or biotinylated peptide (5–20 µg). Biotinylated peptides should be synthesized with a spacer (SGSG) between the biotin and the peptide sequence of interest to avoid steric hindrance in binding assays.
2. Glutathione-sepharose (Pharmacia) or streptavidin-agarose (Sigma).
3. Coupling buffer (phosphate-buffered saline): 50 mM NaH$_2$PO$_4$, 150 mM NaCl, pH 7.4.
4. Wash buffer: 50 mM Tris-HCl, pH 7.4, 1 mM EDTA, 1 mM EGTA, 150 mM NaCl, and 1.0% Triton X-100.

2.3. Generation of Radiolabeled Protein by Coupled In Vitro Transcription/Translation

1. cDNA of interest subcloned into a plasmid (0.5 µg/µL in sterile H$_2$O) with appropriate upstream promoter.
2. [^{35}S] methionine (>1000 Ci/mmol at 10 mCi/ml; New England Nuclear).
3. Promega TNT Coupled Reticulocyte lysate system or individual components.
4. Rnasin ribonuclease inhibitor (40 U/µL; Promega).

2.4. Preparation of Cell Lysates

1. Cell lysis buffer if protein of interest is not easily solubilized (RIPA bufer): 20 mM Tris-HCl, pH 7.4, 150 mM NaCl, 0.1% SDS, 1.0% Triton X-100, 1.0% deoxycholic acid, 5 mM EDTA (optional) containing protease inhibitors.
2. Cell lysis buffer if protein of interest is easily solubilized: 20 mM Tris-HCl, pH 7.4, 150 mM NaCl, 5 mM EDTA (optional), 0.1–1% Triton X-100 containing protease inhibitors.

2.5. In Vitro Binding, Washing, and Data Analysis

1. Appropriate cell lysate OR radiolabeled protein.
2. Binding buffer: 50 mM Tris-HCl, pH 7.4, 1 mM EDTA, 1 mM EGTA, 150 mM NaCl, 0.5% Triton X-100, and protease inhibitors.
3. 4°C rotating platform.
4. Wash buffer (low stringency): 50 mM Tris-HCl, pH 7.4, 1 mM EDTA, 1 mM EGTA, 150 mM NaCl, 1% Triton X-100.
5. Wash buffer (high stringency): 50 mM Tris-HCl, pH 7.4, 1 mM EDTA, 1 mM EGTA, 1 M NaCl, 1% Triton X-100.
6. SDS-PAGE apparatus and material for western blots (if cell lysates are used) or phosphorimaging screen (if radiolabeled protein is used).

3. Methods

3.1. Expression of GST Fusion Protein

1. Generate the bacterial expression plasmid by subcloning the cDNA of interest in frame into the appropriate pGEX vector (Pharmacia) using common restriction endonuclease sites. After confirming the cDNA sequence, transform the plasmid into BL21 (DE3) pLys S *E. coli* (Life Technologies).
2. Grow a single colony of bacteria overnight in 50 mL of LB + 50 μg/mL ampicillin at 37°C in a shaking incubator.
3. Transfer one-fourth of the starter culture into to a 1-L flask of LB plus 50 μg/mL ampicillin; grow at 37°C to an optical density of 0.6 (~3 h).
4. Induce protein expression by addition of 1 m*M* IPTG (final concentration) for 3 h at 37°C and purify according to the manufacturer's instructions (Pharmacia).

3.2. Coupling of GST Fusion Protein or Biotinylated Peptide to Affinity Beads

1. Generate a bed volume of 40 μL of glutathione-sepharose (Pharmacia) or streptavidin-agarose (Sigma) in a 1.6-mL microfuge tube.
2. Wash the beads three times with cold phosphate buffered saline; centrifuge 30 s between washes and completely aspirate the wash buffer.
3. Add 5–20 μg of purified GST-fusion protein or biotinylated peptide to the beads and tumble at 4°C for 3 h (biotinylated peptides can be incubated for shorter lengths of time).
4. Wash the beads three times with wash buffer to remove unbound protein or peptide, and centrifuge between washes (*see* **Note 3**).

3.3. Preparation of Cell Lysates

1. Wash cultured cells with cold phosphate-buffered saline to remove cellular debris and residual medium.
2. Add cold cell lysis buffer (~500 μL/100-mm dish) and lyse cells by dounce homogenization; transfer cell lysate to clean ultracentrifuge tube.
3. Incubate lysate on ice for 20 min.
4. Clear lysate by ultracentrifugation at 40,000*g* for 20 min at 4°C; remove supernatant for binding experiments.

3.4. Preparation of Radiolabeled Proteins Using In Vitro Transcription/Translation

1. Remove reagents from –80°C freezer and thaw on ice.
2. Prepare reaction mixture according to manufacturer's guidelines. For a 50-μL reaction, add 25 μL reticulocyte lysate, 2 μL reaction buffer, 1 μL polymerase, 2 μL amino acid mix (minus methionine), 1 μL RNasin, 4 μL (1–2 μg) DNA template, and 14 μL sterile water.
3. Add 2 μL [^{35}S]methionine.
4. Incubate reaction at 30°C for ~90 min; analyze 3–5 μL of the sample by SDS-PAGE and phosphorimaging.

3.5. In Vitro Binding

1. Briefly centrifuge tubes containing immobilized fusion protein or biotinylated peptide; resuspend resin in ~500 μL of cold binding buffer.
2. Add cell lysate (200 μg–1 mg total protein) to each affinity resin for a final volume of 600 μL or add 5μL of radiolabeled protein generated by coupled in vitro transcription/translation.
3. Tumble the binding reaction for 2–8 h at 4°C (*see* **Notes 3** and **4**).

3.6. Removal of Nonspecific Protein Association

1. Centrifuge samples for 1 min at 4°C.
2. Remove supernatant (unbound fraction); this can be saved for analysis.
3. Wash the beads three times using 500 μL of high stringency wash buffer at 4°C.
4. Wash the beads three times using 500 μL of low stringency wash buffer at 4°C.
5. After aspirating the final wash, elute the bound fraction using 30 μL of SDS-PAGE sample buffer.
6. If you used whole-cell lysates for the binding assay, analyze the bound fraction by western blot analysis using the appropriate antibody. If the binding assay was performed using radiolabeled protein, analyze by SDS-PAGE and phosphorimase analysis. In either case, include an input sample and negative controls on the same gel (*see* **Note 4**).

3.7. Interpretation of Results

Before performing in vitro binding experiments, it is important to generate appropriate positive and negative controls to interpret your results correctly. As a rule, always include GST alone and an unrelated GST-fusion protein as negative control. If possible, include a GST fusion protein known to associate with your protein of interest to serve as a positive control. For biotinylated peptide experiments, the same general guidelines apply, using known binding peptides as positive controls, and unrelated, scrambled, or mutated peptides as negative controls. In addition, to further characterize your binding efficiency, include an input sample from the cell lysate or the radiolabeled protein on the gel. This simple step will allow you to estimate the efficiency of the protein interaction and will also confirm whether your antibody and western blotting procedures were successful in the absence of significant binding. Finally, and most important, in vitro binding assays are only the first step in the characterization of potential protein–protein interactions. These assays should not be used independently as a measure of in vivo protein association, but instead used as the initial step in the characterization of potential interactions. Further in vivo assays including co-immunoprecipitations and co-localization experiments are necessary to determine whether the proteins associate in vivo.

3.8. Troubleshooting

1. Certain GST fusion proteins are difficult to express, or may be found in insoluble inclusion bodies. If this occurs, reduce the induction time to 30 min or lower the

induction temperature to 28°C. Alternatively, use denaturing conditions to solubilize the GST fusion protein but realize that some GST fusion proteins are not easily refolded once they are denatured. There is an excellent discussion of strategies for solubilizing GST fusion proteins provided by the manufacturer.

2. Depending on the protein(s) of interest, it may be necessary to alter the cell lysis buffer or to include 0.1% nonfat dry milk to decrease the amount of nonspecific association with the beads.

3. For high affinity protein–protein interactions, it is important to include high-stringency washes. However, for low-affinity protein interactions, eliminate the high-salt wash and replace with a less stringent wash buffer.

4. Promega sells reagents for nonradioactive, biotin-coupled in vitro transcription/translation. This protocol may be useful when the protein of interest lacks a significant number of methionine residues.

4. Notes

1. Prepare fresh PMSF in 100% ethanol immediately before each experiment.
2. Purified GST-fusion protein should be stored in aliquots at –80°C.
3. The unbound fraction from the in vitro binding experiment can be precipitated using 2 vol of ice-cold acetone (2 h at –20°C) and analyzed next to the bound fraction. Make sure to completely remove all acetone from precipitated protein to prevent smearing of the gel.
4. Once finished with immunoblotting, stain the membrane with Coomassie blue to confirm that you added equal amounts of the GST fusion protein in each experimental sample.
5. Gloves should be worn for all experimental procedures.
6. All buffers should be chilled to 4°C before experiments, and all experiments should be performed at 4°C.
7. Biotinylated peptides should be stored as powder in dessicant at –20°C. Before each experiment, quickly weigh peptide and resuspend in appropriate volume of autoclaved deionized H_2O.
8. Before performing GST fusion protein experiments, perform a protein assay and confirm that the fusion protein is intact by SDS-PAGE and Coomassie staining.
9. Successful in vitro binding using GST fusion proteins or biotinylated peptides is highly dependent on selecting proper solubilization, binding, and washing conditions. In most cases, these variables must be adjusted empirically for each protein–protein interaction.

References

1. Fanning, A. S. and Anderson, J. M. (1999) PDZ domains: fundamental building blocks in the organization of protein complexes at the plasma membrane. *J. Clin. Invest.* **103,** 767–772.
2. Kornau, H. C., Seeburg, P. H., and Kennedy, M. B. (1997) Interaction of ion channels and receptor with PDZ domains proteins. *Curr. Opin. Neurobiol.* **7,** 368–373.
3. Cantiello, H. F. (1996) Role of the active cytoskeleton in the regulation of the cystic fibrosis transmembrane conductance regulator. *Exp. Physiol.* **81,** 505–514.

4. Short, D. B., Trotter, K. W. Reczek, D., Kreda, S. M., Bretscher, A., Boucher, R. C., et al. (1998) An apical PDZ protein anchors the cystic fibrosis transmembrane conductance regulator to the cytoskeleton. *J. Biol. Chem.* **273,** 19,797–19,801.

5. Sun, F., Hug, M. J., Lewarchik, C. M., Yun, C., Bradbury, N. A., and Frizzell, R. A. (2000) E3KARP mediates the Association of ezrin and PKA with CFTR in airway cells. *J. Biol. Chem.* **275,** 29,539–29,546.

6. Hall, R. A., Ostedgaard, L. S., Premont, R. T., Blitzer, J. T., Rahman, N., Welsh, M. J., et al. (1998) A C-terminal motif found in the beta2-adrenergic receptor, P2Y1 receptor and cystic fibrosis transmembrane conductance regulator determines binding to the Na+/H+ exchanger regulatory factor family of PDZ proteins. *Proc. Natl. Acad. Sci. USA* **95,** 8496–8501.

7. Wang, S., Raab, R. W., Schatz, P. J., Guggino, W. B., and Li, M. (1998) Peptide binding consensus of the NHE-RF-PDZ1 domain matches the C-terminal sequence of cystic fibrosis transmembrane conductance regulator (CFTR). *FEBS Lett.* **427,** 103–108.

8. Reczek, D., Berryman, M., and Bretscher, A. (1997) Identification of EBP50: a PDZ-containing phosphoprotein that associates with members of the ezrin-radixin-moesin family. *J. Cell Biol.* **139,** 169–179.

9. Bretscher, A., Reczek, D., and Berryman, M. (1997) Ezrin: a protein requiring conformational activation to link microfilaments to the plasma membrane in the assembly of cell surface structures. *J. Cell Sci.* **110,** 3011–3018.

10. Yun, C. H., Oh, S., Zizak, M., Steplock, D., Tsao, S., Tse, C. M., et al. (1997) cAMP-mediated inhibition of the epithelial brush border Na+/H+ exchanger, NHE3, requires an associated regulatory protein. *Proc. Natl. Acad. Sci. USA* **94,** 3010–3015.

11. Brandt, S. R., Yun, C. H., Donowitz, M., and Tse, C. M. (1995) Cloning, tissue distribution, and functional analysis of the human Na+/H+ exchanger isoform, NHE3. *Am. J. Physiol.* **269,** 198–206.

12. Yun, C. H., Lamprecht, G., Forster, D. V., and Sidor, A. (1998) NHE3 kinase a regulatory protein E3KARP binds the epithelial brush border Na+/H+ exchanger NHE3 and the cytoskeletal protein ezrin. *J. Biol. Chem.* **273,** 25,856–25,863.

13. Weinman, E. J., Minkoff, C., and Shenolikar, S. (2000) Signal complex regulation of renal transport proteins: NHERF and regulation of NHE3 by PKA. *Am. J. Physiol.* **279,** F393–F399.

14. Minkoff, C., Shenolikar, S., and Weinman, E. J. (1999) Assembly of signaling complexes by the sodium-hydrogen exchanger regulatory factor family of PDZ-containing proteins. *Curr. Opin. Nephrol. Hypertens.* **8,** 603–608.

15. Hwang, J. I., Heo, K., Shin, K. J., Kim, E., Yun, C., Ryu, S. H. et al. (2000) Regulation of phospholipase C-beta 3 activity by Na+/H+ exchanger regulatory factor 2. *J. Biol. Chem.* **275,** 16,632–16,637.

16. Kocher, O., Comella, N., Gilchrist, A., Pal, R., Tognazzi, K., Brown, L. F. et al. (1999) PDZK1, a novel PDZ domain-containing protein up-regulated in carcinomas and mapped to chromosome 1q21, interacts with cMOAT (MRP2), the multidrug resistance-associated protein. *Lab. Invest.* **79,** 1161–1170.

17. Custer, M., Spindler, B., Verrey, F., Murer, H., and Biber, J. (1997) Identification of a new gene product (diphor-1) regulated by dietary phosphate. *Am. J. Physiol.* **273,** F801–F806.

18. White, K. E., Biber, J., Murer, H., and Econs, M. J. (1998) A PDZ domain-containing protein with homology to Diphor-1 maps to human chromosome 1q21. *Ann. Hum. Gen.* **62,** 287–290.

19. Sudol, M. (1994) Yes-associated protein (YAP65) is a proline-rich phosphoprotein that binds to the SH3 domain of the Yes proto-oncogene product. *Oncogene* **9,** 2145–2152.

20. Mohler, P. J., Kreda, S. M., Boucher, R. C., Sudol, M., Stutts, M. J., and Milgram, S. L. (1999) Yes-associated protein 65 localizes p62(c-Yes) to the apical compartment of airway epithelia by association with EBP50. *J. Cell Biol.* **147,** 879–890.

21. Moyer, B. D., Denton, J., Karlson, K. H., Reynolds, D., Wang, S., Mickel, J. E., et al. (1999) A PDZ-interacting domain in CFTR is an apical membrane polarization signal. *J. Clin Invest.* **104,** 1353–1361.

26

CFTR-Associated ATP Transport and Release

Marie E. Egan

1. Introduction

After the identification of the cystic fibrosis transmembrane conductance regulator (CFTR) gene, numerous expression studies verified that CFTR is a cAMP-dependent chloride channel *(1–3)*. Given that chloride impermeability is the signature of CF-affected epithelium, these data were completely consistent with previously described findings. However, a number of other characteristics of CF-affected epithelia such as abnormal sodium transport could not explained by CFTR's chloride channel activity. In an attempt to reconcile this apparent discrepancy, further electrophysiologic studies were performed and demonstrated that CFTR has a variety of secondary functions including that of channel regulator *(4)*. CFTR has been shown to regulate and/or modulate the epithelial sodium channel *(4–7)*, and the outwardly rectifying chloride channel *(4,8–10)*. The mechanism(s), by which CFTR can interact or affect these other channels is unknown. While trying to identify the exact mechanism(s) investigators have examined whether CFTR could affect ATP transport to the extracellular surface *(11,12)*. Alterations in extracellular ATP could explain many of the secondary abnormalities observed in CF-affected epithelia. For instance, extracellular ATP has been shown to have a variety of effects on airway epithelial cells, including altering ciliary beat, and stimulating submucosal gland secretion *(13)*. Furthermore, in experimental models it has been shown to activate of a variety of "non-CFTR" chloride channels *(13–16)* and regulate the epithelial sodium transport *(13)*. It has been postulated that CFTR (1) could affect ATP transport by acting as a transporter or pump for ATP, (2) could conduct ATP directly or could be associated with an ATP channel or pore, (3) or could affect the release of vesicles that contain ATP *(17)* (**Fig. 1**).

From: *Methods in Molecular Medicine, vol. 70: Cystic Fibrosis Methods and Protocols*
Edited by: W. R. Skach © Humana Press Inc., Totowa, NJ

A   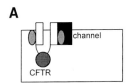   **B**   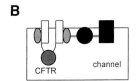   **C**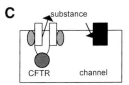

Fig. 1. CFTR interactions. (**A**) Direct interaction: CFTR may couple directly to the channel protein to form a complex. (**B**). Indirect interaction: CFTR may associate with membrane-bound proteins such as cytoskeletal elements, which then interface ion channels. (**C**) Indirect interaction: CFTR may couple by transport of a regulatory substance.

In order to study this hypothesis, a variety of assays were developed to measure extracellular ATP, including ATP release assays utilizing either ^{32}P-labeled ATP or bioluminescence, single-channel patch clamping to detect ATP conduction, and atomic force microscopy to identify surface release. The assays will be discussed in the order they are mentioned. It should be noted that CFTR-mediated ATP release is a fairly controversial area of investigation. Numerous laboratories have studied this question and have arrived at very different answers (*18–25*).

1.1. Release Assays

A number of methods assay for the extracellular release of ATP. Initially, Schweibert et al. described an assay that indirectly measured the release of radiolabeled ^{32}P-ATP (*18*). The method takes advantage of an ATP-scavenging enzyme, hexokinase, which is added to the assay solution. It is believed that once ATP is released from cells, the hexokinase uses the ATP to form glucose 6-phosphate. This transforms the very active ATP and its radioactive label into a stable ^{32}P-labeled glucose 6-phosphate that can then be assayed and quantified (**Fig. 2A**). There are a number of limitations to this assay. First, the measurement is an indirect measure of ATP release, therefore a large number of control measurements need to be performed to validate the assay (which will be discussed at length under **Subheading 3.**). Most important, it must be demonstrated that the ^{32}P measured is actually associated with the generation of glucose 6-phosphate and not nonspecific detection. It should also be mentioned that the use of radioactivity can be costly and requires special handling by experienced laboratory personnel.

Subsequently, a bioluminescence assay for the detection of ATP release was developed that eliminated the need for radioactivity (*26*). It also gets rid of the potential for variability of ATP loading, and the need to permeabilize the cells to enhance ATP loading (as is needed in the ^{32}P ATP assay). ATP bioluminescence assay takes advantage of a luciferase-luciferin reagent that catalyzes ATP to yield a photon that can be measured in a luminometer (**Fig. 2B**). It is believed that one ATP molecule is equivalent to one photon created by the luciferase-

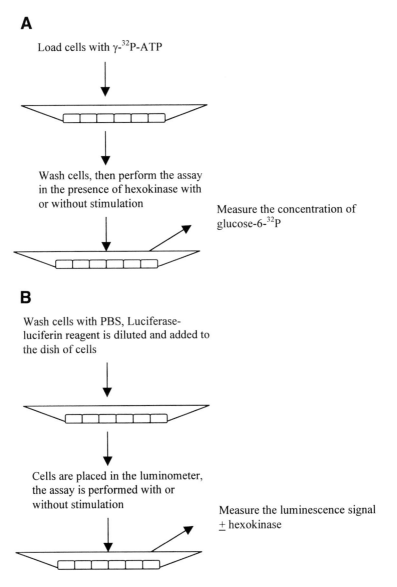

Fig. 2. **(A)** γ-^{32}P-ATP release assay: a schematic of the release assay. **(B)** Luciferase-luciferin ATP release assay: a schematic of the bioluminescence assay

luciferin reaction. Although the assay is very straightforward (*see* **Subheading 3.**), the interpretation of the results can be complicated if the examiner is not careful to control for the effects of technical manipulation on the cells. Extreme care needs to be taken with regard to how cell cultures are handled, how solutions are added to and removed from the cells, and the osmolarity of solutions that are used in the assay. The time-course of the release need to be established. Paired analyses examining the effects of study conditions on release, as well as the effects of agonists on release, need to be ascertained. Lastly, the dynamics of the release and metabolism need to be assayed.

1.2. Patch Clamp Studies

As stated above, the exact mechanism responsible for the CFTR-mediated ATP release is unknown. One possibility is that ATP release is actually secondary to ATP conduction through the conduction pore of CFTR or through a closely associated pore. Using the single-channel patch clamp technique, a number of investigators have been able to identify ATP conduction in epithelial cells and heterologous cells that appears to be associated with CFTR expression *(18,20,22)*. In this assay excised inside-out patches of cell membrane are examined under conditions that would activate CFTR. In a number of experimental protocols, patches are examined with pipet and bath solutions that contain symmetrical chloride concentrations. After CFTR channel activity is established, anion substitutions are performed whereby ATP is substituted for chloride. Channel activity is then reexamined *(18)*. Alternatively, investigators have started with pipet and bath solutions that contain equal concentrations of ATP bilaterally. Anion substitutions are then performed, adding chloride to the bath solution *(20)*. Lastly, channel activity can be assessed having both anions present in different concentrations and calculating reversal potentials for each permeant anion. When channel activity is assessed, both reversals should be evident *(20,22)*. Unlike the ATP release assays, cells are not kept intact.

1.3. Atomic Force Microscopy

One other assay that has been used to examine ATP release from airway epithelial cells is atomic force microscopy (AFM). Schneider et al., have developed ATP-detecting AFM microscopy tips *(21)*. By modifying the AFM scanning probe they were able to demonstrate the use of the AFM as both a morphological instrument and as a biosensor to detect extracellular ATP directly. Commercially available AFM tips were functionalized by adding the myosin (520 kDa) subfragment S1 (105 kDa), which contains the reactive ATPase portion of myosin to the tip before use. This technique was used successfully to detect ATP that accumulated on the surface of an airway epithelial cells expressing CFTR (S9 cell-line). This result confirmed the theory of active ATP secretion by these cells and, furthermore, the ATP concentration along the surface was shown to be influenced by stimulation and inhibition of CFTR. This technique allows for a continuous live update of surface topography as well as a direct measurement of the microenvironment along the surface of the cell membrane in living cells under physiological conditions.

2. Materials

Preparation of cells for all mentioned assays: The quality and characteristics of the cells used for these assays can influence the outcome of studies dramatically. ATP release appears to be dependent on the cell culture conditions and the degree of cellular differentiation. Therefore, all epithelial cell lines are grown on an extracellular matrix such as collagen (Vitrogen diluted with phosphate buffered saline 1/15) or a combination of distilled H_2O, fibronectin (10 µg/mL), bovine serum albumin (BSA) (100 µg/mL), and collagen (6 mg/mL). In addition, a feeding schedule is established and cells are grown to near confluence prior to the assay. A medium that allows for optimal growth and differentiation should be selected for each cell type and/or cell line. Cells are maintained in a 5% CO_2/95% air incubator at 37°C. For patch clamp studies and atomic force microsopy, cells are passaged onto glass cover slips or chips coated with fibronectin, BSA, and collagen as described above and are studied 1–3 d after passage.

2.1. Release Assays

2.1.1. ³²P ATP Release Assay

1. Cells grown to 50% confluence.
2. $\gamma^{32}P$ ATP (3000 Ci/mmol specific activity) (NEN-Dupont Boston, MA).
3. Streptolysin O (1 U/mL) (Sigma, St, Louis, MO).
4. Buffer solution: 140 m*M* NaCl, 100 m*M* PIPES, 5 m*M* glucose, 2.7 m*M* KCl, 2.7 m*M* EGTA, 1 m*M* Na_2-ATP, pH 7.4.
5. Ringer's solution: 140 m*M* NaCl, 1.5 m*M* $CaCl_2$, 1 m*M* $MgCl_2$, 5 m*M* glucose, 5 m*M* HEPES, 5 m*M* K_2HPO_4/KH_2PO_4 (pH 7.4).
6. Hexokinase (type IV isolated from Baker's yeast, 1 U/mL, Sigma).
7. cAMP stimulation cocktail CPT-cAMP, or forskolin (Sigma).
8. Glibenclamide (Sigma).
9. Anion-exchange column containing resin AG 1-X2 (Bio-Rad, Richmond CA).
10. Alkaline phosphatase (1U/mL) (Sigma).

2.1.2. ATP Bioluminescence Assay

1. Cells grown to 75–100% confluence.
2. Sterile serum-free culture medium Optimtm-I (Gibco-BRL, Gaithersburg, MD).
3. Filtered Ringer's solution:140 m*M* NaCl, 1.5 m*M* $CaCl_2$, 1 m*M* $MgCl_2$, 5 m*M* glucose, 5 m*M* HEPES, 5 m*M* K_2HPO_4/KH_2PO_4, pH 7.4.
4. Phosphate-buffered saline (PBS).
5. Luciferase-luciferin reagent L1761 (isolated from the firefly Photinus pyralis) (Sigma).
6. 35-mm cell culture dishes.
7. cAMP stimulation cocktail CPT-cAMP, or forskolin (Sigma).
8. Glibenclamide (Sigma).
9. Turner TD 20/20 luminometer (Turner/Promega, Madison, WI).

2.2. Patch Clamp

1. Cells grown on coated glass chips as described above.
2. Standard NaCl bath: 141 mM NaCl, 2 mM MgCl$_2$, 1 mM EGTA, 0.5 mM CaCl$_2$ (free Ca^{2+} is 110 nM measured by Fura-2), 5 mM HEPES.
3. Standard NaCl pipet: 141 mM NaCl, 2 mM CaCl$_2$, 5 mM HEPES, pH of both solutions adjusted to 7.3 with Tris base.
4. ATP bath solution: the standard bath solution with the folowing substitutions— NaCl is replaced with 40 mM Na-gluconate and 50 mM Na$_2$ATP. CaCl$_2$ is replaced with 0.25 mM Ca gluconate.
5. Nucleotide stock solutions: 10 mM Nucleotide made in appropriate bath solutions and diluted to give the stated concentrations.
6. Sodium-free solutions are made by substituting 145 mMTris-HCl for NaCl or 140 mM Tris-ATP for Na$_2$ATP and Na gluconate.
7. Protein kinase A catalytic subunit (Promega).
8. MgATP, 1 mM (Sigma).
9. Glibenclamide was made as a 100 mM stock solution in dimethyl sulfoxide (DMSO) and ethyl alcohol (EtOH) (1/2) and diluted in the appropriate bath solution.
10. Patch clamp rig, computer, software for data acquisition and analysis.

2.3. Atomic Force Microscopy

1. Cells grown on coated glass chips as described above.
2. Commercially available Si$_3$Ni$_4$ cantilever tips (Digital Instruments, Santa Barbara, CA).
3. Bovine serum albumin (1 mg/mL).
4. Myosin subfragment S1 (Sigma).
5. The cantilever assemblies were mounted on the BioScope (Digital Instruments).
6. HEPES-buffered bath solution: 141 mM NaCl, 2 mM MgCl$_2$, 1 mM EGTA, 0.5 mM CaCl$_2$, 5 mM HEPES, pH 7.4.
7. Glibenclamide stock solution to be diluted into bath solution.
8. Forskolin and 3-isobutyl-1-methylxanthine (IBMX).

3. Methods

3.1. Release Assays

3.1.1. γ-^{32}P ATP Release Assay

1. ATP is loaded into cells grown on collagen at 50% confluence at room temperature using a three-step process
   a. 15-min permeabilization with streptolysin O (1 U/mL) in the buffer solution. The buffer solution should also contain 0.1% BSA and 0.25 m/Ci of γ-^{32}P ATP.
   b. Wash cells vigorously with Ringer's solution three times to remove the streptolysin.
   c. 2-h incubation in Ringer's solution with another 0.25 m/Ci of γ-^{32}P ATP. This allows the cells to recover from the permeabilization and enhances the ATP loading.

2. Release assay:
   a. Before starting the release assay, cells should be washed with Ringer's solution five times.
   b. During the release assay, hexokinase (1–5 U/mL) should be added to the Ringer's solution to yield a Ringer's-plus solution.
   c. The Ringer's-plus solution should be added at time 0 and extracted at time 2.5 min; the procedure should be repeated at time points 5 min, 7.5 min, and 10 min.
   d. The assay should be performed under control conditions and then repeated with cyclic AMP agonists.
   e. The extracted samples are then counted.
   f. 75% of counts complex with glucose as glucose 6-phosphate; 25% of counts are free ^{32}P or labeled phospholipid. This ratio has been established previously through biochemical assay (*see* **Note 1**).

3.1.2. Bioluminescence Assay

The assay needs to be performed in the absence of direct light, there should only be enough light to operate the luminometer and handle the specimens. In addition, all solutions used in this assay need to be sterile. Bacterial contamination can affect the results.

1. Standard curve:
   a. Before starting the release assay, a standard curve must be established in the presence of known amounts of extracellular ATP.
   b. Known concentrations of Mg^{2+}-ATP are diluted in OptiMEM-I medium.
   c. The dishes are placed into the luminometer for study. Luminometer is set at a 40% sensitivity and time points are taken every 30 s (15-s delay period, followed by 15 s of collection).
   d. Luminsecence in arbitrary units are recorded and a standard curve is established.
2. Assay for ATP release:
   a. Before starting, cells should be washed twice with sterile phosphate-buffered saline.
   b. Luciferase-luciferin reagent is diluted 1/20 with either Ringer's solution or OptiMEM-I medium. Then 0.7–1.0 mL of reagent is added to a dish of confluent cells (*see* **Note 2**).
   c. The cells are placed into the luminometer for study. The luminometer is set at 40% sensitivity and time points are taken every 30 s (15-s delay period, followed by 15 s of collection).
   d. Luminsecence in arbitrary units are recorded under basal conditions
   e. Time controls and vehicle controls are performed. The measurement of ATP is the summation of release and degradation. Given that for each cell type there are a number of different release mechanisms and variations in ectoATPases, a time line for each cell type being used should be established.
   f. The assay should be performed under control conditions and then repeated with cyclic AMP agonists (agents include forskolin [10 μM], CPT-cAMP [100–200 μM], 8-Br-cAMP [100–200 μM]).

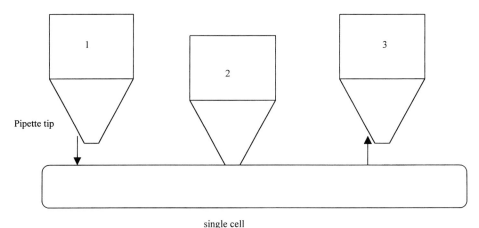

single cell

Fig. 3. Patch clamp technique A schematic of the single-channel patch clamp technique (1) approach a single cell with manufactured microelectrode; (2) touch down onto cell and apply suction to form a high-resistance (gigaohm) seal; (3) quickly retract microelectrode from cell surface to establish an excised inside-out patch.

3.2. Patch Clamp Protocol

Patch clamp technique and pipet manufacturing techniques described by Hamill et al. is followed **Fig. 3** *(27)*. Patch clamp techniques are described in detail in Chapter 4.

1. Cells are visualized with a phase-contrast microscope that is mounted on an air table, and patch pipets are positioned with a micromanipulator.
2. A cell-attached configuration is achieved by having the patch electrode press against the cell membrane of the intact cell, then by applying negative pressure a high-resistance seal, a gigaseal, is formed. When gigaseal formation occurs the pipet is retracted from the cell to obtain excised inside-out patches. The following is a sample protocol that can be followed.
3. Characterization of Cl⁻ currents. The protocol can be started in standard NaCl containing solutions (*see* **Subheading 2.2., item 2**). Excised inside-out patches can be activated with the catalytic subunit of protein kinase A (PKA) (50 nM) and ATP (1 mM). CFTR Cl⁻ channel activity is then assessed and characterized, including single-channel conductance, ATP dependence, anion selectivity, and open probability (*see* **Note 3**).
4. Characterization of ATP currents. The bath solution can then be changed to a chloride-free, Na$_2$ATP bath solution (see **Subheading 2.2., item 4**). Channel activity is then reassessed with regard to single-channel conductance and open probability. In addition, a reversal potential should be determined. If channel activity is present, a current–voltage (I–V) curve should be generated.
5. Inhibition of channel activity: Glibenclamide (100 μM), a blocker of CFTR channel activity, can then be added to the bath to see if there is inhibition of ATP

channel activity. (CFTR generated Cl- currents *[28,29]* and ATP currents *[18,22]* have been shown to be inhibited by glibenclamide.)

6. Reexamination of Cl$^-$ currents: Last, the bath solution is switched back to the standard NaCl-containing solution, and channel activity is reassessed.
7. Data acquisition and analysis. Data are acquired using an integrating patch clamp and data acquisition and analysis system. The following parameters are measured and analyzed: single-channel conductance, mean open and closed times, and opened and closed probability. Current–voltage relationships (I–V curves) are generated, and histograms are constructed by defining one-half of the open-channel current as the threshold.

3.3. Atomic Force Microscopy

Functional tips need to be manufactured and tested before the ATP release assay. For preparation of tips:

1. Commercially available Si_3Ni_4 cantilever tips are initially coated with bovine serum albumin (1 mg/mL) and then with the myosin subfragment S1 by incubation of the 0.06 N/m Si_3Ni_4 tip in a 1 μM S1 solution over 24 h.
2. The cantilever assemblies were mounted on the BioScope, an atomic force microscope, and washed for 5 min by immersion in a HEPES-buffered solution (pH 7.4, room temperature). A thermostatically controlled chamber is used to allow both rapid solution exchange and direct visualization of the cells on an inverted microscope. Functionalized tips are used in a bidirectional scan mode; on the initial pass the cell surface is scanned in contact-mode AFM, allowing a direct topographic display of the cell surface.
3. The subsequent pass of the tip is performed over the same area in "lift mode" to allow detection of ATP in the extracellular microenvironment. The lift mode disengages the tip from the surface and allows direct interactions with the microenvironment rather than with the attractive forces of the cell surface.
4. Test of tip functionalization: 10 μL of an ATP solution (2–200 μM) is added to the chamber (2000 μL vol) and should cause a reproducible detectable deflection of the tip. The functionalized tips should give a dose-dependent response in a concentration range from 10 to 500 nM (*see* **Note 4**).
5. Monolayers of epithelial cells (CF-affected or CF-corrected cells) can be initially scanned with functionalized tips to demonstrate areas of active ATP secretion that will appear as " hot spots" (**Fig. 4**).
6. Following confirmation of "hot spots" along the cell surface, 10^{-4} M glibenclamide *(21)* can be added to the bathing media. The ATP signal is then reassessed. If the signal decreases, this suggests that there is a decrease in ATP release. This might suggest a decreased concentration of extracellular ATP when CFTR activity is inhibited.
7. After the removal of glibenclamide from the bath, cells are exposed to 3-isobutyl-1-methylxanthine (100 μM) and forskolin (10 μM), stimulators of CFTR protein and ATP release. The presence of extracellular ATP should be reassessed.

Cantilever/ bioactive tip

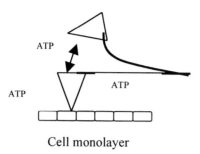

Cell monolayer

Fig. 4. Schematic of the atomic force microscopy biosensor. A functionalized AFM tip will detect ATP releases to the extracellular surface and the tip will deflect as ATP hydrolysis occurs.

4. Notes

1. ^{32}P ATP release assay. When the assay was first developed, a number of experiments were done to determine what percentage of radiolabel was incorporated into glucose 6-phosphate. First samples were mixed with ammonium molybdate and sulfuric acid and then extracted with butanol. The aqueous phase was counted and compared to unextracted samples. After the extraction, 75–80% of counts remained as glucose 6-phosphate. Additional experiments were performed in which samples were loaded onto an anion-exchange resin AG1-X2 (Bio-Rad). The column was then washed (5×) to remove free glucose. Alkaline phosphatase was added to cleave off bound glucose and then ^{32}P was eluted from the column using increasing concentrations of NaCl. This technique yielded simliar results, that is, 75% of ^{32}P was complexed to glucose *(18)*.

2. The choice of regents that you use for bioluminescence is very important. Each manufacturer's reagents are a bit different, so it important to use one brand and work out the controls for the assay. The most reliable results have been obtained using luciferase-lucifrin from Sigma. This reagent should be diluted in either sterile PBS or OptiMEM-I (both solutions are free of endogenous ATP).

3. Patch clamp data are digitalized and stored on videotape. Digitalized data are transferred to computer via an interface (this can be done at the time of acquisition or at a later time). Channel data are viewed on an oscilloscope. Data are analyzed with software such as PClamp (Axon Instruments, Burlingame, CA). Using chloride-free solutions unilaterally can result in the production of significant junction potentials that needed to be factored into all analyses.

4. AFM demonstration of ATP hydrolysis at the surface of a functionalized tip. Previously, Schnieder and colleagues have demonstrated that the deflection signal recorded when scanning with the functionalized tips is due to ATP hydrolysis *(21)*. A series of control studies were conducted using ADP and ATPγS (Sigma), neither of which could cause a cantilever deflection. An additional set of experiments was done with a solution containing 10 n*M* caged ATP, which resulted in no apparent deflection of the tip until exposure to a 100-ms burst of light from a UV light source.

It should be noted that the areas of ATP on the surface do not necessarily appear as single spots but rather as a streaking pattern on the surface of the cells. This is due to the nature of the AFM scan pattern. The tip is not stationary but rather is continuously moving across the surface of the cell in a linear scan pattern. As the tip encounters ATP, hydrolysis occurs and the tip starts to deflect off the surface but continues to move, which appears as a streak.

References

1. Anderson, M. P., Rich, D. P., Gregory, R. J., Smith, A. E., and Welsh, M. J. (1991) Generation of cAMP-activated chloride currents by expression of CFTR. *Science* **251,** 679–682.
2. Bear, C. E., Li, C., Kartner, N., Bridges, R. J., Jensen, T. J., Ramjeesingh, M., and Riordan, J. R. (1992). Purification and functional reconstitution of the cystic fibrosis transmemebrane conductance regulator (CFTR). *Cell* **68,** 809–818.
3. Sheppard, D. N. and Welsh, M. J. (1999). Structure and function of CFTR chloride channel. *Physiol. Rev.* **79,** S23–S45.
4. Schwiebert, E. M., Benos, D. J., Egan, M. E., Stutts, M. J., and Guggino, W. B. (1999) CFTR is a conductance regulator as well as a chloride channel. *Physiol. Rev.* **79,** S145–S166.
5. Stutts, M. J., Canessa, C. M., Olsen, J. C., Hamrick, N., Cohn, J. A., Rossier, B. C., et al. (1995) CFTR as a cAMP-dependent regulator of sodium channels. *Science* **269,** 847–850.
6. Stutts, M. J., Rossier, B. C., and Boucher, R. C. (1997) CFTR inverts PKA-mediated regulation of EnaC single channel kinetics. *J. Biol. Chem.* **272,** 14,037–14,040.
7. Ismailov, I. I., Awayda, M. S., Jovov, B., Berdiev, B. K., Fuller, C. M., Dedman, J. R., et al. (1996) Regulation of EnaC by CFTR. *J. Biol. Chem.* **271,** 4725–4732.
8. Egan, M. E., Flotte, T., Alfone, S., Solow, R., Zeitlin, P. L., Carter, B. J., and Guggino, W. B. (1992) Defective Regulation of outwardly Rectifying Chloride channels by protein kinase A corrected by insertion of CFTR. *Nature* **358,** 581–584.
9. Gabriel, S. E., Clarke, L. L., Boucher, R. C., and Stutts, M. J. (1993) CFTR and outwardly rectifying chloride channels are distinct proteins with a regulatory relationship. *Nature* **363,** 263–268.
10. Jovov, B., Ismailov, I. I., and Benos, D. J. (1995) CFTR is required for protein kinase A activation of an outwardly rectifying anion channel purified from bovine tracheal epithelia. *J. Biol. Chem.* **270,** 1521–1528.
11. Devidas, S. and Guggino, W. B. (1997) The cystic fibrosis transmembrane conductance regulator and ATP. *Curr. Opin. Cell Biol.* **9,** 547–552.
12. Al-Awqati, Q. (1995) Regulation of ion channels by ABC transporters that secrete ATP. *Science* **269,** 805,806
13. Boucher, R. C. (1994) Human airway ion transport. *Am. L. Respir. Crit. Care. Med.* **150,** 581–593.
14. Stutts, M. J., Chinet, T. C., Mason, S. J., Fullton, J. M., Clarke, L. L., and Boucher, R. C. (1992) Regulation of Cl⁻ channels in normal and cystic fibrosis airway epithelial cells by extracellular ATP. *Proc. Natl. Acad. Sci. USA* **89,** 1621–1625
15. Stutts, M. J., Lazarowski, E. R., Paradiso, A. M., and Boucher, R. C. (1995) Activation of CFTR Cl⁻ conductance in polarized T84 cells by luminal extracellular ATP. *Am. J. Physiol.* **268,** C425–C433.

16. Stutts, M. J., Fitz, J. G., Paradiso, A. M., and Boucher, R. C. (1994) Multiple modes of regulation of airway epithelial chloride secretion by extracellular ATP. *Am. J. Physiol.* **267,** C1442–C1451.
17. Higgins, C. F. (1995) The ABC of channel regulation. *Cell* **82,** 693–696.
18. Schwiebert, E. M., Egan, M. E., Hwang, T. H., Fulmer, S. B., Allen, S. A., and Cutting, G. R. (1995) CFTR regulates outwardly rectifying chloride channels through an autocrine mechanism involving ATP. *Cell* **81,** 1063–1073.
19. Abrtaham, E. H., Okunieff, P., Scala, S., Vos, P., Oosterveld, M. J. S., Chan, A. Y., and Shrivastav, B. (1997) CFTR and adenosine triphosphate. *Science* **275,** 1324,1325.
20. Cantiello, H. R. F., Jackson, G. R., Grosman, C. F., .Prat, A. G., Borkan, S. C., Wang, Y., et al. (1998) Electrodiffusional ATP movement through the cystic fibrosis transmembrane conductance regulator. *Am. J. Physiol.* **274,** C799–C809.
21. Schneider, Egan, M. E., Jena, B. P., Guggino, W. B., Oberleithner, H., and Geibel, J. P. (1999) Continuous detection of extracellular ATP on living cells by atomic force microscopy. *Proc. Natl. Acad. Sci. USA* **96,** 12,180–12,185.
22. Sugita, M., Yun, Y., and Forskett, J. K. (1998) CFTR Cl- Channel and CFTR-associated ATP channel: distinct pores regulated by common gates. *EMBO J.* **17,** 898–908.
23. Grygorczyk, R. and Hanrahan, J. W. (1997) CFTR-independent ATP release from epithelial cells triggered by mechanical stimuli. *Am. J. Physiol.* **272,** C1058–C1066.
24. Grygorczyk, R., Tabcharani, J. A. and Hanrahan, J. W. (1996) CFTR channels expressed in CHO cells do not have detectable ATP conductance. *J. Membrane Biol.* **151,** 139–148.
25. Reddy, M. M., Quinton, P. M., Haws, C., Wine, J. J., Grygorczyk, R., Tabcharini, J. A., et al. (1996) Failure of the CFTR to conduct ATP. *Science* **271,** 1876–1879.
26. Taylor, A. L., Kudlow, B. A., Marrs, K. L., Gruenert, D. C., Guggino, W. B., and Schwiebert, E. M. (1998) Bioluminescence detection of ATP release mechanisms in epithelia. *Am. J. Physiol.* **275,** C1391–C1406.
27. Hamill, O. P., Marty, A., Neher, E., Sakmann, B., and Sigworth, F. J.(1981) Improved patch clamp techniques for high resolution current recording from cells and cell free membrane patches, *Pflugers Arch* **391,** 85–100.
28. Sheppard, D. N. and Welsh, M. J. (1992) Effect of ATP-sensitive K$^+$channel regulators on cystic fibrosis transmembrane conductance regulator chloride channels. *J. Gen. Physiol.* **100,** 573–591.
29. Schultz, B. D., DeRoos, A. D., Venglarik, C. J., Singh, A. K., Frizzell, R. A., and Bridges, R. J. (1996) Glibenclamide blockade of CFTR chloride channels. *Am. J. Physiol.* **271,** L192–L200.

III

PATHOPHYSIOLOGY OF CYSTIC FIBROSIS

27

Inflammatory Mediators in CF Patients

Jay B. Hilliard, Michael W. Konstan, and Pamela B. Davis

1. Introduction

Patients with cystic fibrosis (CF) succumb to airway infection and inflammation, and determining the extent and nature of the infecting agents, as well as the extent and nature of the inflammatory response, is critical to understanding the pathophysiology of the disease and how to intervene *(1,2)*. However, for many years this aspect of the disease was glossed over, because the "usual" indicators of infection and inflammation (e.g., leukocyte count, acute-phase reactants, cultures, even cytokine levels), measured in the blood, were unimpressive in CF patients, and correlated poorly with clinical status. Even more detailed investigations into the function of circulating cells of host defense, such as neutrophils, lymphocytes, or monocytes, were not revealing. However, evaluation of infection and inflammation at the infected and inflamed site, that is, in the airways, has proven to be considerably more informative. For example, Berger and colleagues determined that circulating neutrophils from patients with CF behaved normally and could be activated by *Pseudomonas* and ingest and kill the bacteria in the presence of complement, but neutrophils recovered from bronchoalveolar lavage fluid from CF patients often failed to do so *(3)*. He went on to show that, because of the high levels of uninhibited elastase in the airways of patients with CF, either the complement receptors or the complement opsonins were cleaved into nonfunctional states *(4)*. Therefore, once neutrophils arrive at the site of inflammation in the CF lung, they are altered by that environment, to the detriment of the host defense. Thus, sampling the relevant site by bronchoalveolar lavage (BAL) gives useful information not obtainable in other ways. Although expectorated sputum has been used as a noninvasive way of sampling the airway, BAL is considered to yield the most accurate measure of the inflammatory process in the CF airway *(5)*. Therefore, this chapter focuses on the use of BAL in CF research.

From: *Methods in Molecular Medicine, vol. 70: Cystic Fibrosis Methods and Protocols*
Edited by: W. R. Skach © Humana Press Inc., Totowa, NJ

A number of research groups have utilized BAL to study CF lung disease during the last decade. Included are studies that reveal the large extent of infection and inflammation in the CF airway, even in the earliest stages of the disease *(6–12)*, as well as serial lavage studies (sampling the airways of the same patient over time) before and after an anti-infective or anti-inflammatory intervention *(13–15)*. With many new anti-inflammatory and other treatments being proposed for CF lung disease, it is imperative to have a safe and standardized way of sampling the milieu in the lower airways. More recently, the central role of the epithelium in orchestrating the inflammatory response has also become clear, and sampling of epithelial cells in the airway has also become useful in describing the inflammatory state of the patient *(16–18)*. Our center has devised a standardized method of bronchoalveolar lavage (and subsequent processing of the fluid obtained) and epithelial brushing that has provided useful information both for research and for clinical purposes *(3,4,6,16,17,18–24)*. It is particularly important to process and store the fluid in such a way that many different measures can be obtained simultaneously, or so that the fluid can be used at a later time for additional determinations, since the patient has been subjected to an invasive procedure and the maximum information should be extracted from it. When patients are in periods of clinical stability, the procedures described herein give reproducible findings from week to week or month to month. When patients have been treated or have become ill in the interval, values move in the expected directions.

Measurement of markers of inflammation in BAL fluid may be informative, therefore, both for clinical purposes and for research. A variety of markers have been studied, but none in a comprehensive, longitudinal manner so as to validate them as a "gold standard" for assessing the inflammatory response. Markers that may be considered, depending on the clinical or research goal, include total and differential cell counts, elastase and its complexes with inhibitors, pro- and anti-inflammatory cytokine levels, levels of eicosanoids, and the inflammatory state of epithelial cells recovered from the airways. Bacterial counts may also be assessed. In addition, complement fragments and protein markers of transudation, such as albumin, may also be measured. This chapter concentrates on the recovery of BAL fluid and the measurement of total and differential cell counts, active elastase, α_1-antitrypsin, elastase-α_1-antrypsin complexes, cytokines, and eicosanoid mediators. We selected these parameters because measurements of total and differential cell counts and interleukin-8 (IL-8) are commonly used as markers of inflammation in research papers, protease–antiprotease balance may be an important indicator of ongoing lung destruction, and new attention is being paid to lipid mediators with the advancement of the "DHA hypothesis" *(25)*. However, it should be noted that the processing and storage of the lavage fluid that is recommended here may be useful for other lipid mediators (methanol extraction), proteins (storage of cell-free supernatants containing protease inhibitors), and enzymatic activities (storage of cell-free supernatants without protease inhibitors), as well as recovery of cells such as macrophages for culture, neutrophils and lymphocytes for acute studies, and epithelial cells for acute studies or for culture. The processing and storage conditions for each additional assay, however, should be validated separately.

Bronchoalveolar lavage is performed by literally "washing out" the airways and alveoli by instillation and retrieval of saline solution. Since the surface area of the alveoli is much greater than that of the airways, this process results in sampling largely alveolar surface fluid, though by varying the volume of saline instilled, one can change the bronchial and alveolar proportions (larger volumes and more aliquots tend to favor alveolar sampling). Our method of BAL for studies of CF lung disease is designed to preferentially sample the bronchial space. Moreover, the washing process dilutes the epithelial lining fluid (ELF) some 50–100 times. To adjust for this dilution, which can vary from procedure to procedure, a number of methods have been proposed, none of which is ideal. However, we have chosen the urea dilution method to adjust for the dilution *(26)*. Urea is considered to be freely diffusible, and therefore should be at the same concentration in ELF and serum. Measuring urea in serum and BAL fluid simultaneously, therefore, gives a measure of BAL fluid dilution of ELF, provided the dwell time is brief.

The procedure described here has had an excellent track record of safety. More than 300 research procedures have been performed in more than 130 CF patients over a 10-yr period using this procedure. Subjects have ranged from several months to over 40 years of age, with a broad range of disease severity (FEV_1 range from 20% to over 100% of the predicted value). Serial BAL studies are generally limited to subjects with $FEV_1 > 40\%$ predicted, because it is more difficult to get a reproducible BAL in those with more severe lung disease. This same procedure has been used in more than 150 healthy adult volunteers. Despite the fact that the airways of patients with CF are usually infected, the postprocedure incidence of low-grade, self-limiting fever is about 10%, and hypoxia requiring O_2, <2%. There have been no major intraoperative or postprocedural complications. However, this excellent safety record depends not only on scrupulous adherence to the clinical protocol, but also on the skill and judgment of the operator and the assistants. Procedures should not be continued if there is distress on the part of the subject, including, but not limited to, inadequate anesthesia of the airways, oxygen desaturation, tachycardia or tachypnea, or excessive cough.

2. Materials

2.1. Bronchoalveolar Lavage

1. Flexible, fiber-optic bronchoscope with light source, video processor, and video-taping capability.

    a. 4.7–5.0 mm outside diameter (od) for patients ≥ 35 kg (approx 12 yr of age)

    b. 3.5 mm od for patients <35 kg.

2. Sedation medications:

    a. Fentanyl (50 µg/5mL, 100 µg max).

    b. Midazolam (1 mg/mL, 5 mg max).

3. Epinephrine nasal solution (1 mg/mL, 0.5 mg).

4. Topical anesthetics:

    a. Lidocaine HCl, 4% (40 mg/mL) solution. (for aerosol use).

    b. Lidocaine HCl, 2% (20 mg/mL) solution. Prepare 30 mL of 2% solution by diluting 15 mL of the 4% solution with 15 mL of sterile saline (0.9%). Place the 2% solution into 10-cm^3 sterile, disposable syringes (×3).

    c. Lidocaine HCl, 2% jelly.

5. 0.9% NaCl (preservative free), 250-mL bag x1

6. Three-way stopcocks, ×2.

7. 30-cc lure-tip syringes, ×2.

8. 150-cc valveless Buretrol/Add on set (Baxter, #2C7503), ×1.

9. Basic solution/injection tubing set (Baxter, #2C54175), ×1.

10. Aerosol nebulizer.

11. Electrocardiogram (ECG) monitor.

12. Blood pressure monitor.

13. Pulse oximeter.

2.2. Processing Bronchoalveolar Lavage Fluid

1. Methanol (HPLC grade), 40 mL in a glass jar.

2. Phenylmethylsulfonylfluoride (PMSF), 100 mM in isopropanol (HPLC grade).

3. Ethylenediaminetetraacetic acid (EDTA), 200 mM in Hank's balanced salt solution (without Ca^{2+} and Mg^{2+}), pH 8.0.

4. Sterile saline (0.9%), 5 mL.

5. Bactericidal detergent.

6. Ice bucket and ice.

7. Graduated cylinder, polypropylene; 100 cc.

8. Jar, polypropylene, screw-cap; 4 oz.

9. Tube, silanized glass, screw-cap, round-bottom, 50 cc.

10. Polypropylene screw-cap microtubes (2 cc) and centrifuge tubes (50 cc).

11. Polycarbonate centrifuge tubes, round-bottom, 50 cc.

12. Curity gauze sponges, 3in. × 3 in., 12 ply, sterile, (Kendall Healthcare Products, #1903).

13. Gauze pads, sterile, 4 in. × 4 in.

14. Syringes, disposable plastic: 3 cc, 10 cc, and 30 cc.

15. Syringe tip filters, cellulose acetate, 0.22-µm pore size.

Note: Elastase, some cytokines and some eicosanoids adhere to untreated glass. If glassware is substituted for the recommended plastic ware (polypropylene), it must be silanized and autoclaved prior to use.

2.3. Total and Differential Cell Counts

1. Dulbecco's phosphate-buffered saline (D-PBS, 1×, without Ca^{2+} or Mg^{2+}).

2. Bovine serum albumin (BSA) fraction V, 1% in D-PBS: Dissolve BSA, 1 g in D-PBS to a final volume of 100 mL. Prepare fresh as needed. Can be stored frozen (–80°C) in 1–3-mL aliquots for up to 6 mo.

3. Turk's solution: 10 mg crystal violet + 3 mL glacial acetic acid; QS to 100 mL with distilled/deionized water.

4. Trypan blue solution: 0.4% : 400 mg trypan blue + 3 mL glacial acetic acid; QS to 100 mL with sterile saline (0.9% NaCl).

5. Hema 3 Stain Kit (Fisher Scientific, #22-122911).

6. Permount mounting medium.

7. Hematocytometer, Bright Line with improved Neubauer ruling.

8. Cytospin centrifuge (model II or III, Shandon Corporation, Sewickley, PA).

9. Microscope slides, $25 \times 75 \times 1$ mm, frosted.

10. Coplin staining jars.

11. Cover slips, 18×18 mm.

2.4. Measurement of Neutrophil Elastase Activity and Elastase Inhibitory Capacity

1. Dulbecco's phosphate-buffered saline (D-PBS, 1×).

2. BSA, 0.1% in D-PBS: Dissolve BSA (fraction V), 100 mg in D-PBS to a final volume of 100 mL. Prepare fresh as needed.

3. Tris-NaCl substrate solution: Mix 0.2 M Tris and 1 M NaCl in 1 L of deionized/distilled water. Adjust pH to 7.5. Sterile filter and store at 4°C for up to 6 mo.

4. Substrate solution: Dissolve Me-Suc-Al-Al-Pro-Val-pNa (Sigma Chemical, St. Louis, MO, #M 4765), 4.0 mM in 1% 1-methyl-2-pyrrolidinone (Sigma, # M 6762)/Tris-NaCl substrate solution (see above). Dissolve the peptide substrate in the organic solvent prior to adding the Tris-NaCl substrate buffer. Warm the final solution to 25°C. The volume of this solution is dependent on the anticipated number of analyses (standards + samples; 100 µL/well; e.g., 23.6 mg substrate + 100 µL organic solvent + 9.9 mL Tris-NaCl buffer). This solution is stable for up to 3 d when stored in the dark at 4°C.

5. Tris-NaCl Solution: 30 mM Tris and 85 mM NaCl in 100 mL of deionized/distilled water. Adjust pH to 8.0. Sterile filter and store at 4°C for up to 6 mo.

6. Standard purified human sputum elastase stock solution: Dissolve 2 mg of human sputum elastase (Elastin Products, Owensville, MO, # SE563) in 2 mL of Tris-NaCl elastase solution (see above). Store 50-µL aliquots in polypropylene microcentrifuge tubes at –80°C. Frozen aliquots are stable for up to 6 mo.

7. For measurement of the elastase inhibitory capacity of BAL fluid: Standard α_1-antitrypsin (α_1-AT) stock solution (purified human α_1-AT, Calbiochem Biochemicals, San Diego, CA, # 178251); Dissolve α_1-AT, 5 mg in 1 mL of Tris-NaCl standard solution. Store 50-µL aliquots at –80°C for up to 6 mo.

8. Microtiter plates: Ultra low binding 96-well plates (Fisher Scientific, Costar, # 2501).

9. 96-Well plate reader: ThermoMax microplate reader with Softmax software (Molecular Devices, Sunnyvale, CA).

2.5. Measurement of α_1-Antitrypsin and Elastase/α_1-Antitrypsin Complex

1. Dulbecco's phosphate-buffered saline (D-PBS, 1×).
2. BSA, 1.0% in D-PBS: Dissolve BSA (fraction V), 10 g in D-PBS to a final volume of 1 L. Store at 4°C for up to 1 wk.
3. BSA, 0.1% in D-PBS: Dilute the 1.0% solution (see above) in D-PBS. Store at 4°C for up to 1 wk.
4. Substrate buffer: Dissolve 0.05 mM NaCO$_3$ and 1 mM MgCl$_2$ in distilled/deionized water to a total volume of 500 mL. Adjust pH to 9.8 if necessary and sterile filter. Store at room temperature for up to 3 mo.
5. Standard buffer: Dissolve 30 mM Tris-HCl and 85 mM NaCl in distilled/deionized water to a total volume of 100 mL. Adjust pH to 8.0 if necessary and sterile filter. Store at room temperature for up to 3 mo.
6. First antibody (capture antibody): Goat anti-human α_1-AT (IgG fraction) (DiaSorin, Stillwater, MN, # 81902). Assay concentration: 5 µg/mL in D-PBS.
7. Second antibody (α-AT assay only): Rabbit antihuman α_1-AT (IgG fraction) (Boehringer Mannheim Biochemical, Indianapolis, IN, # 605-002). Assay concentration: 0.05 µg/mL in 1% BSA/D-PBS.
8. Second antibody (elastase/ α_1-AT complex assay only): Rabbit anti-human elastase (AHEAb); 250 µg/vial (reconstitute with 1 mL of PBS) (Elastin Products, Owensville, MO, # SP 73) Assay concentration: 0.5 µg/mL in 1% BSA/D-PBS.
9. Third antibody: Goat anti-rabbit IgG/alkaline phosphatase conjugate (Boehringer Mannheim Biochemicals, Indianapolis, IN, # 1-814-206). Assay concentration: Use diluted 1/6000 in 1% BSA/D-PBS.
10. Substrate solution: Sigma 104 phosphatase substrate tablets (*p*-nitrophenyl phosphate, disodium, hexahydrate) (Sigma , # 104-105). Assay concentration: 1 mg/mL in substrate buffer. Prepare solution within 15 min of actual use (*see* **Subheading 3.5., step 11**).
11. α_1-AT stock solution (α_1-AT assay only): Dissolve human α_1-AT (Calbiochem Biochemicals, San Diego, CA, # 178251), 5 mg in 1 mL of standard buffer. Split into 500µL aliquots in polypropylene tubes. Stable for up to 6 months at –80°C. Use to prepare standard solutions for the α_1-AT assay.
12. Elastase/α_1-AT stock solution (elastase/α_1-AT complex assay only): 0.5 mg human sputum elastase (Elastin Products, # SE 563) and 0.82 mg human α_1-AT (Calbiochem Biochemicals, San Diego, CA, # 178251) are dissolved in 2 mL of standard buffer. Elastase forms equal molar complexes with α_1-AT, inactivating the elastase activity *(27)*. Incubate for 30 min at 37°·C. Add an additional 2 mL of standard solution. Add 1 mL of 1% BSA/D-PBS solution for a final elastase equivalent concentration of 100 µg/mL. Split into 50-µL aliquots in polypropylene tubes. Stable for up to 6 mo at –80°C. Use to prepare standard solutions for the elastase/α_1-AT complex assay.
13. Microtiter plates: Nunc Immuno Plate II (Thomas Scientific, Swedesboro, NJ, # 6106-L35).
14. 96-well plate reader: ThermoMax microplate reader with Softmax software (Molecular Devices, Sunnyvale, CA).

2.6. Measurement of Interleukin-8

1. Quantikine Human Interleukin-8 (IL-8) Kit (R&D Systems, Minneapolis, MN, # D8050). Store unopened kits at 2–8°C (up to expiration date). The following components of the kit are stable once opened/reconstituted for up to 1 mo at 2–8°C.

   a. IL-8 microtiter plate: 96-well polystyrene microtiter plate (in strips), coated with murine monoclonal antibody against human IL-8.

   b. IL-8 conjugate: 11.5 mL of polyclonal antibody against IL-8 conjugated to horseradish peroxidase.

   c. IL-8 standard: recombinant human IL-8, 10 ng in a buffered protein base (lyophilized). Reconstitute the IL-8 standard with 5 mL of calibrator diluent RD5P (1×). Allow the vial to sit with gentle agitation for 15 min. Pipet 500 μL of calibrator diluent RD5P (1×) into each of six polypropylene tubes. Prepare serial dilutions of the IL-8 standard by adding 500 μL of standard to the first tube, mixing, then transferring 500 μL to the second tube, and so on. The concentrations of IL-8 in the tubes will range from 1000 to 31.2 ng/mL.

   d. Assay diluent RD1-8: buffered protein base solution, 11 mL.

   e. Calibrator diluent RD5P (5×): buffered protein base solution, 21 mL. To prepare the calibrator diluent RD5P (1×) solution, add 2 mL of calibrator diluent RD5P (5×) to 8 mL of distilled/deionized water.

   f. Wash buffer concentrate (25×): concentrated solution of buffered surfactant. To prepare the wash buffer solution (1×), add 21 mL of wash buffer concentrate (25×) to 504 mL of distilled/deionized water.

   g. Color reagent A: stabilized hydrogen peroxide, 12.5 mL.

   h. Color reagent B: stabilized Chromogen (tetramethyl benzidine), 12.5 mL.

   i. Stop solution: 2 N sulfuric acid, 6 mL.

   j. Plate covers; adhesive strips, ×4.

2. 96-well plate reader: ThermoMax microplate reader with Softmax software (Molecular Devices, Sunnyvale, CA).

2.7. Measurement of Leukotriene B$_4$

1. Leukotriene B$_4$ (LTB$_4$) Enzyme Immunoassay (EIA) Kit (Cayman Chemicals, Ann Arbor, MI, # 520111). Store unopened kits at –80°C (up to expiration date).

   a. LTB$_4$ microtiter plate: 96-well polystyrene microtiter plate (in strips), coated with murine monoclonal antibody against rabbit anti-human LTB$_4$.

   b. EIA buffer concentrate (vial #4): To prepare EIA buffer (1×), dilute the contents of 1 vial with 90 mL of deionized/distilled water. Store at 4°C.

   c. Tween-20 (vial #5a)

   d. Wash buffer concentrate (vial #5): To prepare wash buffer (1×), dilute the contents of 1 vial to a total volume of 2 L with deionized/distilled water. Add 1 mL of Tween-20 (vial #5a). Store at 4°C.

   e. LTB$_4$ standard (vial #3): Reconstitute 1 vial with 900 μL of deionized/distilled water (5 ng/mL LTB$_4$). Store at 4°C for up to 2 wk. To prepare the LTB$_4$ assay standards, obtain 8 polypropylene tubes. Pipet 500 μL of EIA buffer (1×) into 7 of the tubes (#2–8). Add 900 μL of EIA buffer (1×) to the first tube. Add 100 μL of the 5-ng/mL solution to the first tube and mix well. This is a 500 pg/mL solution. Prepare serial dilutions of the 500-pg/mL solution by transferring 500 µL from the first tube to the second tube, and so on, mixing well before each transfer. The concentrations of LTB_4 in the tubes will range from 500 to 3.9 pg/mL. These diluted standard solutions are stable for up to 24 h at 4°C.

    f. LTB_4 acetylcholinesterase tracer (vial #2): Reconstitute one vial with 6 mL of EIA buffer (1×). Store at 4°C for up to 2 wk.

    g. LTB_4 antiserum (vial #1): Reconstitute 1 vial with 6 mL of EIA buffer (1×). Store at 4°C for up to 4 wk.

    h. Ellman's reagent (vial #8): Reconstitute 1 vial with 20 mL of deionized/distilled water. Protect from light and use the day of preparation. It is best to prepare this solution immediately before use.

2. 96-well plate reader: ThermoMax microplate reader (Molecular Devices, Sunnyvale, CA).

2.8. Measurement of Urea Nitrogen in Serum and BAL Fluid for Estimating the Volume of Epithelial Lining Fluid

1. Infinity blood urea nitrogen (BUN) reagent (kinetic) (Sigma, # 64-20). Reconstitute with 10 mL of deionized/distilled water per vial and store at room temperature (20–25°C) during use. Store unused reagent solution at 2–6°C for up to 3 wk.

2. Reconstituted reagent contains the following concentrations of active ingredients: 2-oxoglutarate (16 mM), reduced nicotinamide adenine dinucleotide (NADH, 0.5 mM), urease, jackbean (100,000 U/L), glutamate dehydrogenase, bovine liver (3000 U/L), buffer (pH 8.0 ± 0.1), and stabilizers and fillers

3. Urea standard (100 mg/dL) (Sigma, #16-800).

4. Accutrol glucose/urea standard (Sigma , #A2034).

5. Microtiter plates: ultra-low-binding 96-well plates (Fisher Scientific, Costar, # 2501).

6. ThermoMax microplate reader with Softmax software (Molecular Devices, Sunnyvale, CA)

3. Methods

3.1. Bronchoalveolar Lavage

Safety precautions: The procedure requires four staff in addition to the research subject—the operator (a physician experienced in flexible fiber-optic bronchoscopy), a nurse or respiratory therapist whose sole responsibility is to monitor the subject, a technician to assist the operator with the bronchoscopy and BAL, and a research assistant to help with the collection and processing of the fluid. Subjects are kept without eating or drinking (NPO) for ≥8 h before the procedure (to prevent aspiration), and monitored for heart rate, blood pressure, and oxygen saturation by continuous pulse oximetry during the entire procedure. At any time the subject's safety is believed to be compromised or at risk, the full attention of the physician is directed to the subject and the procedure is terminated if necessary. In order to avoid overdosing with sedatives and anesthetics (including lidocaine), the total permissible dose for the subject's size is calculated in advance of the procedure. The total amount of lidocaine administered (not including the aerosol) should not exceed 7 mg/kg. Guidelines for the sedation medications are given below. Only the maximum amount of these medications is made readily available to the personnel responsible for their administration. Other safety measures are adhered to in accordance with current practice guidelines *(28,29)*.

3.1.1. Pre-Bronchoscopy Setup Procedure

1. Attach one bag of 0.9% NaCl, 250 mL (preservative free), to a Buretrol with extension tubing. Prime the extension tubing. Refill the Buretrol to 50 mL. Add a stopcock to the extension tubing.
2. Attach one 10-cc syringe of 2% lidocaine and an empty 10-cc syringe to a three-way stopcock. Transfer 2 mL of 2% lidocaine into the empty syringe, remove from stopcock, and fill with 8 mL of air. This process will be repeated several times as the contents of this syringe is used to anesthetize the glottis, trachea and lower airways.
3. On a sterile drape, set up the bronchoscope along with lidocaine jelly, 0.5 mL nasal epinephrine solution, one 10-cc syringe of 2% lidocaine, and two 30-cc empty syringes.

3.1.2. Bronchoalveolar Lavage Procedure

1. Attach ECG, blood pressure, and pulse oximeter monitors to the subject.
2. Administer 4% lidocaine (3 mL) by aerosol (this step may need to be forgone in some young children if they react adversely to the taste of this medication).
3. Place the subject in the supine position with a rolled blanket placed underneath the shoulders.
4. Administer sedation intravenously; fentanyl (in 0.5- to 1.0-µg/kg aliquots, max 3 µg/kg not to exceed 100 µg), and midazolam (in 0.025- to 0.05-mg/kg aliquots, max 0.1 mg/kg, not to exceed 5 mg). Note: healthy adult volunteers do not require sedation.
5. Prepare the nasal passages by dripping the nasal epinephrine solution (not to exceed 0.5 mL) onto the nasal mucosa, followed by 2% lidocaine (1–2 mL).
6. Apply 2% lidocaine jelly to the bronchoscope as a lubricant, and insert the bronchoscope into the nose. If the passageway is too tight, more lidocaine jelly can be applied to the bronchoscope as well as around the nares using Q-tips for application. (Rarely is the oral route via a bite block required).
7. When the larynx is in view, gently instill 2 mL of 2% lidocaine (followed by 8 mL of air) through the bronchoscope onto the glottic structures. Repeat to ensure adequate anesthesia to the glottis. Advance the bronchoscope into the trachea, and instill another 2 mL of 2% lidocaine.
8. Guide the bronchoscope through the left mainstem bronchus, administering 2 mL of 2% lidocaine along the way; and then guide the bronchoscope to the lingula, and administer another 2 mL of 2% lidocaine. Lightly wedge the tip of the bronchoscope into the inferior or superior segment of the lingula. (Note: if possible, avoid all suctioning before the BAL).

9. Attach the stopcock from the Buretrol to the bronchoscope and allow 50 mL of saline to infuse by gravity into the airway. Refill the Buretrol to 30 mL.

10. Attach a 30-cc syringe to the stopcock and gently draw the BAL fluid into the syringe, reducing the suction if airway collapse is observed. Change the syringe and infuse the 30-mL aliquot of saline. Again, draw BAL fluid into the second 30-cc syringe.

11. Attach the suction catheter to the bronchoscope and remove excess fluid. Withdraw the bronchoscope from the subject, or continue with the procedure for clinical purposes as required (*see* **Notes 1** and **2**).

3.2. Processing of BAL Fluid

3.2.1. Pre-Bronchoscopy Setup Procedure

1. Preparation of plastic ware. All plastic ware must be prepared at least 1 d before the bronchoscopy. Bulk-processing enough plastic ware for several procedures is recommended.
   a. Soak all plastic ware overnight in bactericidal detergent. Rinse 3× in distilled, deionized water and air dry.
   b. Autoclave or gas-sterilize all plastic ware that will contact the BAL specimen (not necessary for disposable, presterilized plastic ware).

2. Setup bronchoscopy suite immediately before the bronchoscopy:
   a. Place the graduated cylinder, 4-oz jar, glass 50-cc centrifuge tube, and the jar containing methanol (40 mL) in the ice bucket.
   b. On a sterile field using sterile technique, place one sterile 3-in. × 3-in. Curity brand gauze sponge on top of a sterile 4-in. × 4-in. gauze pad, leaving both inside the 4 in. × 4 in. packaging. Saturate the gauze sponge with 5 mL of sterile saline, using a 10-cc syringe. Re-close the packaging to retain sterility.

3.2.2. BAL Fluid Processing

The following method for processing BAL fluid is summarized in **Fig. 1**.

1. Immediately before receiving BAL fluid, remove the gauze sponge from the packaging and place it over the opening of the graduated cylinder.
   a. The sponge consists of three layers of gauze. Peel back the top layer and press the remaining two layers together approx 1 cm into the cylinder opening to form a reservoir for the BAL fluid during filtration. The top layer is used to cover the reservoir before filtering.

2. BAL fluid is received in 30-cc plastic syringes. Record the volume of fluid infused and the total return volume.
   a. Filter the fluid in each syringe through the gauze into the graduated cylinder. Once all the fluid is filtered, gently squeeze the gauze, being careful not to force any mucous plugs into the filtrate.
   b. Record the volume of the total filtrate.

3. Pour the BAL filtrate into the sterile 4-oz jar, from which all subsequent test aliquots are removed. Each aliquot is removed using a sterile syringe.

CF BAL Research Study

Procedure Date: __ __ / __ __ / __ __

Procedure #: __ __ __
Patient Name: _____
Hospital #: _____
DOB: __ __ / __ __ / __ __
Has the subject fasted for at least ___ hours prior to the procedure? ☐ Yes ☐ No
        If No; Reason _____

Instrument: _____
Operator(s): _____
Access route: ☐ oral or ☐ nasal (Left / Right)

Subject
Weight: __ __ __ . __ __ kg or lbs (circle)

4% Lidocaine aerosol: ☐ Yes: ___ cc
                      ☐ No

Topical Lidocaine: _____

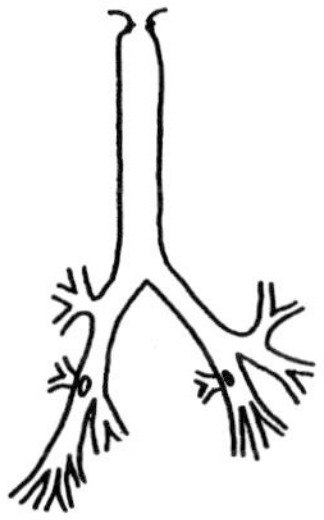

Sedation: _____
          _____

Other drugs: _____

Normal Saline Lavage

	Saline IN	BAL OUT		Saline IN	BAL OUT
1*	___ cc	___ cc		___ cc	___ cc
2	___ cc	___ cc		___ cc	___ cc
3	___ cc	___ cc		___ cc	___ cc
Ttl	___ cc	___ cc	Ttl	___ cc	___ cc
	(primary segment)			(alternate segment)	

* Saline instillation number

Segment location:
_____ | _____
(primary segment) | (alternate segment)

BAL time (24 hr clock):
Start __ __ : __ __   Start __ __ : __ __
Stop: __ __ : __ __   Stop __ __ : __ __
    (primary segment)   (alternate segment)

Post-gauze filtration volume:
    __ __ ml | __ __ ml
(primary segment) | (alternate segment)

Operator(s)
signature: _____ , M.D.

AREA

Findings:
Anatomy:

Secretions:

Mucosa:

Complications:

Comments:

Specimens:

Documentation:

Fig. 1. Standardized method for processing BAL fluid from CF research procedures.

a. Quantitative bacteriology (1 mL in 3-cc syringe).
b. Bacterial culture and sensitivity (1 mL in 3-cc syringe).
c. Total cell count and differential (1 mL in 3-cc syringe).
d. Urea sample (1–3 mL in 3-cc syringe). Filter through a 0.22-μm syringe tip filter into a 2-cc polypropylene tube. Add PMSF, 1 μL/1 mL of sample, and EDTA, 25 μL/1 mL of sample (final concentrations of 100 μM and 5 mM, respectively). Store the sample at –80°C until analysis.
e. Aliquot for assay of lipid mediators: Cyclooxygenase and lipoxygenase pathway metabolite profiles (3–10 mL in 10-cc syringe). Record the exact sample volume. Add methanol (0–4°C) to the filtrate aliquot in the 50-cc, round-bottom, silanized glass centrifuge tube (final methanol concentration, 80% by volume).

- Centrifuge the tube at 300g for 20 min. Discard the pellet.
- Evaporate the supernatant to dryness in a Speed-Vac evaporating system at 0.7 torr vacuum.
- Suspend the residue in 0.5 mL methanol/deionized water (1/1). Transfer the suspension to a 2-cc polypropylene tube and store at –80°C until analysis.

f. Aliquots for cell studies and nonlipid mediators: Suction the total remaining filtrate volume into a 30-cc syringe(s). Record the total volume in the syringe(s).

- Pellet the cells in a 50-cc polypropylene centrifuge tube(s) at 250g for 10 min. Immediately process the cell pellet for leukocyte receptor analysis (*3,4*).
- Further centrifuge the supernatant at 40,000g for 20 min in round-bottom polycarbonate tubes to pellet large cellular debris. Discard the debris and filter the supernatant through a 0.22-µm filter unit. Divide the filtrate into two aliquots. Add PMSF, 1 µL/1 mL of sample and EDTA, 25 µL/1 mL of sample (final concentrations of 100 µM and 5mM, respectively) to one of the aliquots. Further divide both treated and untreated samples into 0.2- to 1-mL aliquots (determined by assay volume requirements) in 2-cc polypropylene tubes. Store all samples at –80°C until analysis.

3.2.3. Deviations from the Standard Protocol

1. Multiple-segment lavages and returns from segments with inadequate volumes:
   a. If plans call for multiple lung segments to be lavaged, prepare additional sets of plastic ware (including filtering gauze). A separate set of plastic ware is required for each segmental BAL fluid, since often the values from different areas of the lung are not the same. Other allocations of BAL fluid may be made at the discretion of the bronchoscopist. In general, a second set of plastic ware should be available in the event a second lavage is required.
   - Additional syringes and processing vessels (e.g., centrifuge tubes) will be needed for removing aliquots from additional BAL samples.
   - The bronchoscopist will determine if aliquots will be removed from secondary segment filtrates for clinical processing. This also applies to primary BAL samples that have inadequate returns (<20% of the instilled saline volume). Minimum aliquot volumes required for each clinical test may be less than those noted here and should be determined at each testing facility.
2. BAL fluid containing obvious blood contamination:
   a. BAL fluid grossly contaminated with blood is unacceptable for further processing.
   b. Interference from occult blood in the clinical assays is nominal and may be ignored.

3.3. Total and Differential Cell Counts

3.3.1. Total Cell Count

1. Load both sides of the hemocytometer with cell suspension. Allow the cells to settle onto the hemocytometer (1–2 min). Count all intact cells within the four major corners of the hemocytometer (each corner measures 1 mm^2). Do not count cells that lie on the top or left boundary line of each square.

a. If the cells are difficult to visualize, mix equal volumes (50 μL) of cell suspension and staining solution (either Turk's or Trypan blue) and recount. Apply an additional dilution factor (ADF) of 2 (below).
b. If the cells are too numerous to count, dilute an aliquot with D-PBS and recount. Correct for this dilution when calculating the total number of cells per milliliter (ADF).
c. Calculate the total number of cells per milliliter:

$$\text{Cells/mL} = (\text{sum of cells from 4 corners})/4 \times 10{,}000 \times \text{ADF}$$

Explanation of equation:
a. sum/4 calculates the average number of cells per corner. The volume of each corner is $1 \times 1 \times 0.1 \text{ mm} = 0.1 \text{ mm}^3 = 0.1 \text{ μL}$.
b. The factor of 10,000 corrects the counts from cells/0.1 μL to cells/1 mL.
c. Additional dilution factors (ADF) must be applied if additional dilutions made, including the use of Turk's or Trypan blue solution.
2. Repeat **step 3** for the other side of the hemocytometer.
3. If the results from the two sides of the hemocytometer are not within 10% of each other, repeat **steps 2** and **3** with a new sample aliquot. Average the results from both sides of the hemocytometer.

3.3.2. Differential Cell Counts

1. Using the concentration of cells determined above, dilute an aliquot of the cells in 1% BSA/D-PBS solution to a final concentration of $1.0–1.6 \times 10^5$ cells/mL (at least 2 mL). If the BAL fluid cell concentration is below 1.0×10^5, do not dilute the sample. Prepare four slides by adding 250 μL of cell suspension to each cytofunnel/slide/cytoclip assembly (see Shandon Cytospin operator's manual for detailed instructions.) If the BAL fluid is being used without dilution or there is only a small quantity available (e.g., infant BAL fluid), make as many slides as possible using the fluid available.
2. Centrifuge (cytospin) the cells at 750 rpm for 5 min onto microscope slides.
3. Carefully remove each slide from its assembly and allow the deposited cells to air dry.
4. Fix the cells to each of the slides using the Hema 3 stain kit fixative (solution 1; *see* instructions supplied with the kit for details). Set two slides aside ("unstained"). Stain the remaining two slides following the Hema 3 stain kit instructions ("stained"). Allow the slides to air dry. If fewer than four slides were made, stain only one of the slides.
5. Apply a drop of Permount mounting medium to the cells on each of the stained slides and cover with a cover slip. Allow to air dry. Do not apply cover slips to the unstained slides.
6. Examine the cells using light microscopy at 200–400× total magnification. Between 200 and 500 cells (not including red cells or epithelial cells) from an array of fields representing the entire cell deposition area are counted and differentiated. Express the results for individual cell types as percent of total cells counted.

3.4. Measurement of Neutrophil Elastase Activity and Elastase Inhibitory Capacity

3.4.1. Neutrophil Elastase Activity

1. Program the plate reader for a kinetic analysis at a wavelength of 405 nm. The read interval is 15 s with a total run time of 5 min. Warm the incubator to 25°C. Set the reader to mix the plate once before reading and set the optical density (OD) limit to 3.000. Input template settings according to the position of samples and standards on the 96-well plate. Store this program as a protocol file.
2. Prepare elastase standards (16, 8, 4, 2, 1, and 0.5 μg/mL) in 0.1% BSA/D-PBS in polypropylene tubes. Warm standards to 25°C. Lower concentrations of standards (0.1–0.5 μg/mL) can be used when samples containing <0.5 μg/mL elastase are measured.
3. Thaw samples and warm to 25°C.
4. Prepare the substrate solution as described above.
5. Place 100 μL of sample, standard, or blank into the preassigned wells of the 96-well plate. Perform each analysis in duplicate or triplicate.
6. Add 100 μL of substrate solution to each well.
7. Read the plate using the protocol file created above (*see* **Subheading 3.4.1., step 1**).
8. If the reaction rate of an unknown sample exceeds the rate of the 16 mg/mL standard, dilute the sample in 0.1% BSA/D-PBS in a polypropylene tube and repeat the assay.
9. Use the Softmax software to construct a linear standard curve (product formation rate vs standard concentration). Determine concentrations of unknown samples from this standard curve. Input dilution factors into the plate reader program if necessary. Conversion to molar units can be made based on the molecular weight of elastase (32 kDa). Normalize results to the volume of ELF.
10. Mark samples as being thawed, then return to storage at –80°C.

   Note: The synthetic substrate, MeO-Suc-Ala-Ala-Pro-Val-pNA is highly sensitive and specific for mammalian elastase *(30)*.

3.4.2. Elastase Inhibitory Capacity

1. Using the standard elastase stock solution, prepare a 20-μg/mL working solution in 0.1% BSA/D-PBS. Calculate the necessary solution volume as 250 μL/sample plus 1000 μL for the controls. Increase the final volume by at least 20% to allow for dead volumes when measuring.
2. Using the standard α_1-AT stock solution, prepare 1 mL of a working solution of 13 μg/mL in 0.1% BSA/D-PBS. To prepare 1 mL of this solution, dilute the standard α_1-AT stock 1/10 (25 μL of stock + 225 μL of 0.1% BSA/D-PBS), then add 26 μL of the diluted solution to 974 μL of 0.1% BSA/D-PBS (*see* **Note 3**).
3. Prepare incubation tubes (in polypropylene) for the positive and negative controls, and the samples as follows (*see* **Note 4**):
   a. Positive controls (in duplicate): 250 μL of elastase working solution + 250 μL of α1-antitrypsin working solution.

   b. Negative controls (in duplicate): 250 μL of elastase working solution + 250 μL of 0.1% BSA/D-PBS.

   c. Samples (single or duplicate): 250 μL of elastase working solution + 250 μL of sample.

   Incubate tubes for 30 min at 37°C. Allow tubes to cool to ~25°C.

4. Program plate reader as described above (*see* **Subheading 3.4.1., step 1**) (*see* **Note 5**).

5. Prepare the substrate solution as described above.

6. Place 100 μL (×4) of each sample, positive control or negative control into the assigned well of the 96-well plate.

7. Add 100 μL of substrate solution to each well.

8. Read the plate using the protocol file created above (*see* **Subheading 3.4.2., step 4**).

9. The negative controls should show the greatest rate (mOD/min) of increase in color formation. The positive controls should develop color at a rate (mOD/min) approx 40% slower than the negative controls. The amount of active elastase in the samples is calculated as

$$X/\text{rate of the sample (mOD/min)} = 20/\text{rate of the positive control (mOD/min)}$$

   Solving for X gives the active elastase (μg/mL) in the incubated sample. Calculate the inhibitory capacity (I) of the original sample as: $I = 20 - X$. To express the elastase inhibitory capacity as α-AT equivalents (μg/mL), multiply (I) by 52/32 (the ratio of the molecular weights of α_1-AT and elastase). Conversion to molar units can be made based on the molecular weight of α_1-AT (52 kDa). For BAL fluid, normalize the results to the volume of ELF (*see* **Note 6**).

10. Mark samples as being thawed, then return to storage at –80°C.

3.5. Measurement of α_1-Antitrypsin or Elastase/α_1-Antitrypsin Complex

1. Program the plate reader for a single-wavelength analysis at 410 nm. Set the reader to mix the plate once before reading and set the optical density (OD) limit to 2.000. Input template settings according to the position of samples and standards on the plate. Store this program as a protocol file.

2. Coat the wells of an EIA plate (96-well) with 100 μL/well of 5-μg/mL goat anti-human α_1-AT (first antibody) and incubate overnight (12 h minimum) at 4°C.

3. Wash the plate three times with 0.1% BSA/D-PBS (200 μL/well/wash).

4. Discard the third wash and block any remaining protein-binding sites with 150 μL/well of 1.0% BSA/D-PBS, incubated at 37°C for 1 h.

5. Repeat **step 2**.

6. Discard the third wash and immediately add 100 μL/well of blank (1.0% BSA/D-PBS), standard, or sample dilution to duplicate wells and incubate for 1 h at 37°C.

7. Repeat **step 2**. Discard the third wash.

8. Add 100 μL/well of 0.5-μg/mL rabbit anti-human elastase (second antibody: elastase/a_1-AT complex assay) or 100 μL/well of 0.05-μg/mL rabbit antihuman α_1-AT (second antibody: α_1-AT assay). Incubate for 1 h at 37°C.

9. Repeat **step 2**. Discard the third wash.

10. Add 100 µL/well of 1/6000 goat anti-rabbit IgG alkaline phosphatase-conjugated antibody (third antibody). Incubate for 1 h at 37°C.
11. Repeat **step 2**. Discard the third wash.
12. Add 100 µL/well of phosphatase substrate solution (1 mg/mL). Incubate at room temperature for 45–90 min in the dark. Plates are ready to read when color begins to develop in the lowest concentrations of standards.
13. Read the plate using the protocol file created above (*see* **Subheading 3.5., step 1**).
14. Calculate sample concentrations using the Softmax software. Construct a sigmoidal shaped standard curve of standard concentration vs absorbance. Determine the concentrations of α-AT or EATC in the BAL samples from the linear range of the standard curve. Correct for the appropriate dilution to obtain final ng/mL values. Conversion to molar units can be made based on the molecular weight of α_1-antitrypsin (52 kDa) or elastase (32 kDa) for the α_1-AT and Elastase/α_1-AT complex assays, respectively. Normalize the results to the volume of ELF (*see* **Notes 7** and **8**).
15. Mark samples as being thawed, then return to storage at –80°C.

3.6. Measurement of Interleukin-8 (31)

1. Program the plate reader for a dual-wavelength analysis at wavelength 450/540 or 570 nm. Set the reader to mix the plate once before reading and set the optical density (OD) limit to 3.000. Input template settings according to the position of samples and standards on the plate. Store this program as a protocol file.
2. Remove the number of microtiter plate strips necessary to accommodate the samples and standards. Arrange the strips in the sample plate. Return any unused strips to the foil pouch and reseal.
3. Add 100 µL of assay diluent RD1-8 to each well.
4. Add 50 µL of standard or patient sample to the appropriate wells.
5. Add 100 µL of IL-8 conjugate to each well. Tap to mix (*see* **Note 9**).
6. Apply adhesive covers to the strips and incubate at room temperature (20–25°C) for 2.5 h.
7. Aspirate the contents of each well (discard aspirates) and wash the wells a total of six times with wash buffer (1×). Following the final wash, aspirate or decant the wash solution and invert the plate onto a clean paper towel.
8. Mix equal volumes of color reagent A and B (substrate solution). Prepare only enough solution for the number of wells (200 µL/well). This solution must be used within 15 min of mixing.
9. Add 200 µL of substrate solution to each well. Apply new adhesive covers to the plate and incubate at 20–25°C for 30 min.
10. Add 50 µL of stop solution to each well. Tap the plate lightly to ensure through mixing.
11. Using the protocol file created above (*see* **step 1**), read the plate within 30 min at 450 nm, with wavelength correction at either 540 or 570 nm. Readings made at 450 nm alone may be higher and less accurate due to optical imperfections in the plate.
12. Calculate sample concentrations using the Softmax software. Construct a four parameter logistic or log-log standard curve of IL-8 concentration vs absorbance.

Determine the concentrations of IL-8 from the linear or near-linear range of the standard curve. If a sample concentration exceeds the range of the standard curve, dilute the sample in calibrator diluent RD5P (1×) and reassay. Correct for any additional dilutions to obtain the final ng/mL concentration. Conversion to molar units is not usually done due to the multiple forms of human IL-8 (72 or 77 amino acids). Normalize the results to the volume of the ELF.

13. Mark samples as being thawed, then return to storage at –80°C.

3.7. Measurement of Leukotriene B_4 (32)

1. Program the plate reader for a single-wavelength analysis at 412 nm (range: 405–420 nm). Set the reader to mix the plate once before reading and set the optical density (OD) limit to 2.000. Input template settings according to the position of samples and standards on the plate. Store this program as a protocol file.

2. Remove the number of microtiter plate strips necessary to accommodate the samples and standards. Arrange the strips in the sample plate. Return any unused strips to the foil pouch and reseal.

3. Wash the plate once with wash buffer (1×). Aspirate or decant the buffer from the wells and invert the plate on a paper towel to dry.

4. Add the samples to the wells as follows:
   a. Add 100 µL of EIA buffer (1×) to each nonspecific binding (NSB) well.
   b. Add 50 µL of EIA buffer (1×) to each maximum-binding (B_0) well.
   c. Add 50 µL of each standard (3.9–500 pg/mL) to each corresponding well.
   d. Add 50 µL of each BAL sample to each corresponding well.
   e. Add 50 µL of LTB_4 acetylcholinesterase tracer to each well *except* the total activity (TA) and Blank wells.
   f. Add 50 µL of leukotriene B_4 antiserum to each well *except* the TA, the NSB, and the Blank wells (*see* **Notes 10** and **11**).

5. Cover the plate with plastic adhesive film and incubate for 18 h at room temperature (20–25°C).

6. Aspirate or decant the contents of the plate and wash the plate five times with wash buffer (1×). Remove the final wash and invert the plate onto a paper towel.

7. Add 200 µL of Ellman's reagent to each well and 5 µL of LTB_4 acetylcholinesterase tracer to the TA wells.

8. Cover the plate with plastic adhesive film and incubate for 60 min in the dark at room temperature.

9. Read the plate using the protocol file created above (*see* **Subheading 3.7., step 1**). The B_0 wells should read in the range of 0.5–0.8 absorbance units (AU). If the wells read <0.5 AU, recover the plate and continue incubating in the dark. Read the plate at intervals of 30 min until the B_0 wells read within the desired range. If the B_0 absorbance exceeds 2.0 AU, wash the plate with wash buffer (1×) and add fresh Ellman's reagent to redevelop (see **Notes 12** and **13**).

10. Calculate results by computer software (Cayman Chemical, Ann Arbor, MI, # 400016) or manually. The steps involved are as follows:
    a. Average the absorbance readings from the NSB wells.
    b. Average the absorbance readings from the B_0 wells.

c. Subtract the NSB average from the B_0 average. The result is the corrected B_0.

d. Calculate the $\%B/B_0$ for the remaining wells. For each well, subtract the average NSB absorbance from the absorbance of the well and divide the result by the corrected B_0. Multiply this result by 100 to obtain $\%B/B_0$.

e. The TA wells are used as a quality control tool. Calculate the actual TA as the average TA absorbance multiplied by 10. The corrected B_0 divided by the actual TA yields the percent bound. This percent bound value should closely approximate the percent bound that can be calculated from the sample.

f. The standard curve is plotted as $\%B/B_0$ vs the log of the concentration for each LTB_4 standard. Use only the linear portion of the standard curve for reading BAL samples (typically where $\%B/B_0$ is between 20 and 80%).

g. Find the LTB_4 concentrations in the samples by comparing the $\%B/B_0$ for each sample to the standard curve and reading the corresponding LTB_4 concentration. Convert the sample concentration to the LTB_4 concentration per milliliter of BAL fluid by correcting for all applied dilutions and for the concentrating effect of the vacuum evaporation on the original BAL fluid aliquot. For example: A 5-mL BAL fluid aliquot is diluted in methanol and vacuum evaporated. The residue is resuspended in 0.5 mL of methanol/water. The 0.5-mL resuspension is diluted 1/10 with EIA buffer (1×) and assayed. The result derived from the standard curve must be multiplied by 10 (for the 1/10 dilution of the 0.5-mL resuspension), and next divided by 10 (for the 5-mL to 0.5-mL concentrating effect of the evaporation step). These numbers are for explanation only. The actual numbers will depend on the initial BAL aliquot volume and the dilution(s) applied to the 0.5-mL resuspension sample. Normalize the results to the volume of ELF.

11. Mark samples as being thawed, then return to storage at –80°C.

3.8. Measurement of Urea Nitrogen in Serum and BAL Fluid for Estimating the Volume of Epithelial Lining Fluid (33)

1. Program the plate reader for a kinetic analysis at a wavelength of 340 nm. The read interval is 15 s with at total run time of 5 min. Warm the incubator to 30°C. Set the reader to mix the plate once prior reading and set the optical density (OD) limit to –1.000. Input template settings according to the position of samples and standards on the 96 well plate. Store this program as a protocol file.

2. Use previously sterile filtered BAL fluid containing 100 µM PMSF and 5 mM EDTA. Bring all samples to room temperature (20–25°C) prior to use.

3. Dilute the 100 mg/dL glucose/urea standard solution with normal (0.9%) saline to a concentration of 40 mg/dL. Perform serial dilutions beginning with the 40-mg/dL solution to prepare 20-, 10-, 5-, and 2.5-mg/dL urea solutions. These solutions (2.5–40 mg/dL) will be the urea standard solutions from which a standard curve will be constructed (see Note 14).

4. Dilute (1/20) all serum samples, the urea standard curve samples, and the Accutol standard. Use normal (0.9%) saline as the diluent. Do not dilute BAL samples.

5. Reconstitute the BUN reagent with 10 mL of distilled/deionized water (Do not reconstitute to 20 mL as instructed on the vial). Warm the BUN reagent to 30°C.

6. Place 50 µL of sample (BAL or serum), urea standard, Accutrol standard, or blank into the assigned wells of a 96-well plate. Perform each analysis in duplicate or triplicate (*see* **Note 15**).
7. Add 150 µL of BUN reagent to each well (*see* **Note 16**).
8. Immediately read the plate using the protocol file created above (**step 1**).
9. Calculate sample concentrations using the Softmax software. Construct a linear standard curve of standard urea concentration vs reaction rate (Vmax). Urea concentrations of unknown samples are based on the Vmax of the samples relative to the standards. Further divide the results for BAL samples by a factor of 20 to adjust for the relative dilution of the serum and standard samples. Verify that the results for the Accutrol standard are within the range stated on the Accutrol bottle.
10. Mark samples as being thawed, then return to storage at –80°C.

3.8.1. Calculation of the ELF Dilution Factor

1. Divide the serum urea concentration by the BAL fluid urea concentration for each subject. This number represents the factor by which the ELF is diluted in the BAL fluid *(26)*.
2. To express the concentrations of the BAL fluid components (e.g., elastase, cytokines, LTB_4, etc.) in terms of their concentrations in the ELF, multiply each measured concentration by the corresponding ELF dilution factor. This applies to BAL fluid concentrations expressed as either molar or mass units.

4. Notes

1. For children less than 35 kg in weight (approx age 12 yr and younger), the procedure must be altered to use a smaller bronchoscope (3.5-mm od). The concentration and instilled amounts of lidocaine is reduced to 1% and 1-mL/aliquot (not to exceed 7 mg/kg). The volume of BAL fluid that is instilled and collected is significantly less. Two or three aliquots of 1 mL/kg (maximum 30-mL/aliquot) are instilled using a syringe (rather than gravity) and aspirated into a suction trap (rather than a syringe). Otherwise the procedure is identical.
2. The procedure is documented on a research form for data entry (*see* **Fig. 2**), as well as by videotape (particularly if a subsequent procedure is planned on the same subject, e.g., to assess the effect of an intervention on BAL measures). Reviewing the videotaping of a previous procedure before a subsequent procedure in the same subject helps the bronchoscopist to return to the same airway segment in a serial lavage study. This is important because of the regional differences in inflammation in the CF airway *(34)*.
3. Elastase forms equal molar complexes with α1-antitrypsin, inactivating the elastase activity *(27)*.
4. Use only polypropylene plastic ware as elastase adheres to glass.
5. Changes in absorbance at 405 (or 410) nm are directly proportional to the rate of *p*-nitroanalide liberation from the peptide substrate. Initial reaction rates are first-order over the range of standard concentrations described.
6. BAL supernatant refers to fluid from BAL samples previously spun at 40,000*g* and sterile filtered. These samples contain no exogenous protease inhibitors. Avoid refreezing and resusing sample aliquots if possible.

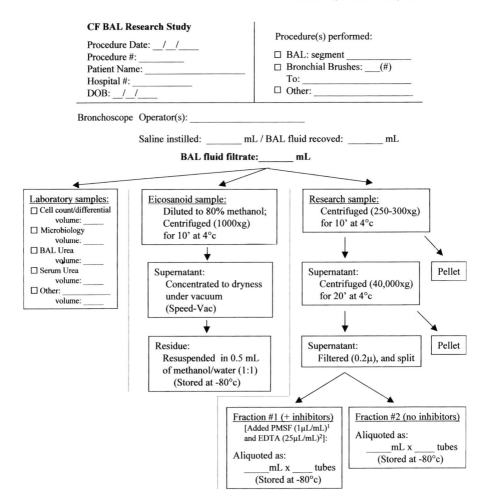

Fig. 2. Standardized form for documenting bronchoscopy and BAL procedures for CF research studies.

7. α_1-AT and Elastase/α_1-AT complexes are measured using separate assays. Each uses different standards, α_1-AT (100, 50, 20, 10, 5, 2, 1, 0.5, 0.2, 0.1, and 0.05 ng/mL in 1% BSA/D-PBS) and elastase/α1-AT complex (50, 20, 10, 5, 2, 1, 0.5, 0.2, 0.1, 0.05, 0.02, and 0.01 ng/mL in 1% BSA/D-PBS), respectively. However, the basic assay methods differ only with respect to the second antibody used. Therefore, a single method is presented with the second antibody difference noted.

8. BAL supernatants dilutions of 1/1000, 1/5000, and 1/10,000 for the α_1-AT assay and 1/200, 1/1000, and 1/2000 for the elastase/α_1-AT complex assay, respec-

tively, are prepared with 1.0% BSA/D-PBS in polypropylene tubes. (BAL supernatant refers to BAL fluid previously spun at 40,000g, sterile filtered, and that contains 100 μM PMSF and 5 mM EDTA.) This step is performed concurrently with **steps 2–4**. Other dilutions may be necessary based on prior patient history or inadequate dilution in a previous assay. Discard used standard aliquots. Avoid using previously thawed sample aliquots if possible.

9. IL-1, IL-6, and IL-10 are routinely measured by similar methodology. Other cytokines of specific interest can be assessed as well.
10. The Blank sample, TA sample, NSB sample, and B_0 sample should be plated in triplicate wells. The standards should be plated in duplicate or triplicate.
11. To minimize assay interferences from the methanol, the BAL samples should be either (a) evaporated to dryness, then resuspended in EIA buffer (1×), or (b) diluted 1/10 in EIA buffer (1×). This decreases the methanol concentration to a noninterfering level for the assay (≤5% of the total volume).
12. Analyze at least two dilutions of each BAL sample (ranging from 1/10 to 1/100).
13. Other eicosanoids, including prostaglandins and leukotrienes, are assayed by similar methodologies.
14. Urea is hydrolyzed to ammonia and carbon dioxide in the reaction catalyzed by urease. The ammonia serves to aminate 2-oxoglutarate to glutamate with concurrent oxidation of nicotinamide adenine dinucleotide (NADH to NAD) in the reaction catalyzed by glutamate dehydrogenase (GLDH). The BUN reagent is formulated in such a way that the decrease in absorbance at 340 nm, resulting from the oxidation of NADH to NAD, is directly proportional to the BUN concentration in the sample *(33)*.
15. Measure corresponding serum and BAL samples in the same assay.
16. The method used to measure BUN in routine clinical laboratories lacks the sensitivity necessary for the dilute BAL fluid.

References

1. Davis, P. B., Drumm, M., Konstan, M. W. (1996) Cystic fibrosis. *Am. J. Respir. Crit. Care. Med.* **154,** 122–1256.
2. Konstan, M. W. and Berger, M. (1993) Infection and inflammation in the lung in cystic fibrosis, in *Cystic Fibrosis* (Davis, P. B., ed.), Marcel Dekker, New York, pp. 219–276.
3. Berger, M., Sorensen, R. U., Tosi, M. F., Dearborn, D. G., Doring, G. (1989) Complement receptor expression on neutrophils at an inflammatory site, the Pseudomonas-infected lung in cystic fibrosis. *J. Clin. Invest.* **84,** 1302–1313.
4. Tosi, M. F., Zakem, H., Berger, M. (1990) Neutrophil elastase cleaves C3bi on opsonized pseudomonas as well as CR1 on neutrophils to create a functionally important opsonin receptor mismatch. *J. Clin. Invest.* **86,** 300–308.
5. Ramsey, B. W. and Boat, T. F. (1994) Outcome measures for clinical trials in cystic fibrosis. Summary of a Cystic Fibrosis Foundation consensus conference. *J. Pediatr.* **124,** 177–192.
6. Konstan, M. W., Hilliard, K. A., Norvell, T. M., Berger, M. (1994) Bronchoalveolar lavage findings in cystic fibrosis patients with stable, clinically mild lung

disease suggest ongoing infection and inflammation. *Am. J. Respir. Crit. Care Med.* **150,** 448–454.

7. Birrer, P., McElvaney, N. G., Rudeberg, A., Sommer, C. W., Liechti-Gallati, S., Kraemer, R., Hubbard, R., Crystal, R. G. (1994) Protease-antiprotease imbalance in the lungs of children with cystic fibrosis. *Am. J. Respir. Crit. Care Med.* **150,** 207–213.

8. Khan, T. Z., Wagener, J. S., Bost, T., Martinez, J., Accurso, F. J., Riches, D. W. (1995) Early pulmonary inflammation in infants with cystic fibrosis. *Am. J. Respir. Crit. Care Med.* **151,** 1075–1082.

9. Balough, K., McCubbin, M., Weinberger, M., Smits, W., Aherns, R., Fick, R. (1995) The relationship between infection and inflammation in the early stages of lung disease from cystic fibrosis. *Pediatr. Pulmonol.* **20,** 63–70.

10. Armstrong, D. S., Grimwood, K., Carzino, R., Carlin, J. B., Olinsky, A., Phelan, P. D. (1995) Lower respiratory infection and inflammation in infants with newly diagnosed cystic fibrosis. *BMJ* **310(6994),** 1571,1572.

11. Noah, T. L., Black, H. R., Cheng, P. W., Wood, R. E., Leigh, M. W. (1997) Nasal and bronchoalveolar lavage fluid cytokines in early cystic fibrosis. *J. Infect. Dis.* **175,** 638–647.

12. Rosenfeld, M., Emerson, J., Accurso, F., Armstrong, D., Castile, R., Grimwood, K., et al. (1999) Diagnostic accuracy of oropharyngeal cultures in infants and young children with cystic fibrosis. *Pediatr. Pulmonol.* **28,** 321–328.

13. Meyer, K. C., Lewandoski, J. R., Zimmerman, J. J., Nunley, D., Calhoun, W. J., Dopico, G. A. (1991) Human neutrophil elastase and elastase/alpha 1-antiprotease complex in cystic fibrosis. Comparison with interstitial lung disease and evaluation of the effect of intravenously administered antibiotic therapy. *Am. Rev. Respir. Dis.* **144,** 580–585.

14. McElvaney, N. G., Hubbard, R. C., Birrer, P., Chernick, M. S., Caplan, D. B., Frank, M. M., et al. (1991) Aerosol alpha 1-antitrypsin treatment for cystic fibrosis. *Lancet* **337(8738),** 392–394.

15. McElvaney, N. G., Nakamura, H., Birrer, P., Hebert, C. A., Wong, W. L., Alphonso, M., et al. (1992) Modulation of airway inflammation in cystic fibrosis. In vivo suppression of interleukin-8 levels on the respiratory epithelial surface by aerosolization of recombinant secretory leukoprotease inhibitor. *J. Clin. Invest.* **90,** 1296–1301.

16. Bonfield, T. L., Konstan, M. W., Burfeind, P., Panuska, J. R., Hilliard, J. B., Berger, M. (1995) Normal bronchial epithelial cells constitutively produce the anti-inflammatory cytokine IL-10 which is down-regulated in cystic fibrosis. *Am. J. Respir. Cell. Mol. Biol.* **13,** 257–261.

17. Bonfield, T. L., Konstan, M. W., Berger, M. (1999) Altered respiratory epithelial cell cytokine production in cystic fibrosis. *J. Allergy Clin. Immunol.* **104,** 72–78.

18. Konstan, M. W. and Berger, M. (1997) Current understanding of the inflammatory process in cystic fibrosis–onset and etiology. *Pediatr. Pulmonol.* **24,** 137–142.

19. Konstan, M. W., Walenga, R. W., Hilliard, K. A., Hilliard, J. B. (1993) Leukotriene B$_4$ is markedly elevated in epithelial lining fluid of patients with cystic fibrosis. *Am. Rev. Respir. Dis.* **148,** 896–901.

20. Berger, M., Norvell, T. M., Tosi, M. F., Emancipator, S. N., Konstan, M. W., Schreiber, J. R. (1994) Tissue-specific Fc gamma and complement receptor expression by alveolar macrophages determines relative importance of IgG and complement in promoting phagocytosis of Pseudomonas aeruginosa. *Pediatr. Res.* **35,** 68–77.
21. Bonfield, T. L., Panuska, J. R., Konstan, M. W., Hilliard, K. A., Hilliard, J. B., Ghnaim, H., Berger, M. (1995) Inflammatory cytokines in cystic fibrosis lungs. *Am. J. Respir. Crit. Care Med.* **152,** 2111–2118.
22. Stone, P. J, Konstan, M. W., Berger, M., Dorkin, H. L., Franzblau, C., Snider, G. L. (1995) Elastin and collagen degradation products in urine of patients with cystic fibrosis. *Am. J. Respir. Crit. Care Med.* **152,** 157–162.
23. Sharma, G. D., Tosi, M. F., Stern, R. C., Davis, P. B. (1995) Progression of pulmonary disease after disappearance of Pseudomonas in cystic fibrosis. *Am. J. Respir. Crit. Care Med.* **152,** 169–173.
24. Chmiel, J. F., Drumm, M. L., Konstan, M. W., Ferkol, T. W., Kercsmar, C. M. (1999) Pitfall in the use of genotype analysis as the sole diagnostic criterion for cystic fibrosis. *Pediatrics* **103,** 823–826.
25. Freedman, S. D., Katz, M. H., Parker, E. M., Laposata, M., Urman, M. Y., Alvarez, J. G. (1999) A membrane lipid imbalance plays a role in the phenotypic expression of cystic fibrosis in cftr(-/-) mice. *Proc. Natl. Acad. Sci. USA* **96,** 13,995–14,000.
26. Rennard, S. I., Basset, G., Lecossier, D., O'Donnell, K. M., Pinkston, P., Martin, P. G., and Crystal, R. G. (1986) Estimation of volume of epithelial lining fluid recovered by lavage using urea as marker of dilution. *J. Appl. Physiol.* **60,** 532–538.
27. Neumann, S., Hennrich, N., Gunzer, G., Lang, H. (1984) Enzyme-linked immunoassay for human granulocyte elastase in complex with α1-proteinase inhibitor in *Proteases: Potential Role in Health and Disease* (Horl, W. H. and Heidland, A., eds.), Plenum Press, New York, pp. 379–390.
28. Committee on Drugs, American Academy of Pediatrics. (1992) Guidelines for monitoring and management of pediatric patients during and after sedation for diagnostic and therapeutic procedures. *Pediatrics* **89,** 1110–1115.
29. Official Statement of the American Thoracic Society. (1992) Flexible endoscopy of the pediatric airway. *Am. Rev. Respir. Dis.* **145,** 233–235.
30. Bieth, J., Spiess, B., Wermuth, C. G. (1974) The synthesis and analytical use of a highly sensitive and convenient substrate of elastase. *Biochem. Med.* **11,** 350–357.
31. R&D Systems, Inc. (1999) Quantikine Human IL-8 Immunoassay, cat. no. D8050. Instruction booklet.
32. Cayman Chemical Company. (1992) Leukotriene B4 Enzyme Immunoassay Kit, cat. no. 520111. Instruction booklet.
33. Sigma Chemical Company. (1999) Infinity BUN Reagent, procedure # 64-UV. Instruction sheet.
34. Meyer, K. C. and Sharma, A. (1997) Regional variability of lung inflammation in cystic fibrosis. *Am. J. Respir. Crit. Care Med.* **156,** 1536–1540.

28

Bacterial Colonization and Infection in the CF Lung

Scott D. Sagel, Elaine B. Dowell, and Frank J. Accurso

1. Introduction

Progressive obstructive pulmonary disease accounts for the majority of morbidity and mortality in cystic fibrosis (CF) *(1)*. Chronic bacterial bronchopulmonary colonization and infection plays a major role in this progression. While the lungs of persons with CF are normal *in utero*, many infants become colonized with a number of bacterial organisms including *Staphylococcus aureus* and *Haemophilus influenzae* shortly after birth *(2–6)*. The role of these organisms in the development of lung disease remains unclear. In time, *Pseudomonas aeruginosa* becomes the predominant bacterial pathogen in older children and is strongly associated with progressive pulmonary decline *(7–9)*. Most CF patients are initially infected with classical, smooth strains of *P. aeruginosa*. During the course of the disease, these bacteria change to a mucoid phenotype with a rough polysaccharide exterior *(10)*. This mucoid exopolysaccharide prevents both phagocytes and antibiotics from being able to penetrate and kill the bacteria and therefore plays a major role in promoting the persistent infection and inflammation that ultimately destroys the lung. *Burkholderia cepacia*, now an increasingly important pathogen, is associated with more advanced lung disease and in some cases is correlated with rapid clinical deterioration *(10,12,13)*. Highly antibiotic-resistant organisms such as *Achromobacter xylosoxidans* and *Stenotrophomonas maltophilia* are also frequently recovered from patients with more advanced disease *(14)*. The incidence of colonization and infection with these and other pathogens is reported annually by the national Cystic Fibrosis Foundation Patient Registry *(15)* and elsewhere *(14)*. It is clear that the presence of these bacterial organisms incites and propagates a chronic inflammatory response that damages the airways and impairs local host-defense mechanisms, resulting in widespread bronchiectasis and respiratory failure.

From: *Methods in Molecular Medicine, vol. 70: Cystic Fibrosis Methods and Protocols*
Edited by: W. R. Skach © Humana Press Inc., Totowa, NJ

Antibiotic therapy has been a mainstay of treatment for CF and appears to be one of the primary reasons for the increased life expectancy of patient with CF over the past 30 years *(16)*. Antimicrobial therapy usually does not eradicate organisms from the lower respiratory tract once chronic infection has been established, but it has been shown to decrease bacterial load *(17)* and decrease the production of microbial virulence factors. Antibiotics also reduce the associated inflammatory response.

Antibiotics are typically prescribed to CF patients for one of the following reasons: (1) intensive therapy, usually inpatient, for treatment of increased respiratory symptoms, termed a pulmonary exacerbation; (2) chronic maintenance therapy in hopes of reducing the frequency and morbidity of pulmonary exacerbations and decline in pulmonary function; and (3) preventive therapy to delay initial lower airway colonization with the most common pathogen, *P. aeruginosa (1)*. Preventive therapy in young patients remains the most controversial of these scenarios. A few European studies found that anti-*Pseudomonas* therapy during early stages of *P. aeruginosa* colonization in the lungs prevented or delayed the development of chronic lung infection *(18,19)*.

In order for clinicians to prescribe appropriate antimicrobial therapy, they must first be able to detect and accurately identify any significant lower respiratory tract pathogens. Controversy exists as to the optimal way to sample the lower respiratory tract. The most frequently obtained diagnostic specimens in CF patients include oropharyngeal swabs, sputum, and bronchoalveolar lavage (BAL). Sputum tends to be the simplest and most appropriate specimen from those subjects who are capable of expectorating. The identification of pulmonary pathogens becomes more difficult in those patients who cannot cough up or expectorate airway secretions.

Oropharyngeal (OP) swabs are routinely used in children with CF who are not capable of expectorating sputum. Ramsey et al. showed that positive throat cultures were highly predictive of the presence of *P. aeruginosa* and *S. aureus* in the lower airways *(20)*. However, in their study, the sensitivity and negative predictive values of OP cultures for *P. aeruginosa* and *S. aureus* were lower, suggesting that a negative throat culture does not rule out the presence of these pathogens in the lower airways. Armstrong et al. also demonstrated that OP cultures lack sensitivity for identifying lower airway *P. aeruginosa* and *S. aureus (21)*. Furthermore, they had a higher incidence of falsely positive OP cultures, resulting in a poor positive predictive value. These authors concluded that OP cultures are poor predictors or markers of lower airway infection. In spite of its insensitivity, most clinicians employ OP cultures as the initial screening source in nonexpectorating CF patients.

Sputum is a very useful specimen, especially from those patients capable of expectorating. In patients with CF, there is a strong correlation between the organisms detected in sputum and those isolated in specimens obtained during thoracotomy *(22)* or by bronchoscopy *(23)*. In patients who cannot spontane-ously produce sputum, inducing sputum can be a helpful diagnostic tool and may reduce the need for more invasive procedures such as a BAL. Sputum induction is performed by inhaling aerosolized hypertonic saline *(24)*. Sputum induction has been useful for the cytological diagnosis of malignancy *(25)*, and for the detection of *Pneumocystis carinii (26)* and tuberculosis *(27)*. It has also become a valid and acceptable method for sampling the airways of subjects with asthma to analyze both cellular and biochemical markers of inflammation *(28–34)*.

Until recently, sputum induction has received little attention in CF. One sys-tematic study found that sputum induction is safe and acceptable in nonexpectorating CF children *(35)*. Another group collected induced sputum samples from those CF patients who could expectorate, yet did not directly compare these results to those obtained from spontaneously expectorated speci-mens *(36)*. Recently, sputum induction was compared with expectorated spu-tum and bronchoalveolar lavage in 10 adults with CF *(37)*. In these subjects, induced sputum yielded similar total cell counts and differentials, and similar detection rates of CF-related bacterial pathogens. We have been routinely applying sputum induction in our younger children with CF who do not typi-cally expectorate. We have found that induced sputum samples are remarkably similar to spontaneously expectorated samples in describing both airway inflammation and infection.

BAL fluid is considered by some to be the optimal specimen for assessing the microbiology of the lower respiratory tract. Unfortunately, the procedure is invasive, expensive, risky, and requires skilled personnel. Serial BALs are par-ticularly difficult to perform. However, BAL may be necessary to definitively detect or exclude lower airway infection, particularly in a patient who does not have established infection and/or does not expectorate. BAL is generally most useful for diagnosing infection and guiding antimicrobial treatment in infants and young, nonexpectorating CF children, especially those being hospitalized for a pulmonary exacerbation.

In addition to the above-mentioned conventional microbiologic techniques, molecular techniques are being also applied to CF specimens. The polymerase chain reaction (PCR) provides the capability to detect pathogens by DNA hybridization even when present in very low numbers. This method has been used to detect *P. aeruginosa* and *B. cepacia* in sputum samples from patients with CF *(38,39)*. DNA probes can accurately differentiate unre-lated *P. aeruginosa* strains that have identical serotype, biotype, and antibiograms. These probes are also useful for demonstrating that mucoid and nonmucoid isolates may be variants of the same strain rather than new acquisi-tions. PCR-based techniques are not yet routine in CF care settings.

In this chapter, the authors describe techniques used for detecting and iden-tifying pulmonary bacterial pathogens. The specific protocol our institution uses for inducing sputum will be provided. This protocol is useful for patients who do not expectorate regularly and in those instances where sputum is required for research purposes. As for procedural issues with bronchoscopy and BAL, we recommend review of Chapter 27.

2. Materials

2.1. Oropharyngeal Swabs (Throat Swabs)

1. BBL™ CultureSwab™ collection and transport system (Becton Dickinson, Sparks, MD).
2. Wooden tongue blade.

2.2. Expectorated Sputum

1. Sterile specimen container.

2.3. Induced Sputum

1. DeVilbiss Ultra-Neb 99 (099HD) ultrasonic nebulizer (Sunrise Medical, Somerset, PA).
2. Disposable medication cup/Aqua Pak.
3. 60cc 3% hypertonic saline, in 15-cc premixed vials (Dey Labs, Napa, CA) ×4.
4. Large-bore corrugated tubing:
   a. 1–2 link segment;
   b. 1–1 link segment;
   c. 1–7 link long segment.
5. Mouthpiece.
6. "T" piece.
7. Nose clip.
8. Electronic timer.
9. Sterile specimen containers.
10. Spirometer.
11. Pulse oximeter.
12. Albuterol metered-dose inhaler (and spacer device).
13. Chair and table.

2.4. Quantitative Microbiology

1. Blood agar (BAP).
2. MacConkey agar (MAC).
3. *B. cepacia* selective agar (BCSA).
4. Mannitol salt agar (MAN).
5. *Haemophilus*-selective agar (HAE).
6. Inhibitory mold agar (IMA).
7. Gram staining reagents.
8. Sterile normal saline.
9. Sterile glass beads.
10. 10% Sputolysin (dithiothreitol).

11. Vortex mixer.
12. Ambient incubators (30°C, 35°C).
13. CO_2 incubator (35°C).
14. Anaerobic incubation system (bags, jars, or chamber).
15. Sterile cotton-tipped swabs.
16. Sterile wooden applicator sticks.
17. Sterile inoculating loops.
18. Sterile 15-mL polystyrene screw-capped tubes.
19. Pasteur pipets.

3. Methods

3.1. Oropharyngeal Swabs (Throat Swabs)

1. Use a sterile prepackaged culture swab with transport medium to obtain the oropharyngeal (throat) specimen.
2. Depress the tongue to adequately expose the oropharynx.
3. The swab must be rubbed over the posterior pharynx and over each tonsillar area. Rotate the swab over these areas for a total of 3–5 s. Any area with exudate should also be touched.
4. Care should be taken to avoid contaminating the swab by touching the tongue or lips.
5. Reinsert the prepackaged swab into the tubing sheath and process according to the manufacturer's instructions.
6. Label the specimen and send to the microbiology laboratory for processing.

3.2. Expectorated Sputum

1. Obtain an expectorated sputum sample in a sterile, leakproof, screw-capped specimen container (minimum volume of sputum, 0.5 mL).
2. Label the specimen and send to the microbiology laboratory for processing.

3.3. Induced Sputum

Our method for inducing sputum has been adapted from a protocol designed by Fahy and colleagues *(40)*. Sputum is induced by administering 3% hypertonic saline (HS) for six 2-min sessions. At our institution, we deliver the HS by an ultrasonic nebulizer, filling the disposable medication cup with 30 cc of 3% HS (two premixed vials) every 6 min during the 12-min induction. Since HS is a known bronchoconstrictive agent *(41)*, sputum induction warrants close supervision during its performance. We ask the subjects to refrain from eating for 1 h before the procedure.

Cytospins of induced sputum specimens from a healthy control subject and a child with CF are displayed in **Figs. 1** and **2**.

3.3.1. Pre-Sputum Induction

1. Calibrate spirometer per ATS standards.
2. Assemble the nebulizer according to the manufacturer's instruction guide.

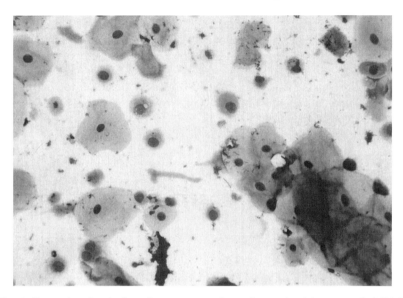

Fig. 1. Cytospin of an induced sputum specimen from a healthy control child. Notice the numerous alveolar macrophages, some of which are vacuolated, interspersed among several squamous epithelial cells.

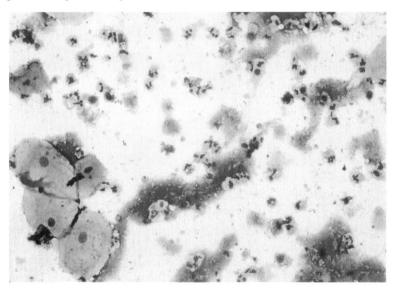

Fig. 2. Cytospin of an induced sputum specimen from a child with CF. Notice the overwhelming abundance of neutrophils, interspersed among a few squamous epithelial cells.

a. We recommend removing the air control valve from the DeVilbiss ultrasonic nebulizer to allow for maximal output.
b. Switch on the nebulizer for a brief period of time to confirm adequate and proper nebulization.

3. Explain to the participants the purpose of the test, how it is to be conducted, possible side effects (e.g., coughing, sore throat, salty aftertaste, chest tightness, wheezing, dyspnea, and nausea), and demonstrate the generation of the nebulization mist.
4. Premedicate all subjects with two puffs of albuterol (180 μg) via a spacer device.
5. Fifteen minutes after giving albuterol, perform three spirometry maneuvers and record the best FEV_1 (L) and corresponding percent predicted on the sputum induction worksheet.
6. Calculate a 10% and 20% fall of the highest postbronchodilator FEV_1 (L) and record both values on the worksheet ($FEV_1 \times 0.8 = 20\%$, $FEV_1 \times 0.9 = 10\%$).

3.3.2. Sputum Induction Procedure

1. Instruct the participants to put on a nose clip and to breathe at their usual rate and volume (tidal volume breathing) from the mouthpiece during the entire procedure except when actively bringing up a sputum sample or performing spirometry.
2. Start inhalation of 3% HS for 2 min.
3. After the 2-min inhalation period, instruct the participants to:
   a. Remove the mouthpiece and expectorate all saliva into a "saliva" container.
   b. Rinse their mouth with water and spit into a disposable cup.
   c. Return the mouthpiece to their mouth and take in a full deep breath and exhale.
   d. Take in a second full deep breath, and when the lungs are fully inflated, hold this breath.
   e. Perform forced expiratory techniques and directed coughing (huff coughs), and expectorate any sputum into a sterile "induced sputum" specimen container.
4. Repeat **steps 2** and **3** for a total of six sessions or a cumulative nebulization time of 12 min.
5. If participants need to expectorate in between the 2-min time frame, instruct the subjects to first rinse their mouth with water and spit into a disposable cup, then expectorate into the induced sputum specimen container.
6. If an adequate sputum specimen is obtained, label it, keep it on ice, and transport it to the microbiology laboratory for processing.

3.3.3. Safety Monitoring During Sputum Induction

1. During sputum induction, we monitor our subjects by:
   a. Chest auscultation at 0, 2, 6, and 10 min into the procedure;
   b. FEV_1 at 0, 4, 8, and 12 min;
   c. Continual oxygen saturation.
2. If the FEV_1 (L) falls by >10% but <20% of the initial postbronchodilator value or if the subject requests, another two puffs of albuterol are administered, and the induction is continued as long as the FEV_1 improves to within 10% of the initial postbronchodilator value.

3. If the FEV_1 falls by >20% or if troublesome symptoms occur (significant wheezing on auscultation, intolerability claimed by the subject, or drop in oxygen saturation to <90%), the induction is discontinued.
4. Discharge criteria:
    a. If the postsputum induction FEV_1 is ≥90% of the initial postbronchodilator value, the induction procedure is completed.
    b. If the postsputum induction FEV_1 remains <90%, despite an additional 2 puffs of albuterol, contact the supervising physician.

3.4. Quantitative Microbiology

3.4.1. Specimen Handling

All respiratory specimens collected from CF patients must be transported to the laboratory as soon as possible, ideally within 30 min. Prolonged delay in specimen transport may adversely affect the laboratory's ability to recover certain CF pathogens. These specimens should be processed in a timely fashion upon receipt in the laboratory. If not processed upon receipt, the specimens should be stored at 4°C. Sometimes, however, it is necessary to transport CF specimens to centers specially equipped and prepared to handle such specimens. Importantly, it has been shown that postal transport of sputa from CF patients does not significantly decrease the microbiological yield (42).

3.4.2. Specimen Processing

Specimens should be processed in a microbiology laboratory in which the recommendations of a consensus conference on CF microbiology are followed. In order to optimize recovery of CF-related bacterial pathogens, the clinician must ensure that the laboratory is aware that the specimen has come from a CF patient. The clinician must also alert the laboratory as to what organisms are suspected. This is particularly important if *B. cepacia* is suspected, since appropriate selective media need to be employed (43). Selective media and specialized conditions have been shown to facilitate detection of CF bacterial pathogens (44–46). Detection of these organisms can be enhanced with prolonged incubation for at least 4 d on these recommended media. This allows slower-growing organisms to become more apparent and is particularly important if the patient is receiving antibiotics.

The most problematic specimens to process for microbiologic purposes are sputa. CF sputum is extremely thick and tenacious, characterized by an abundant concentration of extracellular DNA and increased viscosity (47,48). Further, bacteria are not uniformly distributed in infected sputum (49). Liquefaction and homogenization have been recommended to ensure accurate, representative sputum cultures. Dithiothreitol (DTT) is one mucolytic agent that has been used to liquefy sputum. DTT has been shown to facilitate quantitative cultures of *S. aureus* and *P. aeruginosa* in CF sputum (50). However, in this same study, DTT appeared to inhibit the growth of *H. influenzae*, thus possibly impairing isolation of this organism. In another study, homogenizing sputum with DTT increased the recovery of viable bacteria compared with a mechanical mixing process using sterile glass beads *(51)*. Wong combined DTT liquefaction and dilution to quantitate sputum bacteria and used selective media together with aerobic and anaerobic incubation to facilitate isolation of bacterial organisms *(44)*. This selective technique demonstrated more reliable identification and quantification of the CF-related bacterial pathogens than did routine plating of unhomogenized sputum. This technique was developed because rapidly growing, often mucoid, strains of *P. aeruginosa* may obscure the growth of more fastidious organisms such as *H. influenzae*, and because bacteria are not distributed uniformly in sputum from patients with CF. While DTT remains the most commonly employed mucolytic agent, an Australian group reported that total cell counts and neutrophil counts were significantly increased when using an enzyme mixture for dispersal of CF sputum compared with DTT *(52)*.

The protocols our institution employs for processing and culturing oropharyngeal, sputum, and BAL specimens for CF-related bacterial and fungal pathogens are provided below.

3.4.3. Qualitative Bacterial Culture Setup of Oropharyngeal Specimens

1. Place throat swab in 1.0 mL of sterile saline and vortex well.
2. Discard swab.
3. Using a Pasteur pipet, place 1 drop of the saline mixture onto each of the following media: BAP, MAC, MAN, HAE, BCSA. Streak the plates in 4 quadrants for isolation.
4. Place 1 drop in 3 separate spots on the IMA plate. Do not streak.

3.4.4. Quantitative Bacterial Culture Setup of Sputum Specimens

1. Weigh and record the weight (g) of the specimen.
2. Add an equal volume (in mL) of fresh, sterile 10% Sputolysin (DTT) (diluted 10-fold in sterile normal saline), and 3 sterile glass beads to the sputum specimen.
3. Vortex this sputum mixture vigorously for 30–60 s to liquefy the sputum.
4. Allow the suspended mixture to stand at room temperature for 15 min.
5. Add a further 8 parts of sterile normal saline to the original specimen, making a 1/10 dilution (tube 0).
6. Transfer 1.0 mL of 1/10 dilution to tube with 9 mL of saline. This is a 1/100 dilution (tube 1).
7. Transfer 100 μL of 1/100 dilution (tube 1) to tube with 9 mL of saline. This is a $1/10^4$ dilution (tube 2).
8. Transfer 1.0 mL of $1/10^4$ dilution (tube 2) to tube with 9 mL of saline. This is a $1/10^5$ dilution (tube 3).
9. Transfer 1.0 mL of $1/10^5$ dilution (tube 3) to tube with 9 mL of saline. This is a $1/10^6$ dilution (tube 4).

10. From tube 1, place 1 drop in 3 separate spots onto the IMA plate. Do not streak.
11. From tube 1, inoculate BCSA with 3 drops in the same location and streak in 4 quadrants (streak for isolation).
12. Pipet 10 μL from tube 1 onto a MAN and HAE and streak for quantitation:
    a. Place a sterile inoculating loop into the inoculum and streak in a vertical line down the center of the plate. With the same loop, streak from side to side, crossing the center line. This method is frequently used for quantitation of urine cultures.
13. Pipet 10 μL from tube 2 onto a BAP and MAC—mark each 10^6. Streak for quantitation as described above.
14. Pipet 10 μL from tube 3 onto a BAP and MAC—mark each 10^7. Streak for quantitation as described above.
15. Pipet 10 μL from tube 4 onto a BAP and MAC—mark each 10^8. Streak for quantitation as described above.
16. Make a smear to be gram stained from tube 0 (1/10 dilution).
17. Plates are incubated as follows:
    a. BAP (×3) and MAC (×3) plates at 35°C in a CO_2 incubator for 3 d.
    b. HAE plate at 35°C in an anaerobic incubation system for 2 d.
    c. BCSA plate at 35°C in an ambient non-CO_2 incubator for 2 d, then at room temperature for 2 d more (4 d total).
    d. MAN plate at 35°C in an ambient non-CO_2 incubator for 3 d.
    e. IMA plate at 30°C in an ambient non-CO_2 incubator for 5 d.

3.4.5. Quantitative Bacterial Culture Setup of BAL Specimens

1. Estimate the volume of the BAL specimen.
2. Vortex the specimen at high speed for 30–60 s.
3. Use a 0.5-mL aliquot for cell counts and differentials (cytospins).
4. For quantitative microbiology, partition separate aliquots for bacterial, viral, fungal, or mycobacterial testing as indicated by the ordering physician.
5. For bacterial cultures, pipet 10 μL onto each of the following media: BAP, MAC, MAN, HAE, BCSA. Streak for quantitation as described above.
6. Place 1 drop in 3 separate spots on the IMA plate. Do not streak.

3.4.6. Susceptibility Testing of Bacterial Isolates

Due to the increased longevity of CF patients and the use of multiple and frequent courses of antibiotics, resistant strains of bacteria, especially *P. aeruginosa*, have emerged. We generally evaluate sensitivity patterns in specimens from those patients who are admitted to the hospital for intensive therapy or in those who are not responding to our chosen regimen. With the emergence of multiresistant *P. aeruginosa*, it may be helpful to send specimens to reference laboratories that can perform in vitro synergy studies and help to define better drug combinations *(53)*.

4. Notes

1. Quality control for the nebulizer—Check the ultrasonic nebulizer output on a monthly basis. If the output has significantly decreased, by ≥20%, the transducer may need to be replaced.
2. Acceptability of induced sputum sample—Visual inspection of the sample should reveal mucus clumps or plugs mixed in with the saliva.
3. Wheezing or coughing during sputum induction—we have found symptoms not to be necessarily a result of bronchoconstriction but due to mobilization of secretions into the larger airways and mucus plugging.

References

1. Welsh, M. J., Ramsey, B. W., Accurso, F. J., and Cutting, G. R. (2001) Cystic fibrosis, in *The Metabolic and Molecular Bases of Inherited Disease.* (Scriver, C. R., Beaudet, A. L., Valle, D., and Sly, W. S., eds.), McGraw Hill, New York, pp. 521–588.
2. Balough, K., McCubbin, M., Weinberger, M., Smits, W., Ahrens, R., and Fick, R. 1995. The relationship between infection and inflammation in the early stages of lung disease from cystic fibrosis. *Pediatr. Pulmonol.* **20,** 63–70.
3. Khan, T. Z., Wagener, J. S., Bost, T., Martinez, J., Accurso, F. J., and Riches, D. W. (1995) Early pulmonary inflammation in infants with cystic fibrosis [see comments]. *Am. J. Respir. Crit. Care Med.* **151,** 1075–1082.
4. Armstrong, D. S., Grimwood, K., Carzino, R., Carlin, J. B., Olinsky, A. and Phelan, P. D. (1995) Lower respiratory infection and inflammation in infants with newly diagnosed cystic fibrosis. *BMJ* **310,** 1571,1572.
5. Armstrong, D. S., Grimwood, K., Carlin, J. B., Carzino, R., Gutierrez, J. P., Hull, J., et al. (1997) Lower airway inflammation in infants and young children with cystic fibrosis. *Am. J. Respir. Crit. Care Med.* **156,** 1197–1204.
6. Abman, S. H., Ogle, J. W., Harbeck, R. J., Butler-Simon, N., Hammond, K. B., and Accurso, F. J. 1991. Early bacteriologic, immunologic, and clinical courses of young infants with cystic fibrosis identified by neonatal screening. *J. Pediatr.* **119,** 211–217.
7. Kerem, E., Corey, M., Gold, R., and Levison, H. (1990) Pulmonary function and clinical course in patients with cystic fibrosis after pulmonary colonization with Pseudomonas aeruginosa. *J Pediatr.* **116,** 714–719.
8. Nixon, G. M., Armstrong, D. S., Carzino, R., Carlin, J. B., Olinsky, A., Robertson, C. F., and Grimwood, K. (2001) Clinical outcome after early Pseudomonas aeruginosa infection in cystic fibrosis. *J Pediatr.* **138,** 699–704.
9. Kosorok, M. R., Zeng, L., West, S. E., Rock, M. J., Splaingard, M. L., Laxova, A., Green, C. G., Collins, J., and Farrell, P. M. (2001) Acceleration of lung disease in children with cystic fibrosis after Pseudomonas aeruginosa acquisition. *Pediatr Pulmonol.* **32,** 277–287.
10. Gilligan, P. H. (1991) Microbiology of airway disease in patients with cystic fibrosis. *Clin. Microbiol. Rev.* **4,** 35–51.

11. Tosi, M. F., Zakem-Cloud, H., Demko, C. A., Schreiber, J. R., Stern, R. C., Konstan, M. W., and Berger, M. (1995) Cross-sectional and longitudinal studies of naturally occurring antibodies to Pseudomonas aeruginosa in cystic fibrosis indicate absence of antibody-mediated protection and decline in opsonic quality after infection [see comments]. *J. Infect. Dis.* **172,** 453–461.

12. Tablan, O. C., Chorba, T. L., Schidlow, D. V., White, J. W., Hardy, K. A., Gilligan, P. H., et al. (1985) Pseudomonas cepacia colonization in patients with cystic fibrosis: risk factors and clinical outcome. *J. Pediatr.* **107,** 382–387.

13. Thomassen, M. J., Demko, C. A., Klinger, J. D., and Stern, R. C. Pseudomonas cepacia colonization among patients with cystic fibrosis. A new opportunist. *Am. Rev. Respir. Dis.* **131(5),** 791–796.

14. Burns, J. L., Emerson, J., Stapp, J. R., Yim, D. L., Krzewinski, J., Louden, L., et al. (1998) Microbiology of sputum from patients at cystic fibrosis centers in the United States. *Clin. Infect. Dis.* **27,** 158–163.

15. Cystic Fibrosis Foundation 1999 Registry.

16. FitzSimmons, S. C. (1993) The changing epidemiology of cystic fibrosis [see comments]. *J. Pediatr.* **122,** 1–9.

17. Smith, A. L., Redding, G., Doershuk, C., Goldmann, D., Gore, E., Hilman, B., et al. (1988) Sputum changes associated with therapy for endobronchial exacerbation in cystic fibrosis. *J. Pediatr.* **112,** 547–554.

18. Wiesemann, H. G., Steinkamp, G., Ratjen, F., Bauernfeind, A., Przyklenk, B., Doring, G., et al. (1998) Placebo-controlled, double-blind, randomized study of aerosolized tobramycin for early treatment of Pseudomonas aeruginosa colonization in cystic fibrosis. *Pediatr. Pulmonol.* **25,** 88–92.

19. Frederiksen, B., Koch, C. and Hoiby, N. (1997) Antibiotic treatment of initial colonization with Pseudomonas aeruginosa postpones chronic infection and prevents deterioration of pulmonary function in cystic fibrosis [see comments]. *Pediatr. Pulmonol.* **23,** 330–335.

20. Ramsey, B. W., Wentz, K. R., Smith, A. L., Richardson, M., Williams-Warren, J., Hedges, D. L., et al. (1991) Predictive value of oropharyngeal cultures for identifying lower airway bacteria in cystic fibrosis patients. *Am. Rev. Respir. Dis.* **144,** 331–337.

21. Armstrong, D. S., Grimwood, K., Carlin, J. B., Carzino, R., Olinsky, A. and Phelan, P. D. 1996. Bronchoalveolar lavage or oropharyngeal cultures to identify lower respiratory pathogens in infants with cystic fibrosis [see comments]. *Pediatr. Pulmonol.* **21,** 267–275.

22. Thomassen, M. J., Klinger, J. D., Badger, S. J., van Heeckeren, D. W., and Stern, R. C. (1984) Cultures of thoracotomy specimens confirm usefulness of sputum cultures in cystic fibrosis. *J. Pediatr.* **104,** 352–356.

23. Gilljam, H., Malmborg, A. S. and Strandvik, B. (1986) Conformity of bacterial growth in sputum and contamination free endobronchial samples in patients with cystic fibrosis. *Thorax* **41,** 641–646.

24. Hargreave, F. E., Pizzichini, M. M. M. and Pizzichini, E. (1997) Assessment of airway inflammation, in *Asthma.* (Barnes, P. J., Grunstein, M. M., Leff, A. R., and Woolcock, A. J., eds.), Lippincott-Raven, Philadelphia, pp. 1433–1450.

25. Khajotia, R. R., Mohn, A., Pokieser, L., Schalleschak, J., and Vetter, N. (1991) Induced sputum and cytological diagnosis of lung cancer. *Lancet* **338**, 976,977.
26. Metersky, M. L., Aslenzadeh, J. and Stelmach, P. (1998) A comparison of induced and expectorated sputum for the diagnosis of Pneumocystis carinii pneumonia. *Chest* **113**, 1555–1559.
27. Fishman, J. A., Roth, R. S., Zanzot, E., Enos, E. J., and Ferraro, M. J. (1994) Use of induced sputum specimens for microbiologic diagnosis of infections due to organisms other than Pneumocystis carinii. *J. Clin. Microbiol.* **32**, 131–134.
28. Pin, I., Gibson, P. G., Kolendowicz, R., Girgis-Gabardo, A., Denburg, J. A., Hargreave, F. E., and Dolovich, J. (1992) Use of induced sputum cell counts to investigate airway inflammation in asthma. *Thorax* **47**, 25–29.
29. Fahy, J. V., Liu, J., Wong, H., and Boushey, H. A. (1993) Cellular and biochemical analysis of induced sputum from asthmatic and from healthy subjects. *Am. Rev. Respir. Dis.* **147**, 1126–1131.
30. Spanevello, A., Migliori, G. B., Sharara, A., Ballardini, L., Bridge, P., Pisati, P., et al. (1997) Induced sputum to assess airway inflammation: a study of reproducibility. *Clin. Exp. Allergy* **27**, 1138–1144.
31. Pavord, I. D., Pizzichini, M. M., Pizzichini, E., and Hargreave, F. E. (1997) The use of induced sputum to investigate airway inflammation. *Thorax* **52**, 498–501.
32. Keatings, V. M., Evans, D. J., O'Connor, B. J., and Barnes, P. J. (1997) Cellular profiles in asthmatic airways: a comparison of induced sputum, bronchial washings, and bronchoalveolar lavage fluid. *Thorax* **52**, 372–374.
33. Oh, J. W., Lee, H. B., Kim, C. R., Yum, M. K., Koh, Y. J., et al. (1999) Analysis of induced sputum to examine the effects of inhaled corticosteroid on airway inflammation in children with asthma. *Ann. Allergy Asthma Immunol.* **82**, 491–496.
34. Keatings, V. M., Collins, P. D., Scott, D. M., and Barnes, P. J. (1996) Differences in interleukin-8 and tumor necrosis factor-alpha in induced sputum from patients with chronic obstructive pulmonary disease or asthma. *Am. J. Respir. Crit. Care Med.* **153**, 530–534.
35. De Boeck, K., Alifier, M., and Vandeputte, S. (2000) Sputum induction in young cystic fibrosis patients. *Eur. Respir. J.* **16**, 91–94.
36. Henry, R. L., Gibson, P. G., Carty, K., Cai, Y., and Francis, J. L. (1998) Airway inflammation after treatment with aerosolized deoxyribonuclease in cystic fibrosis. *Pediatr. Pulmonol.* **26**, 97–100.
37. Henig, N. R., Tonelli, M. R., Pier, M. V., Burns, J. L., and Aitken, M. L. (2001) Sputum induction as a research tool for sampling the airways of subjects with cystic fibrosis. *Thorax* **56**, 306–311.
38. LiPuma, J. J., Dulaney, B. J., McMenamin, J. D., Whitby, P. W., Stull, T. L., Coenye, T., et al. (1999) Development of rRNA-based PCR assays for identification of Burkholderia cepacia complex isolates recovered from cystic fibrosis patients. *J. Clin. Microbiol.* **37**, 3167–3170.
39. van Belkum, A., Renders, N. H., Smith, S., Overbeek, S. E., and Verbrugh, H. A. (2000) Comparison of conventional and molecular methods for the detection of bacterial pathogens in sputum samples from cystic fibrosis patients. *FEMS Immunol. Med. Microbiol.* **27**, 51–57.

40. Wong, H. H. and Fahy, J. V. (1997) Safety of one method of sputum induction in asthmatic subjects. *Am. J. Respir. Crit. Care Med.* **156,** 299–303.
41. Schoeffel, R. E., Anderson, S. D., and Altounyan, R. E. (1981) Bronchial hyperreactivity in response to inhalation of ultrasonically nebulised solutions of distilled water and saline. *Br. Med. J. (Clin. Res. Ed.)* **283,** 1285–1287.
42. Hoppe, J. E., Holzwarth, I., and Stern, M. (1997) Postal transport of sputa from cystic fibrosis patients does not decrease the microbiological yield. *Zentralbl Bakteriol* **286,** 468–471.
43. Henry, D. A., Campbell, M. E., LiPuma, J. J., and Speert, D. P. (1997) Identification of Burkholderia cepacia isolates from patients with cystic fibrosis and use of a simple new selective medium. *J. Clin. Microbiol.* **35,** 614–619.
44. Wong, K., Roberts, M. C., Owens, L., Fife, M., and Smith, A. L. (1984) Selective media for the quantitation of bacteria in cystic fibrosis sputum. *J. Med. Microbiol.* **17,** 113–119.
45. Doern, G. V. and Brogden-Torres, B. (1992) Optimum use of selective plated media in primary processing of respiratory tract specimens from patients with cystic fibrosis. *J. Clin. Microbiol.* **30,** 2740–2742.
46. Welch, D. F., Muszynski, M. J., Pai, C. H., Marcon, M. J., Hribar, M. M., Gilligan, P. H., et al. (1987) Selective and differential medium for recovery of Pseudomonas cepacia from the respiratory tracts of patients with cystic fibrosis. *J. Clin. Microbiol.* **25,** 1730–1734.
47. Lethem, M. I., James, S. L., and Marriott, C. (1990) The role of mucous glycoproteins in the rheologic properties of cystic fibrosis sputum. *Am. Rev. Respir. Dis.* **142,** 1053–1058.
48. Picot, R., Das, I., and Reid, L. (1978) Pus, deoxyribonucleic acid, and sputum viscosity. *Thorax* **33,** 235–242.
49. May, J. R., Herrick, N. C., and Thompson, D. (1972) Bacterial infection in cystic fibrosis. *Arch. Dis. Child* **47,** 908–913.
50. Hammerschlag, M. R., Harding, L., Macone, A., Smith, A. L., and Goldmann, D. A. (1980) Bacteriology of sputum in cystic fibrosis: evaluation of dithiothreitol as a mucolytic agent. *J. Clin. Microbiol.* **11,** 552–557.
51. Pye, A., Stockley, R. A., and Hill, S. L. (1995) Simple method for quantifying viable bacterial numbers in sputum. *J. Clin. Pathol.* **48,** 719–724.
52. Cai, Y., Carty, K., Gibson, P., and Henry, R. (1996) Comparison of sputum processing techniques in cystic fibrosis. *Pediatr. Pulmonol.* **22,** 402–407.
53. Saiman, L., Mehar, F., Niu, W. W., Neu, H. C., Shaw, K. J., Miller, G., and Prince, A. (1996) Antibiotic susceptibility of multiply resistant Pseudomonas aeruginosa isolated from patients with cystic fibrosis, including candidates for transplantation. *Clin. Infect. Dis.* **23,** 532–537.

29

Antimicrobial Peptides and Proteins in the CF Airway

Alexander M. Cole and Tomas Ganz

1. Introduction
1.1. CF: The Archetypal Mucosal Disease

Most of the morbidity and mortality of cystic fibrosis (CF) is the result of progressive respiratory damage due to uncontrolled airways infection and inflammation. The genetic cause of CF has been localized to a defective CF transmembrane regulator (CFTR) resulting in a failure of epithelial chloride channel function (*1*). The biological consequences of the genetic defect include abnormal epithelial sodium chloride and fluid transport in epithelia, intracellular pH dysregulation with widespread reductions in sialylation of secreted proteins, and an increase in sulfation and fucosylation of mucus glycoproteins. These biochemical alterations have detectable consequences, including salty sweat and thick mucus. However, the pathogenetic link to the clinically most important aspect of CF, the colonization of respiratory epithelia by bacteria including *Staphylococcus aureus, Hemophilus influenzae,* and most characteristically, mucoid *Pseudomonas aeruginosa*, has not been elucidated. The search for the link between the CF gene defect and the airways colonization was given new impetus by the proposal that the bacterial colonization in CF is due to the abnormal composition of airway surface fluid (*2,3*).

1.2. Antimicrobial (Poly)peptides in Airway Secretions

Airway secretions form a mechanical and chemical barrier to inhaled microbes and form a first line of host defense against microbial invaders. Their antimicrobial properties are due largely to their content of antimicrobial proteins and peptides. Lysozyme and lactoferrin are the most abundant antimicrobial proteins of airway fluid. They are stored in and secreted from serous cells in submucosal glands, and in inflamed secretions they are also secreted from

From: *Methods in Molecular Medicine, vol. 70: Cystic Fibrosis Methods and Protocols*
Edited by: W. R. Skach © Humana Press Inc., Totowa, NJ

neutrophils. Lysozyme and lactoferrin are bactericidal alone for Gram-positive and in concert for some Gram-negative bacteria *(4,5)*. The human β-defensin-1 (HBD-1) is constitutively expressed at low levels in both the lower and upper airways, while HBD-2 is predominantly induced at sites of airway inflammation *(6,7)*. The α-defensin, HNP-1 *(8)* has also been found at varying concentrations in bronchoalveolar lavage (BAL) *(9)* and is likely a degranulation product of transudated neutrophils found in infected airways. Secretory leukoprotease inhibitor is also present at potentially antimicrobial concentrations *(10)*. Anionic antimicrobial (poly)peptides may also contribute to the antimicrobial activity of the airways, and have been detected in ovine and human BAL fluid *(11,12)*. The abundance of antimicrobial peptides and proteins present in airway secretions suggests that the antimicrobial activity of airway fluid results from the combined effects of its many components.

1.3. Synergistic Effects of a Complex Antimicrobial Soup

The mixture of proteins in airway fluid may interact in a complex manner with a net effect that is distinct from individual proteins' separate action. Indeed, studies have revealed a synergistic microbicidal effect of lysozyme with other airway antimicrobials, such as lactoferrin *(4,13)* and anionic peptides *(14)*. Other airway fluid components, including various ions, mucins, and in inflamed fluids also nucleic acids, can bind cationic antimicrobial substances or their microbial targets and modulate the antimicrobial activity of the fluid. Therefore, the putative antimicrobial fluid defect of CF airways could be due to variations in the presence, concentration, and interactions of antimicrobial peptides. In contrast to recent studies that have focused on the antibacterial action of individual components of lower airway fluids *(6,7,15,16)*, the analysis of minimally manipulated airway fluid affords the opportunity to assess the combined antimicrobial activity of multiple components.

1.4. The Influence of Inactive Components on Antimicrobial Activity

Certain factors within airway fluid, including ions and anionic macromolecules, are known to decrease the activity of many antimicrobial peptides. Initial studies on cultured airway epithelial cells revealed that common CF pathogens were killed when added to the apical fluid of cultured normal airway epithelia, but proliferated in the fluid of cultured CF airway epithelia *(3)*. Additionally, the apical fluid concentration of NaCl was elevated in CF airway secretions. The difference in antimicrobial activity between normal and CF epithelia was in part attributed to salt-sensitive factors such as antimicrobial peptides. However, in a slightly different system of cultured epithelia, salt concentrations did not differ between CF and normal cultures *(17,18)*. Rather, in this system CF airway epithelia absorbed airway surface liquid at an elevated rate, which depleted the periciliary liquid layer and subsequently reduced mucus transport *(18)*.

The activity of antimicrobial peptides could be adversely affected regardless of which of these two models applies in vivo. While increased salt concentrations would interfere with the function of many antimicrobial polypeptides, diminished mucociliary clearance would prolong the exposure time of inhaled microbes to antimicrobial substances and could permit microbial adaptation or the emergence of resistant variants. Specific questions that remain to be answered about CF airway fluid include: (1) whether antimicrobial polypeptides are produced in normal or sufficient quantities; (2) which, if any, of the polypeptides are defective; (3) whether the increased production of inhibitory substances (e.g., polyanionic macromolecules) interferes with effective antimicrobial polypeptide activity; and (4) whether the increased production of antimicrobial polypeptides contributes to destructive airway inflammation. Investigations of the antimicrobial activity of natural airway fluid are an appropriate first step in answering these questions.

1.5. Principles of Antimicrobial Fluid Testing

In constructing this chapter, we have followed the traditional biochemical methodology, proceeding from the whole airway fluid and its activity to its biochemical fractionation and the purification and testing of individual components. This approach differs from the most common strategy in the antimicrobial peptide field, in which individual antimicrobial components are purified first and their biological activity is determined later. However, the latter strategy does not adequately address the interactions of the multiple antimicrobial substances in biological fluids and the modulation of their activity by other fluid constituents. To overcome this limitation, the investigator might first directly test minimally manipulated airway fluid for microbicidal activity, and then proceed to fractionation during which the activity of the individual fractions is assayed at each step of the purification until individual active components are pure. The logical final step is the reconstitution of the total activity of the fluid from its individual active components and inactive and modulating fractions.

2. Materials
2.1. Sampling Minimally Manipulated Airway Fluids
2.1.1. Collection Techniques

1. Pediatric #8 French catheters with finger suction control (Safe-T-Vac Suction Catheter Kit, Kendall, Mansfield, MA).
2. 15-mL conical tubes (Fisher Scientific, Pittsburgh, PA).
3. 16-gage needles.
4. Bunsen burner.
5. Laboratory or bedside vacuum port.
6. Whatman #541 filter paper.

7. Ruler with millimeter markings.
8. Sterile scalpels to cut filter paper and catheter tubing.
9. Balance, accurate to 0.1 mg (e.g., Mettler AE100).

2.1.2. Processing

1. Sonicating probe with microtip attachment (BioSonik IV, Bronwill, VWR Scientific, San Francisco, CA).
2. Branson 1200 sonicating water bath (Bransonic Cleaning Equipment, Shelton, CT).
3. Finely crushed ice.
4. Styrofoam float.
5. Mixer, vortex.
6. *N*-acetyl cysteine (NAC) (Sigma).
7. Glacial acetic acid (Fisher).
8. Vacuum centrifuge (e.g., Integrated SpeedVac System ISS110, Savant Instruments, Holbrook, NY).
9. Sterile forceps.

2.2. Identifying Antimicrobial Compounds of Airway Fluid

2.2.1. Batch Separation

1. Glacial acetic acid.
2. Microtip sonicating probe.
3. 1× NB: 75 mM NaCl, 20 mM KCl, 1 mM CaCl$_2$, 0.5 mM MgCl$_2$, 10 mM phosphate buffer, pH 7.3–7.4.
4. 1× Dulbecco's phosphate-buffered saline (PBS), pH 7.4 (Sigma).
5. 25 mM sodium acetate, pH 7.5 (Sigma).
6. Carboxymethyl Macroprep resin (CM resin; Bio-Rad, Hercules, CA).
7. SepPak Vac C4–C18 columns (Waters Corporation, Millford, MA).
8. Methanol (Fisher).
9. Trifluoroacetic acid (Sigma).
10. HPLC-grade acetonitrile (Fisher).
11. 20-cc syringe with luer-lock fitting, to collect eluate from SepPak Vac columns.

2.2.2. Fractionation

2.2.2.1. Molecular Filtration

1. BioGel P-10 resin (Bio-Rad).
2. Urea (Sigma).
3. Glacial acetic acid.
4. 1.0 × 80 cm glass column with frit to support resin (Flexcolumn, Kontes, Vineland, NJ).
5. Peristaltic pump (e.g., Econo Pump, Bio-Rad).
6. Variable-wavelength absorbance monitor (e.g., V^4 Absorbance Detector, Isco, Lincoln, NE).
7. Fraction collector (e.g., RediFrac, Amersham Pharmacia Biotech, Piscataway, NJ).

2.2.2.2. CATION-EXCHANGE HPLC

1. 7.5 × 50 mm Vydac 400VHP strong cation-exchange HPLC column (Western Analytical Products, Murrieta, CA).
2. Variable-speed HPLC pump, controller, absorbance detector, fraction collector, and chart recorder. Our system includes: Waters 600S controller, Waters 626 pump, Waters 490E programmable multiwavelength detector, Waters fraction collector, and Servogor 120 flatbed recorder (Norma Goerz Instruments, Elk Grove Village, IL).
3. HPLC-grade water (Fisher).
4. HPLC-grade acetonitrile (Fisher).
5. Sodium chloride (Sigma).
6. Vacuum centrifuge.

2.2.2.3. REVERSE-PHASE HPLC

1. 4.6 × 250 mm Vydac 218TP reverse-phase C18 HPLC column (Western Analytical Products).
2. HPLC system (*see* **Subheading 2.2.2.2.**).
3. HPLC-grade water.
4. HPLC-grade acetonitrile.
5. Trifluoroacetic acid.
6. Vacuum centrifuge.

2.2.3. Quantitative Techniques

2.2.3.1. LYSOZYME ENZYMATIC ASSAY

1. HPLC-purified human milk lysozyme (Sigma).
2. Lyophilized *Micrococcus lysodeikticus* (Sigma).
3. Low-electroendoosmotic (EEO) agarose (Sigma).
4. 9 × 9 × 1.5 cm square plastic Petri dishes (Nunc, Baxter Scientific Products).
5. Custom-made stainless steel gel punch (3 mm × 5 cm).
6. Gel-leveling table (Research Products, Mount Prospect, IL).
7. 10× magnifier (Bausch and Lomb; Fisher).

2.2.3.2. SEMIQUANTITATIVE AU-PAGE WESTERN BLOT ANALYSIS

1. Hoeffer Mini electrophoresis system with gel casting apparatus (Amersham Pharmacia).
2. 250-V variable-voltage power supply.
3. Solution A: 60% acrylamide, 1.6% *bis*-acrylamide (Sigma).
4. Solution B: 43.2% acetic acid, 4% TEMED (Sigma).
5. Vertical transfer blotting apparatus (Transblot; Bio-Rad).
6. Loading buffer: 9 M urea in 5% acetic acid with methyl green (Sigma). Store at –20°C.
7. Coomassie staining solution: 25% methanol, 5.6% formaldehyde, 0.1% Coomassie Blue R250.
8. Destain solution: 25% methanol, 0.74% formaldehyde.
9. Transfer buffer: 0.7% acetic acid, 10% methanol.

10. Immobilon P^{SQ} PVDF membrane (Millipore, Bedford, MA).
11. Tris-buffered saline (TBS): 500 mM NaCl, 20 mM Tris-HCl, pH 7.5.
12. TTBS = TBS + 0.05% Tween-20.
13. Primary antibody solution in 1× TBS: 1% bovine skin (60 bloom) gelatin (Sigma), 0.01% thimerosal (Sigma), 0.05% Tween-20, 1/1000 dilution of appropriate antibody.
14. Secondary antibody solution in 1× TBS: 1% gelatin, 0.05% Tween 20, 1/2000 dilution of goat anti-rabbit alkaline phosphatase-conjugated antibody (Pierce Chemical, Rockford, IL).
15. Nitroblue tetrazolium (NBT; Sigma): 0.5 g NBT in 10 mL 70% dimethylformamide.
16. 5-Bromo-4-chloro-3-indolyl phosphate (BCIP; Sigma): 0.5 g BCIP in 10 mL 100% dimethylformamide.
17. Developing solution: 198 µL NBT + 99 µL BCIP in developing buffer (100 mM NaCl, 5 mM MgCl$_2$, 100 mM Tris-HCl, pH 9.5).

2.2.4. Depleting and Restoring Cationic (Poly)peptides

1. CM resin (Bio-Rad).
2. Rotisserie mixer (Barnstead Thermolyne, Dubuque, IA).
3. Vacuum centrifuge.

2.2.5. Antimicrobial Assays

2.2.5.1. MICROORGANISMS

We have used *Escherichia coli, Pseudomonas aeruginosa, Salmonella typhimurium, Candida albicans, Staphylococcus aureus, Staphylococcus epidermidis*, and *Bacillus subtilis* for both the standard and micro-CFU assays. All strains can be cultured in 1× trypticase soy broth (TSB; Becton Dickinson, Cockeyswille, MD) and the OD/CFU ratio (given as an approximate value in **Subheading 3.2.6.1.**) should be determined empirically for each strain.

2.2.5.2. CFU ASSAYS

1. Trypticase soy broth.
2. Trypticase soy agar plates (10 cm; Microdiagnostics, Lombard, IL).
3. Thermomixer (Eppendorf Thermomixer R, Brinkmann Instruments, Waterbury, NY).
4. Incubator, 37°C.
5. 10 mM sodium phosphate, pH 7.4 (Sigma).
6. Custom-made glass wand to spread bacterial cultures.
7. Spectophotometer (e.g., Beckman DU-64).
8. 72-well Terasaki microtiter plates (Nalge Nunc, Denmark).
9. Liquid wax (MJ Research, Watertown, MA).
10. 0.01–2-µL capacity micropipettor (Eppendorf).

2.2.5.3. MINIMAL HANDLING ASSAY

1. Low EEO agarose.
2. 37°C waterbath.

3. Trypticase soy broth.
4. 24-chamber tissue culture dish (Corning).
5. 10× dissecting microscope (e.g., Nikon).

3. Methods

3.1. Sampling Minimally Manipulated Airway Fluids

3.1.1. Alternative Collection Techniques to BAL

Bronchoalveolar lavage (BAL) of airway secretions is a standard method of collection adopted by many laboratories studying the processes of airway infection and inflammation. It is clear why this sampling method is so highly regarded: BAL is easily obtainable as a by-product of clinical intervention and relatively large volumes are obtained, which can then be analyzed in multiple assays. Collection of nasal lavage fluid has also been in favor for much the same reasons. However, the main problem plaguing the analysis of BAL and nasal lavage fluids is the inevitable and difficult-to-determine dilution factor. Two methods to collect and process airway secretions that do not dilute the fluid are presented here.

3.1.1.1. NASAL SECRETIONS, A MODEL UPPER AIRWAY FLUID

Nasal fluid has recently been used as a model airway fluid, since the fluid is readily accessible and collection is rapid, efficient, and reproducible. Although lower airway fluid could also be collected by vacuum aspiration during bronchoscopy or after endotracheal intubation, it is difficult to avoid the admixture of local anesthetics or other fluids introduced during bronchoscopy. The alternative method, collection from donors with an endotracheal tube, also modifies the airway fluid, often causing intense coughing and hypersecretion, or microbial colonization and inflammation during more prolonged use.

1. Construct an apparatus to collect nasal fluid (**Fig. 1**). First, cut the tubing of a pediatric #8 French catheter in half on the bias (*see* **Note 1**).
2. Melt two holes in the cap of a 15-mL conical tube using a hot 16-gage needle.
3. Thread cut ends of the catheter tubing through the holes created in the cap.
4. Connect the apparatus to either the standard laboratory or bedside vacuum port.
5. Collect nasal fluid by gently manipulating the tip of the catheter in the nostril approx 1–3 cm from the nasal aperture. Ipsilateral and contralateral stimulation will occur if the catheter tip is moved between nostrils.
6. Stop collection when the secretions are sparse or after approx 10 min.
7. Keep fluid at 4°C for immediate use or at –20°C (or colder) for long-term storage.

3.1.1.2. FILTER PAPER COLLECTION OF UPPER AIRWAY FLUIDS

Although the collection of upper airway fluid by vacuum aspiration can be done with minimal stimulation, the composition of such nasal fluid may not represent that of the baseline unstimulated airway fluid. One method that

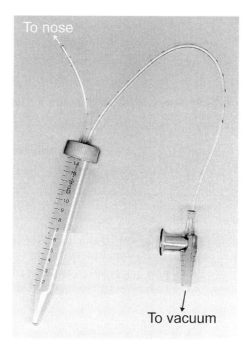

To nose

To vacuum

Fig. 1. Apparatus for collecting nasal fluid.

attempts to diminish the duration and intensity of mechanical stimulation further, the extraction of nasal fluid by filter paper, is presented here. Similar methods can be implemented during bronchoscopy to allow the collection of fluid from the lower airways *(17)*.

1. Cut Whatman #541 filter paper into 0.5 × 3-cm strips and store in an airtight container.
2. Weigh filter paper to the nearest 0.1 mg immediately before use.
3. Gently feed filter paper into the nasal vestibule and press gently against the mucosa for 10 s.
4. Weigh filter paper after fluid collection, preferably in a humidified chamber. The difference in weight of the wet as compared to dry filter paper is a good approximation of fluid volume (1 mg $\simeq$ 1 µL).
5. Store filter paper in a 1.5–2.0-mL microcentrifuge tube at –80°C.

3.1.2. Processing

3.1.2.1. PHYSICAL TECHNIQUES TO FLUIDIZE WHOLE SECRETIONS

Airway fluid contains factors, such as entangled and aggregated mucins and other polyglycosylated proteins, which must be disrupted to obtain a homogenous solution. Except in the most highly particulate mucus-containing samples, sonication can be used to disrupt the mucus clumps.

Method 1: Microtip Sonication

1. Aliquot at least 100 µL into a 1.5-mL microcentrifuge tube. Chill tube in an ice–water slush.
2. Sonicate until fluid, but for no more than three bursts of 10 s each burst.

Method 2: Water Bath Sonication

1. This method is gentler than the microtip sonication and can homogenize <100 µL of airway fluid. Fill a water bath sonicator with ice-cold water.
2. Place tubes in a styrofoam float. Sonicate for 1–2 h.
3. Periodically vortex samples.
4. Maintain temperature of water <8°C throughout sonication by periodically adding finely crushed ice or replacing warm water with ice-cold water.

3.1.2.2. CHEMICAL TECHNIQUE TO FLUIDIZE SECRETIONS

Airway fluid can be treated with *N*-acetylcysteine (NAC; Sigma, St. Louis, MO) at 1% final concentration for 10 min at room temperature to disaggregate mucin beads by reducing the crosslinking disulfide bonds. NAC (1%) had no detectable effect on the growth of Gram-negative (*P. aeruginosa*) or Gram-positive bacteria (*S. aureus*) or on the antimicrobial activity of nasal fluid *(19)*. Additionally, airway fluid also contains several antimicrobial polypeptides that are stabilized by disulfide bonds, such as lysozyme and defensins *(5,20)*. Using lysozyme as a model antimicrobial polypeptide with four disulfide bonds, we also demonstrated that NAC does not disrupt the muramidase activity of lysozyme.

1. Make 20% NAC stock immediately before use (*see* **Note 2**).
2. Add 20% NAC directly to airway fluid at a final concentration of 1% NAC.
3. Vortex gently and incubate at room temperature for 10 min to 1 h, depending on viscosity of fluid.
4. Fluid can be used immediately or stored at –20°C.

3.1.2.3. RECONSTITUTING AIRWAY SECRETIONS FROM FILTER PAPER

1. Calculate volume of airway fluid based on the weight of nasal fluid wicked onto the filter paper strip (*see* **Subheading 3.1.1.2.**).
2. Add 500 µL of 5–10% acetic acid to the microcentrifuge tube containing the filter paper.
3. Vortex vigorously for 10 min.
4. Push the filter paper to the bottom of the tube with a pipet tip and collect the fluid. Wring out the excess fluid using sterile forceps.
5. Repeat **steps 2–4** three times. Pool supernatants into a clean tube. Dry sample by vacuum centrifugation (*see* **Note 3**).
6. Resuspend sample in dH$_2$O to the original calculated volume of fluid.

3.1.3. Analyzing the Antimicrobial Properties of Minimally Manipulated Fluid

Assaying minimally manipulated airway fluid for natural antimicrobial activity is the first step in identifying the active components. Whole airway fluid, collected and processed as presented above, can be admixed with bacteria or fungi and directly subjected to colony-forming unit (CFU) assays (*see* **Subheading 3.2.6.**). The microbicidal profile obtained from analyzing the whole fluid will serve as the basis for following the activity of subsequent purifications.

3.2. Identifying Antimicrobial Compounds of Airway Fluid

Several biochemical properties of antimicrobial peptides facilitate their isolation. They are readily and often selectively soluble in acidic solvents that denature many larger proteins. Most known antimicrobial peptides are cationic at neutral pH, which allow their separation from the anionic molecules by ion-exchange matrices with positive charge selectivity. By definition, antimicrobial peptides are <10 kDa, so they can be separated from larger proteins by molecular filtration or size-exclusion chromatography. In addition, most peptides are amphipathic in solution, i.e., exhibit a conformation that regionalizes hydrophobic side chains. This feature enables separation using organic (reverse-phase) solvents. The following sections present several protocols specifically adapted to take advantage of one or more of these attributes.

3.2.1. Batch Separations

Batch purification can efficiently concentrate peptides of interest and is an effective means to separate antimicrobial peptides from other molecules. Thus, batch methods that require minimal prehandling of human fluids, cells, or tissues are frequently used as the primary mode of separation.

3.2.1.1. ACID EXTRACTION

1. Acidify airway secretions to a final concentration of 5–10% acetic acid.
2. Homogenize using a microtip sonicator at low power for three bursts of 5–20 s each.
3. Incubate at RT for 1 h with intermittent vortexing (*see* **Notes 4** and **5**).
4. Clarify by centrifugation at >14,000*g* for 10 min and discard pellet.

3.2.1.2. SELECTIVE CATIONIC PEPTIDE EXTRACTION

1. Buffer carboxymethyl (CM) resin with 25 m*M* ammonium acetate, pH 6.0, as a 50% slurry (*see* **Note 6**).
2. Dilute airway secretions 5–10-fold in 25 m*M* ammonium acetate, pH 6.0, and add 0.1 vol of equilibrated CM slurry. Incubate end-over-end using a rotisserie mixer overnight at 4°C.
3. Sediment the resin at 300*g* for 5 min. Aspirate and discard supernatant.
4. Wash resin with 25 m*M* ammonium acetate, pH 7.5.
5. Incubate twice with 10–20 bed volumes of 5–10% acetic acid for 2 h each to elute bound peptides and proteins.

3.2.1.3. HYDROPHOBIC EXCHANGE COLUMNS

1. Prime a SepPak Vac C18 column with 20 bed volumes of methanol followed by 40 bed volumes of dH$_2$O/0.1% TFA (*see* **Note 7**).

2. Add 2–10 vol of dH$_2$O/0.1% TFA to homogenized and clarified nasal secretions. Vortex sample and introduce directly to the resin bed. Set buffer flow at a rate of 0.2–1.0 mL/min.
3. Wash column with 40 bed volumes of dH$_2$O/0.1% TFA.
4. Elute the retained peptides with a step gradient of 20, 40, and 60% acetonitrile/0.1% TFA.

Recovered peptides from these three techniques can be dried by vacuum centrifugation and further purified by gel chromatography or HPLC.

3.2.2. Fractionation

3.2.2.1. MOLECULAR FILTRATION

Since antimicrobial peptides are small compared to most proteins, gel filtration (permeation) chromatography can be used as the first purification step. Polyacrylamide matrices that separate molecules with an M_r <10,000 (e.g., BioGel P-10, Bio-Rad) have been most useful in antimicrobial peptide purification and their selectivity is in some cases enhanced by additional interactions of antimicrobial peptides with the matrix, which delay their elution beyond that expected from size considerations alone.

1. Pour a 1 cm × 80 cm BioGel P-10 column equilibrated in 5% acetic acid/3 M urea.
2. Prime column overnight with running buffer (5% acetic acid/3 M urea) at 0.2 mL/min.
3. Resuspend sample in <1 mL of 5% acetic acid/3 M urea and load directly onto resin bed.
4. Set flow at 0.4 mL/min, monitor absorbance at 280 nm, and collect peak fractions (note that the use of acetic acid as a solvent introduces a very high background at 215–225 nm).
5. Dilute target fractions 10-fold in dH$_2$O and concentrate proteins using a SepPak (*see* **Subheading 3.2.1.3.**)
6. Concentrated proteins can be analyzed for antimicrobial activity or subjected to further purification.

3.2.2.2. CATION-EXCHANGE HPLC

Partially purified peptide mixtures subjected to cation-exchange HPLC are bound under aqueous conditions and eluted on an increasing salt concentration gradient.

1. Resuspend partially purified (poly)peptide solution in water and separate for 100 min on a 7.5 × 50 mm Vydac 400VHP strong cation-exchange column using a 10 mM NaCl increment per minute linear gradient in an appropriate buffer (*see* **Note 8**).
2. Monitor absorbance at 205–220 nm and at 280 nm and collect peak protein fractions.
3. Dry fractions by vacuum centrifugation and desalt by SepPak (*see* **Subheading 3.2.1.3.**) for antimicrobial analyses, or subject to reverse phase-HPLC for further purification.

3.2.2.3. REVERSE-PHASE (RP)-HPLC

The most commonly used RP-HPLC matrix utilizes supports to which C4–C18 hydrocarbons are bound and gradients of water-miscible organic solvents are used to elute the bound polypeptides in the "reverse" phase. RP-HPLC is often used to desalt and further purify heterogeneous fractions from cation-exchange HPLC.

1. Resuspend partially purified (poly)peptide solution in 1% acetic acid and separate for 90 min on a 4.6×250 mm Vydac C18 column using a 0.75%/min linear gradient of acetonitrile in 0.1% TFA.
2. Monitor absorbance at 205–220 nm and at 280 nm and collect peak protein fractions.
3. Dry fractions by vacuum centrifugation, resuspend in 0.01% acetic acid or other desired buffer for antimicrobial analyses.

3.2.3. Quantitative Techniques

Several quantitative techniques are useful in following the fractionation of known constituents of airway fluid and other mucosal fluids. Lysozyme, a ubiquitous component of mucosal fluids and often the predominant antimicrobial polypeptide, can be traced and quantified by its enzymatic activity. Specific antibodies are commercially available for many other antimicrobial polypeptides, and a dot-blot or Western blot technique is useful for immunodetection of specific polypeptides in multiple fractions.

3.2.3.1. LYSOZYME ENZYMATIC ASSAY

1. Resuspend 0.5 mg/mL of lyophilized *Micrococcus lysodeikticus* in 66 mM sodium phosphate buffer (Na_2HPO_4/NaH_2PO_4, pH 7.0) with molten 1% low-EEO agarose in 66 mM sodium phosphate *(21)*.
2. Immediately pour 10 mL agarose/*Micrococcus* solution in a level 9×9 cm square Petri dish.
3. Punch 16–25 evenly spaced 3-mm wells in the solidified agarose.
4. Introduce 5 μL of sample or lysozyme standard into each well. Incubate for 3–18 h, depending on concentration of lysozyme.
5. Measure the diameters of zones of clearance relative to lysozyme standards to determine lysozyme enzymatic activity (*see* **Note 9**).

3.2.3.2. SEMIQUANTITATIVE AU-PAGE WESTERN BLOT ANALYSIS

1. Pour a 12.5% acid–urea Hoeffer mini slab gel: For five gels, dissolve 14.4 g urea in 20.3 mL water. Add 10 mL of solution A and 6-mL of solution B, de-gas for 10 min, and add 0.9 mL of 10% APS. Let polymerize for 2 h at room temperature.
2. Prerun gel in 5% acetic acid running buffer for approx 2 h at 90–100 V constant voltage toward the negative electrode.
3. Premix sample and loading buffer, load onto gel, and electrophorese for ~2–3 h at 70–80 V. A duplicate gel may be electrophoresed to identify protein bands by Coomassie staining (**Fig. 2**).

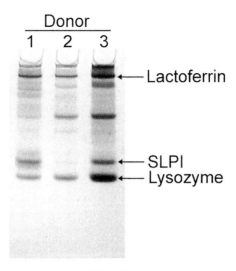

Fig. 2. Coomassie-stained AU-PAGE of 2.5 µL whole nasal fluid from three healthy donors. Three major antimicrobial polypeptides are readily identifiable (SLPI = secretory leukoprotease inhibitor). Note interdonor protein variability.

4. Electroblot onto Immobilon P^{SQ} PVDF membranes in 0.7% acetic acid/10% methanol for approx 30 min at 0.16 A constant current.
5. Place membrane in 3% gelatin/1× TBS and incubate at room temperature for 1 h.
6. Incubate membrane with primary rabbit antihuman antisera diluted 1/1000 in 1% gelatin/TBS overnight at room temperature.
7. Wash membrane three times in TTBS for 15 min each with gentle agitation.
8. Add secondary anti-rabbit antibody coupled with alkaline phosphatase and incubate at room temperature for 1 h.
9. Wash as in **step 7**. Rinse in 1× TBS for 5 min.
10. Add chromogenic developing solution that has been prewarmed to room temperature. Develop membrane to desired intensity and stop reaction by rinsing several times in dH$_2$O.

3.2.3.3. Dot-Blot Analysis

The dot blot, an adaptation of the Western blot technique, immunodetects antimicrobial polypeptides in whole or partially purified airway fluids without gel electrophoresis. This efficient method is particularly suited to identify antimicrobial peptides in multiple patients and in numerous chromatographic fractions. To prevent the loss of protein from the membrane, the protein-binding capacity of the membrane should not be exceeded.

1. Spot 1–2 µL of the tested fluid or protein standard directly onto an Immobilon P^{SQ} PVDF membrane.
2. Let the membrane dry at room temperature (typically 10–20 min).
3. Proceed with **steps 5–10** in **Subheading 3.2.3.2.**

3.2.4. Depleting Airway Fluid of Cationic (Poly)peptides

Airway secretions can be depleted of their cationic peptides while maintaining the in-vivo concentrations of all other components. Subsequent reconstitution of the depleted fluid will determine factors that directly contribute to the activity of airway secretions.

1. Clarify homogenized airway fluid by centrifugation at 10,000g for 10 min.
2. Equilibrate a weak cation-exchange matrix (CM resin) with a buffer that approximates the electrolyte composition of airway fluid (*see* **Note 10**).
3. Sediment the resin at 10,000g for 10 min and remove the overlying buffer.
4. Add clarified airway fluid to the CM matrix at a 4/1 ratio and vortex briefly.
5. Incubate end-over-end for 24 h at 4°C.
6. Remove the CM matrix by centrifugation. Freeze the resulting cation-depleted supernatant at –20°C in aliquots for subsequent experiments.

3.2.5. Restoring the Antimicrobial Activity of CM-Depleted Airway Fluid

Reconstituting CM-depleted airway secretions with purified antimicrobial peptides, either alone or in combination, should restore the fluid's antimicrobial activity. Presented here is an effective method to supplement airway fluid without altering the concentrations of endogenous components.

1. Purify antimicrobial peptides from airway fluid by batch separation and fractionation as described in previous sections (*see* **Note 11** for alternative methods).
2. Dry desired amount of purified antimicrobial peptide by vacuum centrifugation. Take care not to overdry the sample or dry with excess heat.
3. Add CM-depleted airway fluid directly to the dried peptide and resuspend by pipetting gently.
4. Compare depleted and reconstituted fluid in CFU antimicrobial assays.

3.2.6. Antimicrobial Assays to Analyze Peptides and Scant Airway Fluids

3.2.6.1. MICROBES AND CULTURE CONDITIONS

1. Culture microbes (from glycerol stock) 18 h on trypticase soy agar (TSA) plates at 37°C. Store plates for 3–4 wk at 4°C.
2. Inoculate a single colony into 50 mL of TSB and incubate at 250 rpm for 18 h in a 37°C environmental incubator.
3. Subculture the overnight culture 1/100 into 50 mL TSB and incubate at 250 rpm for 2.5 h (37°C) to obtain microbes in mid-logarithmic growth phase.
4. Sediment microbes at 1500g for 10 min.
5. Wash bacteria in 10 mM sodium phosphate, pH 7.4 (NaP), and sediment microbes at 1500g for 10 min.
6. Resuspend microbes in 1–2 mL of 10 mM NaP (*see* **Note 12**), and measure optical density. For bacteria, an OD_{625} = 0.2 was equivalent to 2.5×10^7 CFU/mL. For yeast, an OD_{450} = 1.0 was 2.5×10^7 CFU/mL.

3.2.6.2. STANDARD COLONY-FORMING UNIT ASSAY

1. Dilute bacteria (OD_{625} = 0.2) or yeast (OD_{450} = 1.0) 100-fold in 10 mM NaP.
2. Test sample consists of 72 μL of either bacterial or yeast dilution plus 288 μL of peptide in 10 mM NaP/0.03% TSB or minimally manipulated airway fluid for each condition, to allow triplicates of four timepoints (0, 1, 3, and 24 h incubation). After mixing sample and bacteria, divide equally into three tubes.
3. Incubate tubes at 37°C at 650 rpm in an Eppendorf Thermomixer R.
4. At each timepoint, hand-spread 25 μL in triplicate on TSA plates to count CFUs.
5. Dilute samples that are expected to have >5 × 10^5 CFU/mL in 10 mM NaP prior to plating.
6. Incubate plates overnight at 37°C and count colonies 18–24 h later.

3.2.6.3. MICRO-CFU ASSAY: ANALYSIS OF 1 μL OF BIOLOGICAL FLUIDS

1. Dilute bacteria (OD_{625} = 0.2) or yeast (OD_{450} = 1.0) 100-fold in 10 mM NaP.
2. The test sample consists of 3 μL of either bacterial or yeast dilution plus 12 μL of nasal fluid for each condition, which permits triplicates of four timepoints (0, 1, 3, and 24 h incubation). Separate tubes with 3 μL bacteria or yeast and 12 μL of 1× NB/0.2% TSB are used as controls for microbial growth.
3. Load each well of a 72-well Terasaki microtiter plate with 1.5 μL of liquid wax to prevent evaporation.
4. Load 1 μL of the test sample into each of 12 wells by pipetting directly underneath the liquid wax. The entire plate is incubated at 37°C.
5. Wash wells thoroughly with 47.5 μL of 10 mM NaP to recover the incubated fluid at the specified timepoints, and immediately place the wash fluid on ice.
6. Hand-spread the wash fluid on TSA plates, incubate 18–24 h at 37°C, and count CFUs.

3.2.6.4. MINIMAL HANDLING ANTIMICROBIAL ASSAY

Osmotically fragile bacteria may not survive the physical manipulation of hand spreading onto agar plates. If subjected to an assay that immobilizes the bacteria to prevent mechanical and osmotic stress, the bacteria can recover and proliferate.

1. Standard or micro-CFU assay proceeds as under **Subheadings 3.2.6.2.** and **3.2.6.3.**
2. Instead of hand spreading onto TSA plates, mix 25–50 μL of test sample with 950–975 μL 1% low EEO agarose/3% TSB that is kept fluid at 42°C and immediately pour into one well of a 24-chamber tissue culture dish.
3. Once the agarose has solidified, pour 500 μL of molten 1% agarose over the underlay. This layer serves as a non-nutritive overlay to prevent the growth of large, visually obstructive surface colonies.
4. After 18 h incubation at 37°C, count small colonies formed within the underlay under a 10× dissecting microscope.

4. Notes

1. The nasal end of the catheter should be no longer than 10 cm. The shorter the tubing, the less fluid will unrecoverably stick to the sides of the tubing.

2. Old NAC may become oxidized and thus will lose some of its reducing capability.
3. It may be difficult to resuspend proteins when the sample is dried to completion. Instead, we find that concentrating the sample to 10–50 µL maintains the solubility of most components.
4. Although many peptides and proteins will be extracted by 1 h incubation in acetic acid, longer incubation times have shown increased recovery. Double acid extractions have also proved helpful.
5. When batch-purifying airway secretions, selective precipitation of unwanted proteins can be enhanced further by adding organic solvents such as methanol *(22)*.
6. The CM slurry and airway fluid can alternatively be buffered with 1× PBS or 1× NB. We find that the added salts reduce the binding capacity of the CM resin, but increase the selectivity for bound cationic (poly)peptides.
7. SepPak column extraction can be empirically optimized to remove nontarget proteins by testing alternative hydrophobic supports with straight-chain hydrocarbons ranging from C4 to C18.
8. Examples of running solutions include: 25 mM Tris-HCl, pH 7.4; 50 mM ammonium formate, pH 6.0; and 25 mM sodium borate, pH 9.0.
9. Measure the zones of clearance as quickly as possible, since diffused lysozyme is still active. Alternatively, place the plate at 4°C for 20 min to slow the enzymatic activity before measuring the zone diameters.
10. For nasal fluid, use 1× NB: CM resin, equilibrated with this buffer before binding, did not alter the ionic composition of the nasal fluid.
11. We have utilized baculovirus expression systems for the production of antimicrobial peptides *(23)*. Many antimicrobial peptides, such as the defensins, are stabilized by several disulfide bonds and we found that the baculovirus bioreactor is well suited for the correct folding of these peptides. Large quantities of defensins have also been purified from abundant natural sources, such as CF sputum *(24)* and urine *(25)*. Some human antimicrobial peptides can also be obtained commercially (e.g., HNP-1; Sigma) or synthesized on solid supports (e.g., LL-37, an α-helical peptide).
12. Some bacteria (e.g., strains of *P. aeruginosa*) require buffers with higher electrolyte concentrations. Bacteria can be washed and resuspended in 1× PBS, Hank's balanced salt solution (HBSS), or 1× NB.

Acknowledgments

We thank Yong-Hwan Kim, Dr. Edith M. Porter, Erika Valore, Dr. Lide Liu, and Christina Park for refining many of the techniques presented in this chapter.

References

1. Gregory, R. J., Cheng, S. H., Rich, D. P., Marshall, J., Paul, S., Hehir, K., Ostedgaard, L., Klinger, K. W., Welsh, M. J., and Smith, A. E. (1990) Expression and characterization of the cystic fibrosis transmembrane conductance regulator. *Nature* **347,** 382–386.

2. Goldman, M., Anderson, G., Stolzenberg, E. D., Kari, U. P., Zasloff, M., and Wilson, J. M. (1997) Human β-defensin-1 is a salt-sensitive antibiotic in lung that is inactivated in cystic fibrosis. *Cell* **88,** 553–560.
3. Smith, J. J., Travis, S. M., Greenberg, E. P., and Welsh, M. J. (1996) Cystic fibrosis airway epithelia fail to kill bacteria because of abnormal airway surface fluid. *Cell* **85,** 229–236.
4. Ellison, R. T. and Giehl, T. J. (1991) Killing of Gram-negative bacteria by lactoferrin and lysozyme. *J. Clin. Invest.* **88,** 1080–1091.
5. Raphael, G. D., Jeney, E. V., Baraniuk, J. N., Kim, I., Meredith, S. D., and Kaliner, M. A. (1989) Pathophysiology of rhinitis. Lactoferrin and lysozyme in nasal secretions. *J. Clin. Invest.* **84,** 1528–1535.
6. McCray, P. B. and Bentley, L. (1997) Human airway epithelia express a β-defensin. *Am J Respir. Cell Mol. Biol.* **16,** 343–349.
7. Singh, P. K., Jia, H. P., Wiles, K., Hesselberth, J., Liu, L., Conway, B. D., et al. (1998) Production of β-defensins by human airway epithelia. *Proc. Natl. Acad. Sci. USA* **95,** 14,961–14,966.
8. Ganz, T., Selsted, M. E., Szklarek, D., Harwig, S. S., Daher, K., Bainton, D. F., and Lehrer, R. I. (1985) Defensins. Natural peptide antibiotics of human neutrophils. *J. Clin. Invest.* **76,** 1427–1435.
9. Schnapp, D. and Harris, A. (1998) Antibacterial peptides in bronchoalveolar lavage fluid. *Am. J. Respir. Cell Mol. Biol.* **19,** 352–356.
10. Hiemstra, P. S., Maassen, R. J., Stolk, J., Heinzel-Wieland, R., Steffens, G. J., and Dijkman, J. H. (1996) Antibacterial activity of antileukoprotease. *Infect. Immun.* **64,** 4520–4524.
11. Brogden, K. A., Ackermann, M., and Huttner, K. M. (1998) Detection of anionic antimicrobial peptides in ovine bronchoalveolar lavage fluid and respiratory epithelium. *Infect. Immun.* **66,** 5948–5954.
12. Brogden, K. A., Ackermann, M. R., McCray, P. B., Jr., and Huttner, K. M. (1999) Differences in the concentrations of small, anionic, antimicrobial peptides in bronchoalveolar lavage fluid and in respiratory epithelia of patients with and without cystic fibrosis. *Infect. Immun.* **67,** 4256–4259.
13. Samaranayake, Y. H., Samaranayake, L. P., Wu, P. C., and So, M. (1997) The antifungal effect of lactoferrin and lysozyme on *Candida krusei* and *Candida albicans*. *APMIS* **105,** 875–883.
14. Kalfa, V. C. and Brogden, K. A. (1999) Anionic antimicrobial peptide-lysozyme interactions in innate pulmonary immunity. *Int. J. Antimicrob. Agents* **13,** 47–51.
15. Harder, J., Bartels, J., Christophers, E., and Schroeder, J.-M. (1997) A peptide antibiotic from human skin. *Nature* **387,** 861,862.
16. Zhao, C. Q., Wang, I., and Lehrer, R. I. (1996) Widespread expression of β-defensin HBD-1 in human secretory glands and epithelial cells. *FEBS Lett.* **396,** 319–322.
17. Knowles, M. R., Robinson, J. M., Wood, R. E., Pue, C. A., Mentz, W. M., Wager, G. C., Gatzy, J. T., and Boucher, R. C. (1997) Ion composition of airway surface liquid of patients with cystic fibrosis as compared with normal and disease-control subjects. *J. Clin. Invest.* **100,** 2588–2595.

18. Matsui, H., Grubb, B. R., Tarran, R., Randell, S. H., Gatzy, J. T., Davis, C. W., and Boucher, R. C. (1998) Evidence for periciliary liquid layer depletion, not abnormal ion composition, in the pathogenesis of cystic fibrosis airways disease. *Cell* **95,** 1005–1015.
19. Cole, A. M., Wu, M., Kim, Y.-H., and Ganz, T. (2000) Microanalysis of antimicrobial properties of human fluids. *J. Microbiol. Meth.* **41,** 135–143.
20. Cole, A. M., Dewan, P., and Ganz, T. (1999) Innate antimicrobial activity of nasal secretions. *Infect. Immun.* **67,** 3267–3275.
21. Osserman, E. F. and Lawlor, D. P. (1966) Serum and urinary lysozyme (muramidase) in monocytic and monomyelocytic leukemia. *J. Exp. Med.* **124,** 921–952.
22. Tang, Y. Q., Yuan, J., Miller, C. J., and Selsted, M. E. (1999) Isolation, characterization, cDNA cloning, and antimicrobial properties of two distinct subfamilies of a-defensins from rhesus macaque leukocytes. *Infect. Immun.* **67,** 6139–6144.
23. Valore, E. V. and Ganz, T. (1997) Laboratory production of antimicrobial peptides in native conformation, in *Antimicrobial Peptide Protocols*, vol. 78, (Shafer, W. M., ed.), Humana Press, Totowa, pp. 115–131.
24. Soong, L. B., Ganz, T., Ellison, A., and Caughey, G. H. (1997) Purification and characterization of defensins from cystic fibrosis sputum. *Inflamm. Res,* **46,** 98–102.
25. Valore, E. V., Park, C. H., Quayle, A. J., Wiles, K. R., McCray, P. B., and Ganz, T. (1998) Human β-defensin-1: an antimicrobial peptide of urogenital tissues. *J. Clin. Invest.* **101,** 1633–1642.

30

Bacterial–Epithelial Interactions

Ruth Bryan and Alice Prince

1. Introduction

Airway epithelial cells are often the first cells encountered by inhaled organisms. In addition to providing a physical barrier, these cells orchestrate the initial immune response to the presence of bacteria in the airway. There are increased opportunities for bacterial–epithelial contact in the CF lung due to many factors: the presence of lumenal bacteria trapped behind mucin plugs, decreased bacterial killing, and the increased number of receptor sites on epithelial cells for bacterial attachment. Once organisms are present, epithelial signaling cascades are activated, stimulating NF-κB translocation and the expression of proinflammatory chemokines and cytokines *(1)*.

Several methods are available to examine bacterial–epithelial binding and the consequences of these interactions. Some methodologies are best suited to bring out phenotypic differences among the bacterial strains to compare the effects of specific adhesins or exoproducts. Other techniques are preferred to examine the cell biology of the epithelial response to these organisms, and establish how the bacteria interact with the host, whether they remain solely superficial, intercalate paracellularly, or are invasive. Once organisms or their products contact specific epithelial receptors, several different assay systems are available to identify the signaling systems activated in the epithelial cell and to quantify secreted cytokine or chemokines.

1.1. Adherence Assays

Bacterial attachment to eukaryotic receptors has long been considered a prerequisite to infection, although it is clear that either intact organisms or isolated bacterial gene products are sufficient to initiate inflammatory responses in the host *(2)*. Actual adherence determinations or quantification of epithelial

From: *Methods in Molecular Medicine, vol. 70: Cystic Fibrosis Methods and Protocols*
Edited by: W. R. Skach © Humana Press Inc., Totowa, NJ

responses that are dependent on bacterial binding will have significantly divergent results depending on the nature of the organism to be studied and the types of epithelial tissue to be utilized.

1.1.1. Bacterial Properties

Numerous surface characteristics and exoproducts synthesized by different organisms affect bacterial adherence. The expression of specific adhesins, such as pili or fimbriae, varies depending on the stage of growth (logarithmic or stationary), the type of medium (solid or liquid), and the available nutrients. Some organisms, such as *Haemophilus influenzae,* undergo phase variation, so that surface structures vary even under consistent growth conditions. The expression of many exoproducts relevant to pathogenesis (proteases, neuraminidases, phospholipases) is also dependent on growth conditions and the type of media used *(3,4)*.

1.1.2. Epithelial Properties

The properties of the epithelial cells used in in vitro assays significantly affect binding and cell activation studies. The degree of confluence, age of the monolayer, and cell line passage number may be important, as well as the medium and presence of serum. Cell lines with cystic fibrosis transmembrane conductance regulator (CFTR) mutations may not have growth kinetics identical to control cell lines, even those transfected with appropriate control empty vectors, nor do they necessarily form equivalent tight junctions. Cells collected by bronchoalveolar lavage that are not oriented and may be studied in solution behave significantly differently than highly differentiated polarized monolayers grown on semipermeable supports with an air–liquid interface *(5)*. By their nature, airway epithelial cells are polarized and do not have a random distribution of cell surface receptors. Damaged or regenerating cells have a different distribution of receptors than epithelial cells that are intact *(6)*. It may be necessary to use polarized monolayers with tight junctions to reproduce most accurately the conditions encountered by bacteria in the airways particularly if the relevant receptor is trafficked apically vs baso-laterally *(7)*. To compare the effects of specific bacterial gene products or potential inhibitors of adherence it may be adequate to use nonpolarized, easily grown cells to which the organisms bind readily. It is also important to consider the artifacts introduced by nonspecific bacterial binding to plastic, collagen, or vitrogen. These effects may be pronounced in binding assays performed in small (96)-well plates in which the surface area of the exposed plastic is relatively large compared with the volume of the well, as compared to assays done in larger wells with a smaller surface/volume ratio. Incubation conditions may also influence results. To maintain the viability of some epithelial cell lines, incubation with bacteria is performed at 37°C in 5% CO_2. However, some organisms may grow significantly more (or less) under other conditions.

1.2. Selection of Bacterial Adherence and Uptake Assays

The choice of assay system depends directly on the questions to be addressed: Is the purpose of the assay to compare properties of bacteria? Are the specific characteristics of the epithelial receptors of most interest? Is superficial attachment to be quantified, or is the cell biology of the interaction (invasion, or attachment) of greatest importance? For each of the assay systems described, there are specific advantages or disadvantages depending on the type of information that is required.

1.2.1. Adherence of ^{35}S-Labeled Bacteria

The interaction of organisms and host cells can be readily quantified provided there are adequate means to enumerate the organisms and the host cells. A convenient assay system utilizes organisms labeled by incorporation of radioactively labeled amino acids (^{35}S-methionine), incubation with a confluent culture of epithelial cells, washing to remove non-cell-associated bacteria, and quantification of the number of organisms associated with the epithelial cells *(8)*. This assay detects all organisms associated with the epithelial monolayers or adherent to the wells, including extracellular, adherent bacteria, organisms that have intercalated between adjacent epithelial cells lacking tight junctions, and organisms that have actually invaded or have been ingested by epithelial cells *(9)*.

Organisms grown in minimal media readily incorporate labeled amino acids to sufficient specific activity (CPM/CFU) for detection in a scintillation counter. A standard inoculum or several dilutions are incubated with epithelial monolayers. The incubation time for adherence varies significantly with the strain and species. Control assays to determine the timing, the linear range of the binding assay, and the number of organisms necessary to saturate receptor sites are important *(8)*. Bacterial interactions become a problem when very high inocula are used. Cytotoxic bacteria, such as some *Pseudonomas aeruginosa*, cause significant destruction of the epithelial cells by 45 min of incubation, whereas other strains and species do not. Nonadherent organisms are removed with several phosphate-buffered saline (PBS) rinses, and the cell-associated bacteria are then enumerated by lysing the epithelial monolayers in detergent or 0.2 *N* NaOH and quantifying the scintillations. This standard assay system is convenient for comparing mutants of the same bacterial species (**Fig. 1**) or for testing the efficacy of different compounds in blocking adherence to specific receptors. As the assay can be performed conveniently in 96-well plates, cells in primary culture may be used and sufficient replicates done to ensure the reliability and statistical significance of the results. To establish that the wells contain similar numbers of epithelial cells, control wells are trypsinized and cells counted in a hemocytometer, or the protein content quantified. This assay system is particularly useful to compare the relative adherence of several

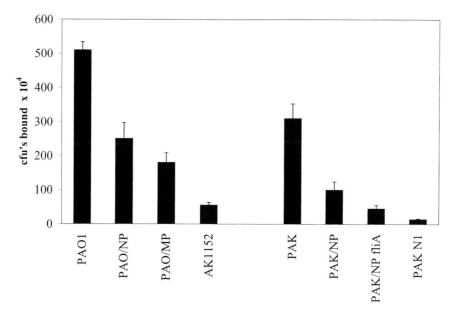

Fig. 1. The effects of mutations in adhesins on the adherence of [35]S *P. aeruginosa* strains to1HAEo- cells is shown: PAO1, wild-type strain; PAO/NP, Pil⁻; PAO/MP, modified pilin, lacks the adhesin domain; AK511, nonmotile PAO1; PAK/NP, Pil⁻, PAK/*fliA*, Fla⁻; PAKN1 (*rpoN*) Pil⁻, Fla⁻.

different bacterial strains with varying properties to the same type of epithelial cells.

1.2.2. Adherence of Bacteria Labeled with Fluorescent Markers

Two techniques are routinely used to quantify epithelial cells that are in contact with fluorescently labeled organisms. Bacteria can be transformed by a plasmid constitutively expressing green fluorescent protein (GFP) and then added to epithelial cells. Epithelial cells with associated GFP-labeled organisms are then identified by flow cytometry. Alternatively, bacteria are first incubated with epithelial cells for desired intervals. The cell-associated bacteria are then identified with antibody to well-conserved superficial bacterial structures such as lipopolysaccharides (LPS) or outer membrane proteins. The primary antibody is tagged with a secondary fluorescent antibody that can be visualized. Epithelial cells with associated fluorescent bacteria are then enumerated by flow cytometry or by fluorescence microscopy. While GFP-labeled bacteria may be intra-, extra- or paracellular, antibody to bacterial structures detects only extracellular organisms unless the epithelial cells are permeabilized. Labeling of organisms between adjacent epithelial cells may or may not be accessible to antibody. Both extracellular and intracellular organ-

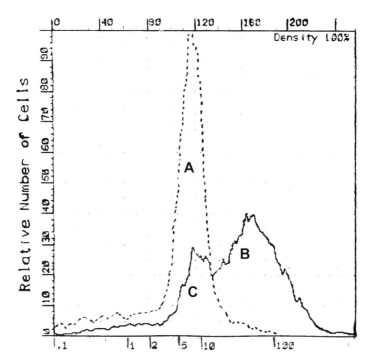

Fig. 2. *P. aeruginosa* adherence to 9HTEo- cells quantified by flow cytometry. The adherent PAO1 were labeled with anti-OMP and FITC-conjugated anti-rabbit IgG. Control cells (A, dotted line) were incubated with antibodies but not bacteria. The population of epithelial cells with adherent bacteria (increased fluorescence) is shown as shifted to the right (B, solid line), as compared with the fraction of that population (C) which did not have associated bacteria.

isms will be labeled if the epithelial cells are permeabilized before immunocytochemical staining with antibody *(10)*.

GFPs that are constitutively expressed on plasmid vectors are commercially available and have "enhanced" fluorescence, optimized for detection within eurkaryotic cells. For flow cytometry, the secondary fluorescent antibody labels must be intense enough to distinguish positive cells from background endogenous fluorescence of the epithelial cells that do not have associated bacteria.

The population of epithelial cells with associated bacteria is differentiated from the uninfected cells by flow cytometry (FACS) (**Fig. 2**). Rabbit anti-sera raised to *P. aeruginosa* outer membrane proteins was used as the primary antibody and goat anti-rabbit FAb2'conjugated with FITC was the secondary label. Different cell types may require specific labeling techniques. Titration studies comparing FACS results with fluorescence microscopy are done to establish how many adherent/ingested organisms are necessary to make an associated epithelial cell "positive" by flow cytometry.

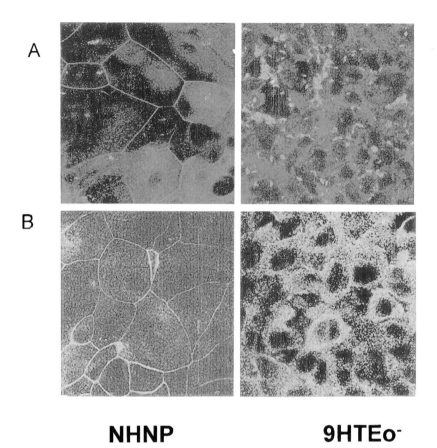

NHNP   9HTEo⁻

Fig. 3. Normal Human Nasal Polyp and 9HTEo- cells imaged by confocal microscopy. (**A**) *P. aeruginosa* association with monolayers. NHNP cells in primary culture
and 9HTEo⁻ cells grown on semipermeable supports are shown following exposure to
1×10^8 CFU/mL of PAO1/GFP for 3 h and imaged 8 μm from the apical surface. The
NHNP cells were also treated with anti-ZO1 and a fluorescent Cy-5 tag to delineate
the cell boundaries. The 9HTEo- cells were treated with anti-fodrin which was visualized with Cy-5. Magnification 100×. (**B**) Demonstration of tight junctions. Monolayers grown under the same conditions as shown in (A) were treated with antibody to
ZO-1, a marker for tight junctions. The images shown were 3 μm from the apical
surface. Magnification 100× *(10)*.

Major advantages of this technique include the ability to enumerate a uniform population of cells that are viable and retain homogeneous characteristics
(11). Bacteria often are associated with dead or dying cells, which may not be
indicative of the cells encountered under in vivo conditions. Unlike
[35]SOlabeling methods, flow cytometry allows a uniform population of epithelial cells to be assessed for bacterial binding or invasion. Only those cells with

the appropriate characteristics are considered, while erroneous binding, such as to plastic, is eliminated.

1.2.3. Fluorescence Microscopy

The interaction of the organisms and the epithelial cells can be visualized using fluorescence labeling and epifluorescent or confocal microscopy. The latter technique is particularly important to establish the intracellular fate of the organisms (**Fig. 3**). As shown, epithelial cells grown on transparent semi-permeable supports at an air–liquid interface can be labeled with antibodies to known intracellular structures for orientation to determine where the bacteria localize. Cells that lack tight junctions (diffuse labeling with anti-ZO-1 antibody) have many paracellular bacteria intercalating between adjacent epithelial cells in a polarized monolayer. The monolayer of nasal polyp cells in primary culture, which have tight junctions and localized anti-ZO1 staining, have few, if any, organisms that have penetrated between cells.

1.2.4. Gentamicin Exclusion Assays

Bacterial–epithelial interactions can also be studied by using antibiotics whose activities are relatively specific for extracellular bacteria, to differentiate between intra- and extracellular organisms *(11)*. Following incubation of a known inoculum of bacteria with epithelial cells, the cells are treated with a cidal concentration (which varies with the organism) of gentamicin to kill extracellular bacteria. The epithelial cells are then washed repeatedly to remove any excess gentamicin, lysed, and viable (i.e., intracellular and thus protected from the antibiotic) bacteria. It is important to perform controls to assess whether cell-bound antibiotic leeches off lysed cells to kill organisms that had been intracellular.

Major variables for this assay system include difficulties assessing how well paracellular organisms, which have intercalated between cells in culture, are protected from the drug.

1.3. Epithelial Responses to Bacteria and Their Secreted Products

In the airway, much of the immediate immune response is due to the activation of epithelial cells by either adherent whole organisms or the interactions of specific bacterial gene products and epithelial receptors. These interactions stimulate transcriptional activation of epithelial immune response genes. For example, piliated (adherent) *P. aeruginosa* recognize asialoGM1 receptors on airway epithelial cells that induce the translocation of NF-κB and transcription of IL-8, a major PMN chemokine *(12)*. This pathway can be monitored by assessing NF-κB activation following the addition of adherent bacteria to monolayers of epithelial cells, or by quantifying IL-8 accumulation in the cell culture supernatant, as described below. Other cytokines can be similarly assayed using this techinque.

1.3.1. Activation of NF-κB

The activation of NF-κB and other transcription factors can be detected by gel shift assays that are labor intensive but provide the most informative data to understand the biology of the system. These experiments must be individualized, probing regulatory DNA sequences from the specific genes being activated under the given experimental conditions. A more convenient system takes advantage of commercially available NF-κB-luciferase reporter constructs, plasmid vectors that contain a TATA box, and several κB-binding sites ligated upstream from the luciferase gene. Epithelial cells are transiently transfected with this reporter construct and another plasmid constitutively expressing the renilla luciferase, which can be detected in the same assay system to act as a control for efficiency of transfection. Epithelial cells are stimulated, allowed to recover, and luciferase activity monitored and compared with unstimulated controls. Known positive and negative controls are important, as NF-κB is readily activated by nonspecific stimuli. A known positive control stimulus is essential to establish the range of NF-κB luciferase activation under these conditions. For example, wild-type *P. aeruginosa,* antibody to asialoGM1 or IL-1β, having been shown by gel shift assay to activate translocation of the p65 component of NF-κB, are included when testing the ability of other strains of bacteria to stimulate NF-κB. Similar reporter constructs are available for other transcriptional activators such as AP-1.

Other considerations for these assays are the efficiency of transfection, which varies significantly from cell line to cell line, and the time allotted for stimulation. Although transfections are most conveniently done in 6-well plates, this results in a "general" response to a stimulus in cells that are not necessarily polarized, and may not reflect the in vivo distribution of relevant receptors.

1.3.2. Measurement of Cytokine or Chemokine Expression—IL-8 Assays

In response to various bacterial stimuli, epithelial cells express a number of different chemokines or cytokines. The expression of IL-8, for example, has been examined following exposure to bacteria, bacterial mutants, or isolated bacterial gene products *(2)*. As IL-8 is a stable secreted product, epithelial cells can be stimulated, washed, and the accumulated IL-8 in the tissue culture supernatant measured at selected time intervals. Again, the nature of the bacterial–epithelial interaction is important, as cytotoxic strains will destroy the integrity of the monolayer, long incubation periods may result in low amounts of IL-8 production, whereas brief exposure to the toxic organisms may result in much greater IL-8 expression. Accordingly, it is important to control for possible variables: size of the bacterial inoculum, length of incubation with the monolayers, timing of harvesting cell culture supernatants. ELISAs for IL-8 are commercially available and include controls.

To determine the effects of potential inhibitors or stimulants of IL-8 expression, epithelial cells are preincubated with the reagent to ascertain that the inhibitor is present when the stimulus is applied. The inhibitor is then re-added following washing of the monolayers, as adherent organisms or ligands that might not be washed away would continue to provide stimulation. Additional controls for the assay system include monitoring unstimulated wells to quantify background IL-8 expression, and assessing control wells with trypan blue after incubation with the bacteria to verify their integrity (>80% should exclude trypan blue). The amount of IL-8 expressed must be standardized, usually by the protein content of the well.

Overall these methods provide the opportunity to assess the nature of the bacterial–epithelial interaction. Adherence assays and fluorescence labeling will provide accurate data to asses the different types of interactions which are occurring, at least in vitro. This is helpful information, as techniques to examine epithelial gene activation may differ depending on the nature of the initial epithelial interaction, if superficial binding occurs, or if the organism is invasive and/or cytotoxic. Bacteria may also secrete or shed components that stimulate epithelial cells independent of whole-organism binding.

2. Materials

2.1. Adherence and Uptake Assays

2.1.1. ^{35}S Adherence Assay

1. 96-well tissue culture plates.
2. Tissue culture media.
3. ^{35}S methionine, (~10 mCi/mL, ~10 nmoles/mL).
4. M9 medium or MAM medium.
5. LB plates.
6. 0.2 N NaOH.
7. Scintillation counter.

2.1.2. Flow Cytometry

1. 24-well tissue culture plates.
2. Tissue culture medium.
3. Paraformaldehyde.
4. GFP expression vector.
5. Antibodies for fluorescence labeling:
   a. Primary antibody—rabbit (or other species) antibody to a superficial, highly conserved bacterial epitope (LPS, outer membrane proteins, or cell wall);
   b. Secondary antibody—goat anti-rabbit IgG FAb2' conjugated to FITC or other fluorescent label for fluorescence microscopy
6. 20-mm HEPES with 0.02% EGTA (Ca^{+2}/Mg^{+2}-free).

2.1.3. Flourescence Microscopy

1. Epithelial cells grown on cover slips in tissue culture wells or on semipermeable supports (Transwells).
2. 3.7% formaldehyde.
3. 0.2% Triton X-100.

2.2. NF-κB Reporter Assays

1. NF-κB luciferase reporter.
2. pRL-TK luciferase control vector.
3. Eukaryotic transfection protocol.
4. Dual-luciferase reporter assay system.
5. Epithelial cells (80% confluent monolayers) in 6 well plates.
6. Luminometer.

2.2.1. IL-8 ELISA

1. 96-well tissue culture plates.
2. IL-8 ELISA kit (commercially available).
   a. 96-well microtiter plates for ELISA.
   b. Monoclonal anti-human IL-8 antibody.
   c. Rabbit polyclonal anti-human IL-8 antibody.
   d. Streptavidin conjugated anti-rabbit IgG antibody.
   e. Biotinylated-horse raddish peroxidase.
   f. Substrate.
   g. Protein assay kit.

3. Methods
3.1. ^{35}S Adherence Assays
3.1.1. Labeling of Organisms

1. From a fresh plate, inoculate 10 mL minimal medium (M9) with bacteria and incubate with aeration at 37°C until late logarithmic growth phase is reached.
2. Add 50 Ci of ^{35}S methionine/mL of culture for 15–30 min. Pellet, wash in PBS, and resuspend in tissue culture media (without antibiotics).
3. Determine the specific activity of the organisms (CPM/CFU) by counting scintillations associated with serially diluted organisms, quantified by plating on LB agar plates. The concentration of the labeled organisms should be 10^6–10^8 cfu/mL.

3.1.2. Preparation of Epithelial Cells for Binding Assays

1. Confluent monolayers of epithelial cells in 96-well plates are prepared and examined for confluence. Controls without epithelial cells should be included to assess adherence to exposed sides of the wells. Enough wells should be prepared to perform each experimental condition at least in triplicate.
2. Using sterile technique, aliquots of the labeled bacteria are added to each well (total volume 100 μL) and incubated. Preliminary assays should be done to ascer-

tain the linear concentration range and optimal incubation periods (usually 30 min–4 h). Shorter times may not achieve saturated binding; longer times may increase epithelial ingestion of the organisms or destruction of the monolayers.

3. Following incubation, non-cell-associated bacteria are removed by three (or more) washes in PBS.
4. The epithelial cells are solubilized overnight in 0.1 mL of 0.2 *N* NaOH.
5. Scintillations associated with the solubilized monolayers and the associated bacteria are counted, as are the aliquots of the labeled inoculum to determine the specific activity and the percent of the added inoculum that was associated with the epithelial cells.

3.2. Assessment of Binding/Ingestion by Flow Cytometry

3.2.1. Construction of Bacterial Strains That Constitutively Express GFP

1. Several commercially available plasmid constructs are available that express enhanced green fluorescent protein (GFP), optimized for detection by flow cytometry. These are used to transform *Escherichia coli*, or used to construct a vector capable of replication in the desired bacterial species. For *P. aeruginosa*, the GFP coding sequence can be introduced into a broad host range vector such as pUCP18, which is then used to transform or electroporate the bacteria.

3.2.2. Assessment of Bacterial Binding Using Fluorescent Labeling

1. Epithelial cell monolayers grown in 12- or 24-well plates are inspected and assessed for confluence. Control wells, which will not have added bacteria, must be included as controls for background fluorescence and for nonspecific antibody binding.
2. Bacteria (either GFP labeled or unlabeled) are added to the monolayers for appropriate incubation periods, determined by binding assays, usually 0.5–4 h at 37°C in 5% CO_2. Nonadherent organisms are removed by several washes with PBS +1 m*M* $CaCl_2$ and 1 m*M* $MgSO_4$.
3. Adherent organisms (if not expressing GFP) are identified by immunofluorescence labeling. Antibody to a superficial and highly conserved bacterial epitope (LPS or outer membranes) is added to appropriate wells in medium or PBS, at a temperature and time that should be determined experimentally (*see* **Notes 1–3**). Unbound antibody is removed with two PBS washes followed by the addition of a secondary antibody conjugated to FITC, TRITC, or other fluorescent marker. It may be sufficient to incubate with the secondary for 15 min on ice. Control wells are incubated with the primary and secondary antibodies alone, to quantify background binding (*see* **Notes 4** and **5**).
4. The monolayers with associated (external) bacteria, now fluorescently labeled, are taken up from the plates (or transwells) in Ca^{2+}/Mg^{2+}-free 20 m*M* HEPES with 0.02% EGTA, triturating with a micropipet tip as necessary. Cells are fixed with the addition of 1% paraformaldehyde and examined by flow cytometry.
5. Details of the bacterial–epithelial interaction are best assessed by confocal microscopy using epithelial monolayers grown on transparent semipermeable

supports. These can be carefully cut out, mounted on a slide, and examined. Fluorescence labeling, as described above, can be performed in the transwells.

6. Intracellular bacteria (if not expressing GFP) can be identified by permeabilizing the epithelial cells. This is done by fixing monolayers in 3.7% formaldehyde, washing in TBS, then permeabilizing the monolayers with 0.2% Triton X-100. A comparison of the number of epithelial cells with and without associated bacteria under permeabilized and nonpermeabilized conditions should indicate how many bacteria are intracellular.

7. To determine if GFP-labeled organisms are extracellular, they can be labeled using primary antibodies, followed by a second fluorescent marker (TRITC, for example). However, it is important to verify that there is little interference between the two different fluorescent indicators, and controls with singly labeled bacteria must be included.

3.3. Determination of NF-κB Activation by Luciferase Reporters

1. The desired cell lines grown in 6-well plates are transiently transfected with an NF-κB-luciferase. Renilla luciferase control vectors are used simultaneously to establish transfection efficiency. Sufficient numbers of wells for triplicate determinations as well as the background activities of unstimulated cells are needed. A number of commercially available kits are available to optimize transfection of eukaryotic cells providing the experimental details including amounts of DNA and transfection conditions.

2. Following transfection (18 h), the transiently transfected epithelial cells are incubated with the desired bacteria or bacterial products, with or without inhibitors. Depending on the nature of the interaction, the stimulus is incubated with the cells for 15 min to 1 h at 37°C in 5%CO_2.

3. The stimulus is removed, cells are refed for 1 h, washed, then lysed. Aliquots of the lysate are removed to measure the two luciferase activities (at different wavelengths), which are stable for several hours in the lysis buffer. Substrate is added immediately prior to detection in the luminometer. The relative amount of renilla luciferase activity is used as a control for transfection efficiency as a basis for the relative activation of the NF-κB associated luciferase.

3.4. Detection of Epithelial IL-8 Expression

1. Epithelial monolayers are grown in 96-well plates to confluence and weaned from serum for at least 18 h before IL-8 assays (see **Note 6**).

2. To quintuplicate wells, bacteria, antibody, or other desired stimuli are added for appropriate incubation periods (usually 30–120 min) at 37°C in 5% CO_2. The effects of inhibitors are tested by preincubating the cells with the inhibitors for 30 min, and replacing the inhibitors during stimulation. Unstimulated controls and wells with inhibitors but no stimuli are always included.

3. Wells are washed three times in PBS and sterilized (if bacteria are added) by the addition of 100 μg/mL of gentamicin, and refed. (Inhibitors are also re-added).

4. Supernatants are removed at desired time points (4–18 h) and assayed by commercial ELISA kits for IL-8 (see **Note 7**).

5. Control wells are lysed and assayed for protein content.
6. Additional control wells for each experimental condition are stained with trypan blue and the number of lysed (nonviable) epithelial cells are quantified. If >20% of the cells are dead, the IL-8 assay is not considered to be valid.

4. Notes

1. Determine if the binding is saturable by doing dose–response curves and binding competition studies. Excess amounts of unlabeled organisms are added to compete for binding with the radioactively labeled bacteria. Many bacteria clump together at high concentrations, which may produce inconsistent binding results.
2. The effects of potential binding inhibitors can be tested by addition to either the monolayers or to the bacteria. Reagents expected to block epithelial sites are added to the monolayers before the addition of bacteria, whereas compounds expected to interact with bacterial components may be more effective if preincubated with the organisms.
3. Transwell clear (Costar) wells are transparent and strong enough to mount and examine by fluorescence/confocal microscopy
4. The amount of antibody binding should increase with time and then reach a plateau. Perform a time-course experiment to determine the minimum amount of time needed to reach that plateau.
5. Nonspecific binding of either the primary or secondary antibodies can be minimized by titrating the concentrations of the antibodies and using the minimum required to reach a plateau, and by blocking with either preimmune antisera or 1–5% BSA.
6. Small amounts of fetal calf serum (0.1%) does not usually increase IL-8 expression, although this may vary significantly in different epithelial cell lines. Some cells in primary culture, such as nasal polyps, may have exceptionally elevated endogenous IL-8, even without serum.
7. The supernatants can be removed from the wells and frozen in tissue culture wells, covered with microplate adhesive film, provided they are protected from any freeze–thaw cycles of a frost-free freezer.

References

1. Prince, A. (2000) Bacterial induction of cytokine secretion in pathogenesis of airway inflammation, in *Virulence Mechanisms of Bacterial Pathogens,* 3rd ed. (Brogden, K. A., et al. eds.), ASM Press, Washington, DC, pp. 189–201.
2. DiMango, E., Zar, H. J., Bryan, R., and Prince, A. (1995) Various *Pseudomonas aeruginosa* gene products stimulate respiratory epithelial cells to produce IL-8. *J. Clin. Invest.* **96,** 2204–2210.
3. Vallis, A. J., Yahr, T. L., Barbieri, J. T., and Frank, D. W. (1999) Regulation of ExoS production and secretion by *Pseudomonas aeruginosa* in response to tissue culture conditions. *Infect. Immun.* **67,** 914–920.
4. Vasil, M. L. and Ochsner, U. A. (1999) The response of *Pseudomonas aeruginosa* to iron: genetics, biochemistry, and virulence. *Mol. Microbiol.* **34,** 399–413.
5. de Jong, P. M., van Sterkenburg, M. A. J. A., Hesseling, S. C., Kempenaar, J. A., Mulder, A. A., Mommaas, A. M., et al. (1994) Ciliogenesis in human bronchial

epithelial cells cultured at the air-liquid interface. *Am. J. Respir. Cell Mol. Biol.* **10,** 217–277.

6. DeBentzmann, S., Roger, P., Dupuit, F., Bajolet-Laudinat, O., Fuchley, C., Plotkowski, M., and Puchelle, E. (1996) AsialoGM1 is a receptor for *P. aeruginosa* adherence to regenerating respiratory epithelial cells. *Infect. Immun.* **64,** 1582–1588.

7. Immundo, L., Barasch, J., Prince, A., and Q. Al-awqati. 1995. CF epithelial cells have a receptor for pathogenic bacteria on their apical surface. *Proc. Nat. Acad. Sci. USA* **92,** 3019–23.

8. Saiman, L., Cacalano, G., Gruenert, D., and Prince, A. (1992) Comparison of adherence of *Pseudomonas aeruginosa* to respiratory epithelial cells from cystic fibrosis patients and healthy subjects. *Infect. Immun.* **60,** 2808–2814.

9. Fleisig, S. M. J., Zaidi, T. S., and Pier, G. B. (1995) *Pseudomonas aeruginosa* invasion of and multiplication within corneal epithelial cells in vitro. *Infect. Immun.* **63,** 4072–4077.

10. Rajan, S., Cacalano, G., Bryan, R., Ratner, A. J., Sontich C. U., van Heerckeren, A., Davis, P., and Prince, A. (2000) *Pseudomonas aeruginosa* induction of apoptosis in respiratory epithelial cells. *Am. J. Resp. Cell Mol. Biol.* **23,** 1–9.

11. Gerceker, A. A., Zaidi, T., Marks, P., Golan, D. E., and Pier, G. (2000) Impact of heterogeneity within cultured cells on bacterial invasion: analysis of *Pseudomonas aeruginosa* and *Salmonella enterica* serovar Typhi entry into MDCK cells by using a green fluorescent protein-labeled cystic fibrosis transmembrane conductance regulator receptor. *Infect. Immun.* **68,** 861–870.

12. DiMango, E., Ratner, A. J., Bryan, R., Tabibi, S., and Prince, A. (1998) Activation of NF-(B by adherent *Pseudomonas aeruginosa* in normal and cystic fibrosis respiratory epithelial cells. *J. Clin. Invest.* **101,** 2598–2606.

31

Thin-Film Measurements of Airway Surface Liquid Volume/Composition and Mucus Transport Rates In Vitro

Robert Tarran and Richard C. Boucher

1. Introduction

Airway surface liquid (ASL) has been reported to vary in height from 5 to 100 μm *(1,2)*, which likely reflects both regional/species variation and differences in methodologies. Potential artifacts may exist during ASL sampling: for example, evaporation may concentrate ASL, yielding abnormally high [ion], and damage to the underlying epithelium may occur during ASL collection (i.e., with filter papers), causing intracellular ions to leak into the ASL *(3)*. The lability of the ASL is inherently due to its minuteness, and hence, discrepancies have arisen in defining ASL volume/composition *(3,4)*.

A powerful aid to studying ASL physiology has been the development of reliable models that approximate airway epithelial morphology in vivo. We have employed a cell culture model that closely mimics human proximal airways surface epithelia, i.e., the possession of ciliated and goblet cells, which produce separate periciliary and mucus layers and exhibit coordinated mucus transport, and we have developed noninvasive techniques to record ASL properties using this model (**Fig. 1**) *(5,6,7)*. In this laboratory in vitro studies of ASL are based on the use of confocal and epifluorescence microscopy to measure ASL height and mucus transport, respectively *(5,6,7)*. These imaging techniques have been performed in parallel with ion-selective microelectrode impalements of ASL (to measure ASL [Cl⁻]), and perfluorocarbons (PFCs) have also been used because they are immiscible with ASL, enabling them to perform the dual functions of preventing ASL evaporation and to serve as a vehicle for drug/compound additions *(6,7)*.

From: *Methods in Molecular Medicine, vol. 70: Cystic Fibrosis Methods and Protocols*
Edited by: W. R. Skach © Humana Press Inc., Totowa, NJ

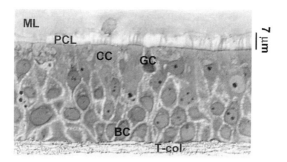

Fig. 1. In vitro model of human tracheo-bronchial epithelia. Cells are grown at an air–liquid interface on semipermeable supports (T-cols) and are typically examined 2–5 wk after seeding. ML, mucus layer; PCL, periciliary liquid layer; GC, goblet cell; CC, ciliated cell; BC, basal cell; T-Col, semipermeable culture insert. Scale bar is 7 μm.

The application of confocal microscopy to ASL physiology is a new and exciting area. Importantly, ASL height can be measured directly by scanning in the vertical (XZ) plane, which gives an index of ASL volume (**Fig. 2**). Thus, the capacity of the underlying epithelia to absorb or secrete ASL can be directly referenced as a function of ASL height. When used in conjunction with double-barreled, Cl⁻-selective microelectrodes, one is also capable of learning whether [ion] (i.e., [Cl⁻]) is directly altered by the epithelia in the process of modifying ASL volume (height) and since double-barreled microelectrodes also monitor the transepithelial potential difference (*Vt*), one can also make direct assessments of ion transport.

1.1. Cell Culture Model of Proximal Airway Surface Epithelia

1.1.1. Cell Isolation

Human airway specimens are obtained from the operating room as per Institutional Review Board-approved protocols and used as soon after excision as possible (typically 1 h, but up to 12 h). Dissected airways are incubated for 2 d in an "isolation cocktail" of buffered culture medium, antibiotics, and protease (*see* **Subheading 2.1.1., item 4**), after which isolated cells are harvested and plated down on (commercially available) collagen-coated, semipermeable tissue culture inserts (*see* **Note 1**).

Cultures are usually confluent within 3–5 d and are then grown with an air–liquid interface (ALI), which means that culture medium is omitted from the mucosal surface after the cultures become confluent, allowing production of native ASL (*see* **Note 2**). These ALI conditions are thought to trigger the cultures to fully differentiate into a layer of ciliated cells interspersed with goblet cells over several layers of [undifferentiated] basal cells by ~2 wk (**Fig. 1**).

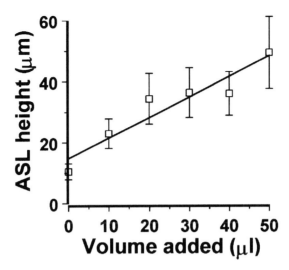

Fig. 2. *XZ* confocal microscopy of ASL: relationship between ASL height and volume. Measurements were made of ASL over human airway epithelial cells cultured on a 12-mm-diameter insert (T-col). After the first dye addition, excess liquid was aspirated and the initial (minimal) ASL height determined. Further 10-μL aliquots of PBS/Texas Red–dextran were added and subsequent ASL heights determined. Data are shown as mean ± standard error ($n = 6$ cultures) and the line is best-fit using linear regression ($r^2 = 0.90$).

Overlying the mucosal-most cells is the ASL, which resembles ASL topography in vivo since it is delineated into an aqueous *sol* layer that baths the cilia (periciliary layer, PCL) and a *gel*-based mucus layer (**Fig. 1**). Perhaps surprisingly, some of these cultures are capable of coordinating ciliary beat to the extent that the cultures spontaneously transport mucus. However, since there is no orifice, this mucus is transported around the culture dish in a circular fashion in the center of the culture where it is visible to the naked eye. Matsui et al. labeled this mucus with fluorescent microspheres *(5,6)*, and under a low-power epifluorescence microscope this mucus appears visually analogous to meteorological images of hurricanes so they have been dubbed "mucus hurricanes" accordingly. Approximately one in three cultures exhibits rotational mucus transport. The reason for this is unclear, since all cultures are ciliated and possess ASL and no difference can be detected in culture morphology or bioelectric properties. Thus, we divide the cultures into two subpopulations following prescreening, and select (cultures) for appropriate experiments on the basis of whether they transport mucus or not.

1.2. Labeling of ASL for Confocal and Epifluorescence Microscopy

Like proximal airways in vivo *(8)*, our airway cultures are predominantly Na$^+$/volume absorbing and deplete ASL volume over time *(6)*. To standardize the starting ASL height/volume, cultures are washed at a predetermined time point to ensure similar starting ASL volumes. This washing may occur 1–2 d before the experiment to allow mucus accumulation and production of "natural" ASL, or may occur immediately before starting the experiment to facilitate mucus-free conditions. Thus, the desired fluorescent probes may be added either (1) days earlier, (2) with the final wash of the mucosal surface following ASL aspiration to minimal levels, or (3) in a bolus of liquid (i.e., 20–50 μL) at the start of the experiment.

1.2.1. Confocal Microscopy of ASL/Cultured Airway Epithelia

In our experiments, we have labeled ASL *sol* with Texas Red conjugated to 10-kDa dextran (**Fig. 2A**) which is freely permeable in the ASL but impermeable across the epithelium (*see* **Note 3**). Changes in ASL height measured in *XZ* mode correspond to changes in ASL volume and can be calibrated as shown in **Fig. 2B**. For confocal microscopy, mucus is labeled with 100-nm fluorescent microspheres that co-localize to "strands" in the mucus layer, allowing an overall impression of mucus location in the ASL. Perusal of the Molecular Probes catalog will yield many other potential ASL-suitable dyes depending on the investigator's individual needs. For example, we have also added fluorescent lipids to see whether they are localized in the ASL.

1.2.2. Epifluorescence Microscopy of Rotational Mucus Transport

For rotational mucus transport measurements under low-power epifluorescence microscopy, larger, 1-μm-diameter microspheres are used since they are better suited for tracking mucus movement. If green fluorescent 100-nm microspheres and Texas Red–dextran have already been added to the ASL for confocal microscopy, blue microspheres may also be added for measuring rotational mucus transport. One-micrometer microspheres are seen as "streaks" when taken as 5-s exposure images acquired with an inverted epifluorescence microscope (**Fig. 3Ai**) (DMIRB and 5× lens, Leica, Germany) and a CCD camera (C5985, Hamamatsu, Japan). Rotational mucus transport rates over the surface of the cultures are measured from these images and the linear velocity of bead transport is normalized to a 1-mm distance from the center of rotation by linear regression analysis after the distance individual streaks have traveled, as assessed using appropriate image analysis software (**Fig. 3Aii**) (i.e., Metamorph, Universal Imaging, USA). Stationary mucus no longer appears as "streaks" and instead can be imaged as plaques of mucus on the surface of cultures (**Fig. 3B**).

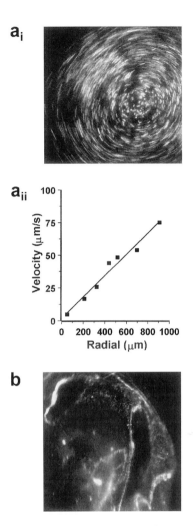

Fig. 3. Epifluorescence microscopy of rotational mucus transport. (a_i) 5-s exposure photograph of rotational mucus transport, seen as streaks of fluorescent microspheres. (a_{ii}) Plot of microsphere velocity against distance from the center of rotation. The line is best-fit using linear regression ($r^2 = 0.97$), and the slope may be used to normalize transport to a set distance from the center (e.g., 1 mm).

1.3. Use of Microelectrodes for ASL Impalement

Double-barreled Cl^--selective microelectrodes are constructed "in house" and have been previously used in this laboratory for intracellular recording (8) and to assess ASL height (9) and composition (6,9). Further information on microelectrodes may be found elsewhere (10). The fabrication of double-barreled Cl⁻-selective microelectrodes is somewhat involved and the success rate varies from 80% of the electrodes being functional down to 0, although with practice one does expect to get some stable electrodes from a batch, and frequently >50% will work. They are sensitive to humidity, and unless they are to be used immediately, care must be taken to keep them free from ambient moisture by storing them in a desiccator under vacuum. Two borosilicate glass capillaries of different thickness (GC120F and GC150F, Clarke, UK) are glued together (**Fig. 4A**) and on a placed horizontal, two-stage electrode puller (P-5, Narishige, Japan). Heat is then applied to the center of the glued-together "preelectrode" (i.e., the dotted line in **Fig. 4A**) and one end of the "pre-electrode" is rotated through 360° to bring the tips of both barrels in close contact. The electrodes are then pulled apart to give two double-barreled electrodes for every pre-electrode (**Fig. 4B**).

The tip of the ion-selective barrel is then filled with an ion-selective resin (available from Fluka) and back-filled with 3 M KCl. The reference barrel is filled with KCl. Both barrels of the electrode are then linked to a high-impedance electrometer (**Fig. 4B**; 10^{15} Ω; model FD 223, World Precision Instruments, USA). We use one that has been designed specifically for use with ion-selective microelectrodes, since Cl⁻ electrodes typically have a high resistances (10^{10}–10^{12} Ω). We use the same electrometer to measure the transepithelial potenial difference (i.e., Vt). since the input signal from the microelectrode can be split to yield both V_{ion} and Vt, but one could also use a simpler, lower-impedance electrometer if Vt alone is to be recorded.

The electrodes are calibrated before each experiment using two standard solutions of known [Cl⁻] (typically 150 and 15 mM Cl⁻) (*see* **Note 4**). An ideal electrode should display a Nernstian shift of 58 mV per 10-fold change in [Cl⁻] and should be relatively drift free (±1 mV drift/h). Electrodes that fall short of this ideal are rejected, since they may lead to unreliable measurements. With double-barreled microelectrodes, the KCl-filled barrel serves as a reference electrode for the ion-selective barrel and to obtain measurements of ASL or mucus [Cl⁻], the microelectrode is positioned with a micromanipulator (Narashigie, Japan). A third macroelectrode (an agar bridge connected to a calomile half-cell) may be placed in the serosal solution to allow simultaneous readings of V_{ion} and Vt if required.

1.4. Perfluorocarbons (PFCs)

PFC is added to the mucosal surface during all ASL measurements to prevent evaporation. Since addition of compounds to the ASL in a liquid vehicle would result in a direct increase in ASL volume, compounds are added as dry powders suspended in PFC (FC-72) and the mass of compound calculated based on the ASL volume per culture following the final rinse as 10 μL. We have recently been experimenting with the use of jet milling to produce ultrafine particles that distribute very well in the PFC.

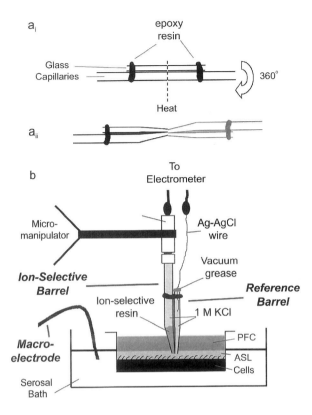

Fig. 4. Fabrication/setup of double-barreled ion-selective microelectrodes. (**a_i**) The "pre-electrode" consists of two glass capillaries glued together with epoxy resin. The pre-electrode is placed into a pipet puller (not shown), heat is applied centrally (i.e., along the dotted line), and one end of the pre-electrode is rotated through 360° to bring the electrode tips close together in the configuration shown in **a_ii**. (**B**) Once the electrodes have been pulled apart, each separate, double-barreled microelectrode is filled with ion-selective resin and KCl and mounted via a micromanipulator to impale the ASL accurately. The reference barrel is connected to the electrometer via n Ag-AgCl wire and the longer, ion-selective barrel is inserted into a pipet holder and also connected to the electrometer. A macroelectrode may also be connected to the electrometer and used in conjunction with the reference barrel to measure the transepithelial potential difference (*Vt*) simultaneously.

Advantage is also taken of the fact that FC-72 PFC has a relatively low boiling point (56°C) compared to FC-77 PFC, which has a much higher boiling point of 97°C. The shorter-lasting FC-72 is typically applied before addition of any compounds (to measure baseline values), while FC-77 is added after addition of the compound to prevent ASL evaporation.

2. Materials

2.1. Cell Culture Model

2.1.1. Cell Isolation Procedure

1. Appropriate human tissue.
2. Lactated Ringer's solution (1000-mL bags, Baxter Healthcare, USA).
3. 50-mL centrifuge tubes.
4. Cold, modified Eagle's medium (obtainable as MEM powder from Gibco, USA, rehydrated and set to pH 7.4 in the presence of 15 mM HEPES) containing DNase (1 µg/mL), antibiotics (100 U/mL penicillin + 100 mg/mL streptomycin, Gibco) and 0.1% Protease (type XIV, Sigma-Aldrich, USA).
5. Rocker/shaker at 4°C.
6. 10% bovine serum (Sigma-Aldrich).
7. Petri dish + concave scalpels.

2.1.2. Cell Culture

1. Bench centrifuge.
2. 15-mL centrifuge tubes.
3. BEGM (*see* **Table 1**).
4. Culture inserts (*see* **Note 1**) and 6-well dishes (2 mL BEGM per well).
5. Phosphate-buffered saline (PBS): 142 mM NaCl, 4.2 mM phosphate buffer, pH 7.4.
6. Tissue culture incubator set at 37°C and gassed with 5% CO_2.

2.2. Fluorescent Imaging of ASL/Mucus Transport

2.2.1. Confocal Microscopy of ASL/Cultured Airway Epithelia

1. Suitable cell cultures.
2. Inverted confocal microscope capable of vertical (XZ) scanning in two wavelengths simultaneously (*see* **Note 5**).
3. PBS as a vehicle for fluorescent dyes: 125 mM NaCl, 4.2 mM KCl, 1.2 mM MgCl$_2$·6H$_2$O, 1.2 mM CaCl$_2$, 9 mM phosphate buffer, adjusted to pH 7.4.
4. Texas Red–dextran (10 kDa, Molecular Probes, USA).
5. 0.1-µm microspheres (green fluorescence).
6. Perfluorocarbon (FC 72 and/or FC 77, electronics grade, 3M, USA).
7. Modified Ringer's solution: 125 mM NaCl, 5.2 mM KCl, 1.2 mM MgCl$_2$, 1.2 mM CaCl$_2$, 10 mM TES, 10 mM glucose, pH 7.4.
8. Image analysis software (Metamorph, Universal Imaging, USA; and Excel, Microsoft, USA).

2.2.2. Epifluorescence Microscopy of [Rotational] Mucus Transport

1. Suitable cell cultures.
2. Inverted Epifluorescence microscope with low-power lens (5× on Leica, may be 4× on other models).

Table 1
Bronchial Epithelial Growth Medium (BEGM)
Components[a]

Class	Component	Final concentration
Hormones	Insuling	5 µg/mL
	Transferrin	10 µg/mL
	Hydrocortisone	0.072 µg/mL
	Epinephrine	0.6 µg/mL
	Epidermal growth factor	0.025 µg/mL
	Triiodothyronine	0.0065 µg/mL
Miscellaneous	L-Glutamine	6 mM
	Phosphoethanolamine	0.5 µM
	Ethanolamine	0.5 µM
	Bovine serum albumin	0.5 mg/mL
	Bovine pituitary extract	0.8% (v/v)
	Retinoic acid	$5 \times 10^{-8}\ M$
Antibiotics	Gentamicin	50 µg/mL
	Amphotericin B	0.25 µg/mL
	Penicillin	100 U/mL
	Streptomycin	100 µg/mL
Inorganics	Iron	$1.5 \times 10^{-6}\ M$
	Magnesium	$6 \times 10^{-4}\ M$
	Calcium	$1.1 \times 10^{-4}\ M$
Buffers	HEPES	22.9 mM
	NaHCO$_3$	11.9 mM

[a]The base medium was a 1/1 mix of LHC basal medium (laboratory of human carcenogenesis; Sigma, USA) and DMEM (Dulbelcco's modification of Eagle's medium; Gibco-BRL).

3. CCD digital camera and image acquisition software.
4. 1.0-µm microsphere (blue or green fluorescence).
5. Perfluorocarbon (FC 72 and/or FC 77).
6. Image analysis software (Metamorph, Universal Imaging, USA; and Excel, Microsoft, USA).

2.3. Double-Barreled Cl⁻-Selective Microelectrodes

1. GC 150F (1.5-mm od) glass capillary tubes (precut to a length of ~7.5 cm) and GC 120F (1.2-mm od) glass capillary tubes (precut to a length of ~3 cm) (Clark, UK).
2. 50% nitric acid (Sigma-Aldrich).
3. Epoxy resin (i.e., Araldite, Copenhagan, Denmark).
4. Horizontal pipet puller.
5. Sialinizing solution (dichlorodimethylsilane vapor, Sigma-Aldrich).
6. 100°C oven.

7. Ion selective resins (e.g., Cl⁻ ionophore I—Cocktail A, Fluka brand, USA).
8. 5-mL syringes and Microfil needles (WPI, USA) for adding selectophores or Hamilton needles (#90029, Hamilton, USA) for adding KCl.
9. Desiccator for storing pipets (at 23°C).
10. High-impedance electrometer (model FD 223, World Precision Instruments, USA).
11. Pipet holder for Cl⁻ barrel (World Precision Instruments).
12. Ag-AgCl wire to connect reference barrel (*see* **Note 6**).
13. Faraday cage/air table for mounting/shielding the microelectrode setup (*see* **Note 7**).
14. Micromanipulator capable of advance the microelectrode in micrometer increments.
15. Macroelectrode (3 *M* KCl in 4% agar in 2-mm polyethylene tubing connected to a calomile half-cell (World Precision Instruments).
16. Perfluorocarbon (FC 72 and/or FC 77).
17. Data acquisition device (chart recorder or PC setup).

3. Methods

3.1. Cell Culture

3.1.1. Cell Isolation Procedure

1. Obtain suitable tissue as soon after surgery as possible (typically 1 h, but up to 12 h). Specimens are transferred to the tissue culture suite moist in sterile saline.
2. Dissect portions of main stem, lobar, and segmental bronchi free of the lungs rinsed in cold lactated Ringer's solution to remove mucus. (Unwanted, nonepithelial tissue, including blood vessels, lymph nodes. and alveolar tissue, is removed).
3. Add dissected airways to 50-mL centrifuge tubes containing the isolation cocktail (MEM, antibiotics, DNase [1 μg/mL] and 0.1% protease [type XIV, Sigma]).
4. Agitate (rocker/shaker [50–60 cycles/min]) for 2 d at 4°C. The tissue/liquid ratio is between 1/7 and 1/10 (vol./vol.).

3.1.2. Cell Harvesting

1. 10% bovine serum is added to the liquid already present in the 50-mL centrifuge tubes to neutralize the protease, and the tissue/media are poured into a Petri dish.
2. Using a convex surgical scalpel blade, the epithelial cells are carefully scraped from the inner, concave lumenal side of the tissues.
3. Collected epithelial cells are then centrifuged at 500*g* for 5 min at 4°C and washed once in cold BEGM. Isolated cells are seeded onto collagen-coated inserts (T-cols, Costar, USA) as primary cultures. A modified bronchial epithelial growth medium (BEGM) plus antibiotics is added serosally (*see* **Table 1**), which is exchanged for fresh medium every 2–3 d.

3.2. Fluorescent Imaging of ASL/Mucus Transport

3.2.1. Confocal Microscopy of ASL (PCL and Mucus Layers)

1. Prewash cultures if required. 3× apical wash with PBS (*see* **Note 8**).
2. Add PBS and fluorescent dyes (e.g., Texas–Red dextran (*see* **Note 5**) and 1% vol/vol 100-nm microspheres). Excess dye may be aspirated to minimal ASL

levels, or a predetermined amount of PBS/dye may be kept on the airway surface (e.g., 50 µL per 12-mm-diameter culture).

3. At the appropriate incubation time after dye addition, add PFC to the mucosal surface to prevent ASL evaporation and place the culture on the scanning stage of the microscope (either confocal or epifluorescence) (*see* **Note 9**).

4. Further compounds may then be added to the ASL suspended in PFC (*see* **Note 10**).

5. Import images into Metamorph (a series of images may be opened linked together as a *Stack*).

6. Use the *Calibrate* function to set the size of the image based on the electronic magnification read from the confocal microscope.

7. Use the region tools to measure height and fluorescence intensity of the regions of interest. Data acquired here may be logged to a spreadsheet such as Excel.

3.2.2. Fluorescent Imaging of Rotational Mucus Transport

1. Prescreen cultures visually, or by phase contrast microscopy for rotational mucus transport.

2. Add a 0.01% (vol/vol) fluorescent microsphere/PBS suspension to the mucosal surface—typically 30–50 µL per 12-mm-diameter T-col.

3. Add PFC to the mucosal surface to prevent ASL evaporation. Note: the working distance of the low-power objective is sufficient to image the microspheres/mucus with the cultures still in their original "long term" culture dishes (*see* **Note 9**). This is advantageous, since the lid of the culture dish does not need to be removed, keeping the cultures sterile.

4. Under a low- power 4–10× inverted epifluorescence microscope coupled to a CCD digital camera and data acquisition software, focus on the microspheres in the rotating mucus while acquiring images over ~0.1 s, then switch to a 5-s exposure to image the "streaks" of moving microspheres.

5. Compounds may then be added to the ASL suspended in PFC (*see* **Note 10**).

6. Import the images into Metamorph (a series of images may be opened as a *Stack*).

7. Use the *Calibrate* function to set the size of the image based on comparison to an image of a reticule scanned under the same power.

8. Use the region tools to measure both the distance a microsphere (streak) has traveled and its distance from the center of the hurricane. Data acquired here may be logged to a spreadsheet such as Excel. Repeat these experiments several times for microspheres at varying distances from the center.

9. In the spreadsheet, plot the total distance the microsphere has moved against the microsphere's distance from the center of the hurricane and, using linear regression, extrapolate to set distance from the center (we use 1 mm) to normalize microsphere movement (*see* **Fig. 3Aii** for an example).

3.3. Fabrication and Calibration of Double Barreled Cl⁻-Selective Microelectrodes

1. Wash the larger (GC 150F) capillaries in 50% nitric acid for 1 h. Remove, rinse in double-deionized water, and dry in a 100°C oven.

2. Glue the large and short barrels together with epoxy resin so that they are symmetrical.

3. The double-barreled "pre-electrode" is then placed in the puller with the heating element centered around the middle of the pre-electrode and turned on, but with no pull. One side of the pre-electrode is rotated through 360°, which brings the barrels of the pre-electrode close together. The pre-electrode is then pulled apart in the conventional manner to yield two double-barreled microelectrodes (*see* **Note 11**). After pulling, the Cl⁻ barrel (which is the longer of the two) is then exposed to vapor from the sialinization solution for ~8–15 s and baked in an oven at 100°C. The sialinization process aids in filling the tip of the microelectrode with the ion-selective resin.

4. The tip of the Cl⁻ barrel (i.e., only the first 2 mm) should be filled with neat resin immediately following removal from the oven. At this almost-complete stage, the electrodes can be stored under vacuum in a standard desiccator for ~3 mo.

5. When ready for use, the reference barrel is filled with 3 M KCl and the Cl⁻ barrel back-filled with KCl.

6. The macroelectrode is made by slowly heating 4% agar while stirring in 3 M KCl. When it has dissolved, it is put into polyethylene tubing (~1–2-mm-inner diameter) via a syringe and then cut off at convenient lengths to reach between the serosal bath and the calomile half-cell (e.g., 5–10 cm).

7. The cultures are prepared in the same way as for confocal microscopy (*see* **Note 9**), with PFC added mucosally and then positioned under the microelectrode, with an macroelectrode (an agar bridge) placed in the serosal solution.

8. With the reference electrode sensing voltage via the electrometer (against the serosally placed macroelectrode), the double-barreled microelectrode is positioned by micromanipulator so that a reading is read as soon as the microelectrode impales the ASL. The electrometer is then switched over to read the [Cl⁻], i.e., $V_{ion}-V_{ref}$. The output may be sent to a chart recorder or PC hookup.

4. Notes

1. We use Transwell Col inserts (T-Cols) which have been collagen-coated by Corning Costar, USA. A variety of different culture inserts are commercially available, and the type of substrate coated on the insert has been shown to affect the ion transport properties of renal epithelial cells (*11*) and may have a similar effect on airway epithelia.

2. The exception to this is when measuring bioelectric properties or removing excess mucus, when 0.2–0.5 mL PBS is added mucosally for a maximum of 30 min and excess solution is aspirated after measurements are complete.

3. The fluorescent intensity of Texas Red–dextran slowly degrades at 37°C. Hence, a greater amount of dye (2 mg/mL) will need to be added for longer-duration experiments (i.e., over several days) than if they are to be examined immediately (0.2 mg/mL).

4. An ideal Cl⁻-selective electrode should exhibit a –58-mV shift per decade change in [Cl⁻]. We test our electrodes before and after each experiment using two solutions containing either 15 mM NaCl and 135 mM Na-gluconate or 150 mM NaCl.

5. To image ASL by confocal microscopy, we have had best results with a 63× water immersion lens (1.2 NA; Leica, Germany) which has sufficient working distance to image the cultures/ASL over a serosal bath (vol <100 μL). The culture is placed on a circular cover slip (diameter/width) that has been clamped into a chamber designed to fit onto the stage of our confocal microscope (TCS 4D, Leica, Germany). Since this confocal microscope is no longer in production, we will not discuss this chamber in further detail. We image ASL at room temperature and since the PFC blocks all ASL evaporation, we do not humidify the chamber.

6. To chloride the silver wire, silver wire is cleaned with ethanol and connected to a cathode which, together with an anode, is dipped into a 10% bleach solution (diluted with H_2O) and ~10 mA of current is passed between them until the wire blackens, which should happen in a few seconds. The blackened wire can then be soldered onto an annulus sized to fit onto one of the electrometer probes.

7. We have found an air table to be most useful in damping vibrations and reducing electrical noise during recordings under thin-film conditions. This apparatus is not always necessary and, like the Faraday cage, can be considered optional, depending on the levels of noise in the laboratory where the experiments are to be performed.

8. To remove mucus from ALI cultures, ~0.5 mL PBS is added mucosally and aspirated. This procedure is repeated three times. In cases of excessive mucus production, the cultures may be incubated with 0.5 mL PBS and 1 mM dithiothryitol for ~15 min, followed by the 3× PBS rinse.

9. Our cultures are maintained under sterile conditions. However, the cultures risk exposure to pathogens (i.e., mold spores, bacteria) during all our experiments, which destroys the cultures. The best approach to protect against infection has been to transfer the cultures from their "long-term" culture dishes (where they are kept in BEGM) into a secondary dish containing serosal TES-buffered Ringer's and 10 mM glucose (with PFC kept on the mucosal surface to prevent evaporation). From this second dish they can be impaled by microelectrodes or transferred to the stage of the confocal microscope. After the experiment, the cultures are washed several times in PBS and then transferred back to the "long-term" culture dish and BEGM. Serial experiments over several days on one culture are more risky since the mucosal surface cannot be washed during the experiment since this will alter the ASL, but with careful rinsing of the serosal surface and transference between long term and temporary culture dishes after every time point we have routinely studied cultures over 4–5 d with no sign of infection.

10. Typically, the faster evaporating FC 72 will initially be added to cover the ASL, and once basal measurements have been made and the FC 72 has evaporated to minimal levels (which can be assessed visually), compounds are added to the apical surface in more FC 72. If the compounds have been added coarsely (e.g., are ground with a mortar and pestle and then sonicated before addition to the ASL in the PFC. An example of masses/volumes added would be to prepare 0.1 mg in 200 μL FC 72 and to aliquot a smaller amount into the ASL, such as 0.001 mg in 2 μL FC 72.

11. A short, blunt microelectrode is preferred to a long, tapering microelectrode since it results in a larger tip diameter and requires less resin to fill it, both of which lower the impedance of the Cl⁻ barrel. If the microelectrode has a slow response time (>10 s), the tip can be broken slightly under a low-powered dissecting microscope by gently touching the flat side of a scalpel blade against the tip which lowers the resistance of the microelectrode and may improve both its response time and sensitivity. Care must be taken since too great a decrease in tip resistance will result in the ionophore leaking out from the tip, which ruins the microelectrode.

References

1. Sims, D. E. and Horne, M. M. (1997) Heterogeneity of the composition and thickness of tracheal mucus in rats. *Am. J. Physiol.* **273**, L1036–1041.
2. Rahmoune, H. and Shephard, K. L. (1995) State of airway surface liquid on guinea pig trachea. *J. Appl. Physiol.* **78**, 2020–2024.
3. Hanrahan, J. W. (2000) Airway plumbing. *J. Clin. Invest.* **105**, 1343,1344.
4. Wine, J. J. (1999) The genesis of cystic fibrosis lung disease. *J. Clin. Invest.* **103**, 309–312.
5. Matsui, H., Randell, S. H., Peretti, S. W., Davis, C. W., and Boucher, R. C. (1998) Coordinated clearance of periciliary liquid and mucus from airway surfaces. *J. Clin. Invest.* **102**, 1125–1131.
6. Matsui, H., Grubb, B. R., Tarran, R., Randell, S. H., Gatzy, J. T., Davis, C. W., and Boucher, R. C. (1998) Evidence for periciliary liquid layer depletion, not abnormal ion composition, in the pathogenesis of cystic fibrosis airways disease. *Cell* **95**, 1005–1015.
7. Tarran, R., Grubb, B. R., Parsons, D., Picher, M., Hirsh, A. J., Davis, C. W., and Boucher, R. C. (2001) The CF salt controversy: Implications for therapies designed to correct abnormalities in CF airway surface liquid based on in vivo and in vitro studies. *Molecular Cell*, **8**, 149–158.
8. Boucher, R. C. (1994a) Human Airway Ion Transport. *Am. J. Resp. Crit. Care Med.* **150**, 271–281.
9. Johnson, L. G., Dickman, K. G., Moore, K. L., Mandel, L. J., and Boucher, R. C. (1993) Enhanced Na⁺ transport in air-liquid interface culture system. *Am. J. Physiol.* **264**, L560–L565.
10. Amman, D. (1986) *Ion-Selective Microelectrodes: Principles, Design and Application.* Springer-Verlag, Berlin.
11. Helman, S. I. and Liu, X. (1997) Substrate-dependent expression of Na⁺ transport and shunt conductance in A6 epithelia. *Am. J. Physiol.* **273**, C434–C441.
12. Willumsen, N. J., Davis, C. W., and Boucher, R. C. (1989) Intracellular Cl⁻ activity and cellular Cl⁻ pathways in cultured human airway epithelium. *Am. J. Physiol..* **256**, C1033–C1044.

III

PATHOPHYSIOLOGY OF CYSTIC FIBROSIS: ANIMAL MODELS OF CYSTIC FIBROSIS

32

Murine Models of CF Airway Infection and Inflammation

James F. Chmiel, Michael W. Konstan, and Melvin Berger

1. Introduction

The agarose bead model of chronic *Pseudomonas aeruginosa* infection was first described by Cash and colleagues in 1979 *(1)*. In this model, *P. aeruginosa* is embedded in agarose beads and instilled into the airways of animals by transtracheal injection. Embedding the bacteria in agarose beads is important because otherwise, animals rapidly clear many bacteria that are pathogenic to humans. The agarose beads are believed to prevent access of neutrophils to the organisms, thus delaying clearance of the infection. This results in a prolonged neutrophilic influx into the airway lumen and peribronchial space similar to that found in the airways of patients with cystic fibrosis (CF). There may be limited extension to adjacent alveoli, but typically there is no dissemination of the infection. Because of the chronic neutrophilic infiltrate that is predominately located in and around the airway, this model mimics the endobronchial pseudomonas infection seen in CF patients, and thus has been used extensively in CF research.

Most of the morbidity and almost all of the mortality in CF is due to progressive lung disease *(2)*. The sequence of pathophysiological processes that lead to end-stage lung disease is not completely understood in CF. The pulmonary disease in most patients with CF is characterized by a noninvasive, chronic endobronchial bacterial infection, most notably with *P. aeruginosa*. CF patients initially are infected with nonmucoid strains of *P. aeruginosa*. However, over time, a change to the mucoid phenotype occurs as *P. aeruginosa* shifts from "smooth" or long O-side-chain lipopolysaccharide (LPS) to "rough" or short O-side-chain LPS and produces mucoid exopolysaccharide (MEP) *(3)*. Although it is not clear how initial, transient infections shift into a chronic state

From: *Methods in Molecular Medicine, vol. 70: Cystic Fibrosis Methods and Protocols*
Edited by: W. R. Skach © Humana Press Inc., Totowa, NJ

in which *P. aeruginosa* infection can no longer be eradicated, it seems quite likely that large amounts of extracellular MEP function to protect pseudomonas deep inside microcolonies or biofilms in much the same way that embedding in agarose beads protects the organisms from eradication by host defenses. In any case, once the *P. aeruginosa* becomes chronic, a vicious cycle of airway obstruction, infection, and inflammation eventually ensues and ultimately leads to destruction of the airways and death of the individual *(4)*. The chronic inflammatory response in CF is characterized by massive numbers of neutrophils in and around the airways. While neutrophils help to contain infection in normal hosts, in CF patients they are present in great excess and are more injurious than protective *(4)*. DNA from decomposing neutrophils causes the CF sputum to become tenacious. Neutrophils also release huge amounts of elastase that quickly overwhelm host antiproteases. Elastase has many adverse effects including digestion of elastin resulting in bronchiectasis, impairment of opsonophagocytosis of bacteria, stimulation of mucin gland secretion, and increased production of neutrophil chemoattractants *(5)*. The presence of chemoattractants in the airway fuels neutrophil influx and potentiates the vicious cycle of obstruction, infection, and inflammation *(5)*.

Although Cash and colleagues originally developed the agarose bead model of chronic endobronchial pseudomonas infection for use in rats *(1)*, others have adapted it for use in diverse species including cats *(6)*, guinea pigs *(7)*, nonhuman primates *(8)*, and mice *(9)*. The adaptation of this model for use in mice is important because so much is known about the immunological response of many strains, not to mention the availability of knockout, transgenic, and other mutant mice, including those with defects in the cystic fibrosis transmembrane conductance regulator (CFTR). These genetically manipulated mice allow one to study the effect of a preexisting abnormality on the pulmonary inflammatory response in the intact animal. While tissue culture and molecular methods are powerful tools for studying isolated events, they have limited usefulness in the evaluation of contributions from whole organ systems. van Heeckeren and colleagues demonstrated that CFTR-knockout mice infected with pseudomonas embedded in agarose beads had increased mortality, more severe weight loss, greater neutrophil influx, and increased concentrations of pro-inflammatory cytokines in bronchoalveolar lavage fluid than similarly infected wildtype littermates without any alteration in the bacterial burden *(10)*. The development of genetically manipulated mice has strengthened the CF researcher's armamentarium. As more varieties of these mice become available, the agarose bead model of chronic pseudomonas infection will take on increased importance.

The agarose bead model of chronic pseudomonas infection has been used to study the immunopathogenesis of disease and to investigate the impact of therapeutic interventions. Winnie and colleagues used this model to demonstrate that cats infected with pseudomonas-embedded agarose beads initially developed serum antibodies that promoted phagocytosis of *P. aeruginosa* but then subsequently shifted to nonopsonic antibodies that inhibited phagocytosis, similar to those that had been previously reported in CF patients *(6)*. Bacterial virulence factors have also been intensely studied in this model, including multiple *P. aeruginosa* exotoxins and the mucoid phenotype itself. Studies using the agarose bead model in rats demonstrated that a shift in *P. aeruginosa* to the mucoid phenotype from the nonmucoid phenotype occurred several months after initial infection *(11)*. This shift was accompanied by characteristic changes in the restriction length polymorphism patterns of the bacteria, suggesting rearrangement of the pseudomonas chromosome *(11)*. Through increased understanding of the interaction between host and bacteria, development of improved therapies will become possible. Konstan and colleagues used the agarose bead model in rats to demonstrate that ibuprofen reduced pulmonary inflammation without increasing the burden of bacteria *(12)*. This led to a 4-yr clinical trial in CF patients in which high-dose ibuprofen was shown to be associated with a slower deterioration in pulmonary function compared to placebo *(13)*. Initial drug dosing regimes were first determined in rats using this model *(12)*. Ibuprofen is now an established clinical therapy in CF, and the agarose bead model was instrumental in the development of this therapy. Chmiel and colleagues demonstrated that the administration of exogenous interleukin-10 (IL-10) to mice infected with *P. aeruginosa* embedded in agarose beads was associated with improved survival, less drastic weight loss, and decreased neutrophil influx without an alteration in the bacterial burden as compared to placebo-treated mice *(14)*. Yu and colleagues used a model of repeated aerosol administration of *P. aeruginosa* to IL-10-knockout mice every 72 h over 3–6 wk to demonstrate that the absence of IL-10 was associated with increased mortality and increased histopathological changes *(15)*. The primary advantage of this model over the agarose bead model is that no survival surgery is required. The primary disadvantages of the aerosol model are that the precise dose of bacteria delivered to the airways is more variable and that the animals must receive multiple inoculations.

The use of the agarose bead model of chronic endobronchial *P. aeruginosa* infection has made large contributions to CF research. As more sophisticated molecular methods and new therapies are developed, the use of this model will likely increase. While technically challenging, this model of chronic pseudomonas infection is a powerful tool for CF research. Since preclinical studies in intact organisms always will be required in the translation of basic science research to clinical trials in CF, more investigators should become familiar with the methodology of the agarose bead model of chronic pseudomonas infection.

Outlined below is our protocol for establishing a chronic endobronchial *P. aeruginosa* infection in mice. This is the method that works best in our laboratory. Also presented are our protocols for obtaining specimens for assessing various outcome measures. These include bronchoalveolar lavage for analysis of inflammatory mediators, total and differential cell counts, histological preparation and analysis of lung tissue for area of inflammation, and quantitative bacteriology.

2. Materials

2.1. Embedding of Pseudomonas in Agarose Beads

2.1.1. Preparation of P. aeruginosa

1. *P. aeruginosa* (such as laboratory nonmucoid isolate, PA01, or mucoid clinical isolate M5715) from a freezer stock (*see* **Note 1**).
2. Tryptic soy broth, 50 mL in a 250-mL Erlenmeyer flask (×2).
3. Culture plates of trypticase soy agar with 5% sheep blood (blood agar plates).
4. Inoculating loops.

2.1.2. Production of Pseudomonas-Laden Agarose Beads

1. Tryptic soy broth culture of *P. aeruginosa* (Density as in **Subheading 3.1.1., step 4**).
2. Phosphate-buffered saline (PBS), 500 mL in a sterile 1-L glass bottle (×2).
3. Heavy white paraffin oil, 150 mL in a 600-mL glass beaker with a sterile 50-mm magnetic stir bar.
4. 2% type I low-electroendosmosis agarose (Sigma Chemical, St. Louis, MO) in PBS, 50 mL in a 100-mL Erlenmeyer flask.
5. 0.5% sodium deoxycholate (SDC) in PBS, 250 mL in a sterile 500-mL glass bottle.
6. Sterile PBS, 149 mL in a 200-mL sterile glass bottle.
7. Crushed ice.
8. Rectangular plastic container, 10.25 in. × 6.25 in. × 2.5 in.
9. Sterile borosilicate culture tubes, 10 × 75 mm.
10. Sterile 5-mL plastic pipets.
11. Sterile 25-mL wide-mouth glass pipets.
12. Sterile 500-mL separatory funnel with stopcock and glass stopper.
13. 60-mL syringe attached to $1^{1}/_{2}$ in. of flexible plastic tubing that is connected to a 1-mL plastic pipet (cut $5^{1}/_{2}$ in. in length) that is placed through the center of a rubber stopper of the proper size to occlude the top of the separatory funnel in place of the glass stopper.
14. 125-mL Erlenmeyer flask for waste.
15. Sterile 25-mL Erlenmeyer flask with a sterile 15-mm magnetic stir bar.
16. Microscope slides and cover slips.
17. Lazy L Spreaders (Midwest Scientific, Valley Park, MO).
18. Blood agar plates.

19. Ring stand with support for the separatory funnel.
20. Sterile aluminum foil (one 9 × 13 in sheet).
21. Vacuum aspirator setup.
22. Bunsen burner.
23. Magnetic stir plate.
24. Polytron® homogenizer (Brinkmann Instruments, Westbury, NY).
25. Microscope with video monitor (13-in. screen) (final magnification approx 350×).

2.2. Inoculation of Mouse Airways with Agarose Beads

1. Working bead stock produced under **Subheading 3.1.**
2. Sterile PBS for dilutions.
3. Avertin anesthetic: 1 g 2,2,2-tribromoethanol, 1 mL *tert*-amyl alcohol, 48 mL 0.9% normal saline.
4. 0.25% bupivacaine diluted 1/10 in sterile saline.
5. Foil-covered polypropylene centrifuge tube (50 mL) containing a 15-mm magnetic stir bar.
6. Silk suture, 4.0, tied into a 2 in. loop.
7. Shoulder roll (2 pieces of 2 in. × 2 in. gauze rolled tightly together and secured by tape).
8. Tape.
9. Male mice, 8–10 wk old (*see* **Note 2**).
10. Surgery table for restraining mice (1 in. × 8 in. × 8 in. board built up to a 30° angle with two small hooks inserted at the head of the table).
11. Angiocatheters, 22-gage × 1 in. (1 each/mouse).
12. Tuberculin syringe (1 each/mouse).
13. Providone-iodine prep pads.
14. Hot bead sterilizer.
15. 3-mL syringes with attached 26-gage needle (1 per every 5 mice).
16. Sterile 25-mL Erlenmeyer flask with sterile 15-mm magnetic stir bar.
17. Blood agar plates.
18. Sterile borosilicate culture tubes, 10 × 75 mm.
19. Lazy L Spreaders (Midwest Scientific, Valley Park, MO).
20. Sterile surgical instruments:
    a. 11.5-cm scissors for cutting fur and skin;
    b. 12-cm micro-Adson tissue forceps for holding skin and fur;
    c. 8.9-cm microdissecting scissors for blunt dissection;
    d. Extra delicate microdissecting forceps (×2) for blunt dissection.
21. Small animal scale.
22. Magnetic stir plate.
23. Polytron® homogenizer (Brinkmann Instruments).
24. Warm packs equilibrated to 37°C, wrapped in disposable underpads, and placed in a clean, empty cage bottom (used for the recovery of the animals).

2.3. Bronchoalveolar Lavage

1. 200 mM Ethylenediaminetetra-acetic acid (EDTA) in saline.
2. 100 mM Phenylmethylsulfonyl fluoride (PMSF) in isopropanol.
3. Crushed ice.

4. 3-mL syringes with 26-gage needles loaded with Avertin anesthetic.
5. Sterile gauze pads, 2 in. × 2 in.
6. Providone-iodine prep pads.
7. Tuberculin syringe with 27-gage needle (1 per mouse).
8. Sterile cotton swabs.
9. Silk suture, 4.0, cut 3 in. in length (1 per mouse).
10. Needles, 20-gage × 1 in. (1 per mouse).
11. Tuberculin syringe loaded with 0.5 mL of sterile 0.9% normal saline (6 per mouse).
12. Polypropylene microcentrifuge tubes (1.5 mL) for processing blood and aliquoting lavage fluid.
13. Polypropylene centrifuge tubes (3 mL).
14. Microscope slides and cover slips.
15. Hema 3® Stain Set (Fisher Scientific, Pittsburgh, PA).
16. Hot bead sterilizer.
17. Dissecting board with 5 18-gage needles for immobilizing the mouse.
18. Sterile surgical instruments:
    a. Same as under **Subheading 2.2., item 20**;
    b. Microdissecting hemostat.
19. Sterile bead tip feeding needle, 22-gage × $1^{1}/_{2}$ in. (1 per mouse); (Harvard Apparatus, South Natick, MA).
20. Piece of wood, 1 in. × 2 in. × 3 in.
21. Hemocytometer.
22. Electronic timer.
23. Cytospin centrifuge with slide carriers.

2.4. Quantitative Histopathology

1. 2% paraformaldehyde stock in PBS, 150 mL, equilibrated to 50–55°C in a water bath.
2. 5% agarose stock in PBS, 100 mL, autoclaved at 250°F, 18 psi, for 20 min, and then equilibrated to 50–55°C in a water bath.
3. PBS, 150 mL, equilibrated to 50–55°C in a water bath.
4. 1% paraformaldehyde in PBS, 1500 mL in a 2-L flask on ice.
5. Heparinized normal saline (2 U heparin/mL 0.9 % saline), 150 mL in a 250-mL glass beaker.
6. 3-mL syringe with 26-gage needle loaded with Avertin anesthetic.
7. 250-mL Erlenmeyer flask.
8. Sterile gauze pads, 2 in. × 2 in.
9. Providone-iodine prep pads.
10. Sterile cotton swabs.
11. Silk suture, 4.0, cut 3 in. in length (1 per mouse).
12. 20-gage needle, 1 in. in length.
13. Plastic specimen cups (100 mL) with screw tops (1 per mouse).
14. 3-mL syringe with luer lock.
15. Nonsterile gauze pads, 2 in. × 2 in. (2 per mouse).
16. Hot bead sterilizer.

17. Dissecting board with 5 18-gage needles for immobilizing the mouse.
18. Sterile surgical instruments (same as **Subheading 2.3., item18**).
19. Sterile bead tip feeding needle, 22-gage $\times$ $1^1/_2$ in. in length (1 per mouse); (Harvard Apparatus).
20. Piece of wood, 1 in. $\times$ 2 in. $\times$ 3 in.
21. Razor blades or scalpel.
22. Pathology pads.
23. Pathology cassettes.
23. Microscope with video monitor (13-in. screen) (final magnification approx 140$\times$).
24. Acetate sheet cut (18.5 cm $\times$ 18.5 cm) to fit over video monitor screen.

2.5. Quantitative Bacteriology of Lung and Spleen Homogenates

1. Sterile glass bottles (50 mL) containing 35 mL sterile PBS (2 per mouse).
2. Sterile PBS, 10 mL in a sterile, plastic 50-mL conical centrifuge tube with a screw cap (2 per mouse).
3. Ethanol 100%, 150 mL.
4. 3-mL syringe with 26-gage needle loaded with Avertin anesthetic.
5. Sterile 2 in. $\times$ 2 in. gauze pads.
6. Providone-iodine prep pads.
7. Tuberculin syringe with 27-gage needle (1 per mouse).
8. Sterile cotton swabs.
9. Sterile silk suture, 4.0, cut 3 in. in length (2 per mouse).
10. Hot bead sterilizer.
11. Sterile Petri plates, 30 mm (1 per mouse).
12. Sterile gauze pads, 2 in. $\times$ 2 in. (2 per mouse).
13. Sterile borosilicate culture tubes, 10 $\times$ 75 mm.
14. MacConkey agar plates.
15. Lazy L Spreaders (Midwest Scientific, Valley Park, MO).
16. Dissecting board with 5 18-gage needles for immobilizing the mouse.
17. Sterile surgical instruments:
    a. Same as **Subheading 2.2., item 20.**
    b. 8.9-cm microdissecting scissors for spleen removal;
    c. Extra delicate microdissecting forceps ($\times$2) for spleen removal.
18. Polytron® homogenizer (Brinkmann Instruments, Westbury, NY).
19. Bunsen burner.

3. Methods

3.1. Embedding of Pseudomonas in Agarose Beads

3.1.1. Preparation of P. aeruginosa

1. Four days before the day on which beads will be made, thaw *P. aeruginosa* from a freezer stock and plate in duplicate on blood agar plates. Incubate at 37°C for 24 h.
2. Three days before the day beads will be made, subculture *P. aeruginosa* in duplicate on blood agar plates and incubate at 37°C for 24 h.

3. Two days before the day beads will be made, subculture *P. aeruginosa* by removing one inoculating loopful of *P. aeruginosa* from the blood agar plate that was inoculated the previous day, and transfer it to into 50 mL of sterile tryptic soy broth in a 250-mL Erlenmeyer flask. Incubate at 37°C in a shaking water bath.

4. Twenty to 24 h later (once the bacteria have grown to plateau phase, approx 2 × 10^9 CFU/mL) (*see* **Note 3**), subculture *P. aeruginosa* by removing one loopful of broth from the flask inoculated the previous day and placing it into a second 250-mL Erlenmeyer flask containing 50 mL of sterile tryptic soy broth on the day before making agarose beads. Incubate the flask in a 37°C shaking water bath.

3.1.2. Production of Pseudomonas-Laden Agarose Beads

1. Autoclave the two 1-L bottles containing 500 mL of PBS, the 600-mL glass beaker containing 150 mL of heavy white paraffin oil, the 500-mL bottle containing 250 mL of 0.5% SDC, and the Erlenmeyer flask of 2% agarose at 250°F, 18 psi, for 20 min.

2. Equilibrate heavy paraffin oil, 0.5% SDC, and agarose in a stationary 50–55°C water bath for at least 2 h. PBS should be kept at room temperature.

3. Place the beaker of warm mineral oil with sterile stir bar into the empty rectangular plastic container on top of the magnetic stir plate and stir rapidly, achieving a vortex 2 cm in depth; do not yet add ice.

4. Twenty to 24 h after the broth culture was inoculated the previous day (plateau phase for *P. aeruginosa*), add 5 mL of pseudomonas-infected tryptic soy broth to the Erlenmeyer flask containing 50 mL of warmed agarose. Swirl to mix thoroughly (*see* **Note 4**). Return the flask to the 50–55°C stationary water bath.

5. Pass a 25-mL wide mouth glass pipet quickly through the flame of the Bunsen burner three times. With the pipet, withdraw 27 mL of the bacteria/agarose mixture and rapidly eject the mixture into the stirring mineral oil to form discrete beads.

6. Stir pseudomonas/agarose/mineral oil mixture for 11 min. During this time, gradually increase the speed on the magnetic stir plate so that the stir bar is spinning as rapidly as possible without losing the vortex or effective spinning (*see* **Note 5**).

7. After 11 min, begin adding 10–20 g of ice to the ice boat around the beaker every 20 s for 7 min more. Continue to increase the speed of the magnetic stir plate to maintain effective mixing.

8. While the pseudomonas/agarose/mineral oil mixture is cooling, remove the glass stopper from the separatory funnel with stopcock and add 250 mL of 0.5% SDC. Replace the glass stopper. Cover the stem of the separatory funnel with sterile aluminum foil. Gently rotate the separatory funnel while it is being held nearly horizontal, so that the entire inside of the separatory funnel is coated with the SDC. Be sure not to contaminate the stem of the separatory funnel (*see* **Note 6**).

9. After the bacteria/agarose/mineral oil mixture has cooled for 7 min, in rapid succession: quickly turn off the stir plate, remove the glass stopper from the separatory funnel, pour the mixture into the separatory funnel, and replace the glass stopper.

10. Agitate gently by shaking the contents of the separatory funnel while it is being held horizontally.

11. Allow the beads to settle (10–20 min). If the beads do not begin to settle after 4–6 min, grasp the stem of the separatory funnel, which is encircled by the sterile aluminum foil, lift up and pull forward on the stem, then gently pull down and push back on the stem. Repeat 2×.

12. Aspirate as much as possible of the supernatant from above beads using a sterile 5-mL pipet connected to the vacuum aspirator. Be careful not to remove any beads.

13. Add approx 250 mL of PBS to the separatory funnel. Do not agitate. Allow the beads to settle (8–12 min). Aspirate the excess supernatant from above the beads. Repeat the PBS washes three additional times (*see* **Note 7**).

14. After the last wash, aspirate off PBS until approx 5 mm remains above the level of the settled beads. Remove the aluminum foil from around the stem of the separatory funnel.

15. Rapidly transfer the lower two-thirds of the beads to a 125-mL Erlenmeyer flask: Remove the glass stopper and replace it in the opening of the separatory funnel with a rubber stopper connected to the air-filled 60-mL syringe. Force air into the funnel by depressing the plunger of the syringe, then quickly open the funnel stopcock, and rapidly expel the lower portion of the beads into a 125-mL flask (*see* **Note 8**). Close the stopcock when approx 15 mL of the bead mixture remains in the separatory funnel. Discard the beads in this flask, because they are too large for mouse airways.

16. Remove the rubber stopper from the separatory funnel and refill the 60-mL syringe with air. Again, occlude the opening of the separatory funnel with the rubber stopper. Rapidly expel the remaining beads into a sterile 25-mL Erlenmeyer flask with magnetic stir bar by repeating the procedure described above. This now constitutes the working bead stock (*see* **Note 8**). This should provide beads of the appropriate size for mouse airways. Place the working bead stock on a magnetic stir plate and spin so that the beads are uniformly distributed throughout. Remove a small aliquot of the working bead stock and place on a microscope slide and cover with a cover slip. Measure the beads microscopically (*see* **Note 9**). Beads should range from 10 to 250 μm, with an average of 100 μm (*see* **Note 10**).

17. *Quantify bacterial dose in the working bead stock:* Remove 1 mL of the working bead stock (while spinning on a stir plate), and add to 149 mL of sterile PBS in a sterile bottle. Homogenize this diluted bead prep for 60 s with a Polytron homogenizer at its maximal allowable setting, being careful not to spill any of the homogenate. Make serial 10-fold dilutions in sterile PBS in sterile borosilicate tubes of the bead homogenate and plate in duplicate on blood agar plates with Lazy L Spreaders. Store the working bead stock with the stir bar at 4°C for use the following day. At 24 h, count the number of colonies and calculate the number of CFU/mL of working bead stock. This allows adjustment of the actual volume instilled into the mice to give uniform inocula in different experiments, and also allows quality control of the bead preparation process.

3.2. Inoculation of Mouse Airways with Agarose Beads

1. Remove working bead stock, which was produced the previous day, from the 4°C refrigerator and allow it to come to room temperature.

2. Prepare Avertin anesthetic by vortexing together 1 mL of *tert*-amyl alcohol, 1 g of 2,2,2-tribromoethanol, and 48 mL of normal saline in a foil-covered 50-mL conical centrifuge tube. Draw up the necessary amount (0.6 mL × number of mice) of Avertin into 3-mL syringes to anesthetize all mice.

3. Place working bead stock on the magnetic stir plate and stir so that all beads are evenly distributed throughout the stock. Dilute agarose bead working stock in sterile PBS in a sterile 25-mL Erlenmeyer flask containing a magnetic stir bar such that each mouse will receive 3–5 × 10^4 CFU in 20 μL. This now constitutes the inoculating bead prep.

4. Place inoculating bead prep on magnetic stir plate and stir rapidly to keep the slurry uniform as serial samples are removed for inoculating the mouse airways.

5. Anesthetize the mouse with 0.015 mL of Avertin/g body weight (*see* **Note 11**).

6. Secure the mouse to the surgery board by placing the loop of 4.0 suture through the hooks at the head of the surgery board and over the upper central incisors of the mouse. Place the shoulder roll beneath the animal and gently pull down on the tail and tape it to the surgery board.

7. Clean the ventral aspect of the mouse from the tip of the jaw to the xiphoid process with a providone-iodine prep pad.

8. Using the micro-Adson forceps, lift up on the fur and skin just cephalad to the sternum and make a small V-like incision in the midline over the trachea with the large (11.5 cm) scissors. The tissue fascia and the large submandibular salivary glands should now be visible. Lift up on the salivary glands with the micro-Adson forceps and cut the fascia caudal to the salivary glands with the large scissors. The strap muscles overlaying the trachea can now be visualized. Bluntly dissect away the strap muscles and surrounding fascia with the two curved microdissecting forceps.

9. Pull back the plunger on a tuberculin syringe so that the tip of the rubber stopper of the syringe is at 0.1 mL. Place the syringe hub into the spinning inoculating bead prep and load the hub of the tuberculin syringe with 25 μL of agarose bead slurry by gently pulling further back on the plunger (filling two-thirds of the syringe hub, *see* **Note 12**). Blot the tip of the syringe on a sterile nonabsorbent flat surface to remove any excess bead slurry, and set aside (the small amount of air behind the agarose bead slurry in the syringe allows this to deliver 20 μL of the slurry to the animal).

10. With the microdissecting forceps, retract the strap muscles so that the trachea is easily visualized. Insert the angiocatheter with stylette in place (bevel up) between two cartilaginous rings in the mid trachea. Advance the stylette and catheter just enough (3 mm) so that the tip of the plastic catheter enters the tracheal lumen. Remove the stylette and advance the catheter into the lower trachea, directing it toward the right mainstem bronchus (*see* **Fig. 1**). The catheter is in the lumen of the right mainstem bronchus when a slight increase in resistance to the advancement of the catheter is felt (*see* **Note 13**). Connect the tuberculin syringe containing the agarose bead slurry to the angiocatheter and rapidly instill the beads into the right mainstem bronchus by quickly depressing the plunger on the syringe. The small amount of air in the syringe behind the agar beads allows

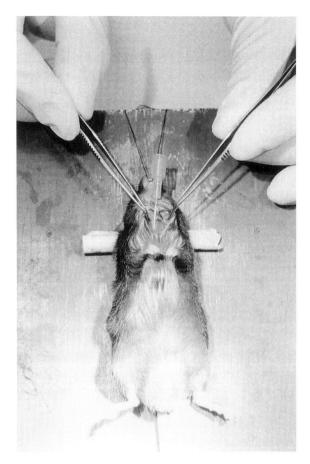

Fig. 1. Surgical site demonstrating the appropriate placement of the 22-gage angiocatheter for inoculating the right mainstem bronchus of the mouse with agarose beads. The incision is enlarged and the salivary glands are retracted for better visualization for photographic purposes.

for all but approx 5 μL of the inoculum to be delivered into the animal's airway. Remove the angiocatheter. Provide postoperative analgesia at the surgical site by applying 0.1 mL of 1/10 bupivacaine topically. There is no need to close the surgical incision, as it will heal quickly. The incidence of local infection is negligible.

11. Remove the animal from the surgery table and allow it to recover on the warm packs wrapped with underpads. Be sure to reposition the animal frequently until it awakens from anesthesia. Once the mouse is awake, place it in a clean cage with sterile food and water. Mice should be weighed and examined daily until sacrificed (*see* **Note 14**).

12. Surgical instruments should be sterilized between animals with a hot bead sterilizer.

13. Once all surgeries are completed, confirm that the calculated dose was indeed delivered to the mice by adding 1 ml of the bead prep (still stirring on the mag-

netic stir plate) to 149 mL of sterile PBS, homogenizing, and plating on blood agar plates as described under **Subheading 3.1.2., step 17**. This also allows one to determine if any contamination of the inoculating bead prep occurred.

3.3. Bronchoalveolar Lavage (see Note 15)

1. Anesthetize the mouse with Avertin, 0.015 mL/g body weight, via i.p. injection (*see* **Subheading 3.2., steps 2** and **5**).
2. Secure the mouse to surgery board with 18-gage needles. Place one needle through each leg and one through the upper lip.
3. Clean the entire ventral surface of the mouse with a providone-iodine prep pad.
4. Lift up the animal's fur and skin at the tip of the xiphoid process with the micro-Adson forceps and make a small incision with the large scissors.
5. Make an incision through the fur and skin from the tip of the xiphoid process in the midline over the sternum to the tip of the jaw using the large scissors. Do not yet enter the abdomen or thorax.
6. Make a lateral incision through the fur and skin from the tip of the xiphoid process along the lowest rib to the back on each side with the large scissors. Retract the overlying fur and skin with the micro-Adson forceps so that the rib cage and upper abdomen are exposed. Again, do not yet enter the thorax or abdomen.
7. Lift up on the xiphoid process with the micro-Adson forceps and make a small cut in the abdominal wall with the large scissors. Cut the abdominal wall laterally from the xiphoid process to the back along the rib cage bilaterally. The diaphragm should be easily visible from below.
8. Lift up the xiphoid process with the micro-Adson forceps and make a small nick in the diaphragm just beneath the sternum with the large scissors. The heart and lungs should fall away from the diaphragm.
9. While still lifting the xiphoid process, cut the diaphragm away from the rib cage with the large scissors by cutting laterally along the lower ribs. Be sure to keep the scissors abutted to the rib cage so as not to accidently cut the lungs.
10. Make a 5–10 mm cut through the xiphoid process and lower sternum along the mid sternal line with the large scissors.
11. Lifting up on the rib cage with the micro-Adson forceps, place the 27-gage needle (bevel up) connected to a tuberculin syringe into the right ventricle and exsanguinate the mouse. Process the blood for peripheral white blood cell count or allow it to clot and save the serum for other studies.
12. Completely divide the thorax by cutting along the mid sternal line with the large scissors.
13. Pin back the rib cage with the two 18-gage needles used to hold down the front legs. Using a sterile 2 in. × 2 in. gauze pad, retract the abdominal contents downward and pin down the gauze using the two18-gage needles holding the hind legs.
14. Loosen the lungs from the parietal pleura with a sterile cotton swab. Transect the inferior vena cava with the microdissecting scissors. Remove the thymus with the microdissecting forceps.
15. Bluntly dissect out the trachea with the two curved microdissecting forceps. Be sure to carefully remove any fascia holding the trachea to the esophagus.

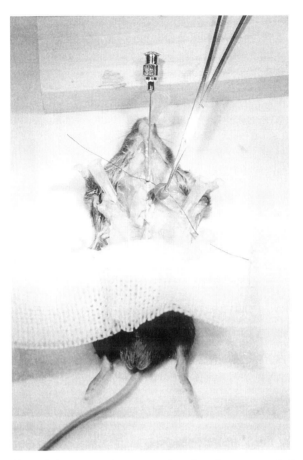

Fig. 2. Dissection of the mouse demonstrating the placement of a bead tip feeding needle for bronchoalveolar lavage. The lungs are inflated with 0.5 mL of 0.9% saline for better visualization for photographic purposes.

16. Place a 3 in. piece of 4.0-silk suture between the esophagus and trachea. Make a small nick between two cartilaginous rings in the mid trachea with a 20-gage needle. Gently enlarge the opening with the tip of the 20-gage needle so that it is just large enough to accommodate the bead on the feeding needle. Pass the feeding needle through the incision and advance into the lower trachea. Secure the feeding needle in place by bringing the suture up and around the trachea and needle shaft and tying. Place the piece of 1 in. × 2 in. wood at the mouse's head and rest the hub of the feeding needle on this.
17. Lift the heart off of the lungs by grasping it with a hemostat and resting the hemostat on the piece of wood (*see* **Fig. 2**).
18. Perform six 0.5-mL normal saline lavages: Connect the syringe of 0.5 mL of PBS to the hub of the feeding needle. The full 0.5 mL of saline should be gently instilled into the mouse airways, allowed to dwell for 3 s, and aspirated back by

applying gentle pressure on the plunger. Be sure that all five lobes of the lung inflate evenly. It is important not to pull back too forcefully, as this will result in trauma. Note the volume returned to the syringe. This should be repeated five more times. Pool the lavage fluid from all six syringes into one 3-mL polypropylene tube (*see* **Note 16**) for each mouse. It is important to keep the lavage fluid on ice at all times until processed.

19. Sterilize the surgical instruments between each animal with a hot bead sterilizer.
20. Gently mix the lavage fluid for each mouse. Remove a 250-μL aliquot of the lavage fluid and process for cell count and differential (*see* **Note 17**).
21. Centrifuge the remaining lavage fluid at 400g for 10 min at 4°C to pellet the white cells.
22. After centrifugation is complete, remove the supernatant from the cell pellet and place in another 3-mL polypropylene tube. Add 25 μL of EDTA/mL of lavage fluid and 1 μL of PMSF/mL of lavage fluid to the supernatant to give final concentrations of 5×10^{-3} M and 1×10^{-4} M respectively. Gently vortex to mix. Aliquot lavage fluid (200-μL aliquots) into small (1.5 mL) polypropylene Eppendorf tubes and freeze at –70°C until the desired ELISAs are performed for various mediators such as cytokines (*see* **Notes 18** and **19**).
23. Using the 250-μL aliquot removed in **step 20**, determine total white cell counts using a standard hemocytometer and make slides for differential counts by cytospinning 200 μL of lavage fluid at 60g for 5 min (sample may need to be diluted). There should be at least 40,000 cells on each slide for each animal. Stain cells with the Hema 3 Stain Set and determine the percentage of various white cells.

3.4. Quantitative Histopathology

1. Combine 125 mL of the 2% paraformaldehyde stock, 50 mL of the 5% agarose stock, and 75 mL of PBS in a 250-mL Erlenmeyer flask to make a 1% paraformaldehyde, 1% agarose in PBS solution. Keep the mixture in a 50–55°C stationary water bath during entire procedure.
2. Aliquot 60 mL of the ice cold 1% paraformaldehyde into the 100-mL plastic specimen cups. Keep the specimen cups on ice.
3. Begin the procedure exactly as described for bronchoalveolar lavage in **Subheading 3.3., steps 1–16** (*see* **Note 20**).
4. Gently remove the heart lung bloc. To do this, sever the trachea above the insertion site for the bead tip feeding needle. Using the bead tip feeding needle as a handle, bluntly dissect away any tissue connected to the heart lung bloc (*see* **Note 21**).
5. Rinse the exterior of the heart lung bloc by gently immersing in heparinized saline.
6. Draw up 3 mL of the 1% paraformaldehyde, 1% agarose in PBS solution into a 3-mL syringe. Using the luer lock, connect the syringe to the hub of the bead tip needle. Holding the syringe and heart-lung bloc vertically, gently instill enough of the paraformaldehyde/agarose solution to completely fill all lung lobes (approx 1 mL). Be careful not to overinflate the lungs (*see* **Note 22**).
7. Holding the heart-lung bloc over a specimen cup, transect the trachea distal to the bead tip feeding needle. Place the heart-lung bloc in a specimen cup containing

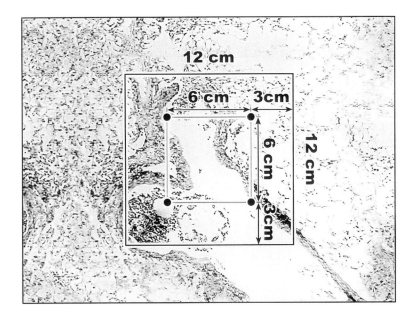

Fig. 3. Diagram of the grid used for point counting. The grid is drawn on an acetate sheet that is cut to size such that it can be affixed to the monitor screen. The border of the histological section represents the entire monitor screen. The grid is shown over-laying a typical histopathological section of the lung (magnification 140×). Two beads can be visualized in the airway lumen.

60 mL of ice-cold 1% paraformaldehyde. Place two nonsterile 2 in. × 2 in. gauze pads over the heart-lung bloc to completely submerge it. Tighten the cap on the specimen cup. Place one heart-lung bloc from each mouse into a separate specimen cup. Keep on ice until the procedure is completed.

8. Store the specimens at 4°C for 5–7 d.
9. After 5–7 d, remove the heart from the heart-lung bloc and discard. Divide each lung lobe through its sagital axis with a razor blade or scalpel. Discard the proximal portions of each lobe. Place the distal lung sections of each lung lobe on a pathology pad in a labeled pathology cassette and immerse in the 1% paraformaldehyde until they are embedded in paraffin using the standard procedure of the pathology department. After embedding, each lung lobe should be sectioned saggitally in 5-μm slices and stained with hematoxylin-eosin. Make slides of entire sagital sections from each lung lobe.
10. Draw a 12 cm × 12 cm grid square on the acetate sheet and place one dot in each corner of the grid square (*see* **Fig. 3**). The dots should be 3 cm from the nearest horizontal and vertical lines of the square, and there should be 6 cm between any two adjacent dots in either the vertical or horizontal direction. Center the acetate sheet over the video microscope monitor screen and affix with transparent tape. The square should be large enough so that the magnified tissue on the monitor screen contained within the square equals between 0.75 and 0.90 mm of actual

tissue. The total magnification from microscope slide to the monitor screen should be approx 140×.

11. Begin by moving the microscope stage so that the farthest left most portion of the tissue specimen on the monitor screen just touches the inner side of the left line of the grid square on the acetate sheet affixed to the monitor screen. Next, move the microscope stage such that the tissue image on the monitor screen moves vertically. Initially move the microscope stage such that all four dots of the grid are no longer overlaying any tissue. Move the microscope stage back in the opposite direction just until at least one point overlays any part of the tissue specimen as visualized on the monitor screen. This is the starting point for the first grid. Determine whether this point falls on a normal lung structure (parenchyma, airway lumen, bronchial wall, vessel, connective tissue, or artifact) or on an area of inflammation (parenchymal inflammation, airway exudate, or peribronchial inflammation). Continue to move the microscope stage in the same direction so that the tissue image moves in the same vertical direction. Move the tissue specimen visualized on the monitor screen one grid square at a time. To do this, note where the horizontal line nearest the direction of movement (i.e., bottom line if you are moving downwards) intersects with a structure on the monitor screen. Move the stage in the same direction so that the opposite horizontal (top) line of the grid square intersects the structure at the same point. With each one grid square movement, record whether each of the points in the grid square fall over a normal lung structure or over an area of inflammation. Continue to move the stage in this direction grid by grid until all points in the square fall off the tissue. Move the microscope stage so that the tissue image on the monitor screen moves one grid square to the right. To do this, note where the right vertical line of the grid square intersects with a structure on the monitor screen and move the stage so that the left vertical line of the grid square intersects with the structure at the same point. Next, move the microscope stage so that the tissue image moves in the opposite vertical direction as previously. Continue moving the tissue image in this fashion (vertically and to the right) until the entire area of each section has been assessed. Perform the grid point counting maneuver on the one best tissue specimen obtained in close proximity to the cut edge and the one best specimen obtained halfway lateral from the cut edge for each lung lobe for each mouse. To determine the areal percent inflammation, total the points falling over inflamed areas and divide by the total number of points counted for all sections from all lung lobes for each mouse (*see* **Note 23**). Typically more than 1000 points are counted for each animal.

3.5. Quantitative Bacteriology of Lung and Spleen Homogenates

1. Begin the procedure exactly as described under **Subheading 3.3., steps 1–14**. Be sure that the surgical instruments used for cutting the fur and skin of the mouse do not come in contact with the surgical instruments used to remove the lungs.

2. Using sterile microdissecting forceps, gently retract the right lung downward by lightly grasping the right mainstem bronchus. Slide a sterile suture beneath the right mainstem bronchus and tie off the bronchus. Completely sever the right

mainstem bronchus proximal to the surgical tie with microdissecting scissors (*see* **Note 24**). Rinse the exterior surface of the tied-off right lung in 35 mL of sterile PBS in a sterile glass bottle. Gently blot the lung on a sterile gauze pad. Trim away the excess suture. Place the right lung in a sterile 30-mm Petri dish. Sterilize the instruments in a hot bead sterilizer. Repeat the procedure for the left lung and place the left lung with the right lung in the Petri dish (*see* **Note 23**). Determine the lung weight with a balance. Place both the right and left lungs in the same sterile 50-mL conical centrifuge tube containing 10 mL of sterile PBS.

3. Using the large scissors and the micro-Adson forceps, make a vertical midline incision through the abdominal wall. Using a second set of sterile microdissecting scissors and forceps, remove the spleen. Be sure that the instruments used to remove the spleen do not come in contact with the other instruments. Rinse the spleen in sterile PBS in a separate sterile glass bottle. Blot dry on sterile gauze. Place the spleen in a second sterile 50-mL conical centrifuge tube containing 10 mL of sterile PBS. Sterilize the instruments in a hot bead sterilizer. Keep the specimens on ice or at 4°C until processed.

4. Homogenize the lungs completely (30–60 s) with a sterile Polytron homogenizer. Make serial 10-fold dilutions in sterile PBS (10^1–10^7) in sterile borosilicate tubes and spread the dilutions of the lung homogenate in duplicate on MacConkey agar plates. Sterilize the Polytron homogenizer between each specimen by flaming the probe after dipping it into 100% ethanol. Incubate the plates at 37°C. Check the plates at 24 and 48 h and determine the number of colony forming units contained within the lungs from each mouse.

5. Homogenize the spleens completely with a sterile Polytron homogenizer. Make serial 10-fold dilutions (10^1–10^3) in sterile PBS in sterile borosilicate tubes and spread the lung homogenate in duplicate on MacConkey agar plates.

6. Proceed as outlined in **step 4** for lung homogenates (see **Note 25**).

4. Notes

1. The protocols described above outline our method for using *P. aeruginosa* in this model, but other investigators have also studied *B. cepacia* (*9*). The agarose bead model of chronic endobronchial infection can be adapted for use with many bacteria including *S. aureus* and *H. influenzae*.

2. It is important to realize that the strain of the host species may also greatly affect the manifestations of inflammation. It is well documented that various strains of mice differ in the characteristics and kinetics of the inflammatory response to *P. aeruginosa* (*16–18*). We have found that BALB/C mice tend to develop little respiratory tract inflammation after inoculation with *P. aeruginosa*, whereas C3H/FeJ mice become severely ill and die shortly after inoculation with the dose described here. In our hands, C57Bl/6 and C57Bl/10 mice appear to have intermediate response, with respect to areal percent inflammation and survival, to pseudomonas infection. We like to use CD-1 mouse to evaluate the effect of an anti-inflammatory therapy. This mouse is generally larger for a given age, thus making the surgery technically easier. The CD-1 mouse has been previously shown to tolerate a large inflammatory response without resulting in great mor-

tality (*9*). This makes it suitable to study the impact of various interventions on inflammation.

3. A growth curve will need to be performed to determine when the bacteria reach plateau phase. This varies by strain of *P. aeruginosa*.

4. If sterile agarose beads are to be produced as a control, add 5 mL of sterile PBS (equilibrated to 37°C) to the melted agarose and swirl.

5. Be sure not to increase the speed so quickly that effective spinning is lost. When movement of the stir bar becomes erratic and begins to lift off the bottom of the glass beaker, the beads will clump and be unusable.

6. If the inside of the separatory funnel is not completely coated with the SDC, the beads will adhere to the glass.

7. The purpose of the four PBS washes is to remove any tryptic soy broth, soluble culture constituents, and nonembedded *P. aeruginosa* from the surface of the beads.

8. The beads must be expelled from the separatory funnel with air pressure from the 60-mL syringe and not just by gravity. Otherwise, the liquid will drain first, and the beads will clog the stopcock.

9. The beads are measured using a video monitor screen in line with a microscope. A measuring grid drawn on an acetate sheet is placed over the monitor screen and typically 50 beads are measured. The final magnification from the microscope slide containing the beads to the monitor screen is 350×.

10. In preparing agarose beads for use in mice, we use only those beads contained in the top 15 mL of the settled beads in the separatory funnel. This allows for the selection of appropriately sized beads (approx 10–250 μm) for mouse airways. When we establish pseudomonas infection in rats, all beads in the separatory funnel are collected and used, since rats have larger airways.

11. If the animal is not adequately anesthetized as determined by toe pinch, an additional 0.005 mL of Avertin/g of body weight may be given. This can be repeated as necessary until adequate sedation is achieved.

12. Before beginning any studies, it will be necessary to verify how much the syringe hub is filled by 25 μL. Once this is established, drawing up this amount as described in this section should be practiced until it can be reliably reproduced.

13. We perform inoculations into the right mainstem bronchus of the mouse. Instilling beads into the trachea will allow a bilateral infection to be established. However, in our experience, bilateral infection may result in excessive mortality.

14. In using this model it is important to look for systemic effects of inflammation and to determine the incidence of bacteremia. Besides survival, we also recommend that the animals be weighed and examined daily, as body weight provides a good marker of overall well-being. Finally, we suggest that a full necropsy with cultures of spleen homogenates be performed on any mouse that dies before planned sacrifice. It is important to determine if a mouse died of overwhelming pneumonia or other effects of the intrapulmonary process itself, from systemic effects of mediators produced in the lung, from dissemination of the infection with sepsis, or from an abnormality of the gastrointestinal tract, such as obstruction.

15. Bronchoalveolar lavage, quantitative histopathology, and quantitative bacteriology are performed on separate animals. Performing more than one outcome measure on a given mouse will increase the variability of subsequent outcome measurements.

16. Always use polypropylene tubes for processing bronchoalveolar lavage fluid. Cytokines adhere to polystyrene and glass.

17. Bronchoalveolar lavage fluid cell count with differentials can be determined at any point during the infection and provide useful information.

18. We typically measure TNF-α, IL-1β, IL-6, mip-2, and KC in the bronchoalveolar lavage fluid. The mouse does not make the same neutrophil chemoattractant C-X-C cytokine, IL-8, as the human, but employs other C-X-C chemokines including mip-2 and KC.

19. We typically determine cytokine concentrations 3 d after inoculation. At later time points, the concentrations of cytokines decrease as the infection wanes. As cytokine concentrations fall toward the sensitivity of the assay, interpretation becomes difficult. Measuring the cytokine concentrations earlier in the course of the infection has the added advantage of avoiding censoring of the data due to animal death.

20. While differences in quantitative histopathology between two experimental groups begin to become evident early during the course of infection, they usually do not reach statistical significance until more than 7 d after the inoculation. For this reason, we typically sacrifice animals for histopathology 10 d after inoculation.

21. When removing the heart-lung bloc, be careful not to put too much traction on the trachea or it will tear.

22. It may be difficult to instill the paraformaldehyde/agarose solution into lung lobes that are completely filled with inflammatory exudate. The difficult lobe can be inflated with the fixing mixture by gently milking the bronchus that supplies the involved lobe. It may first be necessary to tie off the bronchi to less involved lobes that have been already filled with the paraformaldehyde/agarose mixture with a short piece of 4.0-silk suture to prevent over distension of these lobes.

23. Despite the performing unilateral endobronchial inoculations, all outcome measures are determined for both the right and left lung due to the small but real amount of spillover of agarose beads that may occur from the right lung into the left lung.

24. Be sure not to nick any part of the gastrointestinal tract accidently, as this will contaminate the lung.

25. It is important to perform quantitative bacteriology on spleen homogenates for at least those mice whose lungs are being used for quantitative bacteriology. This allows determination of the incidence of bacteremia. It would be ideal to perform quantitative bacteriology on the spleen homogenates from all mice, but this may not be possible if a large number of animals are being sacrificed. Postmortem quantitative bacteriology should be performed on homogenates of spleens from all animals that die before the day of sacrifice for the same reason.

Acknowledgments

The authors wish to thank Kathleen Hilliard for her photographs shown in Figs. 1 and 2.

References

1. Cash, H. A., Woods, D. E., McCullough, B., Johanson, W. G., Jr., and Bass, J. A. (1979) A rat model of chronic respiratory infection with *Pseudomonas aeruginosa. Am. Rev. Respir. Dis.* **119,** 453–459.
2. Davis, P. B., Drumm, M., and Konstan, M. W. (1996) Cystic fibrosis: State of the art. *Am. J. Respir. Crit. Care Med.* **154,** 1229–1256.
3. Hancock, R. E. W., Mutharia, L. M., Chan, L., Darveau, R. P., Speert, D. P., and Pier, G. B. (1983) *Pseudomonas aeruginosa* isolates from patients with cystic fibrosis: A class of serum sensitive, nontypable strains deficient in lipopolysaccharide O side chains. *Infect. Immunol.* **42,** 170–177.
4. Konstan, M. W. and Berger, M. (1993) Infection and inflammation in the lung in cystic fibrosis, in *Cystic Fibrosis* (Davis, P. B., ed.), Marcel Dekker, New York, NY, pp. 219–276.
5. Konstan, M. W. and Berger, M. (1997) Current understanding of the inflammatory process in cystic fibrosis: Onset and etiology. *Pediatr. Pulmonol.* **24,** 137–142.
6. Winnie, G. B., Klinger, J. D., Sherman, J. M., and Thomassen, M. J. (1982) Induction of phagocytic inhibitory activity in cats with chronic *Pseudomonas aeruginosa* pulmonary infection. *Infect. Immun.* **38,** 1088–1093.
7. Pennington, J. E., Hickey, W. F., and Blackwood, L. L. (1981) Active immunization with lipopolysaccharide pseudomonas antigen for chronic pseudomonas bronchopneumonia in guinea pigs. *J. Clin. Invest.* **68,** 1140–1148.
8. Chung, A. T., Moss, R. B., Leong, A. B., and Novick, W. J., Jr. (1992) Chronic *Pseudomonas aeruginosa* endobronchitis in rhesus monkeys: I. Effects of pentoxyfylline on neutrophil influx. *J. Med. Primatol.* **21,** 357–362.
9. Starke, J. R., Edwards, M. S., Langston, C., and Baker, C. J. (1987) A mouse model of chronic pulmonary infection with *Pseudomonas aeruginosa* and *Pseudomonas cepacia. Pediatr. Res.* **22,** 698–702.
10. van Heeckeren, A., Walenga, R., Konstan, M. W., Bonfield, T., Davis, P. B., and Ferkol, T. (1997) Excessive inflammatory response of cystic fibrosis mice to bronchopulmonary infection with *Pseudomonas aeruginosa. J. Clin. Invest.* **100,** 2810–2815.
11. Woods, D. E., Sokol, P. A., Bryan, L. E., Storey, D. G., Mattingly, S. J., Vogel, H. J., and Ceri, H. (1991) In vivo regulation of virulence in Pseudomonas aeruginosa associated with genetic rearrangement. *J. Infect. Dis.* **163,** 143–149.
12. Konstan, M. W., Vargo, K. M., and Davis, P. B. (1990) Ibuprofen attenuates the inflammatory response to *Pseudomonas aeruginosa* in a rat model of chronic pulmonary infection: Implications for antiinflammatory therapy in cystic fibrosis. *Am. Rev. Respir. Dis.* **141,** 186–192.
13. Konstan, M. W., Byard, P. J., Hoppel, C. L., and Davis, P. B. (1995) Effect of high-dose ibuprofen in patients with cystic fibrosis. *N. Engl. J. Med.* **332,** 848–854.
14. Chmiel, J. F., Konstan, M. W., Knesebeck, J. E., Hilliard, J. B., Bonfield, T. L., Dawson, D. V., and Berger, M. (1999) IL-10 attenuates excessive inflammation in chronic pseudomonas infection in mice. *Am. J. Respir. Crit. Care Med.* **160,** 2040–2047.
15. Yu, H., Hanes, H., Chrisp, C. E., Boucher, J. C., and Dretic, V. (1998) Microbial pathogenesis in cystic fibrosis: Pulmonary clearance of mucoid *Pseudomonas*

aeruginosa and inflammation in a mouse model of repeated respiratory challenge. *Infect. Immun.* **66,** 280–288.

16. Morissette, C., Skamene, E., and Gervais, F. (1995) Endobronchial inflammation following *Pseudomonas aeruginosa* infection in resistant and susceptible strains of mice. *Infect. Immun.* **63,** 1718–1724.

17. Sapru, K., Stotland, P. K., and Stevenson, M. M. (1999) Quantitative and qualitative differences in bronchoalveolar inflammatory cells in *Pseudomonas aeruginosa*-resistant and susceptible strains of mice. *Clin. Exp. Immunol.* **115,** 103–109.

18. Tam, M., Snipes, G. J., and Stevenson, M. M. (1999) Characterization of chronic bronchopulmonary *Pseudomonas aeruginosa* infection in resistant and susceptible inbred mouse strains. *Am. J. Respir. Cell Mol. Biol.* **20,** 710–719.

33

Analysis of Lipid Abnormalities in CF Mice

Steven D. Freedman, Paola G. Blanco, Julie C. Shea,
and Juan G. Alvarez

1. Introduction

Patients with cystic fibrosis (CF) and pancreatic disease show changes in fatty acids levels in blood plasma and mucus that are indicative of essential fatty acid deficiency. This has been attributed to many causes, including low fat intake, alterations in fat absorption, increased lipid turnover in cell membranes, increased oxidation of fatty acids, or other disorders of lipoprotein metabolism *(1)*. Recent studies have demonstrated that these alterations are still present in the absence of malnutrition *(2)*. Some investigators believe that the abnormal fatty acid pattern observed in cystic fibrosis might be related to a defect in the CF gene; however, it still remains unclear how this may lead to the phenotypic expression of the disease.

In order to determine whether a defect in fatty acids is present in cystic fibrosis transmembrane conductance regulator (CFTR)-regulated tissues, pancreatic acini consisting of acinar and proximal duct cells were prepared from *cftr–/–* mice and wild-type control animals *(3)*. An increase in membrane-bound arachidonic acid (AA) levels and a decrease in docosahexaenoic acid (DHA) levels was found in *cftr–/–* mice compared to wild-type control animals. This fatty acid imbalance was observed only in CFTR-regulated organs *(3)*. With the exception of a twofold increase in phospholipid-bound docosatetraenoic acid (22:4n – 6) observed in pancreas and lung from *cftr–/–* mice, no other significant lipid changes in *cftr–/–* mice compared with wild-type controls were detected. As proof of concept that this fatty acid abnormality is important in the phenotypic expression of disease, correction of this fatty acid defect with high doses of orally administered DHA resulted in reversal of the pathological manifestations of CF in the exocrine pancreas.

From: *Methods in Molecular Medicine, vol. 70: Cystic Fibrosis Methods and Protocols*
Edited by: W. R. Skach © Humana Press Inc., Totowa, NJ

Taken together, these data indicate that a CFTR dysfunction is associated with a defect in fatty acid metabolism and that this defect plays a role, in part, in the expression of disease. These studies require the use of cell purification techniques combined with lipid extraction and analysis by micro high-performance thin-layer chromatography (HP-TLC) and gas chromatography/mass spectrometry that are described in more detail below.

1.1. Parameters Affecting Lipid Analysis

One of the principal problems encountered in lipid analysis is lipid peroxidation. Since glycerolipid-bound fatty acids, including AA and DHA, contain four and five *bis*-allylic methylene groups, respectively, glycerolipids can undergo lipid peroxidation. This can be prevented by flushing each tube containing the lipids with nitrogen and by storing these tubes at –80°C. In addition, lipid peroxidation can also be prevented by adding antioxidants, e.g., 1 mM butylated hydroxytoluene. Since DHA is dissolved in Peptamen® (Nestle Clinical Nutrtion) and administered to mice in special feeders that are exposed to room air, oxidation of DHA can also occur under these conditions. However, Peptamen contains 3 mg of vitamin E and 34 mg of vitamin C per 100 mL, which are known antioxidants. The relative weight of vitamins E and C to DHA in the Peptamen/DHA emulsion was 0.9% and 10.2%, respectively. This relative excess of vitamin E would prevent DHA oxidation during exposure of the emulsion to air during feeding.

1.2. Interpretation of Banding Patterns

Membrane lipids can be separated by high-performance thin-layer chromatography (HP-TLC) as phospholipids, free fatty acids, monoglycerides, diglycerides, triglycerides, and cholesterol esters *(4)*. Analysis of the total lipid extract by HP-TLC allows the determination of whether cell lipids are intact or hydrolyzed. The presence of hydrolyzed lipids in a sample, e.g., phospholipids, does not allow the analysis of phospholipid-bound fatty acids. Fatty acid methyl esters prepared following tranesterification of glycerolipids, and, in particular, AA and DHA, can also be analyzed by HP-TLC *(see* **Fig. 1**) *(4)*. This provides a rapid quantitative test for the determination of the AA/DHA ratio by HP-TLC reflectance spectrodensitometry. However, since co-migration of fatty acid methyl esters by HP-TLC with the corresponding standards does not guarantee that the observed bands on the HP-TLC plate correspond to those fatty acids, the use of gas chromatography/mass spectrometry (GC/MS) is required to confirm these results. GC/MS, in addition to providing high-resolution means for the separation of fatty acids, also provides for the identification of each particular fatty acid.

1.3. Application of Fatty Acid Analysis

There are many studies in which the analysis of fatty acids is important. These include studies of cell membrane composition, analysis of fatty acids in

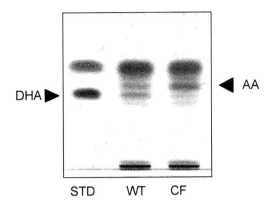

Fig. 1. HP-TLC analysis of preparations of pancreatic acini from wild-type (WT) and *cftr⁻/⁻* (CF) mice. STD refers to standards including DHA. The arrowheads indicate the position of AA and DHA. Levels of AA are increased while DHA levels are decreased in *cftr–/–* mice.

plasma, analysis of rates of incorporation of fatty acids in vitro and in vivo, analysis of secreted substances such as lung surfactant, and measurement of fatty acid proinflammatory mediators such as arachidonic acid.

2. Materials
2.1. Tissue Preparation
1. Krebs-Henseleit bicarbonate medium (KHB):
   a. Mix the following (final concentrations): 13.9 mM glucose (0.25%), 32 mM NaHCO$_3$ (0.27%), 0.1 mg/mL soy bean trypsin inhibitor, 109 mM NaCl, 4.7 mM KCl, 1 mM phosphate buffer, 1.2 mM MgCl$_2$, 1.3 mM CaCl$_2$, 4.5 mM HEPES.
   b. Oxygenate for 10 min with 95% oxygen, 5% CO$_2$.
   c. Adjust pH to 7.4.
   d. After oxygenating add 5 mg BSA/1 mL (0.5%).
2. KHB collagenase solution: Add 1000 U of collagenase to 10 mL of KHB (pH 7.4).

2.2. Lipid Extractions and Transmethylation
1. Chloroform/methanol (C/M) (2:1, v/v).
2. Heptadeconoic acid (17:0) internal standard solution: dissolve 1 mg of 17:0 in 1 mL of C/M, 2:1.
3. 0.5 N sodium methoxide (Supelco).
4. Boron trifluoride (BF$_3$) (Supelco).
5. *n*-Hexane (Sigma GC grade).
6. Saturated NaCl: dissolve 25 g of NaCl in 100 mL of distilled water.

2.3. Aminopropyl Column Chromatography
1. Aminopropyl column (Supelco).
2. Chloroform.

3. Hexane.
4. Chloroform/isopropanol (2:1, v/v).
5. 2% acetic acid in diethylether.
6. Chloroform/methanol/0.1 *N* sodium acetate (60/30/4.5, v/v/v).

2.4. Thin-Layer Chromatography

1. Chloroform.methanol (1.1, v/v).
2. Chromatography plates (HP-K Silica gel plate, 5 × 5 cm, Whatman).
3. Chromatography tank (12 × 15 cm).
4. Chloroform/ethenol/triethylamine/water (30/34/30/8, v/v/v/v).
5. Hexane/ether (100/4.5, v/v).
6. 10% copper sulfate, 8% phosphoric acid.
7. Camag plate heater III (Camag Scientific).
8. Spectrodensitometer (Shimadzu CS-9000).

2.5. Gas Chromatography/Mass Spectrometry

1. GC/MS chromatograph with WCOT capillary column (Supelco-wax-10, 30 m × 0.53 mm id, 1-μm film thickness (Hewlett-Packard).

3. Methods
3.1. Wild-Type and CF Knockout Breeding and Genotyping

1. Wild-type, C57-BL6, and CFTR (+/–), exon 10 UNC knockout mice were procured from Jackson Laboratory.
2. CF mice were obtained by mating male and female mice heterozygotic for the CF gene defect. As expected, approx 25% of the litter was affected by the disease.
3. Tails were clipped at 14 d of age and processed for analysis of the genotype.
4. At 23 d of age C57 WT mice and CFTR (-/-) were weaned and placed on water and Peptamen (Nestle Clinical Nutrition, Deerfield, IL) for 1 wk.
5. Mice were euthanized with carbon dioxide and the pancreas was removed for further analysis.

3.2. Cell and Tissue Preparation

1. Sacrifice animal.
2. Remove pancreas. Place in small weighing boat and add 1–2 drops of KHB-collagenase solution.
3. Mince tissue extensively.
4. Transfer tissue to a 25-mL Erlenmeyer flask and add 8 mL KHB-collagenase solution.
5. Oxygenate for 5 min and cover tightly with a stopper.
6. Incubate in 37°C shaker for 5 min at 175 oscillations/min.
7. Remove flask and mechanically disrupt tissue by holding flask followed by 50 quick snaps of the wrist. If all the connective tissue appears to be dissolved and cells appear to be in a homogenous suspension, proceed to the next step. If not, incubate in 37°C shaker for another 5 min and repeat mechanical disruption.

8. With a 10-mL pipet, slowly layer cell suspension over 2 mL of KHB containing 4% BSA in a 15-mL conical tube.
9. Centrifuge 2 min at 200*g* at room temperature in an IEC clinical centrifuge.
10. Aspirate and discard supernatant.
11. Wash cell pellet with 5–10 mL of KHB containing 4% BSA.
12. Repeat centrifugation for 2 min.
13. Aspirate and discard supernatant.
14. Add 100 μL of KHB (containing 0.5% BSA) to cell pellet and transfer to Eppendorf tube using a P-1000 pipetman. Cut the tip of the pipet so it is easier to transfer all the cells.
15. Homogenize on ice with an eppendorf pestle for ~30 s until the cells are completely homogenized.
16. Dilute homogenate up to 500 μL with KHB.
17. Transfer the homogenate to a glass tube and proceed with lipid extraction.

3.3. Lipid Extraction and Transmethylation

3.3.1. Lipid Extraction

1. Add 6 volumes of chloroform:methanol (C/M) 2:1, v/v, to cell homogenate using a P-1000 pipetman.
2. Vortex for 10 s.
3. Centrifuge at 800*g* for 4 min at room temperature.
4. Aspirate lower phase using a Pasteur pipet. Before crossing the interface, blow out a bubble to prevent contamination of the upper phase.
5. Add 30 μL of a 1-mg/mL solution of the heptadecanoic acid (17:0) internal standard to each lower phase. The internal standard solution is prepared by dissolving 1 mg of 17:0 in 1 mL of C/M, 2:1, v/v.
6. Tubes are placed in a 100°C heat block and the lower phase evaporated to dryness with nitrogen gas.

3.3.2. Transmethylation

1. Add 0.5 mL of 0.5 *N* sodium methoxide (Supelco) to the dry residue. Vortex for 5 s. Place screw cup top coated with Teflon and place in a heating block at 100°C for 3 min.
2. Remove from heating block and allow to cool to room temperature. Add 0.5 mL of boron trifluoride (BF_3) (Supelco).
3. Vortex for 5 s.
4. Place in a heating block at 100°C for 1 min.
5. Remove from the heating block and allow tube to cool to room temperature. Add 0.5 mL of *n*-hexane (Sigma GC grade).
6. Vortex for 5 s.
7. Place in heating block at 100°C for 1 min.
8. Remove from the heating block and cool to room temperature. Add 6.5 mL of a saturated solution of NaCl.
9. Centrifuge at 800*g* for 3 min.
10. Transfer the supernatant to a new glass conical test tube. Do not take the lower phase.

3.4. Aminopropyl Column Chromatography

Aminopropyl column chromatography is utilized to separate lipids in the extract in different lipid classes (6) following extraction, as described under **Subheading 3.3.1.**

1. Add 200 µL of chloroform to the dried lipid residue from **Subheading 3.3.1.**
2. Vortex for 5 s.
3. Fill aminopropyl column with hexane. Elute hexane from the column by simple gravity, applying air pressure, or using a vacuum manifold. Repeat this procedure once again. Make sure that the solvent level is above the column packing interface. Addition of hexane allows for the conditioning of the column.
4. Load lipid extract dissolved in chloroform onto column. Allow sample to elute by gravity. Stop elution when solvent level is 1–2 mm above the column packing interface.
5. Elute with 2 column volumes of chloroform/isopropanol 2/1, v/v (use a Pasteur pipet) and collect in a glass test tube labeled Fraction I. Stop elution when solvent level is 1–2 mm above the column packing interface.
6. Elute with 2 column volumes of 2% acetic acid in diethyl ether and collect in a glass test tube labeled Fraction II.
7. Elute with 2 column volumes of methanol and collect in a glass test tube labeled Fraction III.
8. Elute with 2 column volumes of chloroform/methanol/0.1 N sodium acetate (60/30/4.5, v/v/v) and collect in a glass test tube labeled Fraction IV.
9. Evaporate all four fractions to dryness under nitrogen and 100°C.
10. Add 3 mL of C/M, 2/1, v/v, to Fraction IV.
11. Vortex for 5 s.
12. Add 0.5 mL of distilled water.
13. Vortex for 5 s.
14. Centrifuge at 800g for 4 min.
15. Aspirate lower phase using a Pasteur pipet.
16. Add 30 µL of internal standard stock solution (1 mg/mL in C/M, 2/1, v/v) to each fraction.
17. Evaporate to dryness under nitrogen at 100°C.

3.5. Micro High-Performance Thin-Layer Chromatography (HP-TLC)

3.5.1. General Procedure

1. Wash plates by continuous development overnight in chloroform/methanol, 1/1, v/v.
2. Dry plates thoroughly using a hair dryer or vacuum oven.
3. Mark lanes on the plate using a pencil. Lanes should be 3–4 mm from the bottom of the plate, about 5 mm wide, and separated from each other by at least 2 mm.

As indicated previously, HP-TLC can be applied to the analysis of phospholipids and neutral lipids and to the analysis of fatty acid methyl esters.

3.5.2. Analysis of Phospholipids and Neutral Lipids

1. Evaporate a 50-μL aliquot of the lipid extract to dryness under nitrogen at 100°C. Redissolve dried residue in 5 μL of C/M, 1/1, v/v.
2. Streak 5 μL of the phospholipid and neutral lipid standard mixture (1 mg/mL in C/M, 1/1, v/v) or 5 μL of sample(s) onto the designated lanes of a Whatman HP-K silica gel plate, 5 × 5 cm.
3. Dry plate for 1 min using a hair dryer or vacuum oven.
4. Predevelop in C/M (1/1, v/v) to about 1 cm from the lower edge of the plate. Add 5 mL to a 12 × 15 cm tank (enough of C/M [1/1] to cover the bottom of the tank).
5. Dry plate for 1 min using a hair dryer or vacuum oven.
6. Develop in chloroform/ethanol/triethylamine/water (30/34/30/8, v/v/v/v) to 3.5 cm.
7. Dry plate for 1 min using a hair dryer or vacuum oven.
8. Empty the mobile phase from the tank and rinse with a 2–4 mL of hexane/ether. Then add hexane/ether.
9. Develop in hexane/ether (100/4.5, v/v) to the top of the plate.
10. Dry plate for 1 min using a hair dryer or vacuum oven.
11. Dip plate in a 10% solution of copper sulfate 8% phosphoric acid for 2 s.
12. Dry plate for 1 min using a hair dryer or vacuum oven.
13. Place plate on a Camag Plate Heater III at 185°C for 5 min.
14. Scan plates in the reflectance mode at 400 nm using a spectrodensitometer.

3.5.3. Analysis of Fatty Acid Methyl Esters

1. Evaporate fatty acid methyl ester extract to dryness under nitrogen at 100°C.
2. Redissolve residue in 50 μL of C/M, 1/1.
3. Streak 4 μL of the fatty acid methyl ester standard mixture and 4 μL of the sample(s) onto the designated lanes of a Whatman HP-K silica gel plate, 5 × 5 cm.
4. Dry for 1 min using a hair dryer or vacuum oven.
5. Predevelop in C/M (1/1, v/v) to about 1cm from the lower edge of the plate.
6. Dry for 1 min using a hair dryer or vacuum oven.
7. Develop in hexane/ether (100/4.5, v/v) to the top of the plate.
8. Dry for 1 min using a hair dryer or vacuum oven.
9. Dip plate in a 10% solution of copper sulfate 8% phosphoric acid for 2 s.
10. Dry for 1 min using a hair dryer or vacuum oven.
10. Place plate on a Camag Plate Heater III at 185°C for 3 min.
11. Scan plates in the reflectance mode at 400 nm using a spectrodensitometer

3.6. Gas Chromatography/Mass Spectrometry

1. Inject 1 μL of the fatty acid methyl ester sample solution into a Hewlett-Packard GC/MS chromatograph mounted with a WCOT capillary column (Supelco-wax-10, 30 m × 0.53 mm id. 1-μm film thickness).
2. Use initial and final temperatures in the column of 150 and 250°C, respectively programmed to increase at a rate of 10°C/min.
3. Fatty acid methyl ester peaks are identified by mass spectrometry and quantified using methylheptadecanoate as the internal standard.

References

1. Roulet, M., Frascarolo, P., Rappaz, I., and Pilet, M. (1997) Essential fatty acid deficiency in well nourished young cystic fibrosis patients. *Eur. J. Pediatr.* **156,** 952–956.
2. Henderson, J. W. R., Astley, S. J., McCready, M. M., Kushmerick, P., Casey, S., Becker, J. W., et al. (1994) Oral absorption of omega-3 fatty acids in patients with cystic fibrosis who have pancreatic insufficiency and in healthy control subjects. *J. Pediatr.* **124,** 400–408.
3. Freedman, S. D., Katz, M. H., Parker, E. M., Laposata, M., Urman, M. Y., and Alverez, J. A. (1999) A membrane lipid imbalance plays a role in the phenotypic expression of cystic fibrosis of cftr –/– mice. *Proc. Natl. Acad. Sci. USA* **96,** 13,995–14,000.
4. Alvarez, J. G. and Storey, B. T. (1995) Differential incorporation of fatty acids into an pcroxidative loss of fatty acids from phospholipids of human spermatozoa. *Mol. Reprod. Dev.* **42,** 334–346.

34

Bioelectric Measurement of CFTR Function in Mice

Barbara R. Grubb

1. Introduction

Cystic fibrosis (CF) mice have a defect in cAMP-mediated Cl^- conductance in epithelial tissues. Physiological study of these mice requires techniques that can quantitate epithelial ion transport in affected tissues. A variety of epithelial tissues, including airway (nasal, trachea, bronchi), gallbladder, pancreas, intestine, and reproductive tissues, have been studied in normal and CF mice. These studies have pointed out some major similarities as well as differences between the normal human and murine physiology and disease (for review, *see* **ref. *1***). In addition, ion transport studies in the CF mouse have been useful in determining the therapeutic efficacy of various treatment modalities.

The "gold standard" for studying ion transport across freshly excised (or cultured) epithelial tissue is the measurement of transepithelial bioelectric properties in an Ussing chamber. This technique, described in a now classical paper published 50 yr ago, was named after H. H. Ussing *(2)*. Other than changes in the surface area of the preparation studied (~500-fold smaller preparations for some of the murine tissue than for frog/toad skin as studied by Ussing), the basics of the technique employed today are largely unchanged from those described 50 yr ago. The principle behind the technique involves the observation that many epithelia (resting or stimulated) exhibit transepithelial electrical potential differences (PD). The bioelectric correlate of this active ion transport can be measured in a specially designed chamber (Ussing chamber). (Many ion transport processes do not involve generation of a transepithelial PD, and thus cannot be studied electrically in a Ussing chamber. For these preparations, isotopic flux of the ions of interest must be measured.) In the case of frog skin (the tissue studied by Ussing), the PD (often more than 100 mV, outside of skin negative) was found to reflect the inward active transport of Na^+. Cl^- ions also

From: *Methods in Molecular Medicine, vol. 70: Cystic Fibrosis Methods and Protocols*
Edited by: W. R. Skach © Humana Press Inc., Totowa, NJ

move across the skin, but this movement was entirely passive in response to the electrical potential generated by active Na^+ transport. Ussing and his colleague Zerhan devised an ingenious method to study selectively active ion transport across the frog skin without passive ion transport complicating interpretation of their results. For their method, the tissue is sandwiched between two chamber halves (Ussing chamber, **Fig. 1**) in which buffer of identical composition is placed on both sides of the tissue. Thus, each half-chamber communicates with the other via tissue at a common orifice. An agar bridge connected to a calomel electrode is placed as closely as possible to each side of the tissue. The transepithelial electrical PD across the tissue sensed by this pair of bridges in series with calomel electrodes is measured with a voltmeter. Another agar bridge is placed in each chamber half as far as possible from the epithelial preparation (**Fig. 1**). The distal end of these bridges is placed in a saturated KCl solution containing a AgCl electrode. An external transepithelial current (the current source can be a simple battery with a variable resistor, however, we use a commercially available instrument) is then applied to the tissue (via this pair of electrodes) to reduce the spontaneous PD to zero. The current passing across the tissue (at zero PD) is known as the short-circuit current (I_{sc}). The I_{sc} has been found to equal the sum of the ions actively transported across the tissue. (In most studies, the serosal side serves as ground, the PD is usually negative. The I_{sc} has the same polarity as does the PD, but the I_{sc} is often reported as positive.).

Since the I_{sc} is a measure of the sum of all active ion transport processes, it does not identify which ions are being transported. As an example, the normal neonatal mouse distal colon has a basal I_{sc} of approx 50–55 $\mu A \cdot cm^2$ (**Fig. 2A**). This I_{sc} could reflect the secretion of an anion or the absorption of a cation. Thus, other protocols are necessary to determine which ions contribute to the I_{sc}. The most direct means utilizes radioactive tracers. While this approach has been used in the mouse intestine *(3)*, the small surface area of most murine preparations makes tracer fluxes difficult (*see* **Note 1**). As an alternative, drug and ion substitution protocols have been used with good success to determine the ionic origin of the basal and stimulated I_{sc} in murine tissue. The apical application of amiloride (a drug that blocks Na^+ absorption) rapidly decreases the magnitude of the basal I_{sc} in both the normal and the CF preparations (**Fig. 2A,B**). Thus, this protocol indicates that a large part of the basal I_{sc} in these neonatal colonic preparations is due to Na^+ absorption.

In the mouse distal colon, forskolin increases cAMP, activates cystic fibrosis transmembrane conductance regulator (CFTR) in the apical enterocyte membrane, and stimulates Cl^- secretion, which is associated with a marked increase in I_{sc} in the normal neonatal distal colon (**Fig. 2A**). Forskolin is completely without effect on the CF tissue lacking apical CFTR (**Fig. 2B**). Bumetanide, a drug that blocks basolateral Cl^- entry, rapidly decreases the

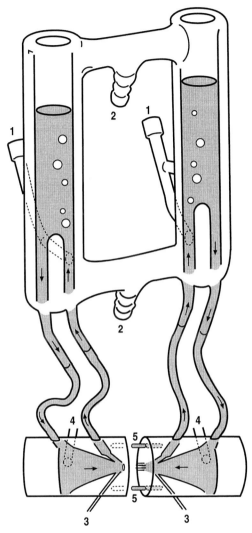

Fig. 1. Schematic drawing of Ussing chamber setup used for murine tissue. The shaded area is the region in which the buffer circulates. Gas line (O_2/CO_2) is attached to 1. The gas bubbles oxygenate the tissue and circulate the buffer in the direction of the arrows. The water bath (set at 37°C) is attached to the glass water jacket at 2. Agar PD bridges (3), which are placed in the KCl reservoir containing the calomel electrode (not shown), are inserted as close to the tissue as possible. The agar current bridges (4) are placed in a reservoir containing the AgCl electrode (not shown). Metal guide pins (5) in one chamber half fit into a hole in the opposite half, thus allowing perfect alignment of the halves. Once the tissue is placed in the Ussing chamber, the chamber halves are placed in a stand that holds the halves together (not shown).

magnitude of the forskolin response in the normal tissue, providing evidence that the stimulated I_{sc} is due to Cl$^-$ secretion. This drug has no effect on the CF

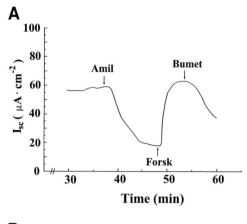

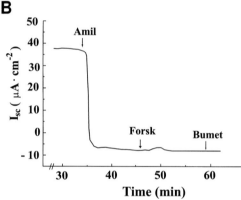

Fig. 2. Actual recorder trace from an Ussing chamber preparation of murine neonatal normal (**A**) and CF (**B**) distal colon. When (Amil) 10^{-4} M amiloride is applied to the apical bath, the I_{sc} of both preparations falls to nearly zero (slightly below zero in the CF preparations, *see* **ref. 7** for an explanation). As amiloride blocks electrogenic Na^+ absorption, these data indicate that most of the basal I_{sc} reflects this process. Forskolin, (Forsk, 10^{-5} M bilateral) a drug that increases cAMP and thus Cl^- secretion through CFTR, induces a prompt increase in the I_{sc} in the normal preparation and no significant response in the CF. The increase in I_{sc} (and a hyperpolarization in PD if tissue were studied open-circuit) is consistent with secretory flow of anions. Then, the preparations are treated with bumetanide (Bumet, $10^{-4}M$ basolateral). Bumetanide blocks the activity of the basolateral Na/K/2Cl co-transporter. Thus, basolateral Cl entry is inhibited, which in turn inhibits the forskolin-induced apical Cl secretion in the normal preparations, which is reflected in a fall in the I_{sc} in the normal distal colon.

tissue (**Fig. 2B**). As further evidence that the forskolin-stimulated I_{sc} in the normal gut is due to Cl^- secretion and not Na^+ absorption, if all Na^+ is removed from the apical side (i.e., the lumen), the forskolin response is not attenuated

(4). However, if Cl$^-$ is removed basolaterally or bilaterally, the forskolin response in the normal tissue is significantly attenuated *(4)*. Therefore, without the use of tracer studies, taken together, drug addition and ion substitution experiments give good evidence that the intestine of the CF mouse exhibits no stimulated anion secretion *(5)*. Thus, with minor modifications and using the dissection techniques described below, the Ussing chamber technique has proven extremely useful in characterizing ion transport defects in the CF mouse as well as other mutant mice.

2. Materials

2.1. Chambers

In our laboratory, chambers having variously sized apertures to accommodate different size tissues, are used: 0.25 cm^2 for intestine (adult); 0.025 cm^2, trachea, nasal epithelia, gallbladder; 0.014 cm^2 bronchi, neonatal intestine, and neonatal trachea. Our chambers are fabricated from Lexan by the university's machine shop. Unlike most other chamber designs, the lumen of our chambers is not cylindrical. Rather, it is conical in shape, the apex of the cone being proximal to the tissue (**Fig. 1**). The advantage of this chamber geometry is that bubbles will not lodge near the tissue, but rather, spontaneously rise to the distal end of the chamber (away from the tissue) and are eliminated via gas lift circulators. This feature is especially important when studying tissue with very small surface areas. The volume of the conical portion (**Fig. 1**) is ~4 mL for the chambers with an aperture of 0.25 cm^2 and ~2 mL volume for all other sizes. A glass reservoir (made by the university's glass shop) is attached to the Lexan portion of the chamber via Tygon tubing. The total volume of buffer in the chamber and reservoirs is 10 mL for most experiments. The glass reservoirs are water-jacketed and the temperature of the water maintained at 37°C with a water bath.

2.2. Agar Bridges

Bridges are made of polyethylene (PE) tubing filled with 3% agar dissolved in 0.9% NaCl. The PD bridges (**Fig. 1**) are made from PE 160 tubing for the chambers of 0.25–0.025 aperture and PE 60 for the smallest aperture chambers. Bridges through which current is passed (**Fig. 1**) should be made from larger-diameter PE tubing (PE 200 or more). As relatively small PDs will be generated by the neonatal tissue (usually 0.1–3 mV), it is imperative that the system be as stable and as noise-free as possible. This requirement necessitates making agar bridges that are completely bubble-free. To make the agar bridges, 3% agar in 0.9% NaCl (or 3 *M* KCl) is heated carefully to boiling. When the tiny bubbles have dissipated, the hot agar is aspirated into a syringe and loaded into the bridges. The bridges are placed in a 0.9% NaCl solution at room temperature for storage. As soon as the agar in the bridges has hardened, the tips at both ends are cut on a diagonal to expose as much surface area as possible and remove any bubbles that may have lodged in the tips. With care, these bridges can be reused many times unless radioactive tracers are used (*see* **Note 2**).

2.3. Electrodes

The calomel electrodes, available commercially (Fisher), are filled with 3 *M* KCl and placed in a small reservoir (we use a 20-mL scintillation vial) filled with 3 *M* KCl. The distal ends of the PD bridges are also placed in the small calomel reservoir. The calomel electrodes are interfaced to a commercially available voltage clamp (we use Physiologic Instruments), which will automatically clamp the PD to zero and record the I_{sc}.

The AgCl electrodes, for passing the current, can be easily made by dipping a length of pure silver wire (Fisher) into Clorox for 20 min. Then a wire with a banana plug on the end is soldered to the coated silver wire. The silver wire electrode is placed in a small 3 *M* KCl reservoir and the distal end of each current bridge is also placed in this reservoir. The banana plug is connected to the proper location on the voltage clamp. (Instructions are supplied with the commercially available clamps as to where to plug the various electrodes.)

2.4. Solutions

As the most common solutions used are Krebs bicarbonate buffer, Na^+-free bicarbonate buffer, and Cl^--free bicarbonate buffer, detailed recipes for making these buffers are given.

1. Krebs bicarbonate Ringer's (KBR): KBR is easily and quickly made by combining four stable stock solutions. Stock 1: 134.4 g NaCl/L of distilled H_2O. Stock 2: 20.9 g K_2HPO_4 + 2.73 g KH_2PO_4/250 mL distilled H_2O. Stock 3: 12.2 g $MgCl_2 \cdot 6\ H_2O$ + 8.88 g $CaCl_2 \cdot 2H_2O$/250 mL distilled H_2O. Stock 4: 42.01 g $NaHCO_3$/L of dH_2O.
   To make the KBR, fill a 1000-mL volumetric flask ~three-fourths full of dH_2O. Add 50 mL of stock 1, and 5 mL of stocks 2 and 3. Then gas with 95% O_2/5% CO_2 for approx 5 min. Then add 50 mL of stock 4 and fill to volume. When added in this order, none of the compounds will precipitate. The pH of this buffer (as well as the Na^+ and Cl^--free buffers) will be 7.4 when gassed with 95% O_2–5% CO_2.
2. Na^+-free buffer: Add 22.4 g N-methyl-D-glucamine (NMDG) to 250 mL dH_2O. Adjust pH to 7.4 with HCl. Add this solution to a 1-L volumetric flask and fill three-fourths full of dH_2O. Add 5 mL of stocks 2 and 3 (*see* **item 1**) and gas with 95/5. Add 25 mL of NMDG bicarbonate and bring final volume to 1 L. (The NMDG bicarbonate stock is made by dissolving 19.5 g NMDG in 100 mL dH_2O. Gas this stock with 100% CO_2 for at least several hours [overnight is best] before use.)
3. Cl^--free buffer: Add 25.81 g/L of Na gluconate (D-gluconic acid sodium salt) to ~750 mL of dH_2O in a 1-L volumetric flask. Add 0.144 g $MgSO_4$. Add 1.29 g

Ca^{2+} gluconate (D-gluconic acid hemi-calcium salt) (*see* **Note 3**). Add 5 mL of stock 2 (*see* **item 1**). Gas with 95/5. Add 50 mL stock 4 (*see* **item 1**). Bring up to volume with dH$_2$O.

3. Methods
3.1. Tissue Dissection and Preparation

Careful dissection and mounting the tissue are amongst the most critical steps to good bioelectric measurements.

3.1.1. Adult Intestine

Intestinal preparations from the adult mouse are relatively easy to dissect and mount. The designated region of the intestine is removed from the animal after euthanization, flushed with cold oxygenated Krebs bicarbonate Ringer's (KBR), excised along the mesenteric border, and cut into pieces ~1–2 cm long for mounting on the Ussing chamber (*see* **Note 4**). A parafilm O-ring is placed on the chamber prior to tissue placement (*see* **Note 5**). The O-rings have been found critical to minimize edge damage resulting from compressing the tissue between the chamber halves. The tissue is then carefully laid mucosal side up on the O-ring and gently stretched across six stainless steel pins, which are located ~1 mm outside the aperture. (The intestine of the adult mouse is the only preparation in which the tissue is placed across steel pins.) Then another O-ring is placed on top of the tissue and the two chamber halves are gently pressed together.

3.1.2. Neonatal Intestine

As both the human CF infant and the neonatal CF mouse exhibit meconium ileus *(5)*, there is much interest in studying the intestine of the neonatal CF mouse. We have been very successful in the study of the neonatal intestinal preparation in Ussing chambers *(6)*. Again, proper dissection and mounting of the tissue are critical for a viable preparation. After decapitation of the neonatal mouse (we have studied mouse pups as young as 1 d prebirth), the abdomen is opened with fine scissors. The designated portion of the intestine is removed and a 2–4 mm piece of intestine is placed on top of a piece of tissue paper (KimWipes, Kimberly-Clark) that has been prewetted with Krebs buffer and positioned on top of a chamber half under a dissecting scope. (The tissue paper prevents the tissue from falling through the aperture and makes positioning easier.) The intestine is then split longitudinally along the mesenteric border with fine scissors, and any fecal contents removed with fine forceps. (The neonatal intestine is very fragile, and flushing to remove fecal contents could cause damage, thus forceps are used.) The opened intestinal preparation (serosal side down) is then positioned precisely over the chamber aperture by moving the paper on which the intestine has been placed over the chamber aperture on which an O-ring has previously been placed (*see* **Note 6**). Then, another O-ring is placed on the apical side of the preparation. This must be done carefully, as once the O-ring has touched the tissue, it should not be moved; otherwise, the mucosal surface will be damaged. Then, the chamber halves are gently squeezed together, placed in a specially designed stand to hold the halves together, and filled with buffer.

3.1.3. Adult Trachea

The same dissection and mounting techniques are used for the adult and neonatal trachea. The muscles, salivary glands, and fascia on the anterior side of the trachea are removed. Once the trachea is cleared of fascia, it is cut longitudinally on the anterior side while still *in situ*. The trachea is then cut transversely as distally as possible. The proximal end near the thyroid is cut and the trachea is then removed from the mouse. With this dissection procedure, the posterior membrane is still intact. We obtain the best transport properties by placing this portion of the tissue over the chamber aperture. Also, by cutting the tissue on the anterior side (leaving the posterior membrane intact), the tissue will lie flatter over the aperture. The tissue is placed mucosal side up on the chamber on an O-ring and then another O-ring is placed on top of the tissue and the chamber halves gently put together.

3.1.3.1. Neonatal Trachea

Dissection and mounting of the neonatal trachea are very similar to that of the adult, with the exception that a smaller aperture chamber (0.0135 cm^2) is used. In addition, the tissue is placed on a Kimwipe (*see* **Subheading 3.1.2.**) before placing the tissue on the O-ring (follow O-ring procedures outlined for neonatal gut).

3.1.4. Nasal Epithelium

In the CF mouse, the nasal epithelium is a particularly good tissue to study, as it exhibits transport defects nearly identical to those of human CF airway tissue (*1*). The success of studying nasal epithelium depends on the ability to dissect undamaged sheets of tissue of sufficient size to fit across the aperture of the Ussing chamber. To remove the epithelial tissue, the skin is cut at the tip of the nose and peeled back to the level of the eyes. This will expose the underlying nasal bones, which are removed by inserting a pair of forceps in the suture where these bones meet the skull and gently pulling each bone downward toward the tip of the nose. After removal of these bones from the left and right sides of the head, two sheets of nasal epithelia, separated by the nasal septum, are visible. The tissue on each side is removed separately by first cutting through the epithelium at the tip of the nose. Then the tissue is freed from the nasal septum by carefully inserting the tip of the forceps between the septum and the epithelium. At the ventral most accessible region of the septum, the tissue is dissected away from the underlying structures, thus freeing the medial edge of the sheet. (When the nasal bones are removed, the lateral border of each sheet is torn away, thus no dissection is required to free the sheet from the lateral (outside) edge of the nasal cavity.) Finally, the tissue at the distal border (skull) of the nasal cavity is carefully pulled free. This procedure is repeated on each side of the nasal cavity, yielding two sheets of epithelia. Each sheet is immediately placed on the small bit of KBR wetted paper (with O-ring underneath) positioned over the aperture of the Ussing chamber half (under a dissecting microscope). The tissue should be mounted serosal side down. It can be difficult to distinguish serosal from mucosal side on this thin tissue. However, with careful observation (under a dissecting microscope) the blood vessels can more clearly be seen on the serosal side. Once the tissue is correctly positioned over the aperture, another O-ring is carefully placed over the top of the tissue, and the two chamber halves are then fitted together.

3.1.5. Gallbladder

The gallbladder is removed intact from the mouse and placed on a hemichamber on which an O-ring and tissue paper have been prepositioned over the aperture. Then, a fine pair of scissors is inserted into the neck of the gallbladder, and the tissue is split open longitudinally. If the gallbladder contains bile, it is flushed from the gallbladder after the tissue is opened. The tissue, serosal side down, is then positioned over the aperture of the chamber, another O-ring placed over the tissue, and the chamber halves are fitted together.

3.2. Bioelectric Measurements

For basal bioelectric measurements (PD, resistance, I_{sc}), tissues are studied in KBR buffer. Glucose (5 mM) is added to the serosal side (as a nutrient source) and 5 mM mannitol is added to the mucosal side to balance the osmolarity. The initial experimental protocol is virtually the same for each of the tissue types being studied.

1. Before the tissue is mounted, the chambers are equilibrated at 37°C in the solution in which the tissues are to be studied (usually KBR). Any electrical PD between the bridges is zeroed out by the voltage clamp. In addition, the solution resistance is zeroed out via the clamp. This step is very important because the tissues usually exhibit small PDs and low resistances and thus any electrical offsets can markedly affect the data. (Most investigators use commercially available voltage clamps, and the instructions for these steps are supplied by the manufacturer.)
2. Once the hemi-chambers are balanced, they are taken down and the tissue is placed between the chamber halves (as described above). The chamber halves are compressed only as much as necessary to prevent leaks. Then buffer is simultaneously placed in each chamber half via a 10-mL syringe connected to a piece of PE tubing (see **Note 7**). The chambers are water-jacketed for warming (37°C)

and oxygenated with 95%O_2/5% CO_2 if a bicarbonate buffer is used. If there is no bicarbonate in the buffer, the tissue should be oxygenated with 100% O_2. This gas, which is bubbled slowly through the gas lifts, also circulates the fluid in the chambers (*see* **Fig. 1**).

3. For most experiments, the tissue is studied under "short-curcuit," i.e., $Vt = 0$, conditions. However, at 1-min intervals (or whatever the investigator chooses), a constant voltage pulse (usually 1–5 mV, depending on the resistance of the tissue), is applied to the tissue. The commercially available clamps can be set to do this automatically. Resistance can thus be calculated by the change in measured ISC in response to the known voltage pulse, according to Ohm's law ($V = IR$), where V is voltage of the pulse in volts, I is the amount by which the short circuit current changes in amperes, and R is resistance in ohms (V/A) (*see* **Note 8**). Data can be output from the voltage clamps to a strip-chart recorder, or a data acquisition system interfaced with a computer.

4. Notes

1. When the tissue is placed in the Ussing chamber, there is some degree of edge damage (despite attempts to minimize it; *see* **Subheading 3.1.**) where the chamber contacts the epithelial tissue. These small exposed surface area preparations are relatively "leaky" due to the larger circumference/surface area ratio (thus greater edge damage), which necessitates the use of much larger quantities of isotopes. This pattern makes tracer measurements somewhat impractical.
2. Bridges should be tested in a buffer-filled chamber in which no tissue is present. If there is no electrical noise and the small offset PD (usually less than 0.5 mV) does not drift more than about 0.2 mV/h, the bridges are suitable for use.
3. This increases the calcium concentration to ~ 5 mM, which overcomes the Ca^{2+} chelating effect of the gluconate.
4. We study our murine intestinal preparations full thickness (not stripped). In species larger than the mouse, it is often desirable to strip the serosal muscle layer from the preparation to allow better access of O_2 and nutrients to the basolateral side of the tissue. However, as we obtain stable preparations and good drug responses in our full-thickness preparations, stripping the muscle layer in mouse intestine does not appear to be necessary.
5. To make the O-rings, three thicknesses of Parafilm (American National Can, Greenwich, CT) are folded and then a custom-made punch is used to make the hole in the parafilm exactly the same size as the chamber aperture. The university's Physics Shop makes these punches for us out of a sharpened stainless steel rod. Another punch of a much larger diameter is used to cut the outside of the O-ring. This outside dimension is not critical. The punch for the outside of the O-ring (~15 mm), is a commercially available cork borer.
6. If this O-ring is colored black using a nontoxic marker, it makes visualization of the aperture under the tissue much easier, and the tissue can be more precisely centered over the aperture of the chamber half. By illuminating the preparation from below (through the chamber) with a fiber-optic light, the aperture can be clearly seen and the tissue placed correctly.

7. It is important with these small pieces of tissue that the buffer be delivered to each side of the chamber simultaneously. If one side is filled before the other, the unequal hydrostatic pressure can dislodge the tissue.

8. The I_{sc} of the tissue is usually expressed per square centimeters of surface area ($\mu A \cdot cm^{-2}$). Thus the measured Is_c is divided by the aperature size (in cm^2). To calculate tissue resistance, the voltage pulse (usually set at 1–5 mV) is divided by the magnitude by which the I_{sc} is changed by the pulse. This I_{sc} value has to be multiplied by 1000 so that the units of both the voltage and I_{sc} are of the same magnitude. Thus, if a 1 mV voltage pulse delivered to the tissue changes the I_{sc} of the tissue by 25 $\mu A \cdot cm^{-2}$, then the tissue resistance would be 40 $\Omega \cdot cm^2$. If one wishes to compare the I_{sc} to an ion flux (assume Na^+), a conversion is necessary. Since the flow of one electrical equivalent of Na^+ ions in solution is equivalent to the flow of 1 faraday (96,500 coulombs) of electrons, and since 1 A = 1 C/s, then 1 μA = 1/96,5000 μ Eq Na/second or 1 μA = 0.0374 μEq Na/h. Thus, by multiplying the I_{sc} (in $\mu A \cdot cm^{-2}$) by 0.0374, the I_{sc} is expressed in terms of an ion flux ($\mu Eq/cm^2\,h^1$).

Acknowledgment

I thank Dr. R. C. Boucher for giving me the unique opportunity to do some of the first bioelectric studies on the CF mouse.

References

1. Grubb, B. R. and Boucher, R. C. (1999) Pathophysiology of gene-targeted mouse models for cystic fibrosis. *Physiol. Rev.* **79,** S193–S214.
2. Ussing, H. H. and Zerhan, K. (1951) Active transport of sodium as the source of electric current in the short-circuited isolated frogskin. *Acta Physiol. Scand.* **23,** 110–127.
3. Sheldon, R. J., Malarchik, M. E., Fox, D. A., Burks, T. F., and Porreca, F. (1989) Pharmacological characterization of neural mechanisms regulating mucosal ion transport in mouse jejunum. *J. Pharmacol. Exp. Ther.* **249,** 572–582.
4. Clarke, L. L., Grubb, B. R., Gabriel, S. E., Smithies, O., Koller, B. H., and Boucher, R. C. (1992) Defective epithelial chloride transport in a gene targeted mouse model of cystic fibrosis. *Science* **257,** 1125–1128.
5. Grubb, B. R. and Gabriel, S. E. (1997) Intestinal physiology and pathology in gene-targeted mouse models of cystic fibrosis. *Am. J. Physiol.* **273,** G258–G266.
6. Grubb, B. R. (1999) Ion transport across the normal and CF neonatal murine intestine. *Am. J. Physiol.* **277,** G167–G174.

35

Xenograft Model of the CF Airway

Mohammed Filali, Yulong Zhang, Teresa C. Ritchie, and John F. Engelhardt

1. Introduction

Mutations in the cystic fibrosis transmembrane conductance regulator (CFTR) result in defective ion transport, leading to thick mucus, impaired mucociliary clearance and decreased bacterial killing in the lung *(1,2)*. Despite recent progress in associating cystic fibrosis (CF) defects with CFTR dysfunction, there are many unanswered questions concerning the roles of CFTR in both normal airway biology and in CF pathology. Before effective therapeutic approaches for CF lung disease will be realized, several remaining challenges must first be overcome. These include a more precise definition of CFTR functions in fluid transport, electrolyte balance, and in the regulation of other epithelial ion channels. Moreover, the heterogeneity of CFTR expression among different cell types and regions of the lung necessitates the identification of pathophysiologic relevant cellular targets for gene therapy approaches for CF. For example, submucosal glands (SMGs) secrete mucous, airway surface fluid, and bactericidal proteins, and are a predominant site of CFTR-expressing cells in the lung. In contrast, cells in the surface airway epithelium show lower levels of CFTR expression *(3)*. The importance of SMGs in the pathoprogression of CF lung disease is still an open question. Hindering a firm answer to this question is a lack of animal models that mimic human CF airways disease at the molecular level and cellular levels.

What characteristics are important in choosing a model system for CF research? The ideal model system would mimic the human CF lung in all aspects, including anatomical structure, cell biology, and physiology, and at the molecular level harbor a defect in CFTR. To date, CF model systems such as transformed airway cells, primary airway cells, in vitro polarized airway

From: *Methods in Molecular Medicine, vol. 70: Cystic Fibrosis Methods and Protocols*
Edited by: W. R. Skach © Humana Press Inc., Totowa, NJ

epithelia, CFTR knockout mice, and human CF bronchial xenografts conform to these expectations to differing extents. Each of these models has proven valuable in a given particular context and experimental setting. For many studies, in vitro models have provided adequate differentiation when cells are grown at the air–liquid interface. However, in vitro models do not have the ideal cytoarchitecture of intact vascularized airways. The CF transgenic mouse model was met initially with great anticipation of its potential utility in understanding the pathophysiology of CF lung disease. However, this animal model has proven to be inadequate for studies of CF pulmonary disease, since it does not exhibit lung pathology *(4–6)*, primarily due to differences in lung cell biology between humans and mice.

To facilitate studies of airway biology and CF pathophysiology, an ex-vivo bronchial xenograft model was developed to supplement other models of the airway *(7–9)*. In recent years significant modifications have refined and improved this model and widened its application for CF research. By means of these improvements, the modern model system consists of open-ended xenograft airways allowing access to the lumen in vivo. Xenografts are generated by seeding primary bronchial epithelial cells into rat tracheas denuded of viable epithelium. The rat tracheas are then ligated to a sterilized tubing cassette, and pairs of xenografts are implanted subcutaneously on the flanks of immune-incompetent Nu/Nu Balbc mice. The transplantation is performed such that the ends of the tubing protrude from incisions and provide access to the airway lumen for experimentation. Over a period of 4–5 wk, these "open-ended" xenografts develop into a fully differentiated, stratified airway epithelium by morphological criteria. Human proximal airway xcnografts have been generated from multiple tissue sources including nasal, tracheal, and bronchial epithelium. Either normal human or CF lung tissue can be utilized as a source of epithelial cells. Studies evaluating the differentiated state of human bronchial xenograft epithelium have demonstrated native bronchial expression patterns of several cell-specific markers including cytokeratin-14, cytokeratin-18, CFTR, and mucin *(3,9,10)*. Morphometric evaluation by electron microscopy has revealed an indistinguishable distribution of basal, intermediate, goblet, and ciliated cells in native human bronchial tissue and xenografts generated from primary airway epithelial cells derived from the same sample. These results suggest that the mucociliary epithelium generated within "open-ended" human bronchial xenografts closely resembles that found within the native human bronchial airway and substantiates the utility of this model system for the study of human airway biology. Furthermore, since human bronchial xenografts are generated from "cleansed" cultured airway cells, they are ideal for studying primary defects in the absence of secondary complications caused by bacterial infection, which promote airway remodeling.

Since defects in ion and fluid transport are hallmarks of the CF phenotype, the utility of the xenograft model also requires that the bioelectric properties of the xenograft epithelium resemble those of the proximal human airway. Boucher and colleagues at the University of North Carolina have developed an approach for studying transport in an intact proximal airway in vivo through the measurement of potential differences (PD) *(11)*. Similar measurements have been performed in the xenograft model, which facilitated direct comparisons in airway surface fluid volumes and in Na^+ and Cl^- transport between normal and CF bronchial epithelium *(12)*. The usefulness of the human bronchial xenograft model in the evaluation of gene therapies has also been exemplified in studies using recombinant E1-deleted adenoviruses *(3,12–14)*. Several important aspects of recombinant adenoviruses, pertaining to host cell–vector interactions, have been addressed using this model system, including: (1) cell types in the airway that are permissive for adenoviral infection, (2) efficiency and persistence of gene transfer, (3) the expression of viral proteins from these vectors, (4) viral shedding following infection, and (5) complementation of primary defects.

In its current form, human bronchial xenografts represent a fully differentiated, stratified proximal airway epithelium remarkably similar to the native human airway. They are adaptable to a variety of research areas and experimental settings pertaining to CF. In this chapter we describe detailed procedures for the generation of the human bronchial xenograft model system, as well as methods for the experimental analysis of the epithelial potential difference in xenografts.

2. Materials

2.1. Isolation and Culture of Primary Human Normal and CF Bronchial Cells

1. Human lung (ideally lung transplant tissue should be utilized, but lungs can also be harvested within 6 h following death; keep on ice)
2. Medium A: modified Eagle medium (MEM; Life technologies) supplemented with: 50 U/mL of penicillin, 50 µg/mL of streptomycin, 80 µg/mL tobramycin (Eli Lilly), 100 µg/mL ceftazidine (Eli Lilly), 100 µg/mL of primaxin (Merck), 5.0 µg/mL of amphotericin B, 10 µg/mL of DNase I (type II-S, from bovine pancreas; Sigma), 0.5 mg/mL dithiothreitol. (Prepare fresh and keep at 4°C.)
3. Bronchial epithelial growth medium (BGEM): Add the following components of the BGEM singleQuot kit to 500 mL of BEBM (bronchial epithelial basal medium; Clonetics). 2 mL of 13 mg/mL bovine pituitary extract (BPE; 0.052 mg/mL final), 0.5 mL of 0.5 mg/mL hydrocortizone (0.0005 mg/mL final), 0.5 mL of 0.5 µg/mL recombinant human epidermal growth factor (hEGF; 0.0005 µg/mL final), 0.5 mL of 10 mg/mL transferrin (0.01 mg/mL), 0.5 mL of 0.5 mg/mL

epinephrine (0.0005 mg/mL final), 0.5 mL of 5 mg/mL insulin (0.005 mg/mL final), 0.5 mL of 0.1 μg/mL retinoic acid (0.0001 μg/mL final), 0.5 mL of 6.5 μg/mL triiodothyronine (0.0065 μg/mL final).

4. Medium B: BGEM supplemented with 50 μ/mL of penicillin, 50 μg/mL of streptomycin, 80 μg/mL of tobramycin, 100 μg/mL of ceftazidine, 100 μg/mL of primaxin, 5.0 μg/mL of amphotericin B. (Store up to 2 wk at 4°C)

5. Medium C: BGEM supplemented with 50 μ/mL of penicillin, 50 μg/mL of streptomycin, 40 μg/mL of tobramycin, 50 μg/mL of ceftazidine, 50 μg/mL of primaxin. (Store up to 2 wk at 4°C)

6. Medium A supplemented with 0.1% (w/v) protease type XIV (Sigma).

7. Fetal bovine serum (FBS).

8. Ham's F-12 medium (Life Technologies) with or without 10% FBS.

9. 10% trypsin/EDTA (Life Technologies).

10. Trypsin inhibitor buffer: Prepare 1 mg/mL trypsin inhibitor (type I-S from soybean; Sigma) in Ham's F-12 medium (Life Technologies). Filter through 0.2-μm filter and store in aliquots up to 6 mo at –20°C.

11. Cryopreservation medium: medium C containing 10% dimethyl sulfoxide (DMSO) and 10% FBS, 4°C.

12. Dissecting instruments, including forceps, scalpel, and hemostat.

13. 100- and 150-mm tissue culture dishes (uncoated plastic).

14. 15- and 50-mL conical centrifuge tubes.

15. Platform rocker.

16. Tabletop centrifuge.

17. 3-cm^2 piece of 500-μm wire mesh, sterile.

18. 2-mL cryogenic vial.

19. Hemocytometer.

2.2. Xenograft Preparation

2.2.1. Xenograft Cassette Construction

1. Silastic tubing (Dow Corning, cat. no. 602-175).

2. Teflon tubing (Thomas Scientific, cat. no. 9567-K10).

3. Adapter (0.8-mm barb-to-barb connector; Bio-Rad, cat. no. 732-8300).

4. Chromel A steel wire (0.035 in. diameter; Hoskins MFG).

5. Ethicon 2-0 braided silk suture (Ethicon).

6. 100-mm tissue culture plates.

7. Self-sealable sterilization pouch (M.D. Industries, cat. no. S40713).

8. Fisher 344 rat, 200–250 g, male.

9. Sterile surgical instruments (forceps, scissors).

10. 70% EtOH.

11. 2-mL screw-cap tubes (Sarstedt, cat. no. 72.694.006).

12. Cryogenic vials.

13. MEM medium (Life Technologies), chilled at 4°C.

14. Sterile pipet tips.
15. Primary airway epithelial cells at ~80% confluency.

2.2.2. Transplantation of Xenograft Cassettes into Nude Mice

1. Nu/Nu athymic mouse, 20–25 g, male.
2. Disposable underpads (Kendall, cat. no. 949).
3. Sterile drapes.
4. Surgical latex gloves.
5. Proviodone.
6. Cotton gauze sponges (Abco Dealers, cat. no. 052113).
7. Ketamine/xylazine.
8. Instrument pack (sterile; 2 forceps, 1 scissors, and 1 hemostat for each mouse).
9. Disposable skin stapler 35R (American Cyanamid, cat. no. 8035-12).
10. Ham's F-12 medium.
11. 21-gauge × 3/4 in. Butterfly infusion set (Abbott Laboratories, cat. no. 4492).
12. 20-μL pipetman.

2.3. PD Measurements

1. Multi-range, variable-rate infusion pump (Orion Research, cat. no. 001967).
2. pH/mV meter (Orion Research, cat. no. 0525A0).
3. Calomel reference electrodes (Fisher cat. no. 13-620-79) in saturated KCl.
4. 21-gauge × 3/4 in. Butterfly infusion set (Abbott Laboratories, cat. no. 4492).
5. Computer with software for recording mV readings.
6. 10-mL disposable syringes with 21-gauge × $1^1/_2$ in. needles.
7. Manifold pump tubing (PVC Solvent Flexible tubing, Fisher, cat. no. 14-190-139).
8. Silicone tubing (Bio-Rad, cat. no. 7318211).
9. Hemostat.
10. HEPES phosphate buffered ringers solution (HPBR): 10 mM HEPES, pH 7.4, 140 mM NaCl, 5mM KCl, 1.2 mM MgSO$_4$, 1.2 mM Ca-gluconate, 2.4 mM K$_2$HPO$_4$, and 0.4 mM KH$_2$PO$_4$.
11. Chloride-free HPBR: 10 mM HEPES, pH 7.4, 140 mM Na-gluconate, 5 mM K-gluconate, 1.2 mM MgSO$_4$, 1.2 mM Ca-gluconate, 2.4 mM K$_2$HPO$_4$, and 0.4 mM KH$_2$PO$_4$.
12. Ham's F12 medium.
13. PD buffer series:
    a. HPBR.
    b. HPBR, 100 μM amiloride.
    c. Chloride-free HPBR, 100 μM amiloride.
    d. Chloride-free HPBR, 100 μM amiloride, 200 μM 8-cpt-cAMP, 10 μM forskolin.
    e. Chloride free HPBR, 100 μM amiloride, 200 μM 8-cpt-cAMP, 10 μM forskolin, 100 μM UTP.
    f. HPBR.
14. pH/mV meter (Orion Research, cat. no. 0525AO).

3. Methods

3.1. Isolation and Culture of Primary Human Normal and CF Bronchial Cells

3.1.1 Isolation of Airway Cells

1. Perform a dissection of the bronchial airway down to the fifth-order bronchus, in a tissue culture hood, either from a fresh lung transplant or from a postmortem lung that was harvested less than 6 h after death. The dissection should take place on ice and the tissue is then transferred into a beaker containing medium A and maintained at 4°C.

2. Gloves should be worn at all stages of the procedure, and all human specimens should be treated as a potential biohazard.

3. Wash the dissected tissue with medium A using 10 times the volume of the specimen. Strip the excess adventia from the surface of the tissue. Section the bronchial segments onto 1–2-cm rings. The rings are then sectioned longitudinally in order to expose the airway surface. Clear excess mucus from the airway surface.

4. Place cleaned bronchial airway specimens (the equivalent of 10 mL of tissue) into 50 mL conical tubes containing 35 mL of medium A. Incubate the tissue with rocking at 4°C for 30 min.

5. Discard the medium and replace with fresh medium A. Repeat this procedure at least 6 times (*see* **Note 1**).

3.1.2. Dissociation of Airway Epithelial Cells

1. Place washed bronchial segments into a new 50-mL tube containing 35 mL of medium A supplemented with 0.1% protease type XIV. Incubate at 4°C for 36 h in order to liberate the epithelium from the cartilaginous tissue (*see* **Note 2**).

2. Add FBS to the conical tube containing tissue to a final concentration of 10%. Shake the tube gently for 30 s to isolate epithelial cells.

3. Liberated cells in suspension are collected after allowing the tissue segments to settle for 1 min. Transfer suspended cells using a pipet to a new collection tube on ice.

4. Transfer the tissue segments to a Petri dish and scrape with the blunt side of a scalpel to loosen additional epithelial cells. Rinse tissue with Ham's F-12 medium/10% FBS, and add these washed cells to the collection tube (*see* **Note 3**).

5. Centrifuge the combined cells at ~300 g (~1500 rpm) for 5 min in a benchtop centrifuge at 4°C.

6. Decant the supernatant and resuspend the cell pellet in a total of 10 mL of Ham's F-12 medium/10% FBS at 4°C. Pass the suspension through a disposable, sterile cell strainer or through a 500 μM wire mesh to separate dissociated single cells from the fibrous tissue. Collect the effluent containing dispersed cells into a 15-mL conical tube.

7. Wash the cells two more times with Ham's F-12 medium/10% FBS by centrifugation, discarding the supernatants and resuspending the cell pellets.

8. Remove a 10-µL aliquot from the last resuspension for quantitating cells with a hemocytometer, taking care not include red blood cells in the quantification. The typical yield from one lobe of a lung is approx $2–4 \times 10^7$ cells.

3.1.3. Culture of Airway Epithelial Cells

1. Pellet the washed epithelial cells by centrifugation and resuspend final cell pellets in 10 mL of medium B at 37°C. Plate $1-2 \times 10^6$ cells per 100-mm uncoated plastic tissue culture dish, and incubate for 24 h in a humidified 37°C incubator (*see* **Note 4**).
2. On the day following plating, aspirate the culture medium containing nonadherent cells and wash the remaining adherent cells twice with Ham's F-12 medium. Feed the washed cells with a fresh supply of medium B and incubate for an additional 48 h, or longer depending on the degree of bacterial or fungal contamination. If longer culturing in medium B is necessary, the medium should be replaced at 48 h.
3. At 72 h after plating, refeed cells with medium C. At this point, clones of expanding epithelial cells should be visible. The cells are then refed every 3 d with fresh medium C.
4. Cells are typically ready for transplantation into xenografts by 5 d postplating (at ~80% confluency). Care should be taken not to allow cells to become more than 80% confluent or they will begin to differentiate and lose their capacity for subculturing. The cells may also be cyropreserved or passaged at this point.
5. If primary airway cells are to be expanded (typically cells can be expanded 1 time without loss of ability to differentiate in a xenograft model), they should be treated with 0.1% trypsin/EDTA for 1–3 min at 37°C followed by neutralization with trypsin inhibitor buffer. Cells should be closely monitored during trypsinization and harvested immediately once released by gentle tapping of the plate. Cell suspensions are centrifuged to remove trypsin and washed two times in medium C followed by plating at a 1.5 dilution. Cells are then propagated as described above in medium C (*see* **Note 5**).
6. For cyropreservation, epithelial cell pellets are resuspended in 4°C medium C with 10% DMSO, 10% FBS, and aliquoted into 2-mL cryogenic vials for slow freezing at –80°C, overnight. Slow freezing can be performed using isopropanol containing cryopreservation containers (Nalgene). Cells are then moved to liquid nitrogen storage. Typically, one subconfluent 100-mm plate of cells is aliquoted per vial and when subcultured placed into five 100-mm plates (*see* **Note 6**).

3.2. Preparation of Human Bronchial Xenografts

3.2.1. Construction and Preparation of the Xenograft Cassette

1. A xenograft cassette is assembled by connecting tubing and adapters cut to length and secured with sutures as illustrated in **Fig. 1**. The tubing cassette is then placed in a 100-mm tissue culture plate, inserted into a sterilization pouch, and sterilized with gas.

3.2.2. Isolation of Rat Tracheas

1. Euthanize a male Fisher rat by anesthetic overdose or CO_2 asphyxiation and pin the limbs to a Styrofoam bed (*see* **Note 7**).

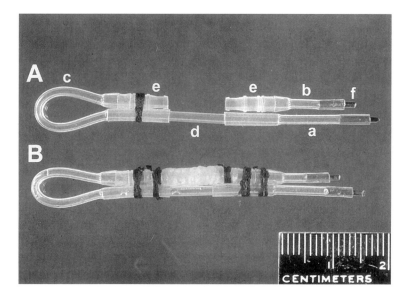

Fig. 1. Construction of xenograft cassettes. Xenograft cassettes are generated from a series of defined types of tubing as illustrated in **A** (a, 1-in. silastic tubing; b, 3/4-in. silastic tubing; c, $1^3/_4$-in. silastic tubing; d, $1^1/_4$-in. Teflon tubing; e, adapter; f, chrome wire plug). A denuded rat donor trachea is connected to a sterilized tubing cassette by a series of sutures as illustrated in **B**.

2. Clean the neck and chest of the rat with 70% ethanol and excise the trachea from the pharynx to the carina (bifurcation of bronchi at the end of the trachea).
3. Immediately place the trachea into a screw-cap vial and keep on ice until all tracheas have been harvested.
4. Denude tracheas of all viable epithelium by applying three cycles of freezing at –80°C and thawing at room temperature.
5. Clean the tracheas of excessive fat and cut to size by sectioning at the first tracheal ring and at the limit of the thirteenth ring. Rinse the lumen of each trachea with 10 mL of cold MEM.
6. Tracheas are matched for length and sorted into pairs placed into the same cryogenic vial. Store the vials at –80°C until needed.

3.2.3. Seeding Tracheas with Primary Airway Epithelial Cells

1. Ligate the rat tracheas to the adapter (e) attached to tubing (b) as shown in **Fig. 1**. To securely tie the trachea to the tubing, wrap the suture around three times, knotting each time. Insert the chrome plug (f) into the end of tubing (b).
2. Using a pipetter, transfer 25 µL containing about $1–2 \times 10^6$ primary airway cells in medium C into the trachea. The tip of the pipetter should be inserted as deeply as possible into the trachea and removed slowly from the trachea as the cells are pipetted.

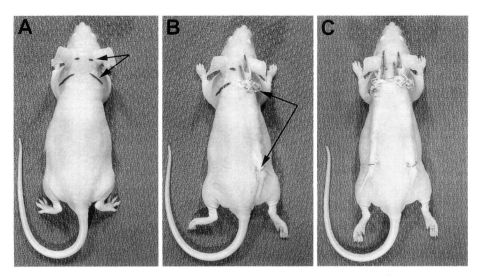

Fig. 2. Transplantation of bronchial xenografts subcutaneously in nu/nu mice. (**A**) The position of four incisions in the skin (arrows). A pocket is formed subcutaneously by blunt dissection, and the xenograft cassette in inserted. Using forceps, the xenograft is guided such that one port exits through the back of the neck and the other port exits through the main incision, as shown in **B**. Surgical staples are used to close incisions (arrows). To maintain the position of the cassettes and prevent subcutaneous migration, staples are also placed to secure the loop (c). (**C**) A mouse with two transplanted xenografts following surgery.

3. Taking care to avoid having the cells leak out the open end of the trachea. Ligate the free end of the trachea to the adapter (e) attached to tubing (c), as illustrated in **Fig. 1**. Secure the trachea to the adapter with sutures, wrapping and knotting the suture three times. Insert the chrome plug into the free end of tubing (a).
4. Adjust the trachea to physiologic length by clamping tubing (a) and tubing (b) with a hemostat. With the trachea held to length with the hemostat, tie two additional sutures as shown in **Fig. 1** to secure the adapters to tubing (d). Tubing (d) is made of rigid Teflon and serves as a stent to stabilize the length of the trachea.
5. Place the xenograft cassettes containing the seeded cells into a 100-mm tissue culture plate. Overlay the trachea with 1–2 mL of medium C to prevent it from drying out. Transfer the plates to a 37°C, 5% CO_2 incubator and incubate for 1–2 h in order to equilibrate the pH before proceeding to transplantation into mice. Transport the xenograft cassettes inside an airtight sterile container that was equilibrated in the same incubator to maintain the CO_2 level prior to transplantation. Alternatively, tissue culture plates harboring xenograft cassettes can be sealed with Parafilm prior to transport. However, if this alternative method is used, care should be taken not to leave the plates out of a 5% CO_2-equilibrated atmosphere for longer than 1 h while performing transplantation.

3.2.4. Transplanting Xenografts into Nu/Nu Mice

1. Anesthesize a male Nu/Nu athymic mouse by intraperitonial injection of 100 mg/kg of ketamine and 20 mg/kg of xylazine in PBS. Once the mouse is anesthetized, place it on a sterile drape, and remove surgical instruments from autoclave pouches.
2. Clean the skin with proviodone then with 70% alcohol. Make four small incisions placed as shown in **Fig. 2**. Two incisions (about 0.16 cm in length) placed high on the neck are just wide enough to pass the tubing ports. Two additional incisions on the flank of the mouse are about 1 cm long.
3. Create a subcutaneous space for placing the xenograft cassette under the skin with blunt dissection. Insert the xenograft cassette into the subcutaneous space, orienting the cassette with the trachea medially. The two ports are guided with forceps so that one exits the main incision and the other exits the smaller, more rostral incision.
4. Use 2–3 staples to close the two largest incisions, and use an additional staple to anchor each xenograft to the skin at the loop of tubing (c) (**Fig. 1**). This anchoring staple must be placed around tubing (c). This can be achieved by pinching the skin and tubing with forceps before anchoring the staple. Do not puncture the xenograft tubing while putting in the staples, as this may result in a leak of material or contamination
5. After transplantation, place the mouse in a sterile cage and monitor until it has recovered from anesthesia. Mice with transplanted xenografts should be housed individually, as they may chew on each other's tubing (*see* **Note 8**).

3.2.5. Maintenance of Transplanted Xenografts

1. Xenograft airways mature into a stratified epithelium by 4–5 wk after transplantation. During this period, xenografts are irrigated weekly for the first 3 wk and twice a week thereafter to remove excess mucous secretions (*see* **Note 9**).
2. To irrigate xenografts, first remove the chrome wire inserts from the two ports of the xenografts. Fill a 1-mL syringe fitted with a 21-gauge needle with warmed Ham's F-12 medium and remove the plunger. Insert the needle into the lateral port of the xenograft.
3. Insert the needle on another (empty) syringe into the medial port of the xenograft. It is easiest to work with butterfly needles to allow for extended working distance and avoid agitating and damaging the xenograft. Apply negative pressure by withdrawing the plunger of this syringe to aspirate the medium under negative pressure from the medium filled syringe. To complete the withdrawal of medium remaining in the xenograft, use the same syringe to aspirate once again. Replace the chrome wire inserts into the tubing ports (*see* **Note 10**).

3.3. In Vivo Trans-Epithelial Potential Difference (PD) Measurements in Xenografts

Transepithelial potential difference (PD) can be used to determine the health and state of differentiation of the xenograft bronchial airway by characterizing electrolyte transport in response to antagonists and agonists of the epithelial

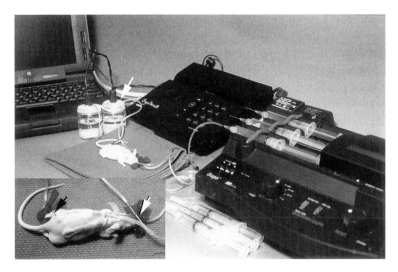

Fig. 3. Equipment and setup for PD analysis. Equipment for PD analysis includes a syringe pump, pH/mV meter, and computer with software for data acquisition (available upon request). The white arrow points to the positive calomel electrode immersed in saturated KCl. Arrows in the inset photograph show the placement of butterfly electrodes, with the positive electrode inserted into the xenograft infusion tubing and the negative electrode inserted subcutaneously in the back of the mouse.

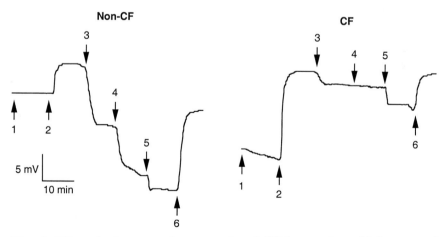

Fig. 4. PD analysis comparing normal and CF human bronchial xenografts. Xenografts were sequentially perfused with (1) HPBR, (2) HPBR with 100 μM amiloride, (3) chloride-free HPBR with 100 μM amiloride, (4) chloride-free HPBR with 100 μM amiloride, 200 μM 8-cpt-cAMP, and 10 μM forskolin, (5) chloride-free HPBR with 100 μM amiloride, 200 μM 8-cpt-cAMP, 10 μM forskolin, and 100 μM UTP, and (6) HPBR. The non-CF graph illustrates a typical recording from a normal human xenograft. The CF graph on the right illustrates typical responses from CF xenografts.

ion channels CFTR and the amiloride-sensitive Na⁺ channel (ENaC) (**Fig. 3**). Using this model, direct comparisons can also be made between normal human bronchial xenograft epithelia and xenograft airways reconstituted with genetically defined CF epithelia to physiologically characterize electrolyte transport defects associated with CFTR dysfunction, as illustrated in **Fig. 4**. Lastly, the PD can be utilized to functionally access the effectiveness of gene therapy approaches after transduction of CF bronchial epithelial cells with viral or nonvectors before or after seeding in xenografts.

1. Four to five weeks following transplantation in Nu/Nu mice, human bronchial xenograft epithelia are fully differentiated and ready for PD analysis. Anesthetize the xenograft-bearing mouse by intraperitonial injection of 100 mg/kg of ketamine and 20 mg/kg of xylazine in PBS. Once the mouse is anesthetized, place it on a sterile drape and remove the chrome wire caps from both ports of the xenograft.
2. Flush the xenograft with 1 mL HPBR as described under **Subheading 3.2.5.**
3. Fill 10-mL syringes with PD buffers and fit them on the syringe pump. A length of manifold pump tubing, which will be placed on the needle of the first syringe, is fitted to silicone tubing, which is placed into the medial port of the xenograft by means of a shortened pipet tip (20–200 μL). For outflow, a butterfly tubing is placed in the distal port.
4. Calomel electrodes, which are immersed in a saturated KCl bath, are connected to the pH/mV meter and to butterfly electrodes.
5. Butterfly electrodes are prepared by filling 21-gauge butterfly tubing with 1 *M* KCl in 3% agarose. Insert the positive butterfly electrode into the perfusion tubing just external to the xenograft port. This is done by directly inserting the 21-gauge needle through the tubing. The negative electrode is inserted subcutaneously in the back of the mouse (*see* **Note 11**).
6. Milli-volt recordings are captured through the pH/mV meter and data-linked directly to a computer, equipped with software to record millivolt measurements at 5-s intervals. (Software will be provided upon request.)
7. Typically, xenografts are sequentially perfused with PD buffers through the syringe pump at flow rate of 200 μL/min for 5 min (*see* **Note 12**).
8. After recording is completed, flush the xenograft with warmed Ham's F-12 medium as described under **Subheading 2.2.5.** Replace the chrome wire inserts into the tubing ports.
9. Repeat **steps 1–8** on the xenograft on the other side of the animal if two are implanted (*see* **Note 13**).

4. Notes

1. Additional washes are required if the lung was derived from a CF patient, due to the high level of bacterial contamination in CF specimens. In this case, we recommend washing CF specimens for 5–6 h and performing washes every 45–60 min. Medium A with twice the listed concentration of antibiotics should be used in all these washes.
2. For CF cells, the antibiotic concentrations in medium A are doubled.

3. The airway tissue may be saved at –80°C for genotyping, if necessary.
4. For CF cells, the antibiotic concentrations in medium B are doubled for the first 24 h.
5. The duration of exposure to medium B will be dependent on the degree of bacterial and fungal contamination in cultures. For heavily contaminated cells, exposure should be maintained for 72 h. However, fungizone is highly toxic to cells and time of exposure should be kept to a minimum unless problems are encountered with contamination. A common source of fungal contamination often stems from tissue harvested in hospital pathology laboratories. Therefore, it is best when possible to acquire tissue directly in the transplantation operating room.
6. Cryopreserved cells should be quick thawed at 37°C and care taken to place cells in growth medium immediately after thawing. It is not necessary to remove DMSO by washing cells, since each plug of cells is diluted into 50 mL of growth medium.
7. All procedures are performed in a laminar-flow hood under sterile conditions.
8. Pathogen-free housing is critical to the success of this model system, since athymic mice are extremely susceptible to infection. All caging, food, and water must be autoclaved. Since these mice are immunocompromised, this is a very important aspect of preventing infection and death.
9. Weekly irrigation of xenografts during maturation is important for maintaining an open, unobstructed lumen in the xenograft airway. Approximately 25–30% of xenografts close during maturation and are not usable for experimentation. Therefore experimental numbers should be increased accordingly.
10. Negative-pressure irrigation is key to avoiding mucus plugs that might otherwise rupture the xenograft under positive pressure.
11. Butterfly electrodes are stored in 1 M KCl at 4°C and can be used up to a year.
12. To change buffers, clamp the solvent flexible tubing with a hemostat to prevent the formation of air bubbles during syringe changes.
13. PD measurements can be performed on the same mice several times, allowing 2–3 d for the animal to recover between recording sessions.

Acknowledgment

This work was supported by the National Institutes of Health grant #NHLBI HL61234.

References

1. Bye, M. R., Ewig, J. M., and Quittell, L. M. (1994) Cystic fibrosis. *Lung* **172(5),** 251–270.
2. Sferra, T. J. and Collins, F. S. (1993) The molecular biology of cystic fibrosis. *Annu. Rev. Med.* **44,** 133–144.
3. Engelhardt, J. F., Yankaskas, J. R., Ernst, S. A., et al. (1992) Submucosal glands are the predominant site of CFTR expression in the human bronchus. *Nat. Genet.* **2(3),** 240–248.
4. Barinaga, M. (1992) Knockout mice offer first animal model for CF [news]. *Science* **257(5073),** 1046,1047.

5. Grubb, B. R., Paradiso, A. M., and Boucher, R. C. (1994) Anomalies in ion transport in CF mouse tracheal epithelium. *Am. J. Physiol.* **267(1, Pt 1),** C293–300.
6. Grubb, B. R., Vick, R. N., and Boucher, R. C. (1994) Hyperabsorption of Na+ and raised Ca(2+)-mediated Cl-secretion in nasal epithelia of CF mice. *Am J. Physiol.* **266(5 Pt 1),** C1478–1483.
7. Engelhardt, J. F., Allen, E. D., and Wilson, J. M. (1991) Reconstitution of tracheal grafts with a genetically modified epithelium. *Proc. Natl. Acad. Sci. USA* **88(24),** 11,192–11,196.
8. Engelhardt, J. F., Yankaskas, J. R., and Wilson, J. M. (1992) In vivo retroviral gene transfer into human bronchial epithelia of xenografts. *J. Clin. Invest.* **90(6),** 2598–2607.
9. Engelhardt, J. F., Yang, Y., Stratford-Perricaudet, L. D., et al. (1993) Direct gene transfer of human CFTR into human bronchial epithelia of xenografts with E1-deleted adenoviruses. *Nat. Genet.* **4(1),** 27–34.
10. Engelhardt, J. F., Schlossberg, H., Yankaskas, J. R., et al. (1995) Progenitor cells of the adult human airway involved in submucosal gland development. *Development* **121(7),** 2031–2046.
11. Boucher, R. C., Bromberg, P. A. Jr., and Gatzy, J. T. (1980) Airway transepithelial electric potential in vivo: species and regional differences. *J. Appl. Physiol.* **48(1),** 169–176.
12. Zhang, Y., Yankaskas, J., Wilson, J., et al. (1996) In vivo analysis of fluid transport in cystic fibrosis airway epithelia of bronchial xenografts. *Am. J. Physiol.* **270(5 Pt 1),** C1326–1335.
13. Goldman, M. J., Yang, Y., and Wilson, J. M. (1995) Gene therapy in a xenograft model of cystic fibrosis lung corrects chloride transport more effectively than the sodium defect. *Nat. Genet.* **9(2),** 126–131.
14. Zhang, Y., Jiang, Q., Dudus, L., et al. (1998) Vector-specific complementation profiles of two independent primary defects in cystic fibrosis airways. *Hum. Gene. Ther.* **9(5),** 635–648.

36

Development of Conditionally Immortalized Epithelial Cell Lines from CF and Non-CF Mice

Calvin U. Cotton

1. Introduction

Mutations in the cystic fibrosis transmembrane conductance regulator (CFTR) gene are responsible for cystic fibrosis (CF) *(1)* and the primary defect in CF is the loss of cAMP-regulated anion conductance in the apical plasma membrane of epithelial cells in affected tissues *(2,3)*. Primary culture of CF epithelial cells and immortalized cell lines derived from CF patients have been particularly useful for studies of cystic fibrosis and CFTR *(4–9)*. A wide spectrum of phenotypic abnormalities associated with mutant CFTR has been described; however, it is unclear how many of these alterations are related to loss of Cl⁻ channel function *(10)*. Most of the studies of CFTR function have been performed using airway and colon carcinoma (T84) cells or heterologous expression systems *(4–9)*. Epithelial cells from other tissues affected by cystic fibrosis have received relatively little attention, primarily due to the lack of access to appropriate human material. The development of the CF mouse has expanded the number of epithelial cell types available for study *(11,12)*.

1.1. Common Methods for Generating Immortalized Cell Lines

The most common method for generation of immortalized cell lines is to isolate primary cultures of the cells of interest and then to introduce either SV40 large T antigen *(5–7,9,13)* or human papilloma virus *(8)* by in-vitro transfection. Since transfection of primary cultures of epithelial cells is relatively inefficient, this approach works well if you can isolate large numbers of cells of interest *(5,7,13)*. It is then necessary to select colonies that have integrated one or more copies of the transgene. In the CF field this approach has been used largely to generate either tracheal *(5–8)* or bronchial *(9)* epithelial cell

From: *Methods in Molecular Medicine, vol. 70: Cystic Fibrosis Methods and Protocols*
Edited by: W. R. Skach © Humana Press Inc., Totowa, NJ

lines from CF and non-CF airways. An alternative approach is to isolate cells from genetically modified mice that carry an SV40 large T antigen *(14)*. In order to develop cell lines from CF mice it would be necessary to cross the mouse line that carries the SV40 large T antigen transgene with the CF mouse line. Murine CF cell lines derived in this manner have recently been described *(15,15a)*.

1.2. Use of the ImmortoMouse to Generate Cell Lines

Jat and co-workers *(16)* developed a transgenic mouse line (H2K^b-tsA58; ImmortoMouse) that carries a thermolabile mutant of SV40 large T antigen under the control of a ubiquitous interferon-inducible promoter. This mouse line has been used to generate several conditionally immortalized cell lines to date *(15–20)*. The major theoretical advantages of cell lines generated in this way are: (1) the ability to immortalize a heterogenous population of cells from an epithelium (e.g., ciliated, goblet, basal cells from the airway), from which clones with specific properties may be selected at a later time; (2) the avoidance of unpredictable characteristics of in-vitro transfection with oncogenes (e.g., variable copy number and multiple sites of integration); and (3) the opportunity to control large T antigen levels and thereby promote differentiation by switching the cells from permissive to nonpermissive culture conditions.

1.3. Generation of CF and Non-CF Cell Lines from the ImmortoMouse

The strategy that we adopted to generate CF and non-CF mouse cell lines was to cross the ImmortoMouse with the UNC CFTR-knockout mouse *(15)*. There are essentially three steps involved in this project: (1) breeding of the ImmortoMouse and the CFTR knockout mouse to obtain second-generation animals that are either CF or non-CF and carry the immortalizing transgene; (2) isolation, culture, and expansion of the epithelial cells of interest; and (3) confirmation of the transport phenotype and characterization of the properties of the cell lines.

2. Materials
2.1. Generation of Mice of the Appropriate Genotype
2.1.1. Animals

1. Female UNC mice heterozygous for the S489X CFTR mutation (UNC; CFTR +/-; C57BL/6j × F129 strain; now available from Jackson Laboratory, Bar Harbor, ME).
2. Male mice, homozygous for the H-2K^b-tsA58 transgene (ImmortoMouse, Charles River Laboratories, Boston, MA).

2.1.2. Genotype Analysis

Tail digestion for DNA extraction:

1. Proteinase K (0.5 mg/mL; Fisher) in NTES buffer (10 mM Tris-HCl, pH 8.0, 2 mM EDTA, 0.4 M NaCl, 0.5% sodium dodecyl sulfate [SDS]).
2. Saturated phenol (Fisher).
3. Phenol/chloroform/isoamyl alcohol (Fisher).
4. Isopropanol.
5. 70% ethanol.
6. Glass micropipets.
7. PCR primers for wild-type CFTR: primer I, 5'-ATA CCG TCC ATC TTG GCA AAG GAG G-3'; primer II, 5'-TTG CTT CAG TCT CTT GAG TAT TAG GAT TGC-3'.
8. PCR primers for the S489X neomycin-disrupted CFTR allele: primer III, 5'-GGG AGA CTT GTG ATT GGA ATA ATT GGA CG-3'; primer IV, 5'-TCC TGC AGT TCA TTC AGG GCA CCG G-3'.
9. PCR primers for the SV40 transgene: primer V, 5'-AGC GCT TGT GTC GCC ATT GTA TTA -3'; primer VI, 5'-GTC ACA CCA CAG AAG TAA GGT TCC-3'.

  PCR amplification:

1. Genomic DNA.
2. PCR primers.
3. Taq polymerase (Boehringer Mannheim Biochemicals, Indianapolis, IN).
4. PCR buffer: 10 mM Tris-HCl (pH 8.3), 1.5 mM MgCl$_2$, 50 mM KCl.
5. Agarose.
6. Ethidium bromide (10 mg/mL).
7. Gel loading buffer: 30% glycerol, 0.25% bromophenol blue.
8. TAE running buffer: 50× TAE; 242 g Tris base, 57.1 mL glacial acetic acid, 100 mL of 0.5 M EDTA (pH 8.0).
9. UV lightbox and camera to photograph gel.

2.1.3. Diet, Bedding, and Cages

1. Sterile Autoclavable laboratory rodent Chow (Purina).
2. Vanilla Peptamen (Clintec Nutrition, DeerField, IL).
3. Bed-O=Cobs cage bedding (Anderson, Maumee, OH).
4. Microisolator cages.

2.2. Tissue and Cell Isolation

2.2.1. Renal Collecting Tubule Cell Lines

1. Stadie Riggs tissue slicer.
2. Hank's balanced salt solution.
3. Collagenase type IV (Worthington Biochemical).
4. DMEM culture medium.
5. Fetal bovine serum.
6. Dolichos biflorus agglutinin (Sigma)
7. 0.1 M NaHCO$_3$.
8. Heated shaking water bath.

2.2.2. Tracheal Cell Lines

1. HEPES-buffered Ringer's solution (HR): 10 mM HEPES (titrated to pH 7.45 with NaOH), 138 mM NaCl, 5 mM KCl, 2.5 mM Na$_2$HPO$_4$, 1.8 mM CaCl$_2$, 1 mM MgSO$_4$, and 10 mM glucose.
2. Protease (type XIV, Sigma) and collagenase (type IV, Sigma).
3. Ca^{2+}- and Mg^{2+}-free Hank's balanced salt solution plus EDTA (5 mM).

2.2.3. Pancreas and Salivary Cell Lines

1. HEPES-buffered Ringer's solution.
2. Collagenase type I and type IV (Worthington Biochemical).
3. Soy bean trypsin inhibitor (Sigma).
4. Nylon filter (149 × 149 μm mesh).
5. Bovine serum albumin.

2.3. Cell Culture and Expansion

2.3.1. Renal Collecting Tubules

1. Tissue culture dishes.
2. Ca^{2+}- and Mg^{2+}-free Hanks balanced salt solution that contains 0.05% trypsin and 0.53 mM EDTA (Gibco-BRL).
3. Collecting tubule culture media. 1/1 mix of Dulbecco's modified Eagle's medium (DMEM) and Ham's F-12 medium (GIBCO-BRL) supplemented with 1.3 μg/L sodium selenite, 1.3 μg/L 3,3',5-triiodo-L-thyronine, 5 mg/L insulin, 5 mg/L transferrin, 25 μg/L prostaglandin E$_1$, 2.5 mM glutamine, 5 nM dexamethasone, 50000 U/L nystatin, 50 mg/L streptomycin, 30 mg/L penicillin G, and 10000 U/L recombinant mouse interferon gamma (INF-γ).

2.3.2. Tracheal Epithelial Cells

1. Tissue culture dishes.
2. Collagen gel-coated dishes (Vitrogen; Collagen Corp.)
3. Ca^{2+}- and Mg^{2+}-free Hank's balanced salt solution that contains 0.05% trypsin and 0.53 mM EDTA (Gibco-BRL).
4. Tracheal cell culture media. Tracheal epithelial cells were maintained in small airways growth media (SAGM, Clonetics), supplemented with 500 mg/L bovine serum albumin, 0.5 μg/L hEGF, 5 mg/L insulin, 6.5 μg/L 3,3',5-triiodo-L-thyronine, 10 mg/L transferrin, 30 mg/L bovine pituitary extract, 0.5 mg/L epineph-rine, 0.5 mg/L hydrocortisone, 0.1 μg/L retinoic acid, 50 mg/L gentamycin sulfate, 50 μg/L amphotericin B, and 10000 U/L IFN-γ.

2.3.3. Pancreatic and Salivary Epithelial Cells

1. Tissue culture dishes.
2. Ca^{2+}- and Mg^{2+}-free Hank's balanced salt solution that contains 0.05% trypsin and 0.53 mM EDTA (Gibco-BRL).
3. Exocrine culture media. 1/1 mix of Dulbecco's modified Eagle's medium (DMEM) and Ham's F-12 medium supplemented with 0.5 mM isobutyl methyl

xanthine, 2 m*M* glutamine, 10 μg/L EGF, 100 mg/L streptomycin sulfate, 60 mg/L penicillin G, 50000 U/L nystatin, 2.5% fetal bovine serum, and 10000 U/L INF-γ.

3. Methods

3.1. Generation of Mice of the Appropriate Genotype

3.1.1. Animals

1. The objective of the breeding program is to generate second generation pups that carry at least one copy of the SV40 transgene and are either non-CF (CFTR +/+, or +/–) or CF (CFTR –/–). A male ImmortoMouse is placed with three female mice heterzygous for the S489X CFTR mutation in a microisolator cage. Multiple breeding cages are established to increase the number of first-generation offspring. When the female mice become pregnant, they are transferred to individual cages and are replaced with new female breeders. About 7–10 d after the pups are born, the animals are marked (toes are cut or ears are punched) for identification and a small piece of the tail is cut (0.5 cm) for DNA isolation and polymerase chain reaction (PCR)-based genotype analysis (*see* **Note 1**). All first-generation pups are expected to be heterozygous for the SV40 transgene and either homozygous wild-type for CFTR or heterozygous for CFTR. Male and female animals that are heterozygous for both traits (i.e., Immorto +/– and CFTR +/–) are selected for breeding.
2. When the first-generation females become pregnant, they are removed to individual microisolator cages with corncob bedding. About 7–10 d after the second-generation pups are born, the animals are marked and a piece of tail is taken for genotype analysis. At this time the solid food is removed and the mother and pups are placed on a liquid Peptamin diet. Second-generation pups that carry the SV40 transgene and are either CF (CFTR –/–) or non-CF (CFTR +/+ or +/–) are selected for tissue removal (*see* **Note 2**).

3.1.2. Genotype Analysis

1. DNA extraction. Place the pieces of tail in 1.5-mL microfuge tubes with 700 μL of NTES buffer plus 0.5 mg/mL proteinase K. Incubate the tail segments overnight at 55°C. Then add 700 μL of saturated phenol and mixed vigorously for 3–5 min. Centrifuge in a microfuge (14,000 rpm) for 10 min and collect the upper aqueous phase in another microfuge tube. Add 700 μL of phenol/chloroform/isoamyl alcohol and mix vigorously. Centrifuge as above and collect the aqueous phase. Add 700 μL of isopropanol to the sample and invert the tube several times to mix. Stir the sample with a glass micropipet to spool the DNA. Rinse the spooled DNA with 70% ethanol, break the tip of the pipet and DNA into a microfuge tube, and allow the DNA to dry. Add 500 μL of sterile distilled water to resuspend the DNA.
2. PCR amplification of mouse tail DNA: Heat DNA sample at 65°C for 15 min and keep all other reagents on ice. Prepare a master mix of all PCR reagents (except DNA sample). The amounts for one reaction are as follows: 39.5 μL sterile water, 1 μL of 3' primer (50 μ*M* stock), 1 μL of 5' primer (50 μ*M* stock), 2 μL dNTP mix

(each dNTP at 2.5 mM), 5 μL of 10× Taq buffer, 2 U of Taq DNA polymerase. Distribute master mix to 600 μL PCR sample tubes (49 μL/tube). Add 1 μL of DNA sample, overlay with mineral oil, and place on ice. Transfer all samples to the PCR thermocycler and amplify for 30 cycles (1 min at 95°C, 2 min at 58°C, and 3 min at 70°C to denature, anneal, and extend, respectively).

3. Analysis of PCR products: The PCR samples are removed, gel loading buffer is added to the sample (10 μL), and a 15-μL sample is run on an agarose gel (1.2% in TAE buffer; ~60 V) and visualized with ethidium bromide (0.5 μg/mL of gel). The predicted PCR product sizes are 500 bp for wild-type CFTR, 650 bp for the neomycin-disrupted CFTR, and 1000 bp for the SV40 transgene.

3.1.3. Mouse Diet and Bedding

1. CFTR (–/–) mice die of intestinal obstruction (*11,21*) shortly after weaning if they are not switched to a liquid Peptamen diet. Peptamen (~100 mL/mother and litter) was provided using a sterile water bottle. The Peptamen was changed daily.
2. Corncob bedding was used in place of the traditional wood shavings and the bedding was changed weekly (*21*).
3. All animals are housed in microisolator cages with no more than four adults/cage. It is important to separate pregnant females before the pups are delivered.

3.2 Tissue and Cell Isolation

3.2.1. Renal Collecting Tubule Cell Lines

1. Preparation of lectin coated plates: Dissolve DBA lectin in sterile 0.1 M NaHCO$_3$ solution (10 μg/mL). Add 8 mL to a 10-cm tissue culture dish and incubate at 4°C overnight. Remove solution and wash with culture medium immediately before use.
2. Tissue digestion and cell isolation: Animals of the appropriate genotype were identified (10 non-CF and 6 CF), sacrificed, and the kidneys were removed and placed in sterile Hank's balanced salt solution (HBSS). A Stadie-Riggs tissue microtome was used to slice each kidney into 100–150-μm sections. The slices were incubated for 30 min in collagenase type IV (0.5%) in HBSS at 37°C. If necessary, small clumps can be dispersed with a 21-gage needle. Centrifuge at 800*g* for 5 min. Wash cell pellet with ice-cold culture medium containing 10% fetal bovine serum and centrifuge again at 800*g* for 5 min. Resuspend pellet in PBS with 5 mM glucose. Centrifuge and resuspend in PBS with 5 mM glucose. Add suspension to lectin (DBA lectin)-coated plates and incubate at 4°C for 45 min. Remove unbound cells by washing three times with PBS (without glucose). Elute cells by adding 10 mls of 150 mM galactose in PBS and incubating for 5 min (scrape if necessary). Centrifuge the cells and resuspend the cells in collecting tubule culture medium and seed culture dishes (*15,20*).

3.2.2. Isolation of Tracheal Epithelial Cells

1. Animals of the appropriate genotype (3 non-CF mice and 2 CF mice) that carried the SV40 transgene were selected. The animals were sacrificed and the trachea removed by blunt dissection and placed in ice-cold HEPES-buffered ringers

solution. Each trachea was cleaned of connective tissue and the tube was opened along the posterior surface and pinned to the bottom of a dissection dish.

2. The tissues were exposed to 0.1% protease and 0.1% collagenase type IV in Ca^{2+}, Mg^{2+}-free HBSS that contained 5 mM EDTA at 37°C for 20 min. The epithelium was freed from the lamina propria by pipetting a steady stream of fluid over the partially digested trachea. Tracheal cells were collected and centrifuged in a microfuge at 14,000 rpm for 30 s. The pellet was resuspended in small airways growth medium (SAGM, Clonetics).

3.2.3. Isolation of Pancreatic Duct Cells

1. Animals of the appropriate genotype (4 non-CF and 4 CF mice) that carried the SV40 transgene were selected. The animals were sacrificed and the pancreas was removed and placed in ice-cold HEPES-buffered Ringer's solution. Tissues were trimmed of connective tissue, placed in a small volume of HEPES-buffer Ringer's solution (1 mL) that contained 0.25 mg/mL collagenase type I, 0.25 mg/mL collagenase type IV, and 0.1 mg/mL soy bean trypsin inhibitor. The glands were minced with scissors to yield small fragments approx 1 mm × 1 mm × 1 mm. An additional 12 mL of the enzyme solution was added to the tissue fragments *(22)*.

2. The digest was placed in a shaking water bath (~70 cycles/min) at 37°C for 45 min. At 15-min intervals, the tissue fragments were disrupted by repeat (8×) passage through a plastic pipet (~0.5-mm diameter tip).

3. At the end of the 45-min digestion period the resulting tissue digest was passed thru a nylon filter (149 μm × 149 μm mesh) and the material trapped by the filter was washed several times, collected and resuspended in exocrine culture medium for culture.

3.2.4. Isolation of Salivary Epithelial Cells

1. Animals of the appropriate genotype (3 non-CF and 3 CF mice) that carried the SV40 transgene were selected. The animals were sacrificed and the submandibular salivary glands were removed and placed in ice-cold HEPES-buffered Ringer's solution. Tissues were trimmed of connective tissue, placed in a small volume of HEPES-buffer Ringer's solution (1 mL) that contained 0.25 mg/mL collagenase type I, 0.25 mg/mL collagenase type IV, and 0.1 mg/mL soy bean trypsin inhibitor. The glands were minced with scissors to yield small fragments approx 1 mm × 1 mm × 1 mm. An additional 12 mL of the enzyme solution was added to the tissue fragments.

2. The digest was placed in a shaking water bath (~70 cycles/min) at 37°C for 60 min. At 15-min intervals the tissue fragments were disrupted by repeat (8×) passage through a plastic pipet (~0.5-mm diameter tip).

3. At the end of the 60-min digestion period the resulting tissue digest was layered over a 4% BSA (in HR) solution and allowed to settle for 10 min on ice. The supernatant was removed and the resulting pellet was resuspended in exocrine medium for culture.

3.3. Cell Culture and Expansion

3.3.1. Collecting Tubule Cells

1. The method of cell isolation used here yields a nearly pure preparation of renal collecting tubule cells. A small number of fibroblasts are also isolated, but they do not survive in the serum-free defined CT media.
2. The cultures are maintained under permissive conditions (33°C plus gamma interferon) until the colonies expand and cover the culture dish. The cells are passaged with low dilution (split 1/2), since viability is compromised if the cultures are sparse (*see* **Note 3**).
3. After 3–4 passages the cultures appear homogenous, and if necessary serum can be added to the medium (5% fetal calf serum) to enhance proliferation. After the first 5 passages the cultures can be split 1:5 or 1:10 at weekly intervals.
4. These cell lines have been maintained in culture for more than 1 yr and continue to grow for more than 50 passages.
5. The cells are cryopreserved (liquid nitrogen) in 10% DMSO/90% fetal calf serum (*see* **Note 4**).

3.3.2. Tracheal Epithelial Cells

1. The method of cell isolation used here yields a highly purified preparation of epithelial cells with some fibroblast contamination. The attachment and proliferation of isolated tracheal epithelial cells is greatly enhanced by seeding the isolated cells on a 1-mm thick collagen gel (Vitrogen).
2. The cultures are passaged with low dilution (split 1:2), and seeded onto new collagen gels for the first three passages. After this time they can be seeded directly onto plastic tissue culture dishes.
3. Fibroblast proliferation is minimal since the culture medium is serum-free. After 3–4 passages, serum can be added to the medium (5% fetal calf serum) to enhance proliferation. After the first five passages the cultures can be split 1:5 every 10–14 d.
4. These cell lines have been maintained in culture for more than 1 yr and continue to grow for more than 50 passages.
5. The cells are cryopreserved in 10% DMSO/90% fetal calf serum.

3.3.3. Pancreatic Duct Cells

1. The method for cell isolation used here yields primarily ductal fragments with significant fibroblast contamination. The pancreatic cells do not grow well in the absence of serum (2.5%), therefore differential trypsinization should be used to eliminate fibroblast contamination.
2. The cultures are exposed to sterile HBSS that contains 0.05% trypsin. The junctions formed between the epithelial cells limit access of trypsin and the nonepithelial fibroblasts detach from the substrate first. It is important to monitor the detachment of the cells carefully and to remove the trypsin after the fibroblasts begin to detach, but before a significant number of the epithelial cells detach.
3. This procedure is repeated several times at 5–7-d intervals to continue to enrich the epithelial preparation. If fibroblast contamination continues to be a problem,

the epithelial cells can be cultured for several weeks in serum-free exocrine media, but their growth is severely slowed.

4. As the cultures proliferate, they can be passaged by low-dilution splits (1:3). After the fifth passage the culture may be split weekly at either 1:5 or 1:10 dilution.
5. These cell lines have been maintained in culture for more than 1 yr and continue to grow for more than 50 passages.
6. The cells are cryopreserved in 10% DMSO/90% fetal calf serum.

3.3.4. Salivary Epithelial Cells

1. The method of cell isolated used here yields primarily ductal and acinar fragments with a modest amount of fibroblast contamination.
2. The same method described above for pancreatic ductal cells is used to remove fibroblasts from the salivary epithelial cell cultures.
3. As the cultures proliferate, they can be passaged by low-dilution splits (1:3). After the fifth passage the culture may be split weekly at either 1:5 or 1:10 dilution.
4. These cell lines have been maintained in culture for more than 1 yr and continue to grow for more than 50 passages.
5. The cells are cryopreserved in 10% DMSO/90% fetal calf serum.

3.4. Genotype and Phenotype Analysis

Once the cell lines are generated and samples have been cryopreserved, it is necessary to confirm the genotype and to characterize the phenotype of the result cell lines.

3.4.1. Genotype Analysis

Essentially the same procedure can be followed to genotype the cell lines that was used to genotype the animals. DNA can be isolated from a cell pellet of cultured cells using the same protocol that was used to isolate DNA from a piece of mouse tail.

3.4.2. Phenotype Analysis

The CFTR gene encodes a cAMP-activated, apical membrane chloride channel, and the transport phenotype of CF cells is the loss of cAMP-stimulated Cl^- permeability. A number of approaches can be used to access the phenotype of the cells, but a description of these methods is beyond the scope of this chapter. ^{36}Cl efflux, SPQ-based Cl^- permeability measurements, patch clamp analysis, and transepithelial short-circuit current measurements, RT-PCR, Western blot, Northern blot verification of CFTR expression are the most widely used. A variety of other features of the cells can also be characterized, including growth rate, sensitivity to nonpermissive growth conditions, formation of electrically resistive epithelial monolayers, establishment of polarity, transport pathways and receptor expression known to be a feature of the native epithelium *(13,15,20,23,24)*.

4. Notes

1. The male ImmortoMouse was used so that we could rapidly increase our colony of double heterozygotes. The female ImmortoMouse is viable and fertile, but we observed that pregnancy tends to exacerbate the thymic hyperplasia that eventually kills the animal. In contrast, we found that the male ImmortoMouse could be breed with multiple females for more than 1 yr.
2. Since only the CFTR –/– pups require a liquid diet, it was not necessary to introduce Peptamin until second-generation pups were born. In order to obtain proper control animals, all mothers and second-generation pups were placed on Peptamin, regardless of genotype. Generally pups were sacrificed between 3 and 6 wk of age for tissue isolation.
3. Each of the epithelial cell lines that we generated exhibits reduced proliferation and viability if they are plated at low density. In general during the first 5 passages the cultures are split either 1:2 or 1:3. After passage 5 the cultures are split 1:5 or 1:10.
4. Each of the cell lines is frozen in liquid nitrogen at ~2 million cells/mL. A variety of cryoprotectants are available, but we found that 10% DMSO/90% fetal calf serum appears to work well.

References

1. Riordan, J. R., Rommens, J. M. Kerem, B. S., Alon, N., Rozmahel, R., Grzelczak, Z., et al. (1989) Identification of the cystic fibrosis gene: Cloning and characterization of complementary DNA. *Science* **245,** 1066–1073.
2. Anderson, M. P., Gregory, R. J., Thompson, S., Souza, D. W., Paul, S. Mulligan, R. C., et al. (1991) Demonstration that CFTR is a chloride channel by alteration of its anion selectivity. *Science* **253(5016),** 202–205.
3. Knowles, M. R., Stutts, M. J., Spock, A., Fischer, A., Gatzy, J. T., and Boucher, R. C. (1983) Abnormal ion permeation through cystic fibrosis respiratory epithelium. *Science* **221,** 1067–1070.
4. Boucher, R. C., Yankaskas, J. R., Cotton, C. U., Knowles, M. R., and Stutts, M. J. (1987) Cell culture approaches to the investigation of human airway ion transport. *Eur. J. Respir. Dis.* **153,** 59–67.
5. Gruenert, D. C., Basbaum, C. B., Welsh, M. J., Li, M., Finkbeiner, W. E., and Nadel, J. A. (1988) Characterization of human tracheal epithelial cells transformed by an origin-defective simian virus 40. *Proc. Natl. Acad. Sci. USA* **85,** 5951–5955.
6. Jefferson, D. M., Valentich, J. D., Marini, F. C., Grubman, S. A., Iannuzzi, M. C., Dorkin, H. L., et al. (1990) Expression of normal and cystic fibrosis phenotypes by continuous airway epithelial cell lines. *Am. J. Physiol.* **259(6 Pt 1),** L496–505.
7. Jetten, A. M., Yankaskas, J. R., Stutts, M. J., Willamsen, N. J., and Boucher, R. C. (1989) Persistence of abnormal chloride conductance regulation in transformed cystic fibrosis epithelium. *Science* **244,** 1472–1475.
8. Yankaskas, J. R., Haizlip, J. E., Conrad, M., Koval, D., Lazarowski, E., Paradiso, A. M., et al. (1993) Papilloma virus immortalized tracheal epithelial cells retain a well-differentiated phenotype. *Am. J. Physiol.* **264(5 Pt 1),** C1219–1230.

9. Zeitlin, P. L, Lu, L., Rhim, J., Cutting, G., Stetten, G., Kieffer, K. A., Craig, R., and Guggino, W. B. (1991) A cystic fibrosis bronchial epithelial cell line: immortalization by adeno-12-SV40 infection. *Am. J. Respir. Cell. Mol. Biol.* **4(4),** 313–319.

10. Schwiebert E. M., Benos, D. J., Egan, M. E., Stutts, M. J., and Guggino, W. B. (1999) CFTR is a conductance regulator as well as a chloride channel. *Physiol. Rev.* **79(1 Suppl),** S145–166.

11. Snouwaert, J. N., Brigman, K. K., Latour, A. M., Malouf, N. N., Boucher, R. C., Smithies, O., et al. (1992) An animal model for cystic fibrosis made by gene targeting *Science* **257(5073),** 1083–1088.

12. Clarke, L. L., Grubb, B. R., Gabriel, S. E., Smithies, O., Koller, B. H., and Boucher, R. C. (1992) Defective epithelial chloride transport in a gene-targeted mouse model of cystic fibrosis. *Science* **257,** 1125–1128.

13. Marino, L. R., and Cotton, C. U. (1996) Immortalization of bovine pancreatic duct epithelial cells. *Am. J. Physiol.* **270** (*Gastrointest. Liver Physiol.* **33**), G676–G683.

14. Hopfer, U., Jacobberger, J. W., Gruenert, D. C. . Eckert, R. L., Jat, P. S., and Whitsett, J. A. (1996) Immortalization of epithelial cells. *Am. J. Physiol.* **270(1 Pt 1),** C1–C11.

15. Takacs-Jarrett, M., Sweeney, W. E., Avner, E. D., and Cotton, C. U. (2001) Generation and phenotype of cell lines derived from CF and non-CF mice that carry the H-2K^b-tsA58 transgene. *Am. J. Physiol.* **280** (*Cell*), 228–236.

15a. Thomas, E. J., Gabriel, S. E., Makhlina, M., Hardy, S. P., and Lethem, M. I. (2000) Expression of nucleotide-regulated Cl currents in CF and normal mouse tracheal epithelial cell lines. *Am. J. Physiol.* **279** (*Cell*), 1578–1586.

16. Jat, P. S., Noble, M. D., Ataliotis, P., Tanaka, Y., Yannoutsos, N., Larsen, L. and Kioussis, D. (1991) Direct derivation of conditionally immortal cell lines from an H-2K^b-tsA58 transgenic mouse. *Proc. Natl. Acad. Sci. USA* **88,** 5096–5100.

17. Chambers, T., Owens, J., Hattersley, G., Jat, P., and Noble, M. (1993) Generation of osteoclast-inductive and osteoclastogenic cell lines from the H-2K^{b}tsA58 transgenic mouse. *Proc. Natl. Acad. Sci. USA* **90,** 5578–5582.

18. Morgan, J. E., Beauchamp, J. R., Pagel, C. N., Peckham, M., Ataliotis, P., Jat, P. S., et al. (1994). Myogenic cell lines derived from trangenic mice carrying a thermolabile T antigen: A model system for the derivation of tissue-specific and mutation-specific cell lines. *Develop. Biol.* **162,** 486–498.

19. Whitehead, R. H., VanEeden, P. E., Noble, M. D., Ataliotis, P., and Jat, P. S. (1993) Establishment of conditionally immortalized epithelial cell lines from both colon and small intestine of adult H-2K^b-tsA58 transgenic mice. *Proc. Natl. Acad. Sci. USA* **90,** 587–591.

20. Takacs-Jarrett, M., Sweeney, W. E., Avner, E. D., and Cotton, C. U. (1998) Morphological and functional characterization of a conditionally immortalized collecting tubule cell line. *Am. J. Physiol.* **275** (*Renal Fluid and Electrolyte*), 802–811.

21. Eckman, E. A., Cotton, C. U., Kube, D. M., and Davis, P. B. (1995). Dietary changes improve survival of the CFTR S489X homozygous mutant mouse. *Am. J. Physiol.* **269** (*Lung Cell. Mol. Physiol.* **13**), L625–L630.

22. Githens, S., Schexnayder, J. A., Moses, R. L., Denning, G. M., Smith, J. J., and Frazier, M. L. (1994) Mouse pancreatic acinar/ductular tissue gives rise to epithe-

lial cultures that are morphologically, biochemically, and functionally indistinguishable from interlobular duct cell cultures. *In Vitro Cell. Dev. Biol.* **30A,** 622–635.

23. Cotton, C. U. and Al-Nakkash, L. (1997) Isolation and culture of bovine pancreatic duct epithelial cells. *Am. J. Physiol.* **272** (*Gastrointest. Liver Physiol.* **35**), G1328–1337.

24. Al-Nakkash, L. and Cotton, C. U. (1997) Bovine pancreatic duct cells express cAMP-and calcium-activated apical membrane Cl⁻ conductances. *Am. J. Physiol.* (*Gastrointest. Liver Physiol.* **36**), G204–G216.

37

Technical Approaches to Analyze the In Vivo Ion Composition of Airway Surface Liquid

Jean-Marie Zahm, Sonia Baconnais, Gérard Balossier, and Edith Puchelle

1. Introduction

Airway surface liquid (ASL) is generally described as a two-layer system formed by a "sol" (or periciliary) and a "gel" layer (overlying the cilia). The ASL, whose total thickness is estimated to be between 10 and 40 μm, contributes to mechanical and antimicrobial defense systems in host airways. In cystic fibrosis (CF), lack of functional cystic fibrosis transmembrane conductance regulator (CFTR) protein may modulate the composition of ASL and lead to an impaired mucociliary clearance associated with inhibition of host defense activity.

The ASL produced in vitro by cultured airway cells possesses antibacterial properties that appear to be highly dependent on the NaCl concentration of the culture medium. The in-vitro measurement of the ionic composition of ASL is generally limited to Na and Cl concentrations evaluated by flame emission spectroscopy and by microlectrodes (1). A prediction of the in-vivo ASL ion composition based on isolated and cultured epithelium is also difficult because it may be not representative of the integrated in-vivo situation.

There is still controversy in the literature at present on the relationship among the ion composition of ASL, the defect in CFTR, and the airway defense capacity in CF. This is probably due to the difficulties encountered in collecting ASL under physiological conditions without causing damage to the airway mucosa. The use of small pieces of filter paper (2–5), a canula (6), or a microcapillary (7) placed in close contact with the mucosa to collect ASL, may stimulate the secretion of ASL and thereby modify the ionic composition of the collected specimen. Moreover, the extraction of ASL from the filter paper or the canula meshes, even if done in mineral oil, risks dehydrating the ASL. It is

From: *Methods in Molecular Medicine, vol. 70: Cystic Fibrosis Methods and Protocols*
Edited by: W. R. Skach © Humana Press Inc., Totowa, NJ

also evident that infected ASL could be contaminated by bacterial and cellular debris that would directly influence its elemental composition, regardless of the sampling technique used.

One approach to improve our understanding of the elemental composition of native ASL would be to collect it under conditions that are as close as possible to the basal physiological state. We have consequently developed a method for collecting ASL from the mouse trachea without causing any epithelial damage to the tracheal surface epithelium, and then analyzed the elemental composition of the ASL. This method is based on the use of a specially designed cryoprobe connected to an apparatus allowing the user to control the contact time and pressure between the probe and the mouse tracheal mucosa *(8)*.

1.1. The Cryoprobe

Difficulties are encountered when collecting ASL under physiological conditions, i.e., without causing damage to the airway mucosa. The cryoprobe has thus been designed to fit within the internal curvature of the mouse trachea. The tip of the probe (**Fig. 1**) has a reduced curvature (radius = 0.6 mm) compared with the internal curvature of the mouse trachea (radius = 1–1.5 mm). Under such experimental conditions, only the extreme distal end of the probe comes in contact with the tracheal mucosa. The top of the probe is made of a receptacle filled with liquid nitrogen, thus permitting the tip of the probe to be maintained at low temperature.

1.2. Apparatus for Collecting ASL

To collect ASL, the cryoprobe is attached to an apparatus specifically developed for controlling the contact pressure and contact time between the cryoprobe and the mouse trachea (**Fig. 2**). This apparatus consists in part of a stage on on which the mouse is placed in the supine position. This stage moves upward or downward at a constant speed of 1 cm/min. The cryoprobe is connected to a microdisplacement transducer, where the displacement measured by the transducer is proportional to the contact pressure of the probe on the mucosa. When the contact pressure between the probe and the trachea reaches 2000 Pa, the displacement of the stage is interrupted for 15 s, allowing the ASL to adhere to the tip of the probe and to be cryofixed. The stage is then moved down to separate the cryoprobe from the trachea. The entire automated procedure is governed by an electronic device.

1.3. Freeze-Drying of the Sample

For analysis of the composition of the ASL, the sample is dehydrated by freeze-drying, which is performed in a vacuum chamber. In order to increase the sublimation of the solidified ASL, the sample is warmed to the yield point

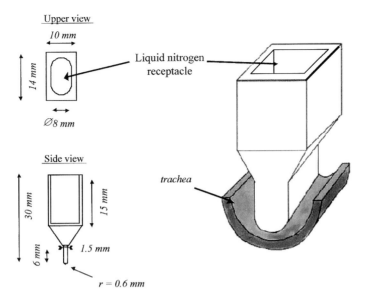

Fig. 1. Representation of the cryoprobe used for collecting airway surface liquid from the mouse trachea.

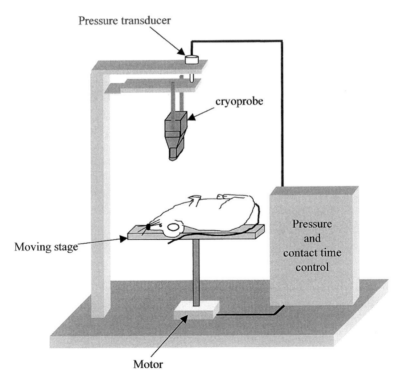

Fig. 2. Representation of the apparatus allowing control of the pressure and contact time between the cryoprobe and the mouse trachea.

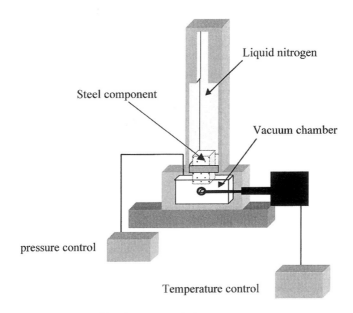

Fig. 3. Freeze-drying apparatus.

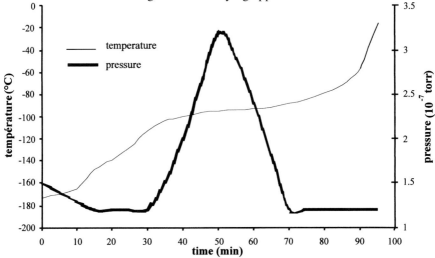

Fig. 4. Variations of temperature and pressure vs time in the vacuum chamber during the freeze-drying procedure.

of the degassing of molecular water determined by pressure variation. Under such conditions, the degassing of water does not disturb the molecular organization of the sample. The main advantage of this process is that the sample can be dehydrated without introducing any artifactual contamination, while keeping the diffusible ions restricted to their original site.

The freeze-drying apparatus is made of vacuum chamber into which the sample is placed. The top of this chamber consists of a steel component, which forms the floor of a receptacle filled with liquid nitrogen (**Fig. 3**). The role of this cooled steel component is to trap the aqueous vapor during the freeze-drying process. An electronic device allows the temperature and the pressure of the vacuum chamber to be controlled. **Figure 4** displays the temperature and pressure variations vs time. At the beginning of the freeze-drying procedure, the increase in temperature is relatively rapid (2°C/min). When the pressure begins to increase, the warming-up process is slowed down (0.2°C/min) until the vacuum pressure returns to its initial value. Thereafter, the increase in temperature up to room temperature is rapid (8°C/min).

2. Materials

2.1. Preparation of Copper Grids

1. Electron microscope copper grid (Maxtaform 200 mesh, Touzard et Matignon, France).
2. Cellulose nitrate (Aldrich, France).
3. Amyl acetate.
4. Ultrapure water (Fluka, France); store at +4°C.

2.2. Collection of ASL

1. Pentobarbital sodium.
2. Straight scissors for experimental surgery (4877, Moria, France).
3. Microscissors for microsurgery (9920, Moria).
4. Dissection forceps with curved serrated jaws (2183, Moria).
5. Ultrapure water (Fluka, France); store at +4°C.
6. Pure methanol (Sigma, France).
7. Liquid nitrogen.

2.3. X-Ray Microanalysis

1. Scanning transmission electron microscope (STEM CM 30, Philips, France).
2. Microanalysis system (S-UTW, Edax International, USA).
3. Cryotransfer system (Gatan 626, Gatan France, France).

3. Methods
3.1. Preparation of Copper Grids

It is important to pay particular attention to the copper grid coating and more specifically to the preparation of the collodion film in order to avoid introducing any artifactual contamination. The coating of these grids is performed 24 h before ASL collection. The collodion consists of cellulose nitrate diluted in amyl acetate (2 g/100 mL), which is then coated on the grids as follows:

1. Spread 20 μL of collodion on the surface of the ultrapure water (30 mL in a glass reservoir 9 cm in diameter).

2. Place the copper grids on the thin film (10 nm) of polymerised collodion. This results in the formation of a homogeneous collodion film on the grid.
3. Place filter paper on the grids.
4. Using forceps, withdraw the copper grids sandwiched between the collodion film and the filter paper.
5. Coat the collodion film on the grid with a 10 nm thick carbon film using a vacuum evaporator.

3.2. Collection of ASL with the Cryoprobe

1. Wash the probe with ultrapure water and then with pure methanol, dry it at room temperature, and cool it by plunging into a liquid nitrogen bath (–180°C) until thermal balance is reached.
2. Anesthetize the mouse with an intraperitoneal injection of 100 μL pentobarbital sodium. Remove the skin and the connective tissue along the trachea. Incise transversally the trachea of the mouse at its upper and lower extremities. Remove approximately one-third of the tracheal wall between the two incisions to provide easy access to the lower part of the internal mucosa. Place the mouse in the supine position on the stage of the apparatus as described in **Fig. 2** (*see* **Note 1**).
3. Move the stage upward while positioning and orientating the open trachea just below the cryoprobe. Stop the raising of the stage when the contact pressure between the probe and the tracheal mucosa reaches 2000 Pa. Wait for 15 s and move the stage downward to separate the cryoprobe from the trachea (*see* **Note 2**).
4. Warm tthe ASL adhering to the cryoprobe o room temperature. Put the tip of the cryoprobe in contact with an electron microscope copper grid that has been previously coated with a collodion membrane and a 10-nm carbon film.
5. The ASL deposited on the coated copper grid is then cryofixed by plunging it into a liquid nitrogen bath. The grid is then stored in liquid nitrogen until analysis (*see* **Note 3**).

3.3. Freeze-Drying

1. Place the sample and the specimen holder (kept at –175°C) into a vacuum chamber at a residual pressure of 10^{-6} torr.
2. To increase the sublimation of the solidified ASL, warm the sample to the yield point of the degassing of molecular water determined by the decrease in the vacuum pressure (*see* **Fig. 4**).
3. Continue warming the sample to room temperature.
4. Transfer the sample and the holder into the electron microscope.

3.4. X-Ray Microanalysis

The X-ray microanalysis technique is dependent on the electron microscope and on the spectrometer used. In our experiments, we use a medium-voltage scanning transmission electron microscope (STEM) equipped with an X-ray energy-dispersive spectrometer (EDXS). This spectrometer was recently upgraded by using an ultrathin window to allow detection of low-Z (atomic number) elements up to $Z = 5$ (boron).

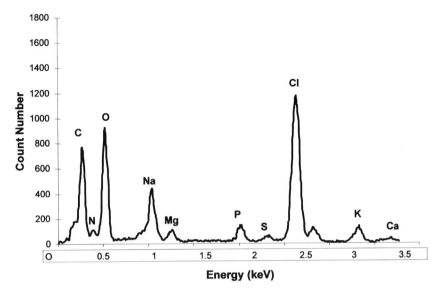

Fig. 5. Typical X-ray microanalysis spectrum after background correction, obtained from a sample of mouse airway surface liquid.

The elemental composition of dehydrated ASL samples is determined using the continuum Hall method *(9,10)*.

The dehydrated ASL is analyzed under the scanning transmission mode, at 100 keV (tilt angle 30°; sample temperature –172°C; spectrum acquisition time 200 s).

A mean value for each of the elemental concentrations of the sample is obtained by scanning the electron probe over a 40-μm² surface and recording 15–20 spectra in different areas of the sample (*see* **Notes 4** and **5**).

The X-ray spectrum is constituted by a continuous background on which the peaks of interest are superimposed. To suppress the background, a top-hat filter is applied to the spectra *(11,12)*. From the final spectrum (see example in **Fig. 5**), we measure the amplitude of the peaks corresponding to the various elements (C, N, O, Na, Mg, Si, P, S, Cl, K, Ca). The amplitude of the peaks measured on the experimental spectrum is then compared to the amplitude of the peaks obtained from calibration spectra.

4. Notes

1. The composition of ASL may be altered by multiple factors, including water loss during sample collection and/or analysis. In fact, in order to limit possible dehydration of the tracheal mucosa before ASL collection, less than 2 min must pass between exposure of the mouse trachea to ambient air following the incision being made and the ASL collected. In addition, the ASL being collected with the cryoprobe is frozen and so water in the air forms a condensate on the ASL. In order to

deposit the ASL on the grid, the sample has to be made fluid once again. The condensed water that had contaminated the ASL is thereafter eliminated during the freeze-drying procedure.

2. This cryotechnique for ASL collection is an efficient and easy method provided the contact pressure and the time of contact of the cryoprobe with the tracheal mucosa are controlled so as to prevent alteration of the surface epithelium integrity. We have demonstrated *(8)* that a contact pressure in the range of 1200–2000 Pa does not alter the epithelial surface or interrupt the ciliary beating frequency. The contact time of the cryoprobe with tracheal mucosa is also an important parameter to take into account in order to maintain the ionic composition of the ASL as close as possible to the normal physiological state. In fact, when in contact with the cryoprobe, the ASL is instantaneously frozen, thus preventing any artifactual ion or water fluxes. Under conditions of prolonged contact times, an increase in Na, Cl, S, K, and Ca concentrations was observed when the contact time of the cryoprobe with the tracheal mucosa was longer than 20 s. This was likely to have been due to the progressive warming up of the probe.

3. To ensure that no contamination is introduced during the copper grid preparation, i.e., during the coating with the collodion membrane and the evaporated carbon film, it is necessary to analyze the coated copper grid by X-ray microanalysis in the absence of any ASL sample. No ions should be detected at concentrations higher than the detection threshold of the apparatus. Before use, the coated copper grids are stored for no longer than 2 d in order to avoid any further risk of contamination.

4. In a general way, X-ray microanalysis uses corrections to take into account the effects of absorption and fluorescence by the specimen. In our case, we are concerned with thin film analysis (thickness lower than 1 μm); these corrections are therefore not necessary for elements with $Z \geq 11$. In the Hall method the elemental concentration $(Cx)_{exp}$ is described by the equation:

$$(Cx)_{exp} = (Cx)_{st} \cdot [(Ix/Ic)_{exp}/(Ix/Ic)_{st}]/[\overline{(Z^2/A)}_{exp}/\overline{(Z^2/A)}_{st}$$

where $(Ix/Ic)_{exp, st}$ are the peak-to-background intensity ratio in experimental and standard spectra, respectively $\overline{(Z^2/A)}_{exp,st}$ are matrix correction factors for experimental and standard spectra, and $(Cx)_{st}$ is the concentration of the element x in a standard specimen.

The main problem when using the Hall method is that the specimen background intensity must be measured precisely. The experimental background is not only due to the specimen itself but is also the result of the fluorescence of the grid, which must be evaluated and subtracted. In our experiments we use pure copper grids. The X-ray spectrum is therefore characterized by the presence of the K_α (8044 eV), K_α and L_α (940 eV) copper peaks in addition to a non-negligible contribution of background. The contribution of the copper peaks and background to the X-ray spectrum is evaluated by measuring the K_α/L_α copper peak ratio and the K_α/background ratio vs the distance between the electron probe and the grid bar. We observe a decrease of the K_α/background ratio when the distance between the probe and the grid bar increases up to 10 μm, and then remains constant for larger distances. This constant K_α/background ratio is the same as that obtained from a pure copper film. Thus, by measuring the K_α peak in an experimental spectrum it is possible to evaluate the copper background intensity and to suppress it.

Another problem related to the copper grid concerns the variations observed in the K_α/L_α copper peaks ratio; these variations are dependent on the distance between the electron probe and the grid bar. Because the K_α peak (1040 eV) of Na is in very close proximity to the L_α peak (940 eV) of Cu, any variation in the K_α/L_α copper peak ratio could affect the quantification of Na. Such variations can occur during the fitting process when we can correct for spectrometer decalibration *(13)*. The L_α copper peak can then be interpreted as an energy-shifted K_α sodium peak. To solve this problem, we introduce an additional synthesized L_α fixed-energy copper peak in the reference library in order to obtain a good fit to the data.

Finally, in order to limit problems with the copper signal, we keep only the experimental spectra recorded when the electron probe is positioned at a distance greater than 10 μm from the grid bars.

5. Calcium standard solutions embedded in resin at concentrations of 50 and 125 mmol/kg of resin (Agar Scientific, Stansted, England) are analyzed to calibrate the spectrometer using the Hall method.

Drops of NaCl (99 m*M*), MgCl₂ (9.9 m*M*), CaCl₂ (80 m*M*), and KCl (10 m*M*) dextran solutions are deposited on the pure copper grid and dehydrated overnight at 40°C. The salt crystals are then analyzed by X-ray microanalysis. The stoichiometry is verified by measuring the $[Na^+]/[Cl^-]$ ratio of pure NaCl, the $[Mg^{2+}]/[Cl^-]$ ratio of pure MgCl, the $[Cl^-]/[Ca^{2+}]$ ratio of pure CaCl₂, and the $[K^+]/[Cl^-]$ ratio of pure KCl for different positions of the salt crystals relative to the grid bar. It also important to check that the collection and analysis method can accurately measure the ion concentrations of native and 1/2 diluted mouse plasma used as standards. Drops of plasma can be cryofixed in liquid ethane, cryosectioned (100 nm at −140°C), deposited on the copper grid, freeze-dried, and analyzed.

References

1. Matsui, H., Grubb, B. R., Tarran, R., Randell, S. H., Gatzy, J.T., Davis, C. W., and Boucher, R. C. (1998) Evidence for periciliary liquid layer depletion, not abnormal ion composition, in the pathogenesis of cystic fibrosis airways disease. *Cell* **95**, 1005–1015 .
2. Boucher, R. C., Stutts, M. J., Bromberg, P. A., and Gatzy, J. T. (1981) Regional differences in airway surface liquid composition. *J. Appl. Physiol.* **50(3)**, 613–620.
3. Joris, L. and Quinton, P. M. (1987) Concentration of elements in airway surface fluid. *Med. Sci. Res.* **15**, 855,856.
4. Joris, L. and Quinton, P. M. (1992) Filter paper equilibration as o novel technique for in vitro studies of the composition of airway surface fluid. *Am. J. Physiol.* **263**, L243–L248.
5. Joris, L., Dab, I., and Quinton, P. M. (1993) Elemental composition of human airway surface fluid on healthy and diseased airways. *Am. Rev. Respir. Dis.* **148**, 1633–1637.

6. Robinson, N. P., Kyle, H., Webber, S. E., and Widdicombe, I. G. (1989) Electrolyte and other chemical concentrations in tracheal airway surface liquid and mucus. *J. Appl. Physiol.* **66(5),** 2129–2135.
7. Govindaraju, K., Cowley, E. A., Eidelman, D. H., and Lloyd, D. K. (1997) Microanalysis of airway surface fluid by capillary electrophoresis with conductivity detection. *An. Chem.* **69,** 2793–2797.
8. Baconnais, S., Zahm, J. M., Killian, L., Bonhomme, P., Gobillard, D., Perchet, A., Puchelle, E., and Balossier, G. (1998) X-ray microanalysis of native airway surface liquid collected by cryotechnique. *J. Microsc.* **191,** 311–319.
9. Hall, T. A. (1979) Biological X-ray microanalysis. *J. Microsc.* **117,** 145–163.
10. Hall, T. A. and Gupta, B. L. (1982) Quantification for the X-ray microanalysis of cryosections. *J. Microsc.* **126,** 333–345.
11. Wagner, D., Puchelle, E., Hinnrasky, J., Girard, P., and Balossier, G. (1994) Quantitative X-ray microanalysis of P, Ca and S in the mucus secretory granules of cryofixed frog palate epithelium. *Microsc. Res. Technol.* **28,** 141–148.
12. Zaluzec, N. J. (1989) Processing and quantification of x-ray energy dispersive spectra in the analytical electron microscope. *Ultramicroscopy* **28,** 226–235.
13. Kitzawa, T., Shuman, H., and Somlyo, A.P. (1983) Quantitative electron probe analysis: problems and solutions. *Ultramicroscopy* **11,** 251–262.

IV

NOVEL THERAPEUTIC APPROACHES FOR CYSTIC FIBROSIS

38

Design of Gene Therapy Clinical Trials in CF Patients

Kimberly V. Curlee and Eric J. Sorscher

1. Introduction

On April 17, 1993, Crystal and co-workers initiated the first human gene therapy trial for cystic fibrosis (CF). In that study, a replication-deficient recombinant adenovirus encoding cystic fibrosis transmembrane conductance regulator (CFTR) cDNA was administered to the nasal and bronchial epithelia of four cystic fibrosis patients (1). Since then, numerous trials have been conducted to evaluate gene therapy in CF, including both viral and nonviral vectors for the delivery of CFTR cDNA. These have primarily been Phase I and II experiments intended to demonstrate safety and feasibility of gene transfer to the nasal and/or bronchial epithelia of patients by either direct application or nebulization (2).

Based on a number of parameters, the majority of these earlier clinical experiments suggest safety of CFTR gene transfer to human lung. Vector constructs do not appear to produce long-term adverse effects in either normal individuals or cystic fibrosis patients. In CF gene therapy protocols using adenoviral vectors, for instance, no evidence has been found to suggest virus recombination, replication, or shedding (2). A number of trials have, however, reported dose-dependent inflammatory responses (e.g., increases in inflammatory cell infiltrates) at high adenoviral titers (1–3). In trials utilizing nonviral delivery systems, safety has been evaluated with clinical parameters including airway symptomatology, changes in lung function, histology, or the systemic inflammatory response. Mild flulike symptoms in a subset of patients receiving aerosolized cationic liposome/DNA complexes were reported in one trial (4). A more substantial syndrome of myalgia, arthralgia, and fever associated with cationic lipid-mediated gene transfer has also been observed (5).

From: *Methods in Molecular Medicine, vol. 70: Cystic Fibrosis Methods and Protocols*
Edited by: W. R. Skach © Humana Press Inc., Totowa, NJ

These initial clinical studies have demonstrated the feasibility of low-level wild-type CFTR gene transfer in vivo. When polymerase chain reaction (PCR)-based methods were used to detect vector-specific mRNA, or when functional endpoints (such as the measurement of nasal potential difference or chloride efflux) were examined, several laboratories reported successful gene delivery *(4,6–11)*. A study by Knowles et al. *(3)*, however, found no evidence to suggest functional correction of chloride transport in any of the patients tested. Wagner et al. *(11)* reported results of a trial using escalating doses of adeno-associated virus (AAV)-CFTR delivery to the maxillary sinuses of 10 patients. Measurements of nasal potential difference suggested some corrective values indicative of functional wild-type CFTR.

2. Materials and Methodological Issues

CF is an autosomal recessive disorder in which heterozygous individuals appear phenotypically normal, implying that a relatively low level of CFTR activity might be enough to produce a therapeutic effect *(2)*. In a study by Dorin et al. (1996), mice with CFTR expression levels between 0% to 100% were examined. CF animals with as little as 5% normal CFTR mRNA levels exhibited 50% of wild-type ion transport activity, and complete rescue from pathophysiologic defects in the intestine *(12)*. Johnson et al. *(13)* tested mixed populations of a CF cell line with varying levels of corrected cells expressing normal CFTR cDNA. Cultures in which as few as 6–10% were corrected with wild-type CFTR showed chloride transport comparable to 100% correction. These results suggest a target threshold in which correction of a minimum of 5–10% of target cells might be sufficient for phenotypic improvement.

The conceptual and practical challenges to successful CF gene therapy in vivo reflect clinical aspects of the disease. For example, preexisting lung disease and lung damage as a result of chronic infection and inflammation (which often begins in infancy) is likely to diminish efficacy of gene transfer. Persistent bacterial infection culminates in the recruitment of neutrophils and macrophages that influence the endogenous levels of cytokines, proteases, oxidants, and α-defensins, and further contribute to tissue destruction. The thick mucosal plugs found in lungs of cystic fibrosis patients represent obvious barriers to gene therapy vectors *(2)*. As epithelial and bacterial cells are lysed, DNA is released, causing airway secretions to become even more viscous and resulting in additional physical barriers to gene transfer *(14)*. Moreover, the human airway epithelium naturally functions to prevent airborne pathogens or other foreign materials from breaching the mucosal barrier. Although adenoviral vectors transduce airway epithelial cells efficiently in vitro, they are less efficient in vivo partly because certain viral receptors are confined to the basolateral cell surface *(15)*. Several clinical protocols have introduced recombinant adenovirus by direct application or aerosolization. In this setting, the vector initially contacts the cellular (apical) surface and must migrate to the basolateral membrane in order to encounter appropriate receptor(s) for internalization. Therefore, in addition to host bacteria, inflammatory cells, and thick mucous, gaining access to the basolateral membrane represents an inherent, cellular barrier to gene transfer in vivo *(16)*.

Inflammatory responses have now been well documented in trials using adenovirus or cationic liposome-mediated gene transfer *(1–3,5)*. It has been suggested that the transient nature of gene expression with adenoviral constructs is due in part to immune clearance of transduced cells *(17)*, necessitating vector readministration. In a dosing experiment by Harvey et al. (1999), transgene expression lasted less than 30 d. A second administration was only effective at intermediate to high doses, and a third administration resulted in no detectable gene expression in vivo. The exact mechanism underlying the refractoriness to repeat administration in the lung is not clear. However, cell-mediated immunity is felt to contribute to gene transfer tachyphylaxis, since expression levels could not be explained solely by production of anti-adenovirus neutralizing antibodies *(16,18)*.

Based on the above considerations, an ideal CF gene therapy vector might be one capable of proficient and persistent transduction after a single administration, without engendering a brisk immune response. Adeno-associated viral (AAV) vectors have been proposed as meeting some of these criteria, since AAV may be less prone to immunologic reactivity. In vitro, AAV vectors have exhibited transduction levels as high as 70%. Studies in New Zealand white rabbits and in Rhesus macques detected vector-derived RNA 6 mo postadministration, with no toxicity or other adverse effects. The clinical data with first-generation AAV vectors points to low transduction efficiency, presumably due to the sequestration of viral receptors at the basolateral cell surface, or the inability of AAV to transduce highly differentiated, quiescent cells *(17)*. It has also been shown that barriers prevent recombinant viral integration into the host genome *(15)*. Recent improvements in preparing high-titer AAV stocks, administering potent serotypes, and use of proteosome inhibition for increasing transduction merit further investigation in CF *(19)*.

2.1. Adenoviral Reagents Useful in Studies of CFTR Gene Transfer

Initial clinical trials of gene therapy in cystic fibrosis utilized replication-deficient adenoviral vectors. These vectors infect nondividing cells, may have natural tropism for airway epithelia, and have been shown capable of CFTR gene transfer **(20)**. Studies with adenovirus in airways of CF mice elicited only partial correction of Cl⁻ transport and no effect on Na⁺ transport, even after multiple administrations of high doses of vector **(21)**. In vivo studies in the cotton rat and in nonhuman primates indicated gene transfer that was as efficient as in other models **(20)**, although studies of repeat dosages in the cotton rat showed reduction in transfer efficiency accompanied by a rise in neutralizing antibodies in the serum *(22)*. Clinical trials in humans have established transgene expression (as judged by total mRNA levels) that in some cases appears to be above a target threshold of 5–10% *(20)*. The actual levels of expression on a per-cell basis in these experiments are more difficult to judge. For example, the number of cells expressing CFTR may be quite small (i.e., expression well below 5–10% of transduced cells), although total CFTR mRNA may be quite high due to markedly elevated per-cell expression.

Factors that influence the safety and the clinical effectiveness of gene therapy procedures include vector dosage and route of administration, the number of administrations, length of exposure, and the particular type of vector being tested. Other considerations include the level and duration of transgene expression in both target and nontarget tissues, the native tissue morphology or function, systemic diffusion of the vector, and the activation of a host immune response against vector, transgene, transgene product, or transduced cells. Adenoviruses elicit dose-dependent immunological reactions that culminate in rapid loss of transgene expression *(16)*. In a study by Zabner et al. (1996), repeated doses of adenovirus escalating to an MOI of 10^{10} were given to patients and the humoral immune response was measured. All patients had preexisting antibodies to adenovirus. In these studies, repeat administrations elicited a concomitant decrease in preexisting expression levels of transgene, a finding attributed to clearance of transduced cells *(23)*. In murine studies, loss of transgene expression after multiple dosings was partly the result of helper T- and B-cell activation against viral capsid proteins *(24)*. Responses to adenovirus in mice with an intact immune system varied with genetic background, suggesting that MHC antigen expression could also influence safety and efficacy *(20)*. Although these earlier studies have been informative concerning the mechanisms underlying the immune response to gene therapy vectors, it is likely that the scope of possible responses in humans will be much more diverse than in inbred mice. It is also likely that primary responses such as those observed with adenovirus will also apply to other vector systems *(24)*.

3. Methods

3.1. Aspects of Study Methodology that Complicate the Predictions of Clinical Safety and Efficacy Based on Preclinical Testing

Although preclinical data are important and necessary for studying the ultimate value of gene therapy in human patients, favorable results in these systems have not been predictive of equivalent success in the clinic. For example, previous studies have shown that both viral and nonviral vectors can be used to deliver CFTR cDNA to the airway epithelia of human patients. However, these studies have not established durable expression, or sufficient levels of expression to provide therapeutic benefit, or substantive alleviation of CF disease manifestations in animal models. The majority of trials performed to date have been Phase I (and address primarily general safety issues). These studies, therefore, have not evaluated clinical improvement, but instead use surrogate endpoints to measure expression of functional CFTR. However, even if a surrogate endpoint indicates positive gene transfer, this does not necessarily correlate with compelling evidence for ultimate alteration of disease status *(20)*. The preclinical experiments that support human gene therapy trials in CF did not predict either the innate refractoriness of human airway cells to gene transfer vectors, or the inflammatory changes that have been observed in human patients. Some of these differences reflect target cell type, cellular organization or differentiation, permissiveness of different species to gene transfer vectors, vector tropism, and immunological responses. The selection of surrogate endpoints and the lack of a complete understanding of the ways in which these endpoints reflect clinical disease status are an important conceptual and practical barrier to progress in CF gene therapy.

Previous studies suggested that gene transfer in vivo that could transduce 5–10% of target cells (leading them to overexpress CFTR) or could produce 5–10% of native levels of CFTR mRNA might have beneficial effects in human subjects *(12,13)*. In the in vitro experiments, cells were organized in a monolayer, were in contact through gap junctions, and "corrected" cells may have expressed atypically high levels of CFTR. Cell culture experiments may therefore not fully reflect the well differentiated airway epithelium in vivo, and conditions that are optimized for gene transfer in cellular (or animal) models may be difficult to replicate in human subjects. It is likely that the fraction of corrected cells necessary to elicit bioelectric improvement in vivo could be considerably higher than what has been modeled in vitro *(2)*. Moreover, the surrogate endpoint used in clinical studies of this type (correction of the Cl⁻ transport defect) may not be an adequate predictor of ultimate therapeutic effects in vivo *(25,26)*.

Gene transfer of viral vectors to the lungs of humans is complicated by difficulties in vector administration, as well as the evaluation and interpretation of data. For example, bioelectric assays in the lower airways are technically complex, and difficult to standardize except in large cohorts of patients and controls. In addition, fundamental differences in CF pathophysiology between animal models and humans are well established. Cystic fibrosis mice are less susceptible to pulmonary disease than humans, possibly because of non-CFTR chloride secretory pathways that exist in murine but not human lower airways *(24)*. Evaluation and interpretation are also confounded by problems detecting transgene in the lung and the requirement for an invasive procedure (bronchoscopy) in order to identify transduced cells. Heterogeneity or patchiness of distribution in the airways, together with tissue sampling error, can further complicate interpretation of gene transfer in CF *(20)*. In preclinical animal studies, extensive regions (or entire lungs) can be sampled and analyzed. The opportunity to tailor dose, rate, or formulation to a specific animal model or vector can be optimized by trial and error in animal models in a fashion that is neither practical nor possible in human clinical trials.

3.2. Methods Relating to Informed Consent, Design, and Interpretation of Study

The media has had a significant impact on familiarizing the public with experimental gene therapy. In an interview of 20 patients preparing to participate in a gene therapy trial, 9 indicated that they had first learned about gene therapy through television, newspapers, or magazines *(27)*. When a fatality resulting directly from gene therapy occurred in September 1999 (in a non-CF patient with ornithine transcarbamylase deficiency), serious concerns were raised regarding the recruitment of patients into experimental trials of gene therapy for genetic or acquired diseases. Even the impact of positive, but preliminary, data on individuals can lead to misinterpretations about what current gene therapy protocols can actually accomplish. Reporting the results of proof of principle in human clinical trials (to both participants and to the general public) should be carefully approached in order to avoid raising unrealistic hopes or expectations. One study of cystic fibrosis patients enrolled in a Phase I gene therapy trial found that the majority had "an emotionally driven optimism about gene therapy" *(27)*. This was interpreted to indicate the possibility of false hopes or unrealistic expectations in patients who enroll in current gene therapy clinical trials.

In part because of clinical toxicities that have been encountered in the area of gene therapy, increasing emphasis has been placed on the clarity, completeness, and language of informed consent documents. The process of consent has traditionally been based on the 1949 Nuremberg Code, which outlined 10 fundamental principles for ethical research involving humans *(28)*, including the mandate that participation be strictly voluntary. According to these guidelines, a satisfactory explanation of the aims and procedures, including any foreseeable risks or inconveniences, should be provided in detail to all prospective subjects *(29)*. In 1966, the Declaration of Helsinki extended the directives set forth in the Nuremberg Code to include disclosure of the right to refuse participation or to withdraw consent at any time.

Events such as the Tuskegee syphilis study prompted the US federal government to enact laws designed specifically to protect individuals enrolled in research studies. A clear distinction between standard care and experimental procedures was delineated based on differences in purpose and predictability. The risks and benefits of standard treatment are well established, and conventional treatment is associated with a reasonable expectation of a favorable outcome. In research, however, the disparity between risks and benefits is usually undetermined, with no guarantee that treatment will be either successful or safe *(29,30)*. Therefore, federal regulations require that informed consent include an explanation of procedures, alternatives, risks and/or benefits, as well as statements regarding a subject's rights to confidentiality and to withdraw at any time *(30)*.

Informed consent in gene therapy protocols is an evolving process. As a prerequisite, competent decision making and voluntariness must be met by a potential subject. If both of these requirements are met, additional information including disclosure of the nature of the research and procedures to be used, alternatives, potential risks and benefits, and the right to withdraw are standard and important aspects of consent *(31)*. These specific areas of the consent process have been particularly scrutinized in gene therapy clinical applications, and substantial questions have been raised. The need to comprehensively review all risks, and clearly state the absence of direct therapeutic benefit to patient volunteers in the majority of early-phase CF and other gene therapy trials, has been emphasized by the FDA, NIH, and other regulatory agencies.

3.3. Future Directions/Conclusion

Based on growing experience from in vitro gene transfer experiments, as well as in vivo studies in animal models and in Phase I and II human clinical trials, gene therapy may someday become a viable method for treating some of the clinical manifestations of cystic fibrosis. However, before this option will be feasible, substantial improvements and modifications in the technology may be necessary. In the case of adenoviral vectors, strategies that increase the efficiency and duration of viral transduction of target cells and facilitate evasion of host immune defense are needed. Conceptual and practical barriers also exist for lipid-mediated gene transfer to the lung. Vectors such as AAV may elicit less inflammatory response, and seem capable of prolonged expression in vivo. AAV-based approaches have shown promise in other diseases, and represent an important area for future clinical testing in CF.

Further understanding of the complex molecular mechanisms underlying cystic fibrosis disease pathology will impel not only the development of more effective gene therapy, but also the establishment of better endpoints to assess functional and clinical intervention *(14)*. The establishment of animal models with complex genetic backgrounds and environmental exposures may provide for better determination of the safety and efficacy of various gene therapy protocols *(24)*. An improved understanding of the cellular response to gene therapy vectors is also emerging. For example, methods to increase transduction efficiency by allowing transient and reversible relaxation of tight junctions (in order to allow access of vectors to the basolateral surface of target cells), or vector modifications that facilitate targeted binding to the apical cell membrane, are important new approaches to improving in vivo transduction efficiency *(2)*. Difficulties with efficient transduction and persistent transgene expression in well-differentiated cells have led to novel, integrating vectors or nucleic acid molecules that might autonomously replicate extrachromosomally *(32,33)*.

While the need for new therapies in cystic fibrosis has not diminished, the complexity of the putative pathogenic mechanisms in the disease has markedly increased. Abnormal chloride transport, defective sodium transport, and absent secretion of bicarbonate have all been suggested as a primary defect in the CF lung disease. The extent to which defective maturational processing of the ΔF508 CFTR is a cause of disease has recently been disputed *(34)*. Despite progress in understanding the cellular biology of CFTR, fundamental aspects involved in CF pathogenesis (e.g., whether the salt content of CF airway surface fluid is high enough to inactivate endogenous antimicrobial peptides) are not known. Moreover, newer disease models that have no discernable relationship to ion transport or salt content (immunologic hyperactivity in the CF lung, membrane lipid composition) have emerged as likely contributors to the disease process. Although the pathogenic chain of events connecting defective CFTR and clinical disease is not known with certainty, there is no question about the primary cause of the disease. While genetic correction of defective CFTR continues to face substantial challenges, it remains an important area of emphasis for the discovery of new therapies in cystic fibrosis.

References

1. Crystal, R. G., McElvaney, N. G., Rosenfeld, M. A., Chu C. S., Mastrangeli, A., Hay, J. G., et al. (1994) Administration of an adenovirus containing the human CFTR cDNA to the respiratory tract of individuals with cystic fibrosis. *Nat. Genet.* **8,** 42–51.
2. Boucher, R. C. (1999) Status of gene therapy for cystic fibrosis lung disease. *J. Clin. Invest.* **103,** 441–445.
3. Knowles, M. R., Hohneker, K. W., Zhou, Z. Olsen, J. C., Noah, T. L., Hu, P. C., et al. (1995) A controlled study of adenoviral-vector-mediated gene transfer in the nasal epithelium of patients with cystic fibrosis. *N. Engl. J. Med.* **333,** 823–831.
4. Alton, E. W., Stern, M., Farley ,R., Jaffe, A., Chadwick, S. L., Phillips, J., et al . (1999) Cationic lipid-mediated CFTR gene transfer to the lungs and nose of patients with cystic fibrosis: a double-blind placebo- controlled trial. *Lancet* **353,** 947–954.
5. Ruiz, F. E., Clancy , J. P., Perricone, M. A., Bebok, Z., Hong, J., Cheng, S. H., et al. Gene transfer of CFTR to lower airways of cystic fibrosis patients and characterization of a clinical syndrome attributable to lipid/DNA administration. (Submitted.)
6. Zabner, J., Couture, L. A., Gregory, R. J., Graham, S. M., Smith, A. E., and Welsh, M. J. (1993) Adenovirus-mediated gene transfer transiently corrects the chloride transport defect in nasal epithelia of patients with cystic fibrosis. *Cell* **75,** 207–216.

7. Caplen, N. J., Alton, E. W., Middleton P. G., Dorin J. R., Stevenson, B. J., Gao, X., et al. (1995) Liposome-mediated CFTR gene transfer to the nasal epithelium of patients with cystic fibrosis. *Nat. Med.* **1,** 39–46.

8. Hay, J. G., McElvaney, N. G., Herena, J., and Crystal, R. G. (1995) Modification of nasal epithelial potential differences of individuals with cystic fibrosis consequent to local administration of a normal CFTR cDNA adenovirus gene transfer vector. *Hum. Gene Ther.* **6,** 1487–1496.

9. Gill, D. R., Southern, K. W., Mofford, K. A., Seddon, T., Huang, L., Sorgi, F., et al. (1997) A placebo-controlled study of liposome-mediated gene transfer to the nasal epithelium of patients with cystic fibrosis. *Gene Ther.* **4,** 199–209.

10. Zabner, J., Cheng, S. H., Meeker, D., Launspach, J., Balfour, R., Perricone, M. A., et al. (1997) Comparison of DNA-lipid complexes and DNA alone for gene transfer to cystic fibrosis airway epithelia in vivo. *J. Clin. Invest.* **100,** 1529–1537.

11. Wagner, J. A., Reynolds, T., Moran, M. L., Moss, R. B., Wine, J. J., Flotte, T. R., et al. (1998) Efficient and persistent gene transfer of AAV-CFTR in maxillary sinus. *Lancet* **351,** 1702,1703.

12. Dorin, J. R., Farley, R., Webb, S., Smith, S. N., Farini, E., Delaney, S. J., et al. (1996) A demonstration using mouse models that successful gene therapy for cystic fibrosis requires only partial gene correction. *Gene Ther.* **3,** 797–801.

13. Johnson, L. G., Olsen, J. C., Sarkadi, B., Moore, K. L., Swanstrom, R., and Boucher, R. C. (1992) Efficiency of gene transfer for restoration of normal airway epithelial function in cystic fibrosis. *Nat. Genet.* **2,** 21–25.

14. Bals, R., Weiner, D. J., and Wilson, J. M. (1999) The innate immune system in cystic fibrosis lung disease. *J. Clin. Invest.* **103,** 303–307.

15. Crystal, R. G. (1999) Bad for cats, good for humans? Modified feline immunodeficiency virus for gene therapy. *J. Clin. Invest.* **104,** 1491–1493.

16. Welsh M. J. (1999) Gene transfer for cystic fibrosis. *J. Clin. Invest.* **104,** 1165,1166.

17. Flotte, T. R. and Carter, B. J. (1998) Adeno-associated virus vectors for gene therapy of cystic fibrosis. *Meth. Enzymol.* **292,** 717–732.

18. Harvey, B.-G., Leopold, P. L., Hackett, N. R., Grasso, T. M., Williams, P. M., Tucker, A. L., et al. (1999) Airway epithelial CFTR mRNA expression in cystic fibrosis patients after repetitive administration of a recombinant adenovirus. *J. Clin. Invest.* **104,** 1245–1255.

19. Duan, D., Yue, Y., Yan, Z., Yang, J., and Englehardt, J. (2000) Endosomal processing limits gene transfer to polarized airway epithelia by adeno-associated virus. *J. Clin. Invest.* **105,** 1573–1587.

20. Wilson, J. M. (1995) Gene therapy for cystic fibrosis: challenges and future directions. *J. Clin. Invest.* **96,** 2547–2554.

21. Grubb, B. R., Pickles, R. J., Ye, H., Yankaskas, J. R. Vick, R. N., Engelhardt, J. F., et al. (1994) Inefficient gene transfer by adenovirus vector to cystic fibrosis airway epithelia of mice and humans. *Nature* **371,** 802–806.

22. Yei, S., Mittereder, N., Tang, K., O'Sullivan, C., and Trapnell, B. C. (1994) Adenovirus-mediated gene transfer for cystic fibrosis: quantitative evaluation of repeated in vivo vector administration to the lung. *Gene Ther.* **1,** 192–200.

23. Zabner, J., Ramsey, B. W., Meeker, D. P., Aitken, M. L., Balfour, R. P., Gibson, R. L., et al. (1996) Repeat administration of an adenovirus vector encoding cystic fibrosis transmembrane conductance regulator to the nasal epithelium of patients with cystic fibrosis. *J. Clin. Invest.* **97,** 1504–1511.
24. Wilson, J. M. (1996) Animal models of human disease for gene therapy. *J. Clin. Invest.* **97,** 1138–1141.
25. Chinet, T. C. (1994) Use of in vivo nasal transepithelial potential difference to evaluate efficacy in CF gene therapy phase I trials. *Eur. Resp. J.* **7,** 1917–1920.
26. Walker, L. C., Venglarik, C. J., Aubin, G., Weatherly, M. R., McCarty, N. A., Lesnick, B., et al. (1997) Relationship between airway ion transport and a mild pulmonary disease mutation in CFTR. *Am. J. Respir. Crit. Care Med.* **155,** 1684–1689.
27. Blair, C., Kacser, E., and Porteous, D. (1998) Gene therapy for cystic fibrosis: a psychosocial study of trial participants. *Gene Ther.* **5,** 218–222.
28. Ellenberg, S. S. (1997) Informed consent: protection or obstacle? Some emerging issues. *Contr. Clin. Trials.* **18,** 628–636.
29. Morin, K. (1998) The standard of disclosure in human subject experimentation. *J. Legal Med.* **19,** 157–221.
30. Tuthill, K. A. (1997) Human experimentation. Protecting patient autonomy through informed consent. *J. Legal Med.* **18,** 221–250.
31. Sugarman, J. (2000) Informed consent in special populations. Ethical Issues in Clinical Trials Conference, University of Alabama, Birmingham, February 25–26.
32. Wang, G., Slepushkin, V., Zabner, J., Keshavjee, S., Johnston, J. C., Sauter, S. L., Jolly, D. J., et al. (1999) Feline immunodeficiency virus vectors persistently transduce nondividing airway epithelia and correct the cystic fibrosis defect. *J. Clin. Invest.* **104,** R55–62.
33. Sverdrup, F., Sheahan, L., and Khan S. (1999) Development of human papillomavirus plasmids capable of episomal replication in human cell lines. *Gene Ther.* **6,** 1317–1321.
34. Kalin, N., Claass, A., Sommer, M., Puchelle, E., and Tummler, B. (1999) DeltaF508 CFTR protein expression in tissues from patients with cystic fibrosis. *J. Clin. Invest.* **103,** 1379–1389.

39

Formulation of Synthetic Vectors for Cystic Fibrosis Gene Therapy

John Marshall and Seng H. Cheng

1. Introduction

Following the identification and subsequent cloning of the gene that is defective in patients with cystic fibrosis (CF), there has been a substantial effort to evaluate gene therapy as a modality for treating this disease. As the primary cause of mortality in CF is respiratory dysfunction, the lung has been the major focus for genetic therapy intervention. Although this organ is relatively accessible for gene transduction—for example, by use of aerosols—it has become evident that there are several barriers to efficient transduction of the airway epithelia. These barriers are often further exacerbated in a diseased CF lung.

Gene transfer vectors that have been evaluated for delivery of the cystic fibrosis transmembrane conductance regulator (CFTR) gene to the airways include recombinant viral (adenovirus, adeno-associated virus, retrovirus) and synthetic, self-assembling (cationic lipids, polymers) vectors. The nonviral or synthetic vectors, the focus of this chapter, are invariably generated through condensation of the negatively charged plasmid DNA (pDNA) by the positively charged polycations to generate macromolecular complexes of variable sizes ranging from ten to several hundred nanometers in diameter. Despite their relatively low efficiency of transfection, at least when compared with viral-based vectors, there is still continued interest in the development of these vectors. This arises primarily from the observations that, unlike viral vectors, synthetic gene delivery systems are not encumbered by host immune-related issues and they are also relatively easier to manufacture in large quantities.

In deciding on the most appropriate synthetic gene delivery vector for use in CF therapy, several factors need to be carefully considered (*1*). Ideally, the synthetic vector formulation should be (1) capable of facilitating efficient gene

From: *Methods in Molecular Medicine, vol. 70: Cystic Fibrosis Methods and Protocols*
Edited by: W. R. Skach © Humana Press Inc., Totowa, NJ

transduction and persistent expression of the transgene product in the appropriate target cells, (2) relatively nontoxic, (3) conducive for use in repeated administrations, and (4) compatible with nebulization to the distal airways. The identification of vector formulations that meet these criteria is not trivial and is compounded by our lack of understanding on how these synthetic gene transfer complexes mediate cellular transfection. Although it is possible to chart the several processes that are necessary in order for productive cellular transfection to occur, it remains unclear which of these are the key limiting events (**Fig. 1**). As such, the development of these synthetic gene delivery vectors has been largely reliant on empirical testing of many different polycations and formulations *(1)*. Despite these impediments, much progress has been made, particularly with cationic lipid-based vectors, to the point where several were deemed sufficiently efficacious to warrant testing in human clinical studies *(2–6)*. The results of these early studies in CF subjects showed that although cationic lipid-based gene transfer to the airway epithelium is possible, the efficiency of gene transduction is low and is associated with mild toxicity. The discordance in the performance and safety of these vectors observed in preclinical studies and in the subsequent human studies also highlighted the importance for use of appropriate test model systems that are more reflective of their performance in humans.

In this chapter we address many of the factors associated with the development and use of cationic lipid-based vectors, with CF gene therapy as the goal. These include methods for formulating and storing the components of this vector system (to reduce undesirable chemical reactions), assays to determine the characteristics of the synthetic vector complexes (to assure reproducibility), formulation modifications that support high concentrations of the complexes (to facilitate aerosolization), methods for delivery, and evaluation of the extent of gene transduction in the lung.

2. Materials
2.1. Formulation and Storage of Cationic Lipids

1. 1,2-dioleoyl-*sn*-glycero-3-phosphatidylethanolamine (DOPE) and 1,2-dimyristyl-*sn*-glycero-3-phosphtidylethanolamine-N-[poly(ethylene glycol)5000] (DMPE-PEG$_{5000}$) were from Avanti Polar Lipids, Alabaster, AL. The GL series of cationic lipids were synthesized at Genzyme Corporation, Cambridge, MA.
2. Chloroform, *t*-butanol.
3. Argon.
4. 20 mm neck, 10 mL serum tubing vials, aluminum crimp (Wheaton, Milville, NJ).
5. Butyl-ʟ stoppers (Helvoet Pharma, Burlington, NJ).
6. Lyophilizer, DuraStop/DuraDry–FTS Systems, (Kinetics Thermal Systems, Stoneridge, NY).

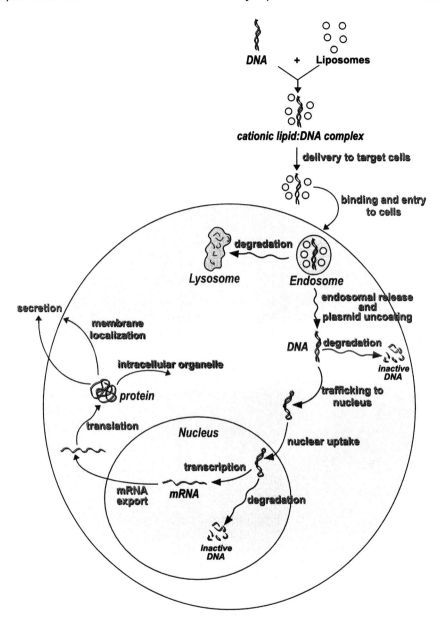

Fig. 1. Schematic of the events associated with lipid-mediated gene transfer.

7. Bath sonicator Labline model T5540, (Barnstead/Thermolyne, Dubuque, IA).
8. 0.2 μm filter.
9. –70°C freezer.
10. Dispensing pump–model 505Di/RL (Watson Marlow, Wilmington, MA).

2.2. Preparation of Cationic Lipid:pDNA Complexes

1. Water for irrigation (WFI) (VMR, Philadelphia, PA).
2. Polystyrene tubes Falcon #2054, (Becton Dickinson, Franklin Lakes, NJ).
3. Multitube vortexer (VWR, Philadelphia, PA).
4. 30°C water bath.

2.3. Physical Characterization of Cationic Lipid:pDNA Complexes

2.3.1. Size of Complexes

1. Nicomp model 380ZLS (Nicomp, Santa Barbara, CA).

2.3.2. Zeta Potential Measurements

1. Nicomp model 380ZLS (Nicomp).

2.3.3. Extent of pDNA Complexation

1. Electrophoresis apparatus (e.g., Horizon 11-14, Life Technologies, Rockville, MD), power source, gel cassette, and comb.
2. Tris-borate-EDTA (TBE) buffer: 45 mM Tris-borate, 1 mM ethylene diaminetetraacetic acid (EDTA), pH 8.0.
3. Agarose gel loading buffer: 25% sucrose (w/v), Orange G in TBE.
4. Ethidium bromide (1 μg/mL) stored as 5 mg/mL aqueous solution.
5. Transilluminator (Fotodyne, Hartland, WI).

2.4. Aerosol Delivery of Cationic Lipid:pDNA Complexes to the Mouse Lung

1. Rhodamine-phosphatidylethanolamine (Avanti Polar Lipids, Alabaster, AL).
2. TOTO-1 (Molecular Probes, Eugene, OR).
3. Octylglucoside.
4. Pari LC Jet Plus nebulizer (Pari Respiratory Equipment, Richmond, VA).
5. Pall BB-50T Breathing Circuit Filter (Pall Biomedical, Fajardo PR 00648).
6. Anderson IACFM cascade impactor. (Anderson Industries, Smyrna, GA).
7. All Glass Impinger (AGI, Ace Glass Vineland, NJ).
8. Spex Fluoromax fluorometer (Spex Industries, Edison, NJ).
9. Female BALB/c mice (Taconic, Germantown, NY).

2.5. Insufflation of Complexes into Mouse Lung

1. Isoflurane (J. A. Webster, Sterling, MA).
2. 2,2,2-Tribromoethanol.
3. *t*-Amyl alcohol.

2.6. Histochemical Staining for Human Placental Alkaline Phosphatase Activity

1. Euthasol.
2. AP Fix buffer: 2% (v/v) formaldehyde, 0.2% (v/v) glutaraldehyde in phosphate-buffered saline (PBS).
3. AP stain buffer: 0.17 mg/mL 5-bromo-4-chloro-3-indoyl-1-phosphate (BCIP) (Promega, Madison, WI), 0.33 mg/mL Nitro blue tetrazolium (NBT) (Promega), 0.02% (v/v) Nonidet-P40 (NP-40) (Sigma, St. Louis, MO), 0.01% (w/v) sodium deoxycholate, 100 mM Tris-HCl, pH 10.0, 100 mM sodium chloride, and 5 mM magnesium chloride.
4. 65°C water bath.

3. Methods

3.1. Formulation and Storage of Cationic Lipids

Several cationic lipids of different structure types have been synthesized and evaluated for use in CF gene therapy. Examples of cationic lipids that have been shown to be particularly active at mediating gene transfection of the lung include DC-Chol *(2)*, DOTAP *(4)*, and the GL series of lipids *(1,6,7)* (*see* **Note 1**). These cationic lipids are invariably formulated with a neutral co-lipid such as dioleoylphosphatidylethanolamine (DOPE) or cholesterol as a dry film. To highlight an example of how such a formulation is generated, we will describe our process for generating GL-67:DOPE lipids (*see* **Note 2**).

1. The cationic lipid GL-67 is weighed out and dissolved in *t*-butanol:water (9:1, v/v) in a volumetric flask to approximately half the final desired volume. The lipid is then sonicated using a bath sonicator (Labline model TS540) until the lipid is completely in solution. An appropriate volume of the *t*-butanol/water is added until the required concentration (10 mM) is reached.
2. An appropriate amount of the neutral lipid DOPE is weighed out and dissolved in *t*-butanol:water (9:1, v/v) in a volumetric flask to approximately half the final desired volume. The lipid is then sonicated as with the cationic lipid above using a bath sonicator until the lipid is completely in solution. An appropriate volume of *t*-butanol:water is then added until the required concentration (20 mM) is attained.
3. The neutral and cationic lipids are combined and quantities (typically 4 μmoles of cationic lipid) are aliquotted into glass vials (20 mm neck, 10 mL serum tubing vials, Wheaton) using a dispensing pump (Watson Marlow, model 505Di/RL). Unsiliconized inert butyl stoppers (Omniflex, Helvoet Pharma) are placed on the tops of the vials but only loosely to allow for subsequent lyophilization.
4. The vials are placed on a shelf in a lyophilizer (DuraStop/DuraDry, FTS Systems), which is then cooled to −30°C for 25 min to freeze the contents. Vacuum is applied and when the pressure reaches below 100 mT, the shelf temperature is raised to −20°C and the lyophilizer maintained at this temperature with the vacuum at 0 mT for 5 h. The shelf temperature is then raised to −5°C and the vials subjected to a further 48–60 h under vacuum at 0 mT to remove any residual solvent.

5. Following lyophilization, the vacuum is released and the lyophilizer is back-filled with argon gas that has been passed through a sterile 0.2 μm filter at 1 atm pressure. Filling the vials with an inert gas such as argon is an important consideration especially for cationic lipids like GL-67 that contain spermine as a headgroup as they are reactive with carbon dioxide. Before opening the lyophilizer, the stoppers are pushed into place by raising the shelves inside such that it pushes against the rack above, resulting in the stoppers becoming fully seated into the vials.
6. The lyophilizer is then opened and the stoppers are sealed in place with an aluminum crimp (Wheaton). The vials are normally stored at –70°C until ready for use.

Some cationic lipids such as those of the GL series contain unprotonated primary amines on their cationic headgroups. These are particularly susceptible to a transacylation reaction when they are co-formulated with a neutral lipid containing an ester-linked acyl chain, such as those in DOPE. The resulting transacylation reaction occurs by nucleophilic attack of the lone pair of electrons of the primary amine on the δ^+ carbonyl group of the ester moiety. This results in the transfer of an acyl chain to the cationic lipid and the generation of an isomeric pair of lysophosphatidylethanolamines. We have determined that this chemical reaction is time, pH, and temperature dependent, and occurs regardless of whether the lipids are in an aqueous suspension or a dry film. Aqueous suspensions of these lipid formulations at room temperature transacylate at a rate of approx 1%/h. However, this reaction can be reduced by storing the dry films at –20°C (conversion at a rate of 2%/mo over 6 mo) and can be effectively negated by storage at –70°C *(7)*. Hence for long term storage of such unprotonated cationic lipids, it is recommended that they be kept as a dry film at –70°C. Following suspension in aqueous solution, the rate of transacylation can be reduced by maintaining the pH at least one unit below the p*Ka* of the primary amine. The primary amines of a cationic lipid possessing a spermine headgroup (such as GL-67) typically have a p*Ka* of approx 10 *(8)*, thus suspension of the cationic lipids in a relatively neutral (pH 7.0–7.4) buffer will be protective.

3.2. Preparation of Cationic Lipid:pDNA Complexes

Cationic lipid and pDNA complexes are normally prepared just prior to use. The cationic lipid and pDNA are hydrated and diluted with sterile water (WFI-VWR) at 4°C to a concentration that is double that required for the final concentration in the complex *(see* **Note 3***)*. All the dilutions and subsequent complex formation are performed in sterile polystyrene tubes (Falcon #2054).

1. Water (WFI) is added to the lipid film (e.g., 2 mL is added to a 4 μmol cationic lipid vial to generate a 2 m*M* suspension) and hydrated for 60 min at 4°C on a multitube vortexer (VWR) set at approximately 1500 cycles/min. Careful visual evaluation of the lipid vial is necessary to ensure that complete hydration has occurred and that the liposomes are in a homogenous suspension.

2. An appropriate volume of the liposome suspension is then aliquotted into poly-styrene tubes (e.g., for 100-μL mouse instillations, 55 μL is aliquotted for each mouse receiving that formulation).

3. The appropriate pDNA concentration, which needs to be determined empirically but typically is in the 0.1–10 m*M* range, is achieved by dilution with water (WFI) at 4°C. A volume of the pDNA equal to the liposome suspension is then aliquotted into polystyrene tubes. The molarity of the pDNA solution refers to the molarity of the nucleotides and is calculated based on an average nucleotide molecular weight of 330 Dalton.

4. Five minutes before mixing, the complex components are warmed to 30°C in a water bath and then an equal volume of the cationic lipid is gently pipetted into the pDNA solution, avoiding subsequent agitation (*see* **Note 4**). The complexes are then allowed to form at 30°C for a further 15 min. Once formed, the com-plexes are stable for up to 4 h at room temperature and can be used for aerosoliza-tion or for direct instillation into mouse lung.

3.3. Physical Characterization of the Cationic Lipid:pDNA Complexes

The extent and nature of the electrostatic interactions between the cationic moiety of the lipid and the anionic phosphates of the pDNA can be variable depending on experimental details such as the temperature and vigor of agita-tion during complex formation, the concentration and purity of the compo-nents, and the resultant charge ratio of the complexes. To determine if the complexes generated are reproducible and conform to those of previous experiments, a number of physical characterizations can be performed *(9–11)*. For example, dynamic light scattering can be used to assess the overall size of the liposomes and lipid:pDNA preparations, agarose gel electrophoresis can be used to measure the extent of pDNA association with the lipids, and freeze-fracture electron microscopy can be used to visualize the size and morphology of the resultant entities formed *(12)*. Electron microscopy is recommended and can yield most informative data. However, it requires highly trained techni-cians and very expensive equipment and is usually contracted out to laborato-ries that specialize in the procedure.

3.3.1. Size of Cationic Lipid:pDNA Complexes

The size of the complexes that are formed is an important consideration for gene transduction. Depending on the desired target for genetic modification, differently sized complexes may be more suitable. Most cationic lipid:pDNA complexes generated by the simple mixing of the two components exhibit mean diameters ranging between 300 and 600 nm. These complexes are unlikely to be effective at penetrating the fenestrations (<100 nm) and transducing the liver hepatocytes. Indeed, it has been shown that intravenous delivery of such complexes invariably results in localization of a proportion of the complexes in the pulmonary capillaries. This may explain why most of the gene transfection associated with systemic delivery of this synthetic vector is primarily in the lung endothelium. However, we have determined that complexes over a broad size range are active when delivered to the lumen of the lung.

The size of the liposomes and cationic lipid:pDNA complexes can be determined by dynamic light scattering using a NICOMP model 380 or similar instrument. For such measurements, cationic lipid:pDNA complexes typically are formed at a cationic lipid concentration of between 100 and 500 μM in water. The temperature is fixed at 25°C, slit width at 250 nm, viscosity set to 1.00, and the index of refraction set to 1.00. Mean diameters are taken from at least three separate readings of 10 cycles. The data are usually presented in terms of either intensity vs mean diameter (i.e., the relative volume of liposomes at a given size distribution) or particle count vs mean diameter (i.e., the number of liposomes detected at a given size distribution). Typically the mean diameter of GL-67:DOPE:pDNA complexes are between 400 and 500 nm, but other cationic lipid:pDNA complexes may range from 100 nm up to 1 μm, depending on the cationic lipid species and also the formulation of the complex. Complexes that are over 1 μm in diameter are likely aggregates resulting from a rapid and irreversible nucleation event. These large complexes, which are visible as a fine precipitate, are not recommended for in vivo studies. With the GL series of cationic lipids, this precipitation can be minimized by the inclusion of a small amount of DMPE-PEG$_{5000}$ in the lipid formulation, as will be described under **Subheading 3.4.1.**

3.3.2. Zeta Potential Measurements

The zeta potential of complexes tends to become more positive as the charge ratio of the cationic lipid:pDNA is increased to greater than 1, reflecting that more of the pDNA is present as a complex with increasing amounts of cationic lipid. Zeta potential measurements can be taken using a NICOMP model 380ZLS particle sizing system. Cationic lipid:pDNA complexes are formed typically at a cationic lipid concentration of between 100 and 500 μM in water (*see* **Subheading 3.2.**). Following complexation, the sample is placed into a standard disposable fluorescence cuvette and the zeta electrode that accompanies the NICOMP is inserted and then placed into the chamber. Zeta potential measurements are evaluated using the default software parameters for aqueous samples. The zeta potential of the cationic lipid:pDNA complexes is dependent on the molar ratio of the cationic lipid:pDNA complexes. GL-67:DOPE liposomes typically have a zeta potential of approximately +55-65 mV. When present as a complex with pDNA, charge neutrality (zeta potential of 0 mV) is attained when the molar ratio of GL-67:pDNA is 1:1.2.

3.3.3. Extent of pDNA Complexation

To determine the extent to which pDNA is involved in a complex with the cationic lipid (at any particular cationic lipid:pDNA ratio), complexes are freshly prepared by adding 15 µL of cationic lipid (at twice the required final concentration) to 15 µL of 400 µM pDNA. Alternatively, aliquots of complexes from samples can be taken and used for gel analysis by loading 1–2 µg of pDNA/well. Following complexation, 5 µL of loading buffer (25% sucrose, Orange G) is added to each 25 µL sample and then loaded into the wells of a 0.75% (w/v) agarose gel. The samples are electrophoresed in Tris-borate-EDTA (TBE) buffer, pH 8.0, containing 0.5 µg/mL ethidium bromide, at approximately 100 V for 1–2 h. The ethidium bromide-stained pDNA is visualized by transillumination on an ultraviolet transilluminator. Because of its size, cationic lipid-complexed pDNA remains in the well. Typically, complexes that are at charge neutrality or that contain an excess of cationic lipid (a positive zeta potential) do not migrate from the well. Free or uncomplexed pDNA, as present in formulations containing an excess of pDNA (a negative zeta potential), will co-migrate with pDNA alone. Quantitation of this band using known standards provides a means to estimate the amount of free pDNA and the extent of pDNA that is present as a complex in the formulation.

3.4. Aerosol Delivery of Cationic Lipid:pDNA Complexes to the Mouse Lung

Aerosol delivery of synthetic vector systems to the lung requires that several physical properties of the complexes be taken into consideration *(13)*. Formulation modifications need to be evaluated to identify those that (1) prevent the degradation of pDNA caused by the shear forces generated during nebulization, and (2) stabilize the complex against lipid-phase separation, which could lead to precipitation. Careful evaluation of the available commercial nebulizers also needs to be performed to identify those that would (1) optimize the delivery time of the aerosolized complexes, (2) ensure the generation of appropriately sized respirable particles, and (3) minimize any changes in the physical characteristics of the complexes (e.g., degradation, aggregation, and precipitation).

3.4.1. Formulation Modifications for Effective Aerosol Delivery

Uncomplexed pDNA is rapidly degraded by the nebulization process. To minimize this loss, the pDNA can be protected by completely complexing it with the cationic lipid *(10,11)*. Formulations of cationic lipid:pDNA complexes that are close to charge neutrality or that have a slightly positive charge ratio should conform to this requirement. The extent of pDNA complexation can be readily assessed by gel electrophoresis (*see above*). Demonstration that the pDNA in the complex is intact can be achieved by adding sodium dodecyl sulfate to 0.4% to disrupt the cationic lipid:pDNA interactions and electrophoresing alongside an uncomplexed pDNA standard.

The concentration of the complexes that could be aerosolized can be limiting (containing less than 0.5 mg/mL of pDNA) due to nebulization-induced aggregation *(10)*. However, we have shown that with GL-67:DOPE:pDNA complexes, the inclusion of a small amount of DMPE-PEG$_{5000}$ can act to stabilize the complexes. By incorporating DMPE-PEG$_{5000}$ at as low as 0.05 molar ratio, formulations of complexes that contain as high as 6 mg/mL pDNA can be generated without aggregation. The inclusion of DMPE-PEG$_{5000}$ in the formulation does not alter the size range or the in vivo activity of the nebulized particles. The development of formulations that support high concentrations of pDNA is important as it facilitates delivery of more complex per unit time.

3.4.2. Analysis of Nebulized Cationic Lipid:pDNA Complexes

With the lung being the target for the aerosolized synthetic vectors, nebulizers need to be evaluated for their ability to deliver the therapeutic within several defined specifications (e.g., particle size, integrity of complexes, rate of delivery). We have determined that the Pari LC Jet Plus nebulizer *(14)* operated at a flow rate of approx 7.8 L/min (provided by a standard air compressor) is capable of delivering 0.62 ± 0.06 mL of GL-67:DOPE:DMPE-PEG$_{5000}$:pDNA complexes/min. The mass median aerodynamic diameter (mmad) of the aerosol droplets generated under these conditions is approx 2.2 μm with a geometric standard deviation (gsd) of 3.0, which is within the respirable range (1–5 μm). Measurement of the aerosol droplet size is normally performed by nebulizing rhodamine-labeled phosphatidylethanolamine-containing complexes into an Andersen 1 ACFM cascade impacter. The complexes that collect on the stages of the impactor are recovered by addition of 1% Triton X-100 and the amount of the fluorescent lipid on the different stages quantitated using a fluorometer (Spex Fluoromax).

Nebulization of GL-67:DOPE:DMPE-PEG$_{5000}$:pDNA (1:2:0.05:1.3 molar ratio) using the Pari LC Jet Plus nebulizer under these conditions does not result in measurable degradation of the pDNA, nor does it alter the ratio of the components of the complexes. There is, however, a slight time-dependent increase in the concentration of the complexes remaining in the nebulizer reservoir, as predicted *(15,16)*. The ratio of cationic lipid and pDNA present in the aerosol can be determined by use of fluorescently labeled lipids and pDNA. For example, the cationic liposomes can be formulated at a 2.5 mol% with rhodamine-phosphatidylethanolamine (Rh-PE) and pDNA can be labeled with TOTO-1 (one TOTO-1 per thousand nucleotides). The ratio of lipid to pDNA in the nebulized complex is determined by collecting the aerosolized complexes on an All Glass Impinger (AGI, Ace Glass) *(11,14)*.

1. The AGI and the Pari LC Jet Plus nebulizer are first weighed prior to commencement of aerosolization.
2. Four milliliters of the complexes is pipetted into the nebulization chamber and the complexes nebulized as described above.
3. The nebulizer is then reweighed to determine the amount of complexes that has been aerosolized.
4. The complexes that are deposited on the AGI are recovered by rinsing the impinger sequentially with 4 mL octylglucoside buffer (100 m*M* octylglucoside in distilled water) 4 mL PBS, and again with 4 mL octylglucoside buffer.
5. The AGI is re-weighed to determine the total volume it contains.
6. The fluorescence of both the Rh-PE and TOTO-1 present in the AGI washes is quantitated using a fluorometer (Spex Fluoromax). By using the constant-wavelength analysis program and standard curves generated using the starting materials diluted in a 1:1 mixture of PBS and octylglucoside buffer, the amounts of lipid and pDNA transferred to the AGI can be quantitated.

The transfection activity of the complexes following nebulization can be assessed by placing a plate of tissue culture cells in an acrylic box connected to the nebulizer and vented through a Pall BB-50T Breathing Circuit Filter (Pall Biomedical, Fajardo PR 00648) *(10)*. Following exposure of the cells to the aerosolized complexes, the cells are grown for a further 48 h, after which they are lysed and the extent of transduction and transgene expression determined.

3.4.3. Nebulization of Cationic Lipid:pDNA Complexes to the Mouse Lung

The ability of aerosolized cationic lipid:pDNA complexes to effect transfection in vivo can be tested in the lungs of mice. As it is difficult to analyze statistically relevant numbers of mice using adapted masks to provide direct aerosol delivery, compounded by the need that they be anesthetized, thus altering respiratory function, use of a whole-body exposure chamber to deliver the complexes to the mice is preferred (*see* **Note 6**).

1. Ten female BALB/c mice (16–18 g) are placed in an acrylic box (approx $20 \times 20 \times 15$ cm) that is connected to the Pari LC Jet Plus nebulizer using anesthesia tubing and vented through a Pall BB-50T Breathing Circuit Filter.
2. Ten milliliters of complex (GL-67:DOPE:DMPE-PEG$_{5000}$:pDNA) is aerosolized using 2 s bursts followed by 4 s rests (total time 20–45 min). The airborne aerosol particles can be seen as a dissipating cloud entering the acrylic chamber, with the mice becoming moist as the droplets coalesce.
3. Following completion of the nebulization process, the mice are normally housed for a further 48 h, after which they are sacrificed and their lungs analyzed for expression of the transgene.

3.5. Administration of Cationic Lipid:pDNA Complexes to Mouse Airway Epithelia

We routinely assess the in vivo transfection activity of the synthetic gene delivery vectors in the lungs of female BALB/c mice (4–6 wk old) by administering a bolus of 100 µL of the complexes via insufflation through the nose *(17)* or by direct injection through a trans-tracheal incision. The instillation technique is the preferred method for complex delivery because it (1) allows a larger cohort of animals to be treated in any given time, (2) results in less animal-to-animal variability in groups of mice receiving the same test article (smaller standard deviations), and (3) generally results in higher levels of transgene expression in the lung (unpublished observations).

3.5.1. Intranasal Instillation of Cationic Lipid:pDNA Complexes

1. Mice are anesthetized by inhalation of isoflurane. The mice (≤ 10 at a time) are placed in a rodent anesthesia machine (Colonial Medical, Franconia, NH) and receive oxygen at 800 mL/min passed over an isoflurane reservoir set to level 5 (results in approx 5% isoflurane content in the air) for 1 min. The animals are kept under anesthesia by maintaining isoflurane at 2.5% in the chamber.
2. Mice are removed individually and instilled immediately by holding the animals upright with their noses up and applying pressure to the lower mandible to immobilize the tongue and prevent the reflex to swallow the complex. The cationic lipid:pDNA complexes (100 µL) are administered dropwise (20–25 µL/drop over 15 s) into the nares of mice using a standard Pipetteman (0–200 µL) with an appropriate tip. Using this procedure, we estimate that approx 70% of the total complexes are delivered into the lung. The mice recover from the anesthesia within 30 s of removal from the isoflurane atmosphere.
3. The mice are routinely housed for a further 48 h, after which they are sacrificed and their lungs assayed for expression of the transgene.

3.6. Staining for the Alkaline Phosphatase Reporter Gene

The *de facto* standard reporter gene for histochemical localization of transfected cells is bacterial β-galactosidase using 5-bromo-4-chloro-3-indoyl-β-D-galactopyranoside (X-gal) as substrate. However, the validity and sensitivity of the results obtained with this reporter has been questioned, and consequently the use of a nonsecreted alkaline phosphatase (NSAP) reporter gene is also recommended *(13,19)* (*see* **Note 5**).

1. Two days post-administration of cationic lipid:pNSAP (NSAP: a nonsecretable form of human placental alkaline phosphatase) complexes, the mice are euthanized with an intraperitoneal injection of euthasol (sodium pentobarbital), the transfected lungs are removed and the trachea catheterized.
2. The lungs are fixed by inflation with AP fix buffer for 10 min at room temperature and 30 cm of water pressure, and then incubated for an additional 60 min at 4°C but without added pressure.

3. Following fixation, the lungs are rinsed three times with phosphate-buffered saline (PBS), placed into 50 mL conical tubes filled with PBS, and heated at 65°C for 30 min to inactivate endogenous phosphatases *(20)*.
4. The lungs are rinsed a further three times with PBS at room temperature, and then both inflated and bathed in AP stain solution at room temperature.
5. Staining proceeds for approx 4 h or until a sufficient degree of staining is achieved, at which point the reaction is terminated by rinsing the lungs three times with 20 m*M* EDTA in PBS. Tissues can then be stored at 4°C in AP fix buffer for later microscopic examination.

4. Notes

1. For optimal transfection of the lung, we have found significantly higher levels of transgene expression using the non-protonated or free-base forms of the GL series of cationic lipids than with the salt forms of the protonated amines *(7)*.
2. Preparation of cationic lipid formulations (*see* **Subheading 3.1.**) should be performed sterilely to minimize contamination by potential pathogens or pyrogens. Glassware should be depyrogenated by heating at 250°C for 6 h. Where appropriate materials should also be autoclaved.
3. Formulation of complexes in excipients, even with the solutes as low as 10 m*M*, results in significantly reduced transgene expression when compared with complexes formulated in water *(7)*.
4. Agitation of the cationic lipid:pDNA mixture during complex formation can lead to a nucleation event that results in aggregation and precipitation of the complexes.
5. Transcriptional activity of the CMV promoter can be enhanced by instilling 100 μL of 20 m*M* sodium butyrate (Sigma) to the mouse. If this is performed 24 h before tissue harvest, a two- to fivefold elevation in transgene expression can be attained, which can be beneficial when using chromatic visualization of transgenes such as BCIP/NBT for NSAP and X-gal for β-galactosidase.
6. Aerosol delivery of complex to mouse lung is very inefficient, with approx 2 μL being deposited onto the airway epithelium for every 10 mL nebulized.

References

1. Marshall, J., Yew, N. S., Eastman, S. J., Jiang, C., Scheule, R. K., and Cheng, S. H. (1999) Cationic lipid-mediated gene delivery to the airways, in *Non-Viral Vectors for Gene Therapy* (Huang, L., Hung, M.-C., and Wagner, E., eds.), Academic Press, San Diego, CA, pp. 39–68.
2. Caplen, N. J., Alton, E. W. F. W., Middleton, P. G., Dorin, J. R., Stevenson, B. J., Gao, X., et al. (1995) Liposome-mediated CFTR gene transfer to the nasal epithelium of patients with cystic fibrosis. *Nature Med.* **1,** 39–46.
3. Gill, D. R., Southern, K. W., Mofford, K. A., Seddon, T., Huang, L., Sorgi, F., et al. (1997) A placebo-controlled study of liposome-mediated gene transfer to the nasal epithelium of patients with cystic fibrosis. *Gene Ther.* **4,** 199–209.
4. Porteus, D. J., Dorin, J. R., McLachlan, G., Davidson-Smith, H., Stevenson, B. J., Carothers, A. D., et al. (1997) Evidence for the safety and efficacy of DOTAP

cationic liposome mediated CFTR gene transfer to the nasal epithelium of patients with cystic fibrosis. *Gene Ther.* **4,** 210–218.

5. Zabner, J., Cheng, S. H., Meeker, D., Launspach, J., Balfour, R., Perricone, M. A., et al. (1997) Comparison of DNA-lipid complexes and DNA alone for gene transfer to cystic fibrosis airway epithelia *in vivo. J. Clin. Invest.* **100,** 1529–1537.

6. Alton, E. W. F. W., Stern, F., Farley, R., Jaffe, A., Chadwick, S. L., Phillips, J., et al. (1999) Cationic lipid-mediated CFTR gene transfer to the lungs and nose of patients with cystic fibrosis: a double-blind placebo-controlled trial. *Lancet* **353,** 947–954.

7. Marshall, J., Nietupski, J. B., Lee, E. R., Siegel, C. S., Rafter, P. W., Rudginsky, S. A., et al. (2000) Cationic lipid structure and formulation considerations for optimal gene transfection of the lung. *J. Drug Targeting.* **7(6),** 453–469.

8. Geall, A. J., Taylor, R. J., Earll, M. E., Eaton, M. A. W., and Blagbrough, I. S. (2000) Synthesis of cholesteryl polyamine carbamates: pK_a studies and condensation of calf thymus DNA. *Bioconjugate Chem.* **11,** 314–326.

9. Eastman, S. J., Siegel, C., Tousignant, J. D., Smith, A. E., Cheng, S. H., and Scheule, R. K. (1997) Biophysical characterization of cationic lipid:DNA complexes. *Biochim. Biophys. Acta* **1325,** 41–62.

10. Eastman, S. J., Tousignant, J. D., Lukason, M. J., Murray, H., Siegel, C. S., Constantino, P., et al. (1997) Optimization of formulations and conditions for the aerosol delivery of functional cationic lipid:DNA complexes. *Hum. Gene Ther.* **8,** 313–322.

11. Eastman, S. J., Lukason, M. J., Tousignant, J. D., Murray, H., Lane, M. D., St. George, J. A., et al. (1997) A concentrated and stable aerosol formulation of cationic lipid:DNA complexes giving high-level gene expression in mouse lung. *Hum. Gene Ther.* **8,** 765–773.

12. Fisher, K. and Branton, D. (1974) Application of the freeze-fracture technique to natural membranes. *Meths. Enzymol.* **32,** 35–44.

13. Cheng, S. H. and Scheule, R. K. (1998) Airway delivery of cationic lipid:DNA complexes for cystic fibrosis. *Adv. Drug Delivery Rev.* **30,** 173–184.

14. Eastman, S. J., Tousignant, J. D., Lukason, M. J., Chu, Q., Cheng, S. H., and Scheule, R. K. (1998) Aerosolization of cationic lipid:pDNA complexes—*in vitro* optimization of nebulizer parameters for human clinical trials. *Hum. Gene Ther.* **9,** 43–52.

15. Mercer, T. T., Tillery, M. I., and Chow, H. Y. (1968) Operating characteristics of some compressed-air nebulizers. *Am. Ind. Hyg. Assoc.* **29,** 66–78.

16. Dennis, J. H., Stenton, S. C., Beach, J. R., Avery, A. J., Walters, E. H., and Hendrick, D. J. (1990) Jet and ultrasonic nebulizer output: use of a new method for direct measurement of aerosol output. *Thorax* **45,** 728–732.

17. Lee, E. R., Marshall, J., Siegel, C. S., Jiang, C., Yew, N. S., Nichols, M. R., et al. (1996) Detailed analysis of structures and formulations of cationic lipids for efficient gene transfer to the lung. *Hum. Gene Ther.* **7,** 1701–1717.

18. Jiang, C., O'Connor, S. P., Fang, S. L., Wang, K. X., Marshall, J., Williams, J. L., et al. (1998) Efficiency of cationic lipid-mediated transfection of polarized and differentiated airway epithelial cells *in vitro* and *in vivo. Hum. Gene Ther.* **9,** 1531–1542.

19. Scheule, R. K., St. George, J. A., Bagley, R. G., Marshall, J., Kaplan, J. M., Akita, G. Y., et al. (1997) Basis of pulmonary toxicity associated with cationic lipid-mediated gene transfer to the mammalian lung. *Hum. Gene Ther.* **8,** 689–707.

20. Cullen, B. R. and Malim, M. H. (1992) Secreted placental alkaline phosphatase as a eukaryotic reporter gene. *Meths. Enzymol.* **216,** 362–368.

40

Adeno-Associated Viral Vectors for CF Gene Therapy

Terence R. Flotte, Isabel Virella-Lowell, and Kye A. Chesnut

1. Introduction

AAV is a nonpathogenic human parvovirus that has a natural mechanism for long-term persistence in human cells. Wild-type AAV is unique in that it undergoes stable integration of its DNA into a specific region of human chromosome 19, the AAVS1 site (1–4), a process that our group has also recently described in vivo in rhesus macques (5). This site specificity appears to be mediated by specific interactions between the nonstructural protein, Rep, and the sequence-specific binding elements within the AAVS1 site (6). AAV vectors have been developed by deleting the two AAV genes, *rep* and *cap* from the viral genome, and substituting transgenes such as *CFTR* (7,8). Since the *rep* gene is deleted, these vectors generally do not integrate in a site-specific manner, yet they do persist long-term in mammalian cells through a complicated process that involves both episomal persistence and random-site integration (9–11).

The packaging capacity of rAAV is rather limited, at only 5 kb, including the AAV inverted terminal repeats (ITRs) that are required *in cis* for replication and packaging of vector genomes. This leaves only 4.7 kb for the coding sequence, promoter, and polyadenylation signal. In the case of CFTR, the coding sequence consists of 4.44 kb of DNA. Therefore, the use of small promoters and/or truncated versions of CFTR has been investigated by several groups. rAAV vectors expressing full-length CFTR have been developed using either the AAV-p5 promoter (12), the HSV-tk promoter or the cryptic promoter sequences present within the ITR (13,14). AAV-CFTR vectors have been shown to be active for stable complementation of the CFTR defect in vitro (13,15,16), and for in-vivo gene transfer in the lungs of rabbits (17,19) and rhesus macaques (10,18). In each of these settings, rAAV-CFTR transduction

From: *Methods in Molecular Medicine, vol. 70: Cystic Fibrosis Methods and Protocols*
Edited by: W. R. Skach © Humana Press Inc., Totowa, NJ

has been stable and has not been associated with acute inflammatory responses or other toxicities.

Based on these data, several phase I trials of rAAV-CFTR in cystic fibrosis (CF) patients were initiated by our group. A total of 50 patients have been treated to date. The first of these trials involving a combined nasal and bronchial administration is still ongoing *(19)*. The results of a second Phase I trial of delivery of rAAV-CFTR to the maxillary sinuses of individuals with CF have recently been reported *(20–22)*. These results indicate that gene transfer occurred in a dose-dependent fashion, with a maximal efficiency of 1 vector genome copy per cell. Gene transfer was stable for up to 70 d after a single instillation. Furthermore, the vector-treated sinuses showed a dose-related increase in cAMP-activated chloride conductance as judged by transepithelial potential difference measurement in vivo. Perhaps even more promising was a trend toward decreased levels of IL-8 in sinus lavage fluid after AAV-CFTR therapy. Additional studies of administration to the sinuses, nose, and lung are ongoing. A preliminary analysis of the bronchoalveolar lavage (BAL) fluid from several of the CF patients involved in the bronchial gene transfer trial has shown inhibition of rAAV, and there is some indication that this effect correlates with the degree of inflammation present in the airways. While these sorts of barriers may be overcome by simply increasing the vector dosage, it is also possible that transient anti-inflammatory therapy may be helpful. Concern has also been raised about the availability of receptors for AAV on the apical surface of bronchial epithelial cells *(23–25)*. However, data from both our own laboratory *(10,17,26)* and that of Dusty Miller *(27)* indicate that pulmonary gene transfer with rAAV is feasible and that it is persistent once it occurs. Ultimately, treating the lungs with this vector may be optimally done at a young age, prior to the onset of severe airway inflammation.

Recent data also indicates that the size limitation of rAAV packaging can be overcome to some extent by the ability of the vector genome to form heterodimers within transduced cells. One scheme that has been recently devised to utilize this in the context of rAAV gene therapy would be to package rAAV-CFTR vectors utilizing the minimal cryptic ITR promoter activity and a second vector containing multiple strong enhancers. Once the dimerization event occurs, the minimal promoter activity of the ITR can be enhanced by approx 1000-fold (John Engelhardt, personal communication). Another option is to package the amino-terminal half of CFTR in one vector along with a splice donor and the 5'-end of an intron, while the second vector contains the 3'-half of the intron, the splice acceptor, and the carboxy-terminal half of the CFTR coding sequence (also personal communication by Engelhardt et al.). In either case, one would still face the issue of inflammatory barriers to CFTR gene transfer in the airway if gene therapy were attempted after lung disease was established.

2. Materials

2.1. Cell Culture

1. Vector plasmid: pSA315, available from UF Vector Core (vcore@mgm.ufl.edu).
2. Packaging plasmid: pDG, available from Jurgen Kleinschmidt.
3. Packaging cells: HEK293, cells available from ATCC.
4. Cell line for titering: C12 (Hela Rep/cap), cells available from ATCC.
5. 15-cm and 96-well tissue culture dishes.
6. Dulbecco's modified Essential medium (DMEM) supplemented with 10% fetal bovine serum (FBS).
7. Penicillin/streptomycin.
8. Phosphate-buffered saline (PBS).
9. Trypsin/EDTA.
10. 2× HEPES-buffered saline (2× HBS), pH 7.05–7.10.
11. 2.5 M CaCl$_2$.

2.2. Plating of 293 Cells

1. Nunc cell factories and accessories (source).
2. Complete medium: DMEM with 5% FBS and 1% PCN-streptomycin (Gibco).
3. Sterile, individually wrapped pipets.
4. Pipet aid.
5. PBS.
6. 10× trypsin/EDTA.

2.3. Cell Transfection

1. Nunc cell factory accessories.
2. Complete medium (DMEM/5%FBS).
3. Sterile, individually wrapped pipets.
4. Pipet aid.
5. 2× HBS.
6. pDG helper plasmid; rAAV plasmid (pSA315).
7. Sterile H$_2$O.
8. 2.5 mM CaCl$_2$.

2.4. Purification of rAAV

1. rAAV cell pellets.
2. Lysis buffer with and without NaCl: 20 mM Tris-HCl, pH 8.0, 150 mM NaCl, 0.5% deoxycholate.
3. Elution buffer: 20 mM Tris-HCl, pH 8.0, 0.5 M NaCl, 0.5% deoxycholate.
4. Benzonase.
5. Saturated MgCl$_2$ (~4.8 M).
6. Microfluidizer.
7. 80-mL Streamline Heparin column and P-500 pump (Pharmacia).
8. AKTA-FPLC (Pharmacia).
9. POROS HE/M column (Boehringer Mannheim).
10. PBS/0.5 M NaCl.

2.5. Dot-Blot Hybridization Assay to Determine the Physical (Particle) Titer of Recombinant AAV and Replication-Competent (Wild-Type) AAV

1. 10× DNase buffer and DNAse I.
2. 10× Proteinase K buffer and proteinase K.
3. dH$_2$O.
4. Phenol/chloroform and chloroform.
5. Glyogen.
6. 3 *M* sodium acetate, pH 5.2.
7. Ethanol.
8. 0.4 *N* NaOH/10 m*M* EDTA solution.
9. 2× SSC.
10. Dot-blot manifold and nylon membrane.
11. Solutions for standard DNA hybridization and probc labcling.
12. X-ray film.
13. PBS.

2.6. Infectious Center Assay for the Determination of the Biological Titer (Infectious Units) of Recombinant AAV and Replication-Competent (Wild-Type) AAV

1. 96-well tissue culture dishes.
2. DMEM containing 10% FBS.
3. G418, 5 mg/mL stock solution.
4. Wild-type adenovirus stock (known titer).
5. Nylon hybridization membranes.
6. Millipore 47-mm filter holder or equivalent.
7. 0.5 *M* NaOH, 1.5 *M* NaCl.
8. 1.5 *M* NaCl, 0.5 *M* Tris-HCl, pH 7.8.
9. Solutions for standard DNA hybridization and probe labeling.
10. X-ray film.
11. PBS.

3. Methods

3.1. Plating of 293 Cells in Cell Factories for Transfection

1. Warm DMEM/5% FBS medium, PBS and PBS/EDTA to 37°C; wipe all bottles with 80% ETOH before placing in hood.
2. Dilute 5 mL of trypsin-EDTA in 45 mL 1× PBS in a 50-mL conical tube.
3. Remove 8 confluent T225 flasks of 293 cells from the incubator; remove medium from the flask and discard; gently wash the monolayer with 25 mL PBS.
4. Add 4 mL diluted trypsin-EDTA and rock until cells begin to dislodge.
5. Add 20 mL of medium and gently pipet the cell suspension to detach any remaining cells.
6. Collect cells from all 8 flasks and pool in a 250-mL conical tubes; remove sample for cell count.

7. Add 1.1 L of complete medium (type) to an aspirator bottle.
8. Add cells to the aspirator bottle and mix gently.
9. Load cell factory as per manufacturer's instruction and incubate at 37°C overnight.

3.2. Transfection of 293 Cells for Packaging of rAAV

1. Thaw 2× HBS and place at 37°C until ready to use.
2. Prepare and prewarm DMEM/5% FBS medium.
3. Calculate DNA and water to add: 1867.5 µg of pDG and 622.5 µg of rAAV per factory in a total volume of 46.7 mL.
4. Add H_2O and DNAs to a 250-mL conical tubes.
6. Add 5.2 mL of 2.5 mM $CaCl_2$ to the 250-mL conical tubes and mix well.
7. Discard medium from cell factory.
8. Add 52 mL of 2× HBS to the 250-mL conical tubes and mix well.
9. Immediately add the transfection mix (DNA/$CaCl_2$/HBS) to the 1.1 L of prepared medium (DMEM, 5% FBS, and 1% PCN/Strep.) and mix well.
10. Pour medium into the aspirator bottle and load cell factory as per manufacturer's instructions.
11. Incubate at 37°C for 60 h.

3.3. Purification of rAAV *(see Note 1)*

1. Decant the cell factory medium and add 500 mL PBS. Rock the cell factory trays gently, then decant PBS.
2. Add 500 mL of 10 mM EDTA in PBS to cell factories and rock gently until cells are released (about 10 min).
3. Decant the cells from one cell factory into two 250-mL conical centrifuge tubes (Corning).
4. Add another 500 mL PBS to the cell factory, rock gently, and decant into a second set tof two 250-mL conical tubes.
5. Spin the cells in all the conical tubes at 1000 rpm for 15 min (Beckman J6-HC).
6. Decant supernatant and resuspend the cell pellet in each tube with resuspended in 15 mL of lysis buffer containing 20 mM Tris-HCl, pH 8.0, 150 mM NaCl, and 0.5% deoxycholate. Mix well; this solution will become very viscous. Combine lysate from all four samples obtained from each individual cell factory.
7. Five cell factories of lysate are pooled at this point (for total volume of 300 mL).
8. Add 30 µL of benzonase (250 U/µL) and 30 µL of saturated $MgCl_2$ (~4.8 M). Mix well and let digest for 30 min at 37°C, mixing once during the digestion.
9. Cells are then disrupted in a single pass through a Microfluidizer (Microfluidics). The system is rinsed with 10 mL of lysis buffer that is added to the pool.
10. The lysate is then loaded immediately onto an 80-mL Streamline Heparin (Pharmacia) column at 3 mL/min using a P-500 (Pharmacia) syringe pump. The column is washed with 800 mL of lysis buffer.
11. The column is then placed on the AKTA-FPLC (Pharmacia) and the "streamline heparin method template" is run (see attached method template). Monitor absorbance at 280λ. Elute with lysis buffer containing 0.5 M NaCl (elution buffer); collect 10-mL fractions.

12. Pool peak fractions, approx 40 mL and dilute to ~150 m*M* NaCl by adding 100 mL buffer containing 20 m*M* Tris-HCl, pH 8.0 and 0.5% sodium deoxycholate (DOC).
13. Load virus on a 1.7-mL Poros HE/M (Boehringer Mannheim) at 2 mL/min (see Poros method template). Wash with 10 column volumes of PBS and elute with PBS/0.5 *M* NaCl, collecting 1-mL fractions. Each batch will be titered before final lot pooling.

3.4. Dot-Blot Hybridization Assay to Determine the Physical (Particle) Titer of Recombinant AAV and Replication-Competent (Wild-Type) AAV

3.4.1. Preparation of Viral DNA for the Slot-Blot Assay and QC-PCR

1. DNAse I (Boehringer Mannheim)/Proteinase K (Boehringer Mannheim): To 4 µL of purified recombinant virus add 20 µL of 10× DNase buffer (50 m*M* Tris-HCl, pH 7.5, 10 m*M* MgCl$_2$), 2 µL of DNAse I (Boehringer Mannheim), 174 µL of dH$_2$O, for a total volume of 200 µL.
2. Incubate at 37°C for 1 h. Then, to the 200 µL DNAse sample add 22 µL protein-ase buffer (10 m*M* Tris-HCl, pH 8.0, 10 m*M* EDTA, 1% SDS), and 2 µL of Proteinase K (18.6 mg/mL, Boehringer Mannheim), for a total volume of 224 µL.
3. Incubate at 37°C for 1 h.
4. To the sample, add an equal volume (224 µL) of phenol/chloroform.
5. Vortex for 5 min and centrifuge for 5 min at 14,000 rpm.
6. Repeat phenol/chloroform extraction and follow with a final chloroform extraction.
7. Precipitate DNA in the presence of glycogen (1 µL of glycogen, 20 µg/µL, Boehringer Mannheim) with 1/10th vol (22.4 µL) of 3 *M* Na-acetate and 2.5 vol of EtOH overnight at −20°C. Centrifuge for 20 min at 14,000 rpm.
8. Wash pellet with 75% EtOH and air dry for 5 min.
9. Resuspend DNA in 40 µL of dH$_2$O.

3.4.2. Dot-Blot Assay

1. Viral DNA prepared above is resuspended in 0.4 *N* NaOH/10 m*M* EDTA. A hybridization standard (rAAV plasmid DNA) is serially diluted twofold and resuspended in the same buffer.
2. The DNA samples are applied to the wells of a dot-blot manifold apparatus set with a prewetted nylon filter. The wells are rinsed with 400 µL of 0.4 *N* NaOH/10 m*M* EDTA. The apparatus is disassembled and the membrane is rinsed in 2× SSC and air-dried.
3. Filters are hybridized with a rAAV-specific ^{32}P-probe. Viral DNA points are compared to the standard curve and the amount of DNA is determined (Prism densitometry software by Graphpad) and rAAV genomes calculated. The num-ber of genomes, corresponding to the number of physical particles, is then com-pared to the infectious particle titer.

3.5. Infectious Center Assay for the Determination of the Biological Titer (Infectious Units) of Recombinant AAV and Replication-Competent (Wild-Type) AAV

1. *Day 1*: Seed a 96-well dish to be 75% confluent on d 2. To titer rAAV we use the C12 cell line; for rcAAV we use 293s.

2. *Day 2*: Infect cells. Set up 10× serial dilutions of the recombinant virus in a separate 96-well dish as follows:
   a. Add 250 μL of media to the first wells, add 225 μL of medium to the following wells.
   b. Add 2.5 μL of virus to the first well and serially dilute 10× by transferring 25 μL per dilution. Be sure to change tips after each dilution. Leave a few wells for "Ad only" control.
   c. Transfer 100 μL of virus from each dilution from the serial dilution dish onto the cell dish.
   d. Dilute wtAd in medium to infect each well in 50 μL (MOI ~5–titrated to give good CPE in 40 h).
3. *Day 4 (40 h postinfection)*: Harvest cells.
   a. Set up the ICA manifold or Millipore filter unit(s); prelabel and prewet filters in PBS, then mount in the unit. Apply 5 mL of PBS to each filter.
   b. Detach cells from the 96-well dish by resuspending each well in its medium by gentle repeated pipetting.
   c. Apply the contents of the entire well to the filter.
   d. Wash the well with PBS and apply it to the membrane.
   e. Mix gently to disperse evenly before applying vacuum.
   f. Allow the filter(s) to air dry for 5 min on Whatman paper.
   g. Denature for 5 min (0.5 M NaOH, 1.5 M NaCl). Blot on Whatman paper.
   h. Neutralize for 5 min (1.5 M NaCl, 0.5 M Tris-HCl, pH 7.8). Blot on Whatman paper.
   i. Rinse in 4× SSC for 30 s.
   j. Air dry for 10 min.
   k. Crosslink DNA either by UV irradiation or microwaving.

3.6. Prehybridization

Prehybridize (7% SDS, 0.25 M phosphate buffer, pH 7.2, 1 mM EDTA, pH 8.0) at 65°C at least 2 h before adding the probe (p$_{32}$ radiolabeled by nick translation). The probe is designed to either target the promoter or gene of interest for rAAV, or the wtAAV fragment for rcAAV titers). Expose to film overnight. Count dots on filters that have between 10 and 300 positive signals.

3.7. Titer

The titer of the preparation is equal to the number of positive cells per filter, multiplied by the dilution factor and 10^3, and is expressed as IU/mL.

4. Notes

1. The production and purification of recombinant AAV is a labor-intensive process that can be fraught with several potential difficulties, yet the production of high-titer, highly-purified rAAV is essential to the performance of valid experiments. Over time, several laboratories have found that contamination of rAAV preparations with replication-competent or wild-type AAV can drastically alter

the biological activity of these preparations. In particular, the AAV *Rep* gene can dramatically impair the expression of foreign transgenes contained within rAAV. Likewise, the presence of any contaminating Ad proteins can increase the immunogenicity of rAAV, which can in turn alter the profile of transgene expression. This is why detailed protocols are presented for the quality control of vector preparations. In addition to the two assays presented, it may also be useful to analyze the vector preparation by polyacrylamide gel electrophoresis followed by silver staining, in order to determine the purity of the preparation at the protein level, i.e., how much contaminating non-AAV protein is present.

In addition, there is growing evidence that certain AAV serotypes may be more useful in the lung than others. The protocol presented here described the production of rAAV particles packaged in AAV serotype 2 capsids. Data from several sources has recently indicated that AAV serotypes 5 and 6 may be more efficacious for transduction of the airways, which might relate to the relative scarcity of heparan sulfate proteoglycan on the apical surface of bronchial epithelial cells.

References

1. Kotin, R. M., Siniscalco, M., Samulski, R. J., et al. (1990) Site-specific integration by adeno-associated virus. *Proc. Natl. Acad. Sci. USA* **87(6)**, 2211–2215.
2. Kotin, R. M., Menninger, J. C., Ward, D. C., et al. (1991) Mapping and direct visualization of a region-specific viral DNA integration site on chromosome 19q13-qter. *Genomics* **10(3)**, 831–834.
3. Kotin, R. M., Linden, R. M., and Berns, K. I. (1992) Characterization of a preferred site on human chromosome 19q for integration of adeno-associated virus DNA by non-homologous recombination. *EMBO J.* **11(13)**, 5071–5078.
4. Samulski, R. J., Zhu, X., Xino, X., et al. (1991) Targeted integration of adeno-associated virus (AAV) into human chromosome 19 (published erratum appears in *EMBO J.* [1992] **11[3]**, 1228. *EMBO J.* **10(12)**, 3941–3950.
5. Hernandez, Y. J., Wang, J., Kearns, W. G., et al. (1999) Latent adeno-associated virus infection elicits humoral but not cell- mediated immune responses in a non-human primate model (In Process Citation). *J. Virol.* **73(10)**, 8549–8558.
6. Weitzman, M. D., Kyostio, S. R., Kotin, R. M., et al. (1994) Adeno-associated virus (AAV) Rep proteins mediate complex formation between AAV DNA and its integration site in human DNA. *Proc. Natl. Acad. Sci. USA* **91(13)**, 5808–5812.
7. Tratschin, J. D., West, M. H., Sandbank, T., et al. (1984) A human parvovirus, adeno-associated virus, as a eucaryotic vector: transient expression and encapsidation of the procaryotic gene for chloramphenicol acetyltransferase. *Mol. Cell Biol.* **4(10)**, 2072–2081.
8. Hermonat, P. L. and Muzyczka, N. (1984) Use of adeno-associated virus as a mammalian DNA cloning vector: transduction of neomycin resistance into mammalian tissue culture cells. *Proc. Natl. Acad. Sci. USA* **81(20)**, 6466–6470.
9. Flotte, T. R., Afione, S. A., and Zeitlin, P. L. (1994) Adeno-associated virus vector gene expression occurs in nondividing cells in the absence of vector DNA integration. *Am. J. Respir. Cell Mol. Biol.* **11(5)**, 517–521.

10. Afione, S. A., Conrad, C. K., Kearns, W. G., et al. (1996) In vivo model of adeno-associated virus vector persistence and rescue. *J. Virol.* **70(5),** 3235–3241.

11. Kearns, W. G., Afione, S. A., Fulmer, S. B., et al. (1996) Recombinant adeno-associated virus (AAV-CFTR) vectors do not integrate in a site-specific fashion in an immortalized epithelial cell line. *Gene Ther.* **3(9),** 748–755.

12. Flotte, T. R., Solow, R., Owens, R. A., et al. (1992) Gene expression from adeno-associated virus vectors in airway epithelial cells. *Am. J. Respir. Cell Mol. Biol.* **7(3),** 349–356.

13. Flotte, T. R., Afione, S. A., Solow, R., et al. (1993) Expression of the cystic fibrosis transmembrane conductance regulator from a novel adeno-associated virus promoter. *J. Biol. Chem.* **268(5),** 3781–3790.

14. Baudard, M., Flotte, T. K., Avan, J. M., et al. (1996) Expression of the human multidrug resistance and glucocerebrosidase cDNAs from adeno-associated vectors: efficient promoter activity of AAV sequences and in vivo delivery via liposomes. *Hum. Gene Ther.* **7(11),** 1309–1322.

15. Egan, M., Flotte, T., Afione, S., et al. (1992) Defective regulation of outwardly rectifying Cl- channels by protein kinase A corrected by insertion of CFTR (see comments). *Nature* **358(6387),** 581–584.

16. Schwiebert, E. M., Flotte, T., Cutting, G. R., et al. (1994) Both CFTR and outwardly rectifying chloride channels contribute to cAMP- stimulated whole cell chloride currents. *Am. J. Physiol.* **266(5 Pt 1),** C1464–1477.

17. Flotte, T. R., et al. (1993) Stable in vivo expression of the cystic fibrosis transmembrane conductance regulator with an adeno-associated virus vector. *Proc. Natl. Acad. Sci. USA* **90(22),** 10,613–10,617.

18. Conrad, C. K., Allen, S. S., Afione, S. A., et al. (1996) Safety of single-dose administration of an adeno-associated virus (AAV)- CFTR vector in the primate lung. *Gene Ther.* **3(8),** 658–668.

19. Flotte, T., Carter, B., Conrad, C., et al. (1996) A phase I study of an adeno-associated virus-CFTR gene vector in adult CF patients with mild lung disease. *Hum. Gene Ther.* **7(9),** 1145–1159.

20. Wagner, J. A., Reynolds, T., Moran, M. L., et al. (1998) Efficient and persistent gene transfer of AAV-CFTR in maxillary sinus (letter). *Lancet* **351(9117),** 1702,1703.

21. Wagner, J. A., Moran, M. L., Messner, A. H., et al. (1998) A phase I/II study of tgAAV-CF for the treatment of chronic sinusitis in patients with cystic fibrosis. *Hum. Gene Ther.* **9(6),** 889–909.

22. Wagner, J. A., Messner, A. H., Moran M. L., Daifuku, R., Kouyama, K., Desch, J. K., Manly, S., et al. (1999) Safety and biological efficacy of an adeno-associated virus vector-cystic fibrosis transmembrane conductance regulator (AAV-CFTR) in the cystic fibrosis maxillary sinus. *Laryngoscope* **109,** 266–274.

23. Teramoto, S., Bartlett, J. S., McCarty, D., et al. (1998) Factors influencing adeno-associated virus-mediated gene transfer to human cystic fibrosis airway epithelial cells: comparison with adenovirus vectors. *J. Virol.* **72(11),** 8904–8912.

24. Duan, D., Yoe, Y., Yau, Z., et al. (1998) Polarity influences the efficiency of recombinant adenoassociated virus infection in differentiated airway epithelia (In Process Citation). *Hum. Gene Ther.* **9(18),** 2761–2776.

25. Bals, R., Xiao, W., Sang, N., Weiner, D. J., Meegalla, R. L., and Wilson, J. M. (1999) Transduction of well-differentiated airway epithelium by recombinant adeno-associated virus is limited by vector entry. *J. Virol.* **73(7),** 6085–6088.
26. Flotte, T. R., Barraza-Ortiz, X., Solow, R., et al. (1995) An improved system for packaging recombinant adeno-associated virus vectors capable of in vivo transduction. *Gene Ther.* **2(1),** 29–37.
27. Halbert, C. L., Slandaert, T. A., Wilson, C. B., et al. (1998) Successful readministration of adeno-associated virus vectors to the mouse lung requires transient immunosuppression during the initial exposure. *J. Virol.* **72(12),** 9795–9805.

Index

A

AAV, *see* Adeno-associated virus
Adeno-associated virus (AAV),
    gene therapy vectors,
  HEK293 cell culture and plating,
    601–603
  integration site, 599
  packaging capacity and options,
    599, 600
  phase I trials, 600
  purification of virus, 601, 603–606
  titering,
    calculations, 605
    dot-blot hybridization, 602, 604
    infectious center assay, 602,
      604, 605
    prehybridization, 605
  transduction efficiency, 577
  transfection, 601, 603
AFM, *see* Atomic force microscopy
Airway surface liquid (ASL),
  antimicrobial peptides and
    proteins in airway
    secretions,
    assays,
      colony-forming unit assays,
        452, 456, 461
      culture, 460, 462
      materials, 452, 453
      microorganisms, 452, 460
      minimal handling assay,
        452, 453, 461
    components, 447, 448

identification,
  acid extraction, 456, 462
  batch separation, 450,
    456, 457
  cation-exchange
    chromatography,
    451, 457
  dot blots, 459
  gel filtration, 450, 457
  hydrophobic exchange
    columns, 456, 457, 462
  lysozyme assay, 451, 458, 462
  materials, 450–452
  reverse-phase
    chromatography,
    451, 458
  selective cationic peptide
    extraction, 456, 460, 462
  Western blot, 451, 452,
    458, 459
principles of testing, 449
restoration of depleted fluids,
  460, 462
salt effects, 448, 449
sampling,
  filter paper collection,
    453, 454
  fluidization of secretions,
    454, 455, 462
  materials, 449, 450
  nasal secretions, 453, 461
  reconstitution from filter
    paper, 455, 462

preparation of bacteria, 498,
501, 502, 511, 512
histopathology, 500, 501,
508–510, 513
inoculation of airways with
beads, 499, 503–505,
511, 512
materials, 498–501
mouse strains, 511
utility with other bacteria, 511
cystic fibrosis role, 495, 496
strains, 495, 496

R, S

Regulatory domain, *see* Cystic
fibrosis transmembrane
conductance regulator
Reticulocyte lysate, *see* Proteasome
SCAM, *see* Substituted cysteine
accessibility method
SPQ, *see* Chloride secretion
Sputum induction culture,
culture, 441, 442
induction protocol, 439
materials, 436
overview, 434, 435
pre-sputum induction, 437–439
safety monitoring, 439, 440
Substituted cysteine accessibility
method (SCAM), cystic
fibrosis transmembrane
conductance regulator,
channel blocker binding site
localization, 166
charge-selectivity filter
localization, 164, 165
endogenous cysteines, 161
messenger RNA preparation,
in vitro transcription, 168–171

materials, 166, 167, 170
RNase-free cDNA template
preparation, 168, 170, 171
methanethiosulfonate reagents for
sulfhydryl modification,
161–163
mutagenesis, 167
plasmids, 166, 167
principles, 160
reactivity interpretation for
residues, 163
secondary structure
elucidation, 164
state-dependent conformational
changes and channel gate
location, 165, 166
substitution tolerance and
cysteine modification,
160, 161
transmembrane segment analysis
rationale, 159, 160
voltage clamp,
conductance measurement,
169–172
materials, 167, 170
sulfhydryl reagant reaction,
170–172
voltage dependence of reaction
rates, 165
Xenopus oocyte preparation,
166–168, 170
Syntaxin 1A,
cystic fibrosis transmembrane
conductance regulator
interactions,
coimmnoprecipitation, 177, 178
COS-7 cell expression of
CFTR, 182
function, 176